Arthroplasty of the Shoulder

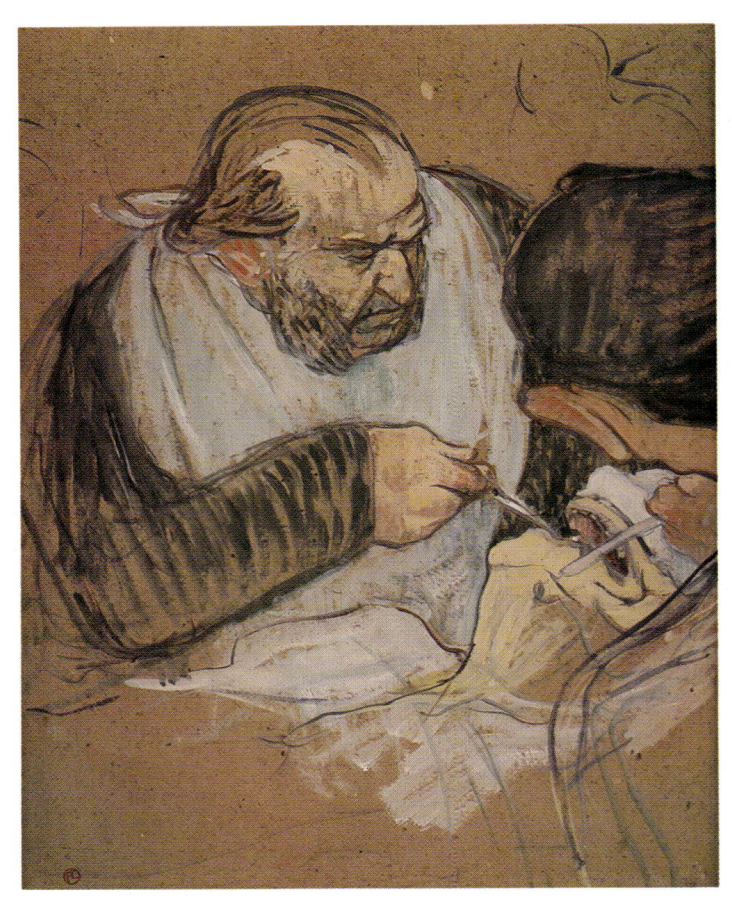

Dr. Jules Pean while operating, 1891, by Henri D. Toulous-Lautrec (1864–1901). (Reproduced with the permission of the Sterling and Francine Clark Art Institute, Williamstown, Massachusetts.)

Arthroplasty of the Shoulder

RICHARD J. FRIEDMAN, M.D., F.R.C.S.(C)
Associate Professor of Orthopaedic Surgery
Medical University of South Carolina
Charleston, South Carolina

1994
Thieme Medical Publishers, Inc., New York
Georg Thieme Verlag, Stuttgart • New York

Thieme Medical Publishers, Inc.
381 Park Avenue South
New York, New York 10016

ARTHROPLASTY OF THE SHOULDER
Richard J. Friedman

Library of Congress Cataloging-in-Publication Data

Arthroplasty of the shoulder / [edited by] Richard J. Friedman.
     p.   cm.
     Includes bibliographical references and index.
     ISBN 0-86577-495-1.—ISBN 3-13-113301-5
     1. Shoulder joint—Surgery. 2. Artificial shoulder joints.
I. Friedman, Richard J.
     [DNLM: 1. Arthroplasty—methods. 2. Shoulder Joint—surgery.
3. Joint Diseases—surgery. WE 810 A787 1994]
RD557.5.A78   1994
617.5′72059—dc20
DNLM/DLC
for Library of Congress   93-8924
                                                                            CIP

Copyright © 1994 by Thieme Medical Publishers, Inc. This book, including all parts thereof, is legally protected by copyright. Any use, exploitation or commercialization outside the narrow limits set by copyright legislation, without the publisher's consent, is illegal and liable to prosecution. This applies in particular to photostat reproduction, copying, mimeographing or duplication of any kind, translating, preparation of microfilms, and electronic data processing and storage.

Important note: Medicine is an ever-changing science. Research and clinical experience are continually broadening our knowledge, in particular our knowledge of proper treatment and drug therapy. Insofar as this book mentions any dosage or applications, readers may rest assured that the authors, editors, and publishers have made every effort to ensure that such references are strictly in accordance with the state of knowledge at the time of production of the book. Nevertheless, every users is requested to carefully examine the manufacturers' leaflets accompanying each drug to check on his own responsibility whether the dosage schedules recommended therein or the contraindications stated by the manufacturers differ from the statements made in the present book. Such examination is particularly important with drugs that are either rarely used or have been newly released on the market.

Some of the product names, patents, and registered designs referred to in this book are in fact registered trademarks or proprietary names even though specific reference to this fact is not always made in the text. Therefore, the appearance of a name without designation as proprietary is not to be construed as a representation by the publisher that it is in the public domain.

Printed in the United States of America.

5 4 3 2 1

TMP ISBN 0-86577-495-1
GTV ISBN 3-13-113301-5

This book is dedicated to my parents, who provided a guiding light; my wife, Vivian, who has added something special to my life; and my daughters, Arielle and Leah, for whom we work to build a better future.

Contents

Contributors xi
Foreword *Carter R. Rowe, M.D.* xv

Preface xvii
Acknowledgments xix

Section I: History

1. History and Development of Shoulder Arthroplasty 1
   Wayne Z. Burkhead, M.D.

Section II: Basic Principles

2. Biomechanics and Design of Shoulder Arthroplasties 27
   Richard J. Friedman, M.D., F.R.C.S.(C)

3. Preoperative Clinical Evaluation 41
   Melvin Post, M.D., and Enrique Grinblat, M.D.

4. Radiology of Total Shoulder Arthroplasty 53
   Piran Aliabadi, M.D., and Barbara N. Weissman, M.D.

5. Anesthesia for Shoulder Arthroplasty 70
   B. Hugh Dorman, M.D., Ph.D., and Gary R. Haynes, M.D., Ph.D.

6. Surgical Anatomy and Technique 80
   Gordon I. Groh, M.D., and Charles A. Rockwood, Jr., M.D.

7. Rehabilitation Following Shoulder Arthroplasty 99
   John J. Brems, M.D.

Section III: Alternatives to Total Shoulder Arthroplasty

8. Synovectomy of the Shoulder 113
   Jan A. Pahle, M.D., and Lasse Kvarnes, M.D.

9. Osteotomy and Resection Arthroplasty of the Shoulder 126
   Karl Tillmann, M.D., Dieter Braatz, M.D., Wolfgang Rüther, M.D., and Jan Backer, M.D.

10. Shoulder Arthrodesis 134
    Robin R. Richards, M.D., F.R.C.S.(C)

Section IV: Indications for Total Shoulder Arthroplasty

11. Glenohumeral Osteoarthritis 147
    Keith Watson, M.D.

12. Total Shoulder Arthroplasty in Rheumatoid Arthritis 158
    Richard J. Friedman, M.D., F.R.C.S.(C)

13. Osteonecrosis 170
    Robert H. Cofield, M.D.

14. Shoulder Arthroplasty for Proximal Humeral Fractures 183
    Gregory P. Nicholson, M.D., Evan L. Flatow, M.D., and Louis U. Bigliani, M.D.

15. Arthritis of Dislocation 194
    John J. Brems, M.D.

16. Massive Rotator Cuff Defects and Glenohumeral Arthritis 204
    Gerald R. Williams, Jr., M.D., and Charles A. Rockwood, Jr., M.D.

17. Shoulder Arthroplasty for High-Grade Tumors 215
    Martin M. Malawer, M.D., and Albert J. Aboulafia, M.D.

Section V: Results and Survivorship of Total Shoulder Arthroplasty

18. Long-Term Results of Total Shoulder Arthroplasty 227
    John D. Henry, M.D., and Thomas S. Thornhill, M.D.

19. Revision Shoulder Arthroplasty 234
    Steve A. Petersen, M.D., and Richard J. Hawkins, M.D.

20. Complications Following Shoulder Arthroplasty 242
    James F. Silliman, M.D., and Richard J. Hawkins, M.D.

21. The Unstable Shoulder Arthroplasty 254
    Bruce H. Moeckel, M.D., Russell F. Warren, M.D., David M. Dines, M.D., and David W. Altchek, M.D.

Section VI: Current Trends in Total Shoulder Arthroplasty

22. Bipolar Shoulder Arthroplasty 265
    Alfred B. Swanson, M.D., and Genevieve de Groot Swanson, M.D.

23. Cementless Shoulder Arthroplasty 281
Wayne Z. Burkhead, M.D.

24. Glenoid Resurfacing in Shoulder Arthroplasty 306
Allen D. Boyd, Jr., M.D., and Thomas S. Thornhill, M.D.

Index 317

Contributors

Albert J. Aboulafia, M.D.
Division of Orthopaedic Oncology
Washington Hospital Center
The Cancer Institute
Washington, D.C.

Piran Aliabadi, M.D.
Visiting Associate Professor Of Radiology
Harvard Medical School
Boston, Massachusetts

David W. Altchek, M.D.
Hospital for Special Surgery
Cornell University Medical College
New York, New York

Jan Backer, M.D.
Dept. of Orthopaedics
Hamburg University
Hamburg, Germany

Louis U. Bigliani, M.D.
Associate Professor of Clinical Orthopaedic Surgery
The New York Orthopaedic Hospital
Columbia-Presbyterian Medical Center
New York, New York

Allen D. Boyd, Jr., M.D.
Associate Professor
Dept. of Orthopaedic Surgery
University of Rochester
Rochester, New York

Dieter Braatz, M.D.
Dept. of Orthopaedics
Hamburg University
Hamburg, Germany

John J. Brems, M.D.
Section of Adult Reconstructive Surgery
Dept. of Orthopaedic Surgery and Program Director of
    Residency Training
Cleveland Clinic Foundation
Cleveland, Ohio

Wayne Z. Burkhead, M.D.
Clinical Associate Professor
Dept. of Orthopaedics
Southwestern Medical School
University of Texas
Dallas, Texas

Robert H. Cofield, M.D.
Consultant in Orthopaedics, Mayo Clinic
Professor, Mayo Medical School
Rochester, Minnesota

David M. Dines, M.D.
Associate Clinical Professor of Surgery (Orthopaedics)
Cornell University Medical College
New York, New York

B. Hugh Dorman, M.D., Ph.D.
Assistant Professor
Dept. of Anesthesiology
Medical University of South Carolina
Charleston, South Carolina

Evan L. Flatow, M.D.
Assistant Professor of Clinical Orthopaedic Surgery
The New York Orthopaedic Hospital
Columbia-Presbyterian Medical Center
New York, New York

Richard J. Friedman, M.D., F.R.C.S.(C)
Associate Professor of Orthopaedic Surgery
Medical University of South Carolina
Charleston, South Carolina

Enrique Grinblat, M.D.
Associate Professor of Orthopaedic Surgery
Rush Medical College
Chicago, Illinois

Gordon I. Groh, M.D.
Assistant Professor
Dept. of Orthopaedic Surgery
University of Colorado
Denver, Colorado

Richard J. Hawkins, M.D.
Clinical Professor
Dept. of Orthopaedics
University of Colorado
Vail, Colorado

Gary R. Haynes, M.D., Ph.D.
Assistant Professor
Dept. of Anesthesiology
Medical University of South Carolina
Charleston, South Carolina

John D. Henry, M.D.
Assistant Professor, Orthopaedic Surgery
Emory University School of Medicine
Atlanta, Georgia

Lasse Kvarnes, M.D.
Deputy Head
Department of Rheumatoid-Orthopaedic Surgery
Oslo University
Oslo, Norway

Martin M. Malawer, M.D.
Professor of Orthopedic Surgery
George Washington University
    School of Medicine
Washington, D.C.

Bruce H. Moeckel, M.D.
Hospital for Special Surgery
Cornell University Medical College
New York, New York

Gregory P. Nicholson, M.D.
St. Vincent Hospital
Indianapolis, Indiana

Jan A. Pahle, M.D.
Director of Orthopaedic Surgery
Dept. of Surgery of Rheumatoid Arthritis
Oslo University
Oslo, Norway

Steve A. Petersen, M.D.
Assistant Professor
Dept. of Orthopaedic Surgery
Wayne State University School of Medicine
Detroit, Michigan

Melvin Post, M.D.
Professor of Orthopaedic Surgery
Rush Medical College
Chicago, Illinois

Robin R. Richards, M.D., F.R.C.S.(C)
Associate Professor of Orthopaedic Surgery
University of Toronto
Toronto, Ontario, Canada

Charles A. Rockwood, Jr., M.D.
Professor and Chairman Emeritus
Dept. of Orthopaedics
University of Texas Health Science Center
    at San Antonio
San Antonio, Texas

Carter R. Rowe, M.D.
Private Practice
Peterborough, New Hampshire

Wolfgang Rüther, M.D.
Dept. of Orthopaedics
Hamburg University
Hamburg, Germany

James F. Silliman, M.D.
Dept. of Orthopaedic Surgery
Southwestern Medical School
University of Texas
Dallas, Texas

Alfred B. Swanson, M.D.
Professor of Surgery
Michigan State University
Grand Rapids, Michigan

Genevieve de Groot Swanson, M.D.
Assistant Clinical Professor of Surgery
Michigan State University
Grand Rapids, Michigan

Thomas S. Thornhill, M.D.
Associate Professor of Orthopaedic Surgery
Harvard Medical School
Boston, Massachusetts

Karl Tillmann, M.D.
Professor
Dept. of Orthopaedics
Hamburg University
Hamburg, Germany

Russell F. Warren, M.D.
Chief of Sports Medicine/Shoulder Service
The Hospital for Special Surgery
Cornell University Medical College
New York, New York

Keith Watson, M.D.
Private Practice
Fort Worth, Texas

Barbara N. Weissman, M.D.
Head, Musculoskeletal Radiology Section, and
Associate Professor of Radiology
Harvard Medical School
Boston, Massachusetts

Gerald R. Williams, Jr., M.D.
Assistant Professor
Dept. of Orthopaedic Surgery
University of Pennsylvania
Philadelphia, Pennsylvania

Foreword

It is a singular privilege to write the foreword for the textbook *Arthroplasty of the Shoulder,* edited by a former orthopaedic resident at the Massachusetts General Hospital who credits me with interesting him in the shoulder. Thank you, Richard, for your long memory and for your continued contributions to the study of the shoulder.

Dr. Friedman has collected an impressive group of contributors concerning every aspect of shoulder arthroplasty. His own background in bioengineering lends itself to his specific interest in the biomechanics and design of shoulder implants. The chapters of this book are well organized and give continuity for indications and alternatives in the treatment as well as the management of revisions, sepsis, and an unstable shoulder after arthroplasty. Included also is a study of end results and survivorship—an emphasis Dr. Codman pleaded for in his classic book *The Shoulder,* written in 1934.

In retrospect, when I was an orthopaedic resident at the Massachusetts General Hospital from 1937 to 1939, the shoulder was of little concern to us, for its problems were few. During my residency I assisted in the repair of only two recurrent dislocating shoulders. Impingement syndrome did not exist as a diagnosis. Perhaps we referred to this as a "sore" shoulder, which usually cleared up if the patient made a few adjustments in his or her activities; certainly it was not a problem that required surgery.

However, over the past 20 years, shoulder problems have been on the increase and are today multiplying rapidly. We may ask "Why?" One of the chief reasons has been the marked increase in the demands placed on the shoulder, beginning with the Little League baseball player and ending up with the professional athlete. Regular seasons have been increased with preseason and postseason extensions and then championships, all of which greatly lengthen the time of the season and the demands placed on the shoulder.

Secondly, we are in an epidemic of body building and physical fitness programs. Patients who are too compulsive can overstretch or tear the shoulder capsule or musculotendinous cuff, resulting in pain and/or instability of the shoulder. Excessive horizontal shoulder exercises can produce an impingement syndrome, which years ago with more normal use of the shoulder was not a problem. Large tears of the rotator cuff and late degenerative changes can be the final stage.

In addition to the increased use of the shoulder, other problems, as outlined in the text, such as rheumatoid arthritis, osteonecrosis, arthritis of dislocation, massive rotator cuff defects and glenohumeral arthritis, fractures, and tumors call for help. In response, orthopaedic surgeons have specialized to perfect procedures and techniques to replace the destroyed shoulder–hence, this book. A closing section covers current trends in shoulder arthroplasty, summarizing up-to-date concepts, with a look toward the future.

Carter R. Rowe, M.D.

Preface

Arthroplasty of the shoulder is a relatively new procedure that has come into its own over the last 20 years. While the first report of a prosthetic shoulder, presented by a French dentist, dates back to the early 1890s, the procedure had its early successes in the 1950s with the Neer hemiarthroplasty. However, it was almost another 20 years before the development of a total shoulder arthroplasty, which only recently has gained widespread acceptance. Arthroplasty of the shoulder is now one of the fastest growing orthopaedic reconstructive procedures being performed today.

This book was written in response to numerous requests from students, orthopaedic residents and fellows, practicing orthopaedic surgeons, and rheumatologists for a comprehensive book on arthroplasty of the shoulder. The goal was to develop one book that would become the definitive work on this subject, covering all aspects of shoulder arthroplasty from diagnosis to treatment outcomes, and that would save the reader from having to search endlessly through various textbooks and journals.

The book begins with a thorough history of the development of shoulder arthroplasties over the last 100 years. The next section covers the basic principles for a successful shoulder arthroplasty, including biomechanics, clinical and radiographic evaluation, anesthesia, surgical anatomy and technique, and postoperative rehabilitation. Various alternatives to a shoulder arthroplasty are proposed for the patient in whom it may not be indicated.

Different diagnoses and indications for shoulder arthroplasty are presented in the following section, encompassing osteoarthritis, rheumatoid arthritis, osteonecrosis, proximal humeral fractures, arthritis of dislocation, massive rotator cuff defects associated with glenohumeral arthritis (a term preferred to cuff-tear arthropathy), and high-grade tumors. Survivorship, complications, and outcome studies are very important in determining the success of a procedure, and these data have been compiled from a comprehensive review of the literature. Finally, special chapters covering controversial issues such as a bipolar shoulder arthroplasty, cementless shoulder arthroplasty, and the indications for glenoid resurfacing are presented.

The contributors to this book are recognized authorities in their field and present an in-depth review of their subject with regards to the current state of the art. The authors have been given the freedom to express their views and opinions based on their extensive experience. It is hoped that the reader will find this book to be a valuable source of information and that it will stimulate further advances in the field of arthroplasty of the shoulder, ultimately leading to improved care of shoulder disorders for patients.

Richard J. Friedman, M.D., F.R.C.S.(C)

Acknowledgments

I want to thank all the wonderful people who helped make this book a reality, including orthopaedic surgeons and residents, Thieme Medical Publishers and their editors, our secretaries, and our families. In particular, I wish to make the following acknowledgments with a deep feeling of gratitude: To John B. McGinty, M.D., who provided the environment and support for this work to take place; to my editors, James Costello, who believed in this project and got it started, and **Stephany Scott**, who carried it through to fruition, for their guidance and many suggestions in the production of this book; to Paul P. Griffin, M.D., and Richard M. Silver, M.D., who reviewed portions of the manuscript; to Allen E. Gross, M.D., who introduced me to orthopaedic surgery in medical school and stimulated my interest and curiosity; to the attending orthopaedic surgeons at Harvard Medical School who guided me through my orthopaedic training; to Carter R. Rowe, M.D., who steered me towards the vast uncharted waters of the shoulder; and to Sylvia Chapman, my trusted and loyal secretary, who has kept some semblance of order to my days.

Richard J. Friedman, M.D., F.R.C.S.(C)

SECTION I
History

1 History and Development of Shoulder Arthroplasty

Wayne Z. Burkhead, M.D.

It is not the critic who counts; not the man who points out how the strong man stumbled or where the doer of deeds could have done them better. The credit belongs to the man who is actually in the arena, whose face is marred by dust and sweat and blood, who strives valiantly, who errs, and comes up short again and again, because there is no effort without error and shortcoming, who does actually try to do the deed, who knows the great enthusiasm, the great devotion, and spends himself in a worthy cause, who—at the worst—if he fails, at least fails while daring greatly. Far better it is to dare mighty things, to win glorious triumphs even though checkered by failure, than to rank with those spirits who neither enjoy nor suffer much because they live in the gray twilight that knows neither victory nor defeat.

—Theodore Roosevelt

From the late nineteenth century to the early 1950s, performance of a successful shoulder arthroplasty was limited much more by sepsis and biomaterial quality than by surgical skill, imagination, or ingenuity. While the shoulder was the first human joint to be replaced with a prosthesis,[1] in 1892, this procedure was still described in 1977 as "an experimental, investigational proposition,"[2] and as late as 1983, Souter[3] stated that "Arthroplasty of the shoulder must still be regarded as being in the developmental, if not frankly experimental stage." As will be seen, many have been in the arena contributing to our understanding of the shoulder. Over the last 35 years, based on this understanding, coupled with the untiring efforts of Charles S. Neer, II (Figure 1–1), shoulder arthroplasty has been elevated from an "experimental proposition" to a well-established component of the orthopaedic surgeons' armamentarium.

The first successful replacement of a human shoulder was performed by the French surgeon Jules E. Pean (Figure 1–2) in March 1892.[1,4,5] Before this, Gluck and others had tried unsuccessfully to replace joints with ivory and animal bone. Pean noted that the ivory used by Gluck was too weak and too resorbable, and had an articulation with too little movement for replacing the shoulder.[4]

Pean's prosthesis, which was designed and created (at Pean's request) by the Parisian dentist J. Porter Michaels, was implanted 26 years prior to the first hip replacement. We are indebted to Lugli[5] for rediscovering Pean's and Michaels' prosthesis at the Smithsonian Institute, for retracing the process, and for presenting the facts of this "exceptional intervention." The prosthesis was made of an iridescent platinum tube with two ridges, having several holes to serve as attachment sites for periosteum and muscle. A rubber ball, hardened by boiling in paraffin, substituted for the humeral head. A deep groove, containing metal loops, attached the ball to the scapula and platinum tube (Figure 1–3). A young man with a massive tuberculous infection presented to the Hospital St. Louis in Paris, near death from a tuberculous abscess of his humerus. A massive débridement of infected bone was followed by implantation of the prosthesis. The muscles were resutured with horse hair. The patient recovered and apparently the prosthesis functioned well. A chronic draining sinus necessitated excision of the implant 2 years postoperatively. Although the prosthesis was in place for only 2 years, it saved the patient's life and spared this 37-year-old patient a certain shoulder disarticulation. With this "exceptional intervention," Pean proved that it was possible to replace an important part of the skeleton, even a diarthrodial joint, as long as the following criteria were met: The device was aseptic, nonresorbable, and well tolerated by the body, and provided a mechanism for the joint to preserve its motion.

Murphy,[6] who reported on several cases in 1913, removed the humeral head in proximal humeral fractures, reshaped it, and then drove in a nail at an angle through the shaft into the head (Figure 1–4). He accompanied this by a fat or fascial transplant as a bearing surface. Though the treatment appears crude, one has to keep in mind that one of the patients was a biplane pilot who crashed into a chicken coop. To put things further into perspective, the physician, John B. Murphy, owned the hospital and the journal in which his article was published.

In 1910 Rovsing[7] reported the use of the proximal part of the fibula to replace a bony defect in the shoulder joint. Albee[8,9] utilized the proximal part of the fibula to reconstruct the arms of World War I veterans. The surrounding muscles were preserved and resutured to the transplanted fibula utilizing kangaroo tendon as a suture material (Figures 1–5, 1–6, and 1–7). Hammond[10] in 1926 presented a case utilizing a fibular autograft for the treatment of a painful ankylosed shoulder after failed surgery for a fracture-dislocation. Satisfactory outcomes utilizing this technique were reported by Groves,[11] Behrend,[12] and others,[13–15] including a 26-year follow-up case by Clark[16] (Figures 1–8 and 1–9). Konig[17] in 1914 utilized an ivory prosthesis to replace the upper end of the humerus.

While his name is frequently associated with simple resection of the upper end of the humerus, Laurence Jones[18,19] of Kansas City, Missouri, described an operation

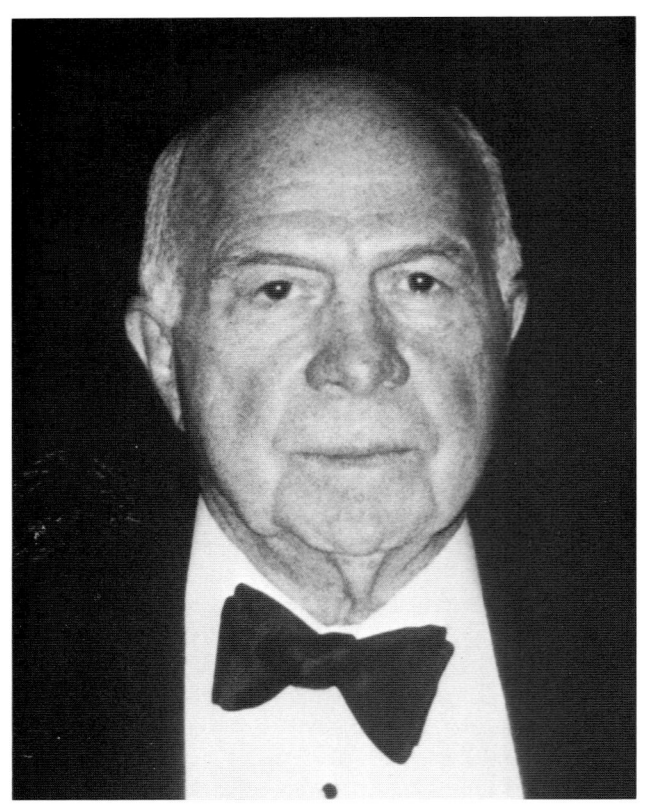

Figure 1–1. Charles S. Neer, II, circa 1987. The great master of shoulder arthroplasty. (Photograph courtesy of Hiro Fukuda.)

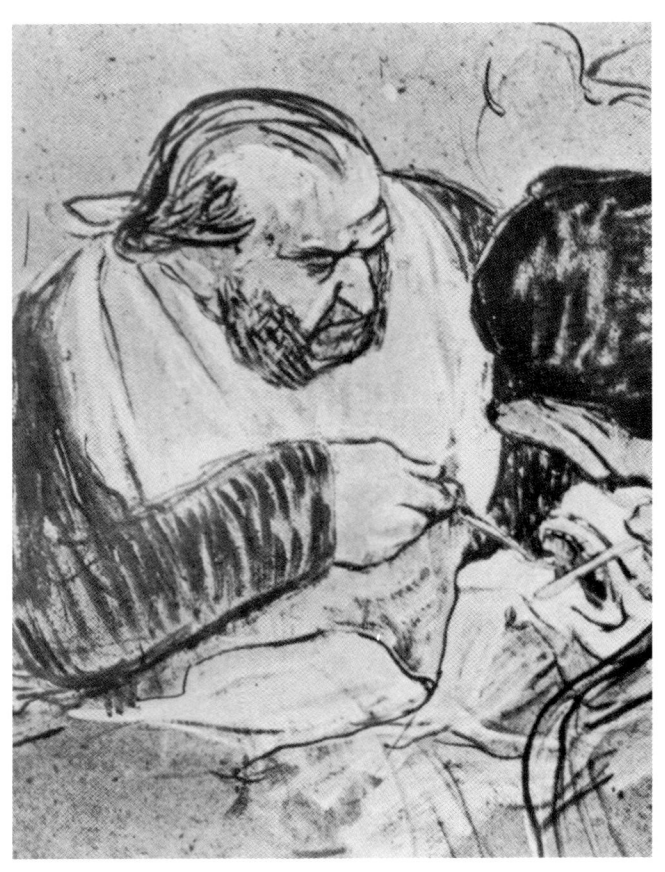

Figure 1–2. Dr. Jules Pean while operating, 1891, by Henri D. Toulouse-Lautrec (1864–1901). (Reproduced with the permission of the Sterling and Francine Clark Art Institute, Williamstown, Massachusetts.)

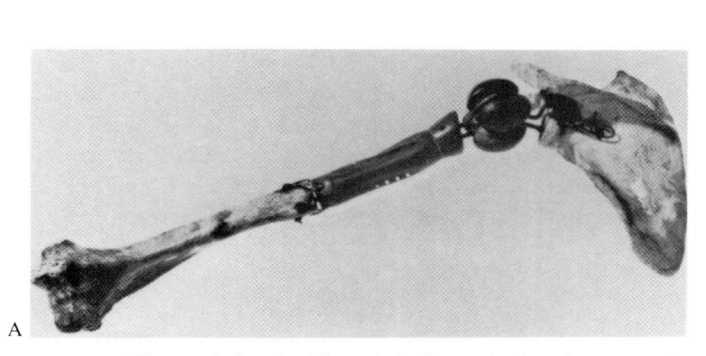

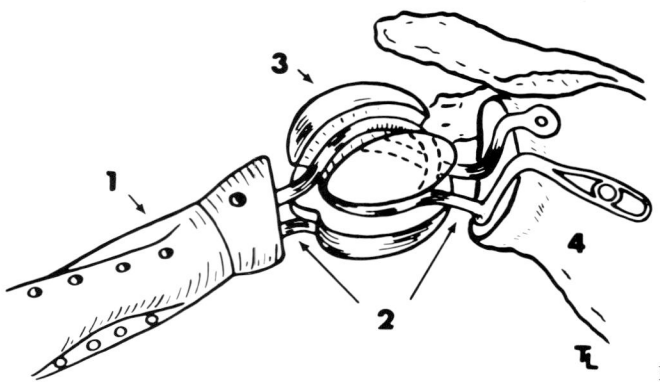

Figure 1–3. **A.** The original prosthesis of Pean, rediscovered by Lugli, on display at the Smithsonian Institute, Washington, DC, Division of Medical Science's National Museum of History and Technology, Washington, DC. **B.** Illustration emphasizing the functional components of Pean's artificial joint: (1) the platinum tube that substitutes for the humeral shaft; (2) two platinum loops connecting the scapula to the paraffin-hardened rubber ball. (Reproduced with permission from Lugli.[5])

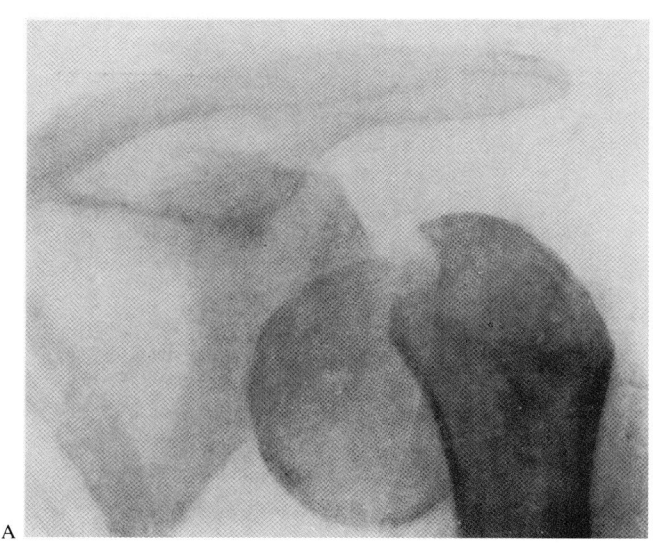

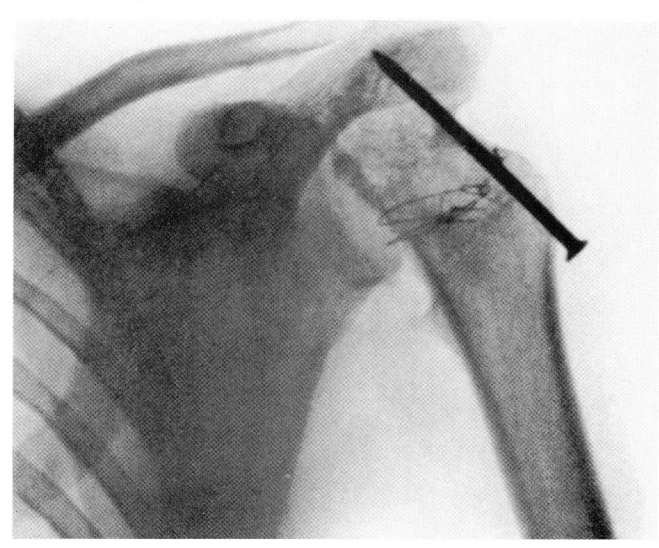

Figure 1–4. **A.** Anterior fracture-dislocation that occurred in a pilot when his biplane crashed into a chicken coop in 1913. **B.** Fixation by John B. Murphy, who reshaped the humeral head and reattached it by means of a nail and wire fixation. The nail was subsequently removed. Function was said to be satisfactory. (Reproduced with permission from Murphy.[6])

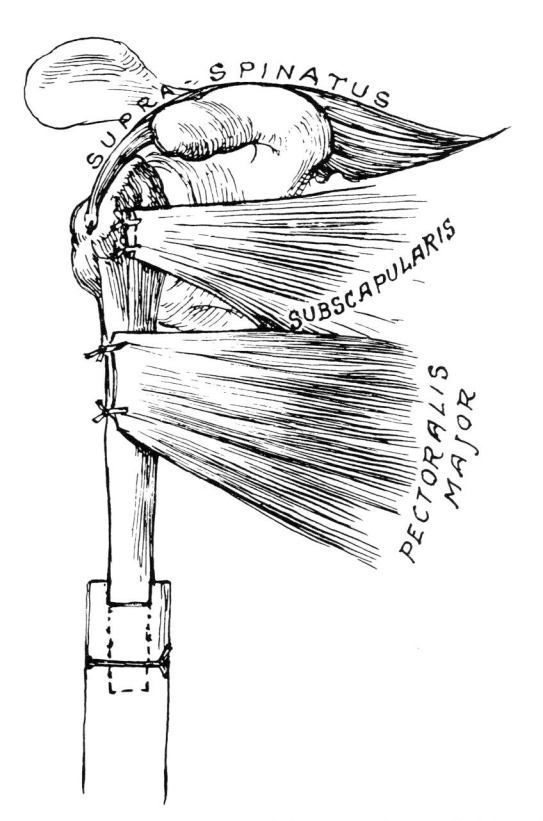

Figure 1–5. Albee reconstructed the arms of wounded American soldiers from World War I utilizing fibular autograft with careful resuturing of the muscle, each fastened into place by means of kangaroo tendon. (Reproduced with permission from Albee.[9])

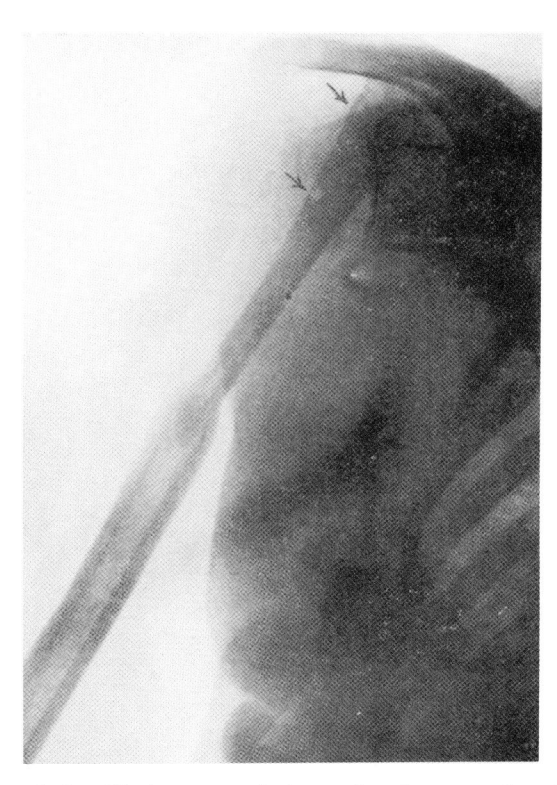

Figure 1–6. Fibular autograft 4 months after operation. The arrows indicate drill holes in the graft through which muscles were attached at their proper place of insertion by means of fine kangaroo tendon.

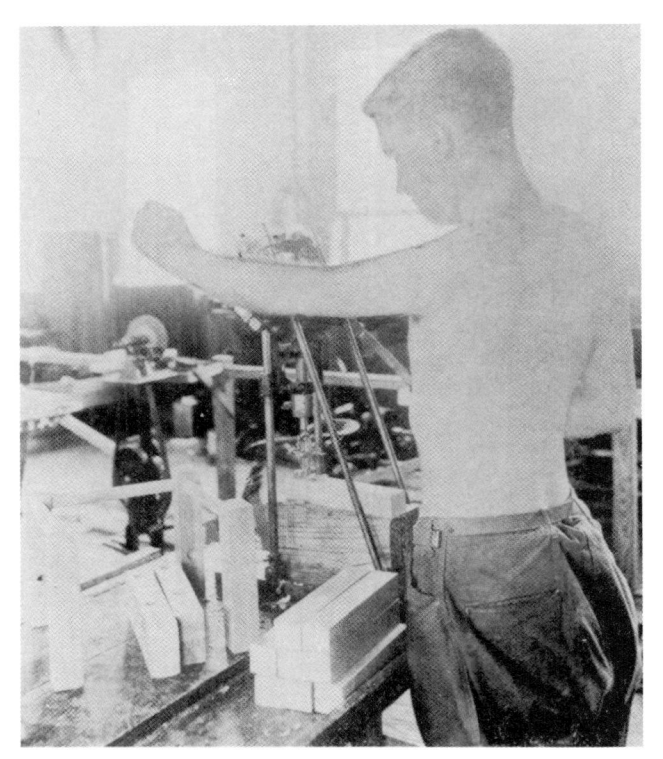

Figure 1–7. Shoulder function after fibular transplantation. What Albee was able to do with the patient's own fibula and kangaroo tendon, we sometimes cannot duplicate with titanium and Dacron. (Reproduced with permission from Albee.[9])

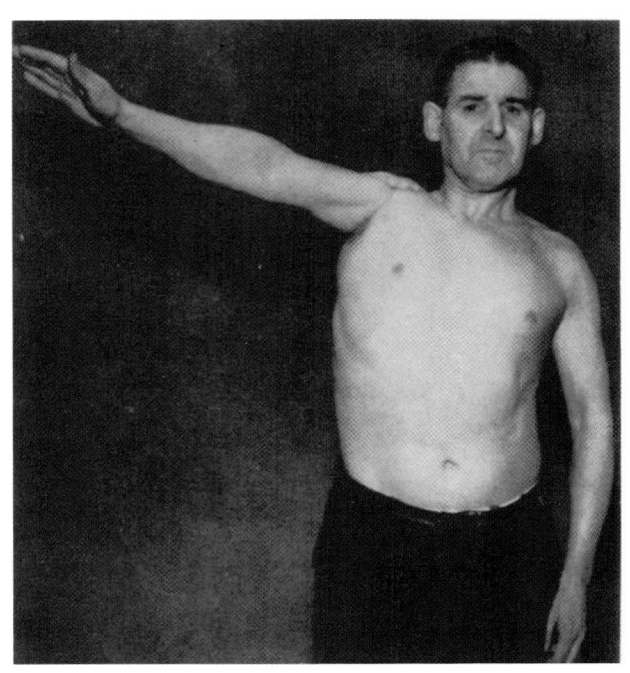

Figure 1–8. At 26-year follow-up, transplanted fibula shows excellent functional result.

that included not only excision of the humeral head, but also resurfacing of the resected end utilizing fascia lata, with a unique method for resuturing the rotator cuff (Figures 1–10 and 1–11). He reported satisfactory results with surprisingly good strength in three patients, utilizing his technique. The figures from his article are oftentimes mislabeled, and most surgical texts have shown the anatomic resuturing of the cuff (Figure 1–11B) as his preferred method. Actually, he found that his patients had improved strength and function if the supraspinatus was resutured in an anterior and more distal position rather than an anatomic position (Figure 1–11A). His rationale for this was based on his belief that the short rotators were indeed important suspensory muscles that also provided compression across the glenohumeral joint. It is well recognized now that his observations were true. However, whether this technique allows the cuff to function more effectively as a compressor has not been proved. The sometimes disappointing results of this procedure in other surgeons' hands may be related to his attention to detail.

In conjunction with excisional arthroplasty, the mainstay of treatment for the painful ankylosed shoulder and rheumatoid arthritis in the 1930s and 1940s was an acromioplasty as described by Smith-Peterson, Aufranc, and Larson,[20] first

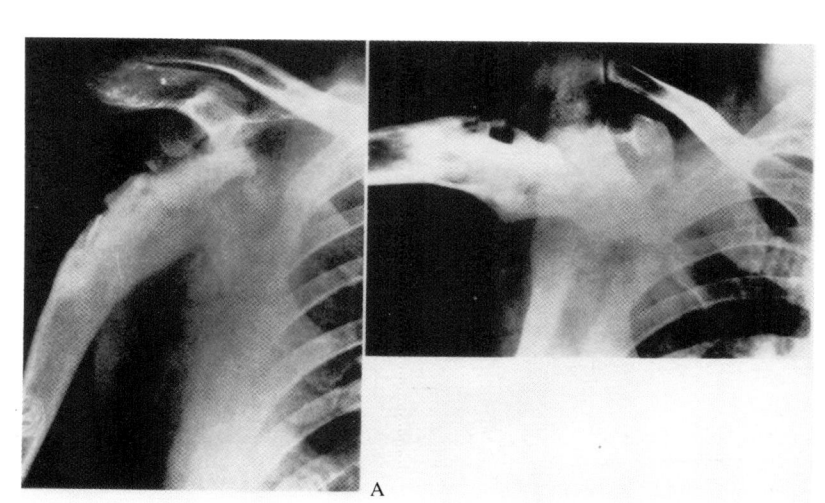

Figure 1–9. At 26-year radiographic follow-up, transplanted fibula demonstrates hypertrophy of the graft. **A.** The arm at the side. **B.** In abduction.

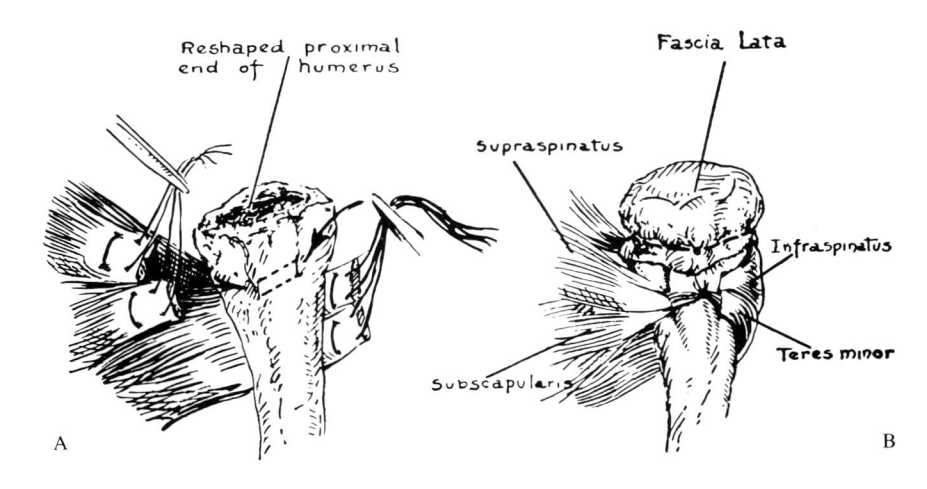

Figure 1-10. A and B. Illustration of reshaping of the end of the humerus, the unique transplantation of the rotator cuff, and the addition of a fascia lata resurfacing on the resected end of the humerus. It should be noted that some of these steps were neglected by subsequent authors. (Reproduced with permission from Jones.[18])

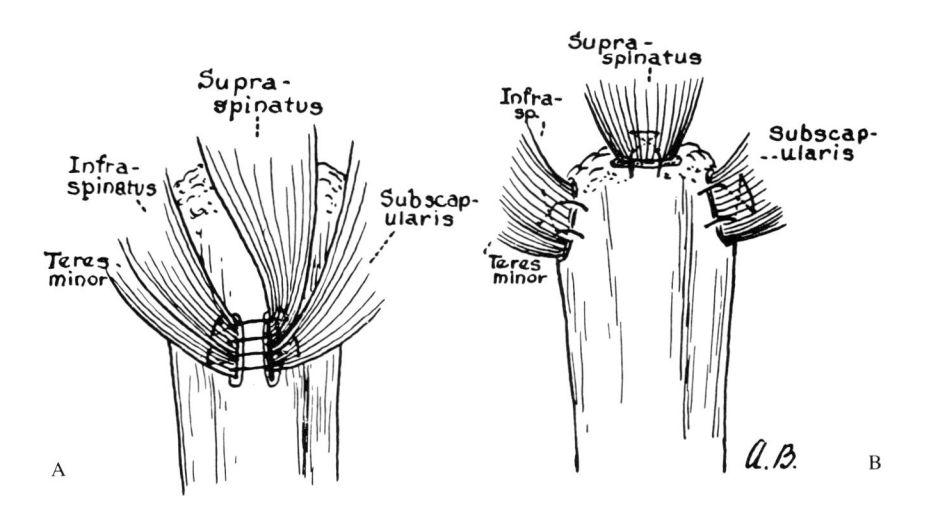

Figure 1-11. A. Illustration from Jones' second article emphasizes distalizing and placing more anteriorly the supraspinatus in resection arthroplasty. This position resulted in complete stability, full range of motion, and good muscle power. B. The anatomic suturing shown gave good stability. It was accompanied only by limited motion and decreased muscle power. (Reproduced with permission from Jones.[19])

performed in September 1935. The most striking effect of this procedure, which accurately should be described as an acromionectomy, was improvement in upper extremity function because of the elimination of pain. All of their 11 patients had satisfactory results, particularly with respect to pain relief. However, there was no increase in glenohumeral joint motion. Improvement in function in all of these cases was felt to be due to an improvement in compensatory scapulothoracic motion. In their technique, the acromioclavicular joint was kept intact but the resection included the remainder of the acromion to the posterior angle. Careful attention to the deltoid repair, which is now well recognized as the single most important step and the number one cause of failure with this technique, was emphasized in their 1943 report.

An acrylic prosthesis for the shoulder was described by Baron and Senn in 1951.[21] The use of an acrylic implant to replace the proximal part of the humerus in fracture-dislocations was reported by Richard et al. in 1952 (Figures 1-12 and 1-13).[22] Unfortunately, because of the wear characteristics of acrylic, anchorage difficulty, and component breakage, this concept was abandoned. A case reported by Lynn et al.[23] illustrated the problems inherent in biomaterials and implant fixation in the late 1940s and early 1950s. Their patient had an acrylic prosthesis attached to a metal stem implanted for a defect in the proximal part of the humerus. Over a 12-year period, the initial prosthesis (Figure 1-14), as well as a subsequent stainless-steel prosthesis, fractured at the head-shaft junction. A final design with a diamond-shaped stem to control rotation was functioning well at the time of the report, 4 years postoperatively. Beginning in 1953, de Anquin[24] performed 11 acrylic shoulder replacements for fracture and had one of the first designs developed to allow tendinous reattachment around the prosthesis. Monteleone[25] added a report of two additional cases of acrylic replacement in 1969 but the results were less favorable than current designs.

The first modern shoulder arthroplasty, with an anatomic shape and manufactured from long-lasting inert biomaterials, appears to have been done on December 12, 1950 by

6 Arthroplasty of the Shoulder

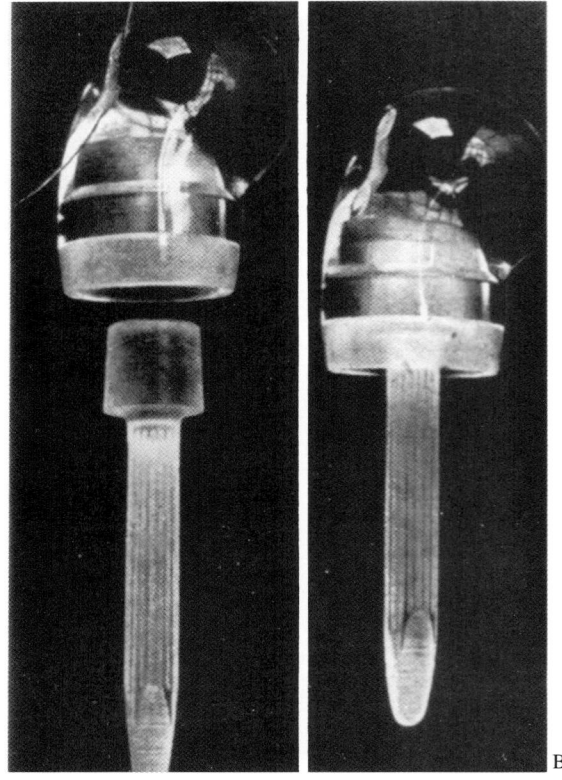

Figure 1–12. A and B. An acrylic prosthesis designed to replace the upper end of the humerus for fractures and fracture-dislocation of the proximal part of the humerus. (Reproduced with permission from Richard et al.[22])

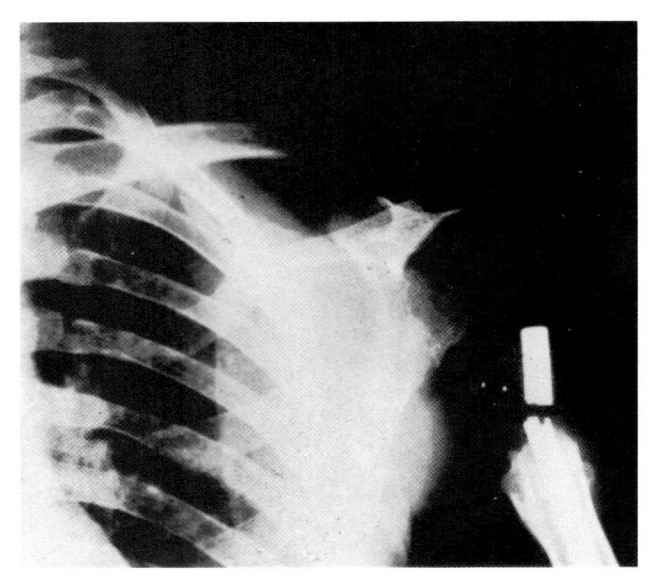

Figure 1–14. Fracture at the junction of an acrylic head with a metal stem component. (Reproduced with permission from Lynn et al.[23])

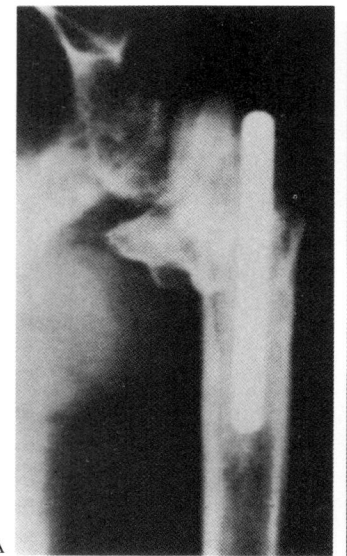

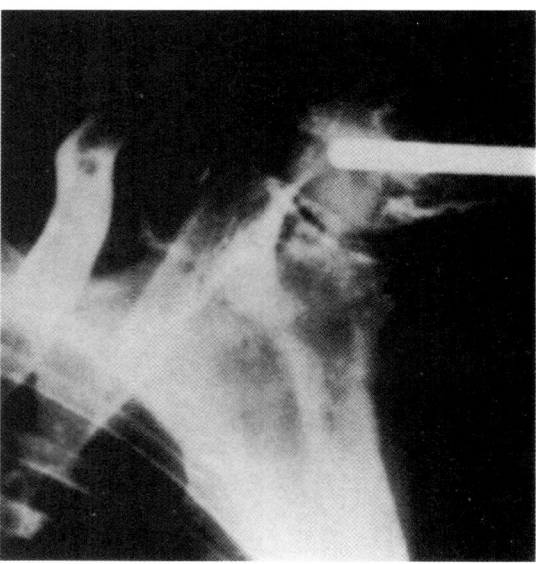

Figure 1–13. A and B. Radiograph of acrylic prosthesis in place with a metal stem. (Reproduced with permission from Wolff R, Kolbel R. The history of shoulder joint replacement. In: Kolbel R, Helbig B, Blauth W, eds. *Shoulder Replacement*. Berlin: Springer-Verlag, 1987:3–13.)

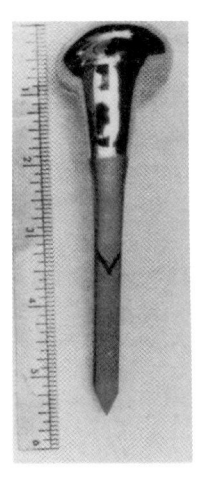

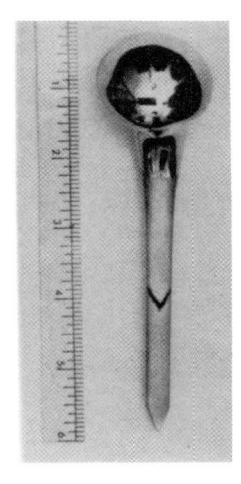

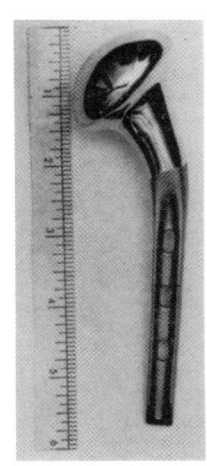

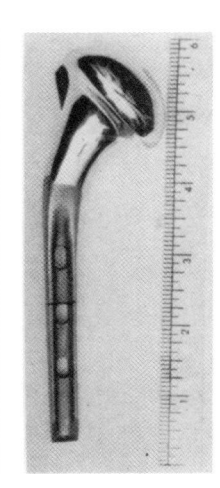

Figure 1–15. Krueger's original vitallium prosthesis. Note the egg-shaped head with rounded corners, similar to modern prostheses. Fenestrations within the stem allow permeation of cancellous bone. (Reproduced with permission from Krueger.[26])

Frederick Krueger.[26] He initially made acrylic replicas from cadaveric humeral heads and then had Austinol Laboratories in New York create a vitallium mold prosthesis based on these replicas (Figure 1–15). The stem was fenestrated to allow intrusion of bone for long-term stability. The prosthesis was implanted into a young sailor who had aseptic necrosis from a traumatic dislocation. In his technique, the head was excised down to the capsule and the rotator cuff tendon attachments preserved. This resulted in a "well functioning and painless shoulder" (Figure 1–16).

In 1953 Neer et al.[27] presented a review of fractures of the neck of the humerus with dislocation of the head fragment. At that time, the best treatment for these unimpacted lesions appeared to be simple excision of the head fragment. However, because of limited motion, fatigue, and pain following this operation, they postulated that the value of a replacement prosthesis was to serve as a fulcrum for motion (Figure 1–17). This was described as "recently revised, without adequate trial, and its true worth remained to be determined."

By April 1955, Neer's prosthesis had been redesigned[28] (Figure 1–18). The articular portion of this prosthesis was formed in the shape of the normal humeral head, with the exception of the superior surface which was flattened to permit seating of the prosthesis into the greater tuberosity. The edges were lipped all the way around so they could be set into bone. The solid proximal body was replaced by a three-flange mechanism with multiple holes for permeation

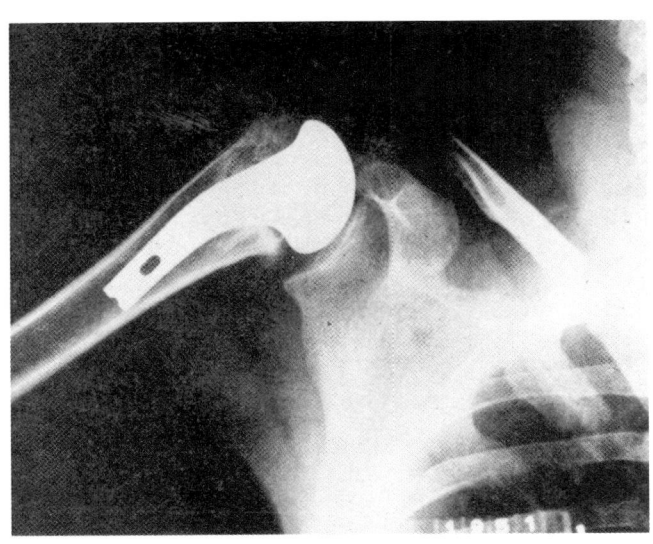

Figure 1–16. Follow-up radiograph of Krueger's patient showing the first modern vitallium prosthesis. (Reproduced with permission from Krueger.[26])

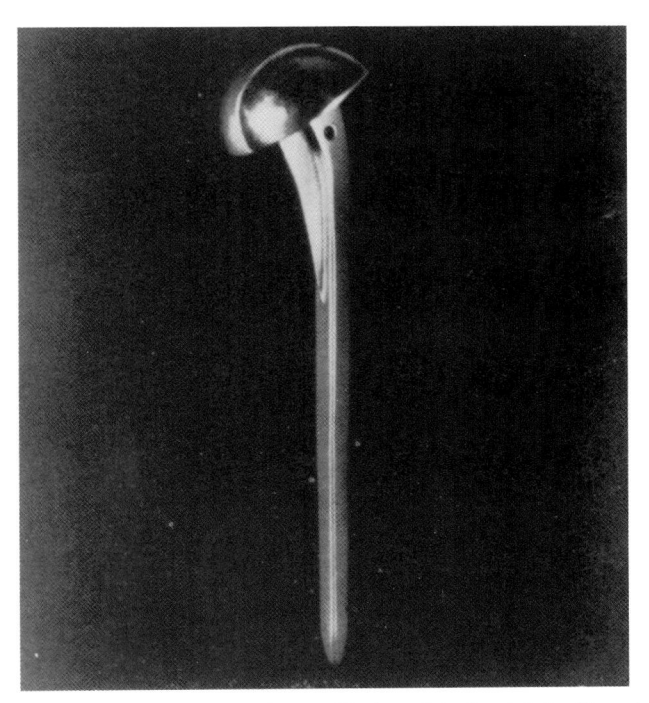

Figure 1–17. Prosthesis featured in the original article by Neer et al.[27] Note the solid body. (Reproduced with permission from Neer et al.[27])

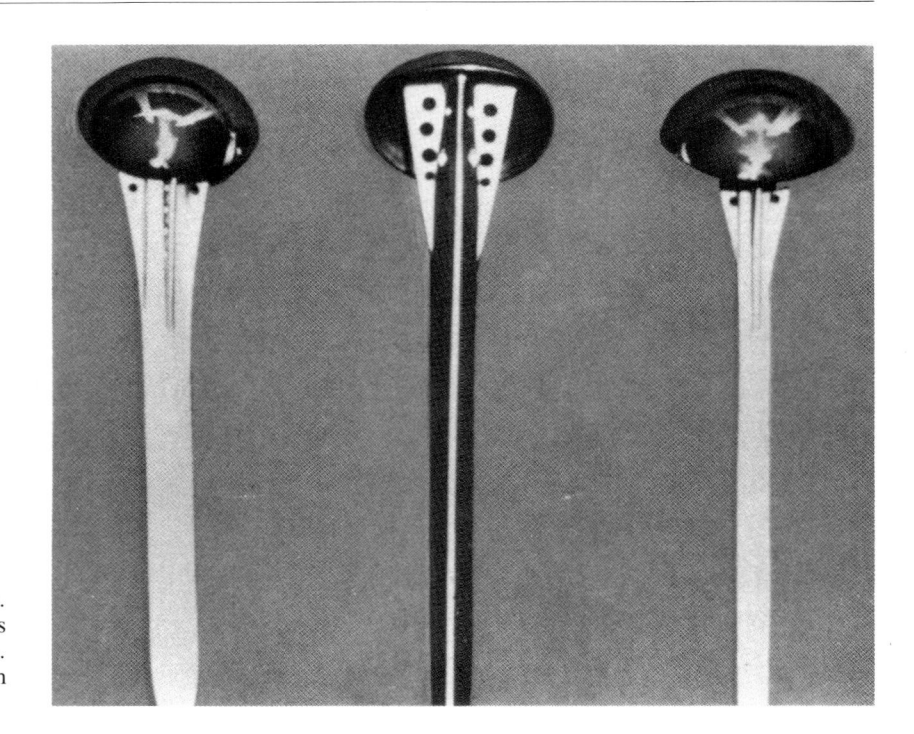

Figure 1–18. Neer I prosthesis. Note the triflange fins and large holes for macrointerlock bone ingrowth. (Reproduced with permission from Neer.[28])

of cancellous bone and rotational stability. A hole was placed in the neck so that the tuberosity fragments could be reattached to each other and the humeral shaft when fresh fractures and fracture-dislocations are being treated.

Neer reported on 12 replacements that were performed from January 1953 to April 1954 at the New York Orthopaedic Hospital-Columbia Presbyterian Medical Center. All the patients in this series had stiff, painful shoulders and avascular necrosis from either previous four-part fractures, fresh four-part fractures, or fracture-dislocations. Following the replacements, all of which were done without bone cement and utilized only three different stem sizes, 11 of the 12 patients were free of pain. Follow-up ranged from 2 to 23 months and revealed good range of motion in 4 patients, excellent in 1 patient, satisfactory in 2, fair in 1, and unknown in 2 patients. Two patients, both of whom had fracture-dislocations neglected for several months prior to surgery, had poor motion. Lack of improvement in motion in these cases of late trauma convinced Neer that early reconstruction of "extra-articular lesions" should be undertaken prior to a point in time when extensive healing could occur. In fact, in his article in 1964, Neer recommended the surgery be done within a 3-day time interval.[29]

By 1956 de Anquin[24] had modified his original acrylic design as well to a metallic noncemented component with a fenestrated stem, similar to that of Krueger and Austin Moore. A subsequent design modification utilizing a polyethylene head failed rapidly and was abandoned.

As of 1964 Neer had applied his technique to 54 patients, with only minor alterations in technique, including the addition of a fourth stem size.[29] The peculiarities of shoulder replacement as opposed to hip replacement were discussed. He noted that the head of the prosthesis should supply a gliding fulcrum that provides leverage but at the same time a loose fit upon the glenoid. The importance of accurate subscapularis repair along with proper retroversion to ensure anterior stability of the prosthesis was also emphasized.

Forty-eight replacement arthroplasties for glenohumeral arthritis were reported by Neer in 1974.[30] All were done as uncemented hemiarthroplasties, except for one patient in whom an all-polyethylene glenoid was utilized with acrylic cement. In this article, Neer described the structural alteration of primary glenohumeral arthritis including "thinning of the articular cartilage, most advanced at the area of maximum humeral contact between 60 and 100 degrees. This is the area of maximum joint reaction force and it was eburnated and sclerotic. Degenerative subarticular cysts, occurred just superior to the midpoint of the articular surface. The largest osteophytes were located at the inferior margin of the joint. The articular surface of the glenoid was smooth but usually consisted of eburnated bone devoid of cartilage. Marginal osteophytes could be palpated in the ligaments of the glenoid." The technique of subscapularis Z-plasty was also described in this article and the recommended retroversion increased from 20 degrees to 30 to 35 degrees.

In this series of patients evaluated 1 to 20 years after surgery, with an average follow-up of 6 years, the results were excellent in 20 patients, satisfactory in 20, and unsatisfactory in 6. There was no evidence of prosthetic stem loosening or subsidence in the medullary canal; no increase in flattening, sclerosis, or enlargement of the glenoid when compared to preoperative films; or any definite resorption or

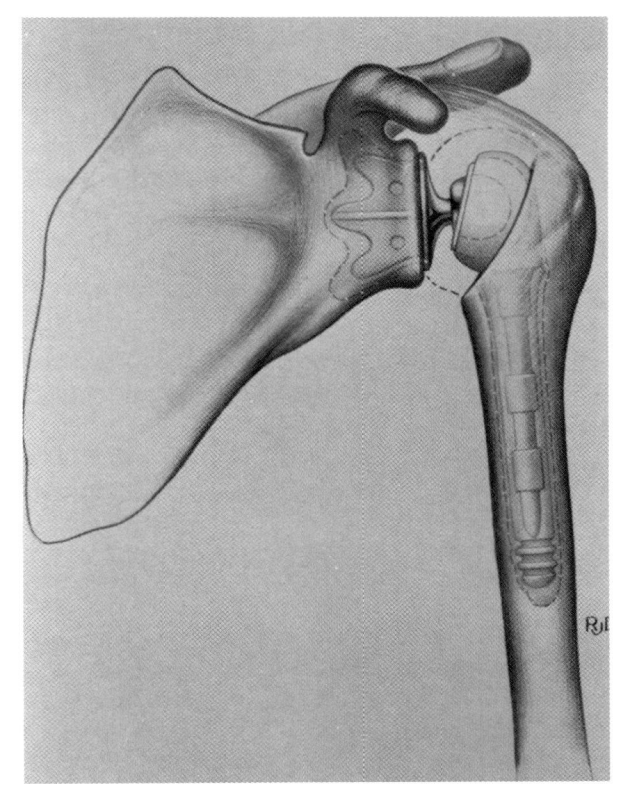

Figure 1–19. Neer Mark III fixed fulcrum prosthesis. Note the reverse ball-and-socket configuration and rotating metallic stem. (Reproduced with permission from Neer.[31])

intrusion of the prosthesis. A postmortem specimen from this series revealed that permeation and filling of the holes in the proximal portion of the prosthesis had occurred, the prosthetic stem was firm, and the glenoid was free of tissue reaction. The first polyethylene glenoid utilized with a modified humeral head prosthesis was used in this series. This study showed that a properly performed hemiarthroplasty combined with release of contractures can be expected to stop the deterioration of the glenohumeral joint, relieve pain, and allow normal use. The articular surface of the glenoid did not appear to be a significant source of pain. Since relief of pain and recovery of function were the rules in his series, it appeared to Neer that there was little reason at that time to recommend a more extensive replacement that might increase complications and lack durability.

Like most pioneers, Neer would develop an idea, test it, and then discard it if it did not prove worthwhile. Between 1970 and 1974, Neer, along with Robert Averill, designed and later modified twice a fixed fulcrum shoulder replacement.[31] The first design was a fixed conventional ball-and-socket joint. The second incorporated a reverse ball-and-socket arrangement with a large ball. The last (the Mark III) (Figure 1–19) was a reverse ball-and-socket joint with a unique dual-compartment humeral component that allowed axial rotation of a metal stem within a polyethylene sleeve. However, even with these ingenious modifications to limit the stress at the bone-cement interface and component articulation, these devices all failed.

It was hoped that a redesigned, nonconstrained prosthesis with a larger and more rounded head and shorter neck would improve the mechanical advantage of the rotator cuff. Neer's desire to keep his prosthesis nonconstrained and his concern about the emerging designs with constraint being developed at that time in Europe and in the United States have proved over time to be well founded. He predicted in the early 1970s that leverage would be transferred to the fixation of the glenoid component in constrained designs, with loosening and fracture occurring in active patients. By 1972 his guiding principles were well established, i.e., minimal bone resection, anatomic design, avoidance of mechanical impingement, and repair and rehabilitation of the soft tissues.

In the early 1970s, Englebrecht, Stellbrink,[32–34] (Figure 1–20) and Kenmore et al.[35] (Figure 1–21) developed polyethylene components to replace the articular surface of the

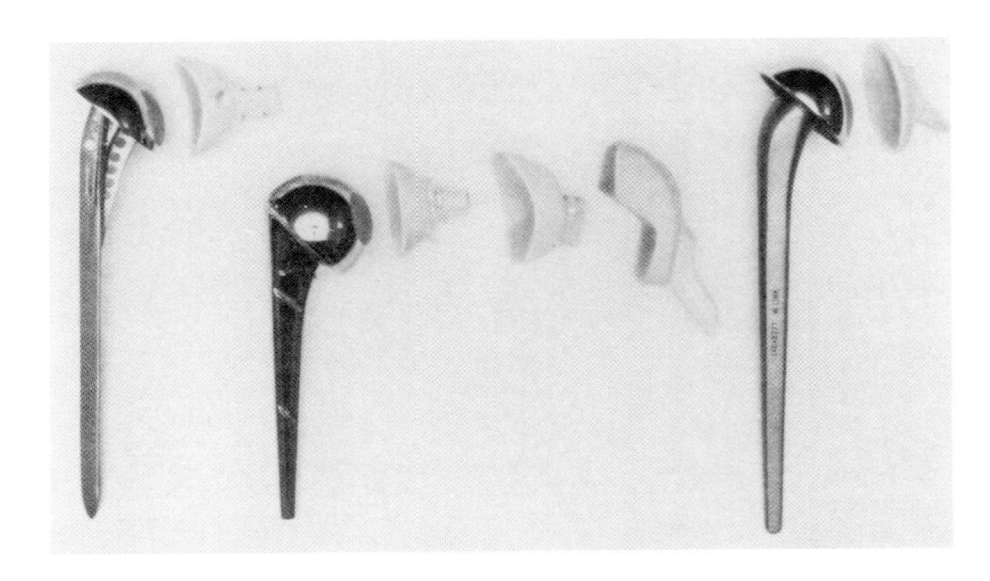

Figure 1–20. A variety of glenoid components with varying degrees of constraint designed by Stellbrink to be used from left to right with Neer, St. Georg, and Link prostheses.

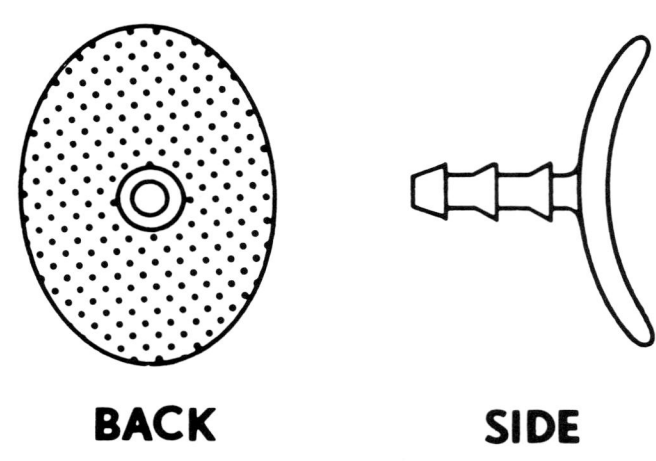

Figure 1–21. A simple glenoid replacement implanted in 1973. This surface replacement was the forerunner of modern surface replacement glenoid components. (Reproduced with permission from Kenmore et al.[35])

glenoid. The components were to be used primarily with the Neer or St. Georg prostheses. The simple, relatively nonconstrained designs have stood the test of time with minor modification. However, to a certain degree, Neer's warnings about treating the shoulder joint like the hip joint with constrained designs fell on deaf ears.

The introduction of methylmethacrylate with Sir John Charnley's successful low-friction arthroplasty, coupled with the vexing problems of the rotator cuff and capsule-deficient shoulder, led many investigators to adopt a constrained ball-and-socket design. Each model had its own unique features to address one of four major areas of concern: (1) reproduction of the force couple normally provided by the rotator cuff, allowing the deltoid to work more efficiently; (2) long-term scapular fixation; (3) maximizing range of motion in a constrained environment; and (4) a "fail-safe" mechanism.

The Bickel shoulder prosthesis (Figure 1–22) was designed at the Mayo Clinic.[36] This cemented prosthesis, incorporating Charnley's low-friction arthroplasty concept of a small metallic ball articulating with a larger-radius polyethylene socket, required extensive excavation of the glenoid vault to seat the glenoid component entirely within the scapula. The operation was described as difficult, with a high complication rate, including glenoid fracture, prosthesis fracture, and early glenoid loosening leading to a reoperation rate of 50% at 5 years.

The Stanmore total shoulder replacement (Figures 1–23 and 1–24), developed by Lettin and Scales,[37] was introduced in 1969 and later modified to displace the instant center of rotation, thereby increasing the range of motion and hopefully decreasing the stress on the component interface.[38] A retaining ring was utilized to provide a restraint to dislocation, and three smooth pegs provided scapular fixation with methylmethacrylate. In a 1982 report,[39] range of motion was "inconsistent and disappointing," and despite the extralong pegs into the scapula, glenoid loosening was a major problem, requiring revision in 10 of 50 shoulders. Whereas the authors believed there was undoubtedly a place for prosthetic replacement of the glenohumeral joint in a small number of patients, they felt it should not be contemplated in younger patients with monoarticular disease.

Recognizing that long-term scapular fixation was of primary concern, Post[40] developed a constrained prosthesis utilizing screw fixation of the glenoid component (Figure 1–25). The addition of screws into the bone-cement-implant composite increased its strength to such an extent that scapular fracture rather than bone-cement interface loosening was of major concern. To avoid scapular destruction, this prosthesis was designed to dislocate at a force less than that required to cause scapular fracture. The initial model (Series I) was made of 316-L stainless steel, with a humeral head component mated to a polyethylene socket, which in turn was inserted into a metal glenoid component designed for attachment to the scapula. A self-locking metal ring completed the assembly (Figure 1–26). In his initial series, 11 of 22 patients required revision within 5 years. While secure scapular fixation was achieved, there were three dislocations, six humeral component fractures, and two humeral components that underwent plastic deformation. In Series II, where the humeral component was changed to a cobalt

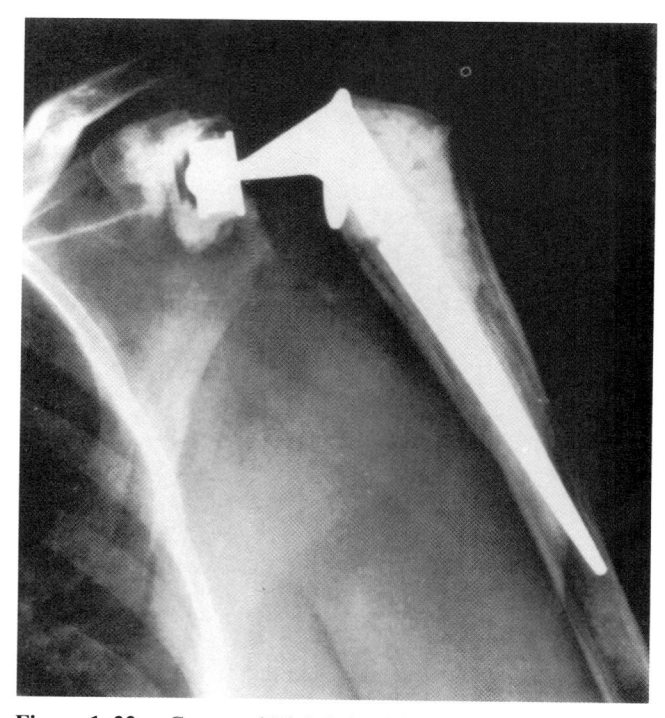

Figure 1–22. Cemented Bickel shoulder prosthesis with a small ball articulating with a medialized glenoid component. The high rate of failure with this prosthesis served as evidence that engineering principles that were successful in the hip such as medialization, a low friction system with a small ball, and constraint could not be applied to the shoulder with the same degree of success. (Reproduced with permission from Cofield.[2])

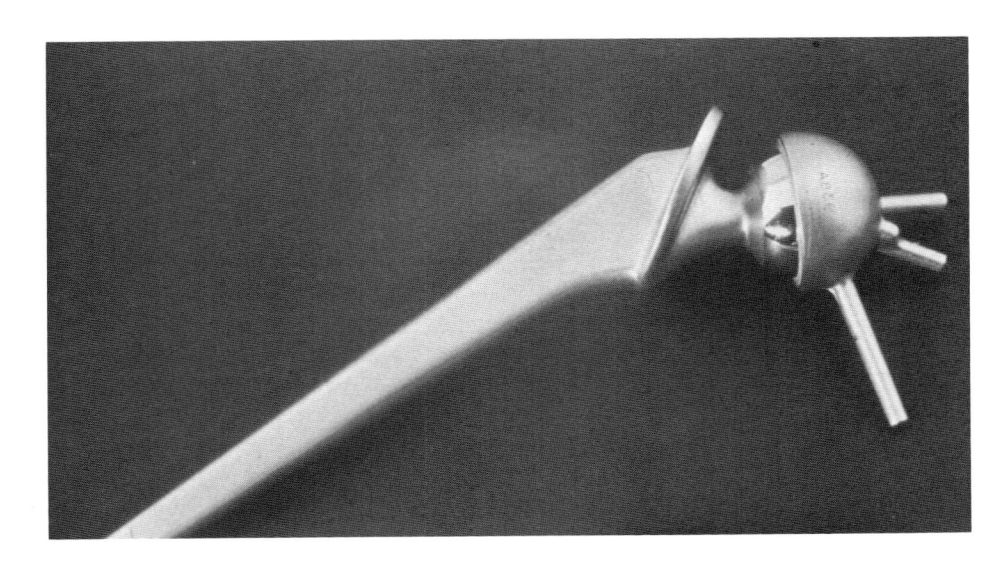

History and Development of Shoulder Arthroplasty   11

Figure 1-23. Stanmore total shoulder prosthesis showing conventional ball-and-socket design similar to total hip prostheses of the same era. (Reproduced with permission from Lettin et al.[39])

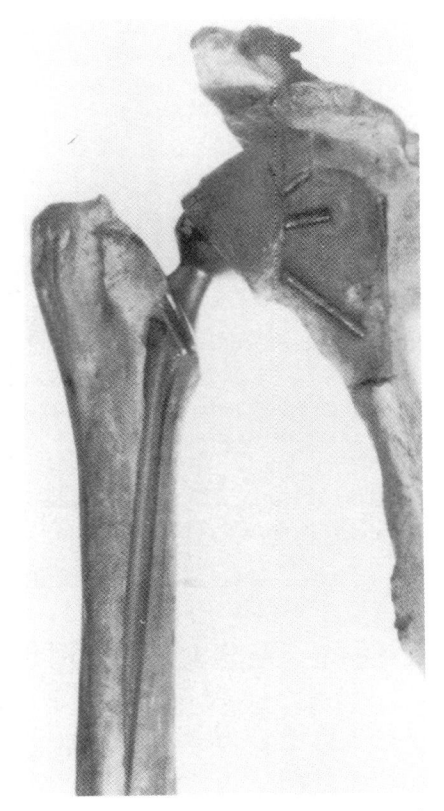

Figure 1-24. Stanmore prosthesis cemented into cadaveric bone. One can see how the tuberosities would impinge against the glenoid and cement mantle with this design. (Reproduced with permission from Lettin et al.[39])

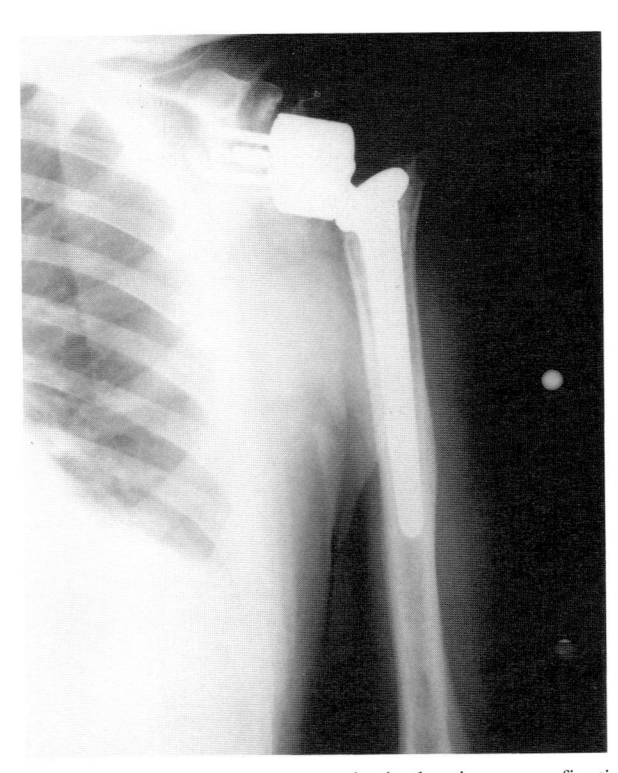

Figure 1-25. Michael Reese prosthesis showing screw fixation combined with cement. Despite excellent scapular fixation, the constrained design of this prosthesis led to early glenoid loosening.

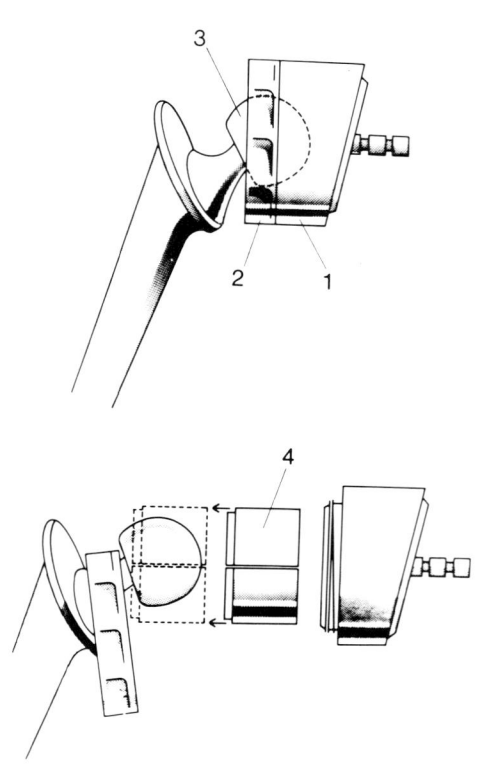

Figure 1–26. Assembly of Michael Reese conventional ball-and-socket joint showing (1) the metallic glenoid fixation device, (2) the retaining ring to prevent dislocation, (3) the spherical humeral head, and (4) the polyethylene liner. A grommet with a wire was later added to prevent backing out of the retaining ring and dislocation. (Reproduced with permission from Post.[42])

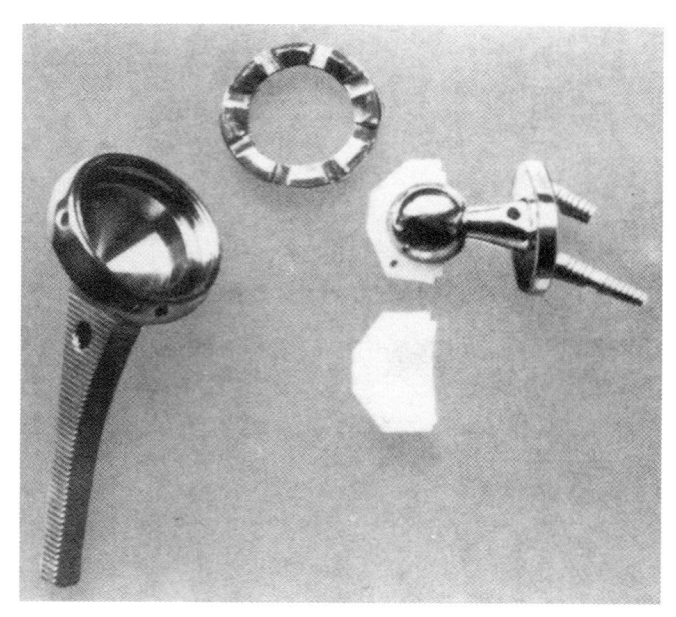

Figure 1–27. Reverse ball-and-socket design with polyethylene liner and retention ring, designed by Reeves, Jobbins, Dowson, and Wright. Note the divergent scapular pegs found in their series to give the best pullout strength for the scapular component. (Reproduced with permission from Reeves et al.[44])

chrome alloy, the initial results seemed encouraging in that only 2 of 22 patients required revision within 3 years. However, subsequent reports revealed a persistently high rate of revision, and therefore this prosthesis and other constrained devices should be looked upon as a salvage procedure at best.[41–43]

The Leeds shoulder of Reeves et al.[44] (Figure 1–27) tried to solve the scapular fixation problem with a divergent threaded peg system, which during in vitro testing resisted pullout better than other designs. Its reverse ball-and-socket articulation had an instant center of rotation coinciding with the anatomic center.

Alternate forms of scapular fixation include a single screw, as recommended by Kessel,[45] as well as fixation with a flange bolted to the base of the spine of the scapula, designed by Kolbel (Figure 1–28).[46–50] The Kessel prosthesis is discussed in Chapter 23. The Kolbel prosthesis has an outrigger which captures the spine of the scapula and limits

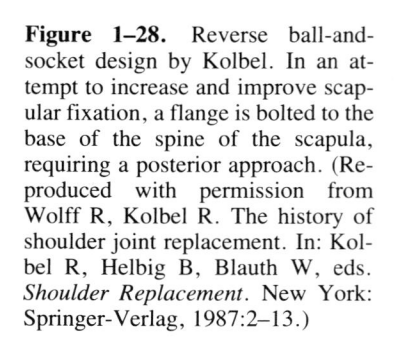

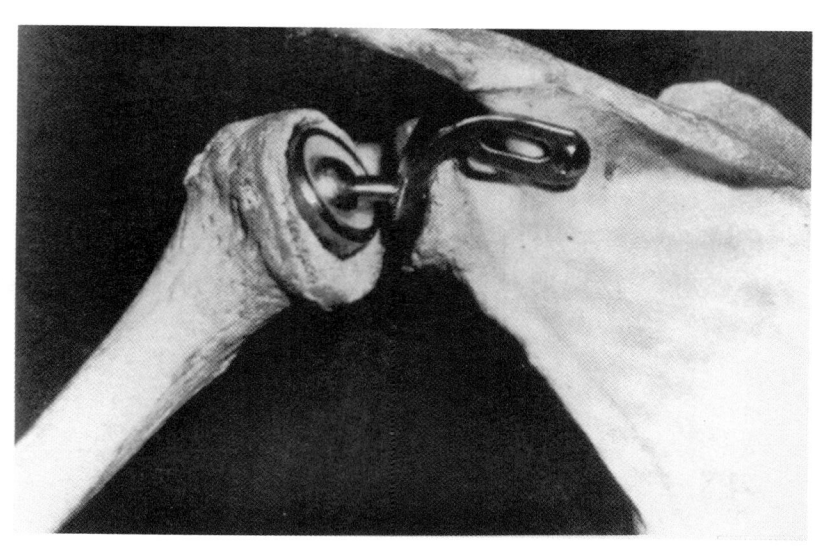

Figure 1–28. Reverse ball-and-socket design by Kolbel. In an attempt to increase and improve scapular fixation, a flange is bolted to the base of the spine of the scapula, requiring a posterior approach. (Reproduced with permission from Wolff R, Kolbel R. The history of shoulder joint replacement. In: Kolbel R, Helbig B, Blauth W, eds. *Shoulder Replacement*. New York: Springer-Verlag, 1987:2–13.)

the transfer of stress to the scapular component via a fail-safe mechanism that allows the component to dislocate at a force of 9 Nm. The joint has a 90-degree range of motion and permits rotation around its long axis. However, it is now only recommended in patients with soft-tissue defects.

A central screw with an articulating sphere similar to Kessel's was placed through a base plate and two more screws were subsequently added in the design by Gerard et al.[51] The polyethylene cup was semiconstrained, attached to a metal stem, and turned in all directions without dislocation. In 1973 he reported on six patients with sufficient follow-up.

The addition of acromial fixation with screws was recommended in a semiconstrained device by Mazas.[52] Fenlin, as well, utilized acromial fixation for difficult revision cases (personal communication, 1992). The DANA (designed after natural anatomy) hooded prosthesis[53,54] as well as the English-McNab[55] prosthesis have a peg for acromial load-sharing.

In an effort to gain motion and decrease the stresses seen on either side of the articulation in a constrained arthroplasty, a reverse ball-and-socket joint was developed by several authors. These include Kessel and Bayley,[45] Reeves et al.[44] (Leeds), Fenlin,[56] Kolbel and Friedebold,[46] Beddow and Elloy[57] (Liverpool), Buechel et al.[58] (floating shoulder), Gerard et al.,[51] and Gristina et al.[59] (trispherical). A metal-to-metal total shoulder prosthesis with a reverse ball-and-socket configuration was developed by Wheble and Skorecki.[60]

Buechel et al.[58] utilized the concept of a floating fulcrum to explain how the rotator cuff and humeral head form an essentially random pivot center when combined with a second socket, i.e., the glenoid. It was postulated that "impingement torque," i.e., the torque created by muscle forces across the glenohumeral joint leading to prosthetic impingement on the coupling between the humerus and glenoid, would eventually lead to failure either at the bone-cement interface or at the humeral glenoid interface. They felt that a prosthesis should provide more motion than the normal glenohumeral joint. In order to achieve this, a reverse ball-and-socket joint was incorporated, utilizing a small ball on the scapular side with a larger ball made of polyethylene on the humeral side. Early results in six patients were encouraging.

Fenlin[56] utilized a reverse large ball-and-socket concept with a fixed fulcrum designed for replacement of the cuff-deficient shoulder (Figure 1–29). The rationale for using a metallic cup and polyethylene ball was that the large ball-and-socket arrangement increased the freedom of motion and the lever arm for the deltoid. With the socket on the humeral side, the potential for dislocation would be less. The early results were excellent; however, the long-term results, as with other fixed fulcrum devices, were poor due to both prosthetic loosening and breakage. Despite the theoretic advantages stated previously, this prosthesis tended to be unstable anteriorly.[61]

Gristina and Webb[62] introduced the trispherical prosthesis (Figure 1–30) for management of these difficult patients. It consisted of vitallium humeral and glenoid components, each incorporating a sphere. These two spheres were then made part of a variable-fulcrum three-bar linkage system with an interposed polyethylene ball. This system was felt to afford a much greater range of motion than a simple ball-and-socket prosthesis. Although pain relief and improved range of motion were uniform, fracture of the glenoid and dislocation of the humeral component–middle ball interface occurred.

Another constrained design, which initially appeared promising and subsequently was abandoned, was that of Zippel.[63] This "dislocation proof" prosthesis transferred the stress to the humeral neck, resulting in fractures of four prosthetic humeral necks.[64–67]

An excellent review by Cofield[2] of the difference between

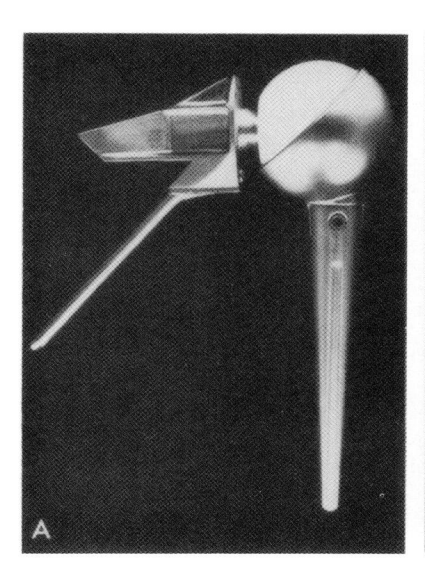

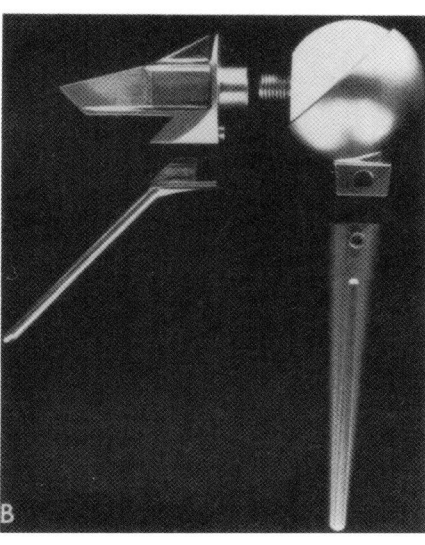

Figure 1–29. A prosthesis with an inherently stable fulcrum, designed by John M. Fenlin, Jr. to allow the deltoid alone to elevate the humerus. Note the large polyethylene ball and metallic socket design. **A.** Assembled. **B.** Disassembled. Note that the anchoring device on the scapular side incorporates a peg for the hard cortical bone along the axillary border of the scapula. (Reproduced with permission from Fenlin.[56])

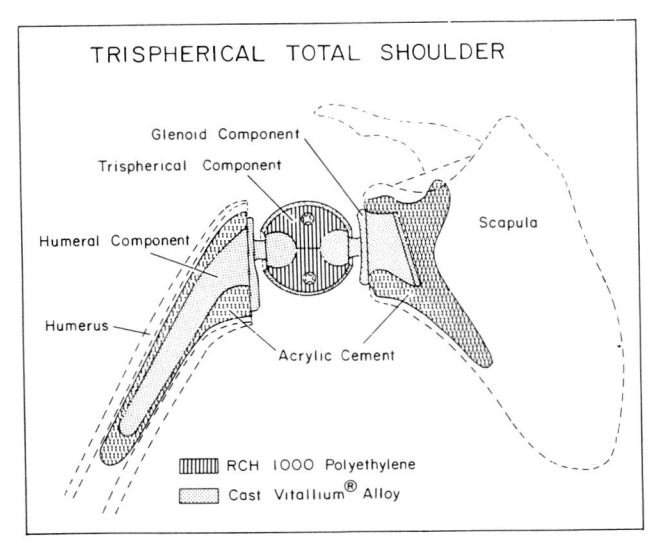

Figure 1–30. The unique double ball-and-socket configuration of the trispherical total shoulder. Note the two discrete ball joints on both humeral and scapular sides, articulating with a central polyethylene ball housed within a separate metallic socket. (Reproduced with permission from Gristina and Webb.[62])

the results of constrained versus nonconstrained designs at one institution was published in 1977. The Neer prosthesis, with its nonconstrained glenoid, proved far superior to either the Bickel or Stanmore prostheses. The results suggested that "emphasis should be placed on the repair of the glenohumeral stabilizing structures rather than on their replacement."[2]

The complications of constrained prostheses were dramatic and occurred in a relatively short period of time. These disappointing results in total shoulder arthroplasty led some investigators back to nonprosthetic reconstructive techniques. The double osteotomy of Benjamin[67,68] involves osteotomies through both the neck of the glenoid and the surgical neck of the humerus (Figure 1–31). The posterior periosteum is spared. Thirteen of 16 patients who had the operation, followed from 1 to 9 years, showed good or excellent pain relief with a substantial increase in active abduction. Tillmann and Braatz[69] confirmed the usefulness of this technique, especially in the older patient. Pain relief appears to occur very quickly, usually within 48 hours after surgery, and is felt to be secondary to a reduction of subchondral hyperemia and interosseous hypertension.

Tillmann and Braatz[69] also described a resection arthroplasty done through a transacromial approach in which a radical synovectomy is performed and the head of the humerus reshaped and covered with lyophilized dura. The rotator cuff was then reconstructed. Nothing was done to the glenoid in these cases. The retroversion on the head was increased by 10 degrees to avoid anterior dislocation, and an abduction splint was worn for 6 weeks postoperatively. Active physiotherapy was required for several months and in some cases as long as 1 year. Postoperatively, patients had less pain, averaging between none and mild, and improved their range of motion by 32 to 35 degrees. Resection arthroplasty was complicated by instability in two patients.

Gariepy[70] recommended glenoidectomy for the management of the rheumatoid patient (Figure 1–31). This procedure includes a release of the capsule, a 7- to 8-mm resection of the glenoid articular surface, exposure of the subdeltoid bursa and biceps sheath if synovectomy is needed in this area, and full removal of pannus. Twelve cases were reviewed with follow-up from 1 to 13 years. Relief of pain was satisfactory in all cases. The best results occurred in patients with no gross deformity of the humeral head and in patients whose systemic disease was not too severe. Wainwright[71] has also used glenoidectomy with good results, as five of six patients achieved good pain relief and improvements in motion. In spite of these favorable reports, as well as good results in his own patients, Souter[3] in 1983 felt that this technique should be considered obsolete.

Glenoid reshaping and grafting have been utilized in conjunction with a proximal humeral replacement by Engelbrecht and coworkers,[34] to avoid glenoid loosening (Figure 1–32). These techniques have included reshaping with a reamer, osteotomy, grafting the superior aspect of the glenoid to prevent superior subluxation, and central expansion with a graft to increase the surface area of a deficient glenoid with capsular insufficiency.

Bateman[72] described a cheilotomy of the shoulder in which the large teardrop or "turkey beard" osteophyte in

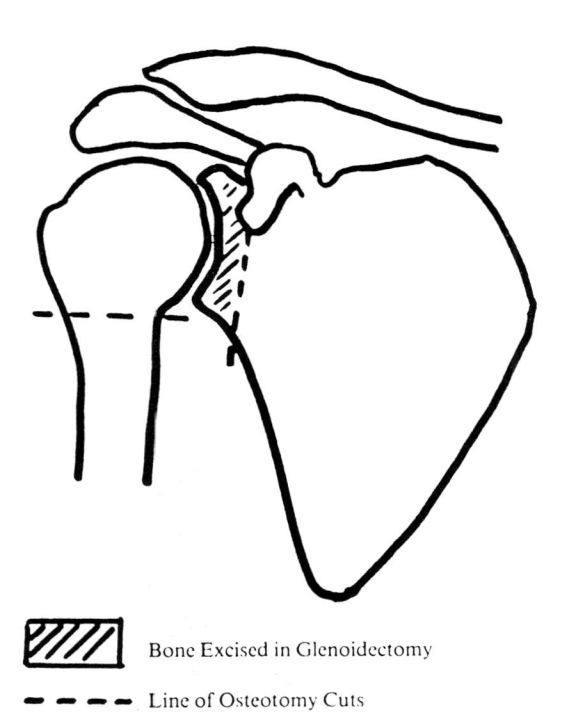

Figure 1–31. Alternatives to total shoulder arthroplasty include glenoidectomy and double osteotomy. The hatched lines indicate bone excised in glenoidectomy. The dotted lines indicate the osteotomy cuts for double osteotomy. (Reproduced with permission from Souter.[3])

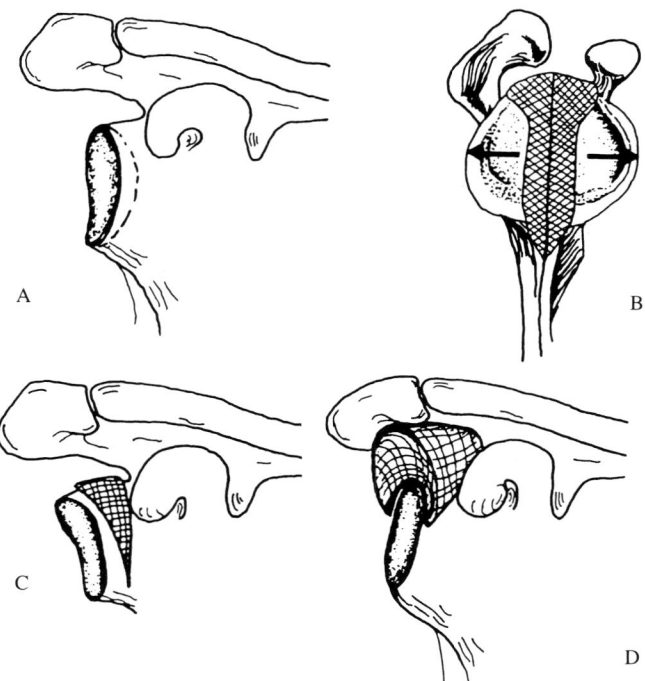

Figure 1–32. Alternatives to total shoulder arthroplasty include glenoid resurfacing with a reamer (**A**), and glenoid expansion with a graft (**B**). **C and D.** The superior osteotomy and interposition graft are designed to block proximal migration of the replaced humerus. (Reproduced with permission from Engelbrecht and Heinert.[34])

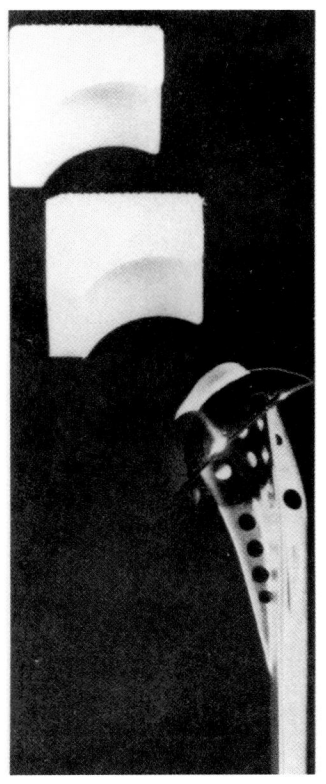

Figure 1–34. Polyethylene subacromial spacer designed to be used with the Neer prosthesis to prevent proximal humeral migration and resurface the "subacromial joint" in rheumatoid arthritis. (Reproduced with permission from Ferlic.[79])

primary glenohumeral arthritis is removed. This relatively conservative procedure, including débridement of the joint, removal of obvious osteophytes, smoothing of the articular surface, and concomitant acromioclavicular joint arthroplasty, gave his patients considerable relief of pain.

Interposition arthroplasty using Silastic (Figure 1–33) was introduced by Swanson[73] in 1973. Varian[74] in 1980 reported dramatic pain relief and improvement in shoulder movement and function, but a report by Spencer and Skirving in 1986[75] confirmed what is now known about Silastic implants, that there is dramatic fragmentation of the Silastic associated with severe cystic changes and destruction of the glenohumeral joint.

Keeping the humeral head down after a shoulder arthroplasty, especially in the rotator cuff–deficient patient, is a tremendous challenge. Although proximal humeral migration was not shown to adversely affect the results of a shoulder arthroplasty in one series,[76] clearly motion would be greater and the muscles would function more efficiently if the instant center of rotation was kept near the anatomic center of the glenoid. Ferlic and Clayton[77–79] utilized a custom metallic and polyethylene spacer (Figure 1–34) to function as an interposition between the humeral head and

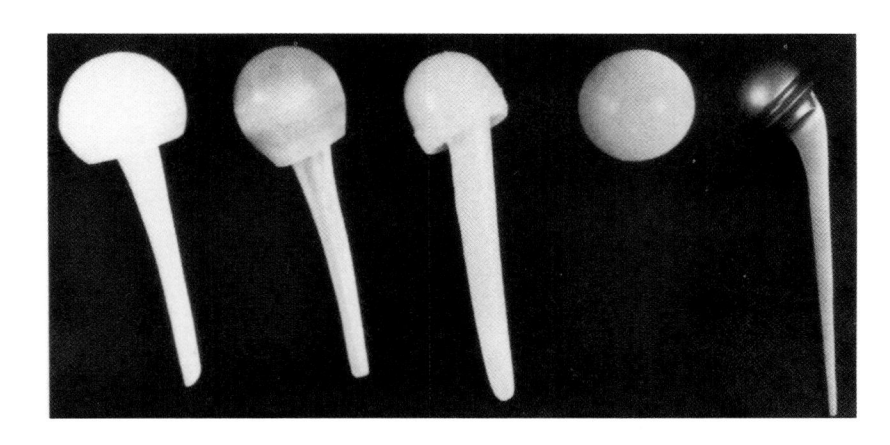

Figure 1–33. Silastic head component and double-cup metal stem head component. (Reproduced with permission from Swanson.[73])

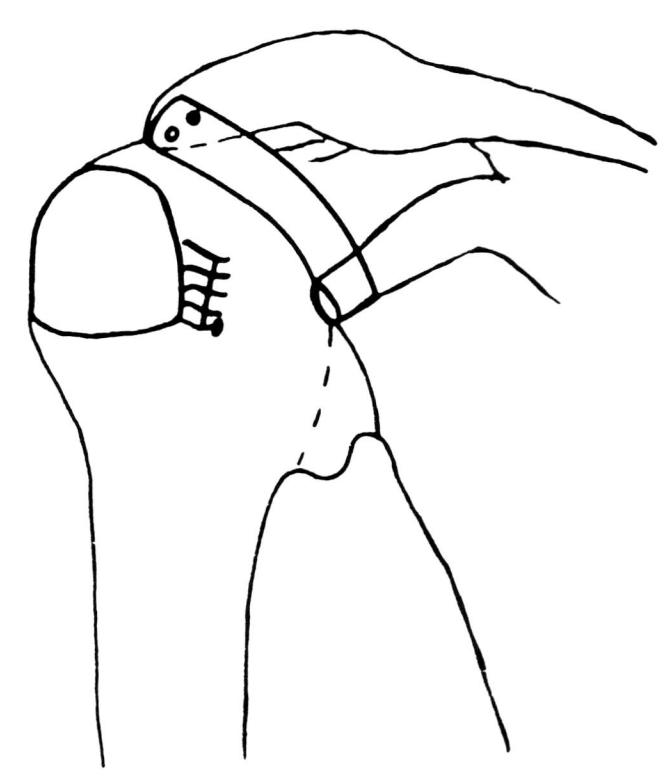

Figure 1–35. A new subacromial articulation is created between a prosthesis, spanning the space between the coracoid and the acromion and the opposing tuberosity. (Reproduced with permission from Grammont.[80])

acromion to prevent superior subluxation of the humerus and decrease pain in the rheumatoid patient.

Another design to resurface the coracoacromial arch developed by Grammont,[80] called the Acropole prosthesis (Figure 1–35), was used to treat the patient with a rotator cuff tear arthropathy. This prosthesis seeks to prevent the upward extension of the humerus, to control pain, and to restore the normal fulcrum of movement beneath the subacromial arch. He recommended this both for patients with a rotator cuff tear arthropathy and for patients with rheumatoid disease. Twelve of these metal-on-metal prostheses were implanted between December 1977 and January 1980. Ten patients achieved complete pain relief; however, active range of motion was poorly enhanced. There were no cases of instability.

In an effort to find a middle ground between minimally constrained prostheses such as the Neer design and the constrained devices previously described, several investigators, in an effort to protect against superior subluxation, developed what Cofield termed "semiconstrained devices." These include the English-McNab prosthesis, which is discussed in Chapter 23, the Mazas (nonretentive) prosthesis, and the hooded version of the DANA shoulder. Mazas and de la Caffiniere[52] reported on 38 cases using a nonretentive but superior lipped glenoid component. Six failures occurred, including five dislocations. Fourteen shoulders remained very stiff. These procedures were done through a posterior approach.

Experience with the DANA hooded component was described by Ellman et al.[81] Twelve patients with a rotator cuff tear arthropathy and irreparable cuff deficiency underwent a shoulder arthroplasty. Range of motion improved, but only modestly and included 70 degrees of abduction, 22 degrees of external rotation, 7 degrees of internal rotation, and only 3 degrees of active forward flexion. Two patients had chronically dislocated shoulders and three had subluxating shoulder joints. Removal of the greater tuberosity in these patients seemed to give better results. However, satisfactory results occurred in only 50% of cases using a hooded prosthesis. Brownlee and Cofield[82] presented a series in 1986 demonstrating that hooded glenoid components offered no advantage in the treatment of a rotator cuff tear arthropathy, as the patients had less motion and more problems with instability than did those who had had conventional shoulder replacement arthroplasty with rotator cuff reconstruction.

Amstutz[53,54] developed the DANA total shoulder (Figure 1–36) based on the work of Maki and Gruen,[83] and recognized that while a 44-mm radius of curvature as described by Neer was the average, there were multiple variations on either end of the spectrum in regards to head diameter, head height, and radius of curvature. This prosthesis was the first to utilize different-sized glenoid-bearing surfaces matched

Figure 1–36. The DANA total shoulder system, designed by Harlan Amstutz, was the first to offer multiple head sizes and multiple glenoid sizes. A hooded, semiconstrained glenoid was also available. (Reproduced with permission from Amstutz et al.[53])

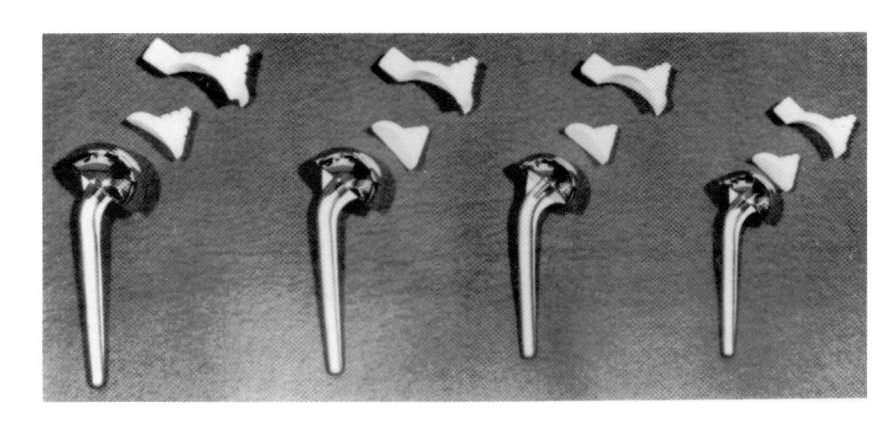

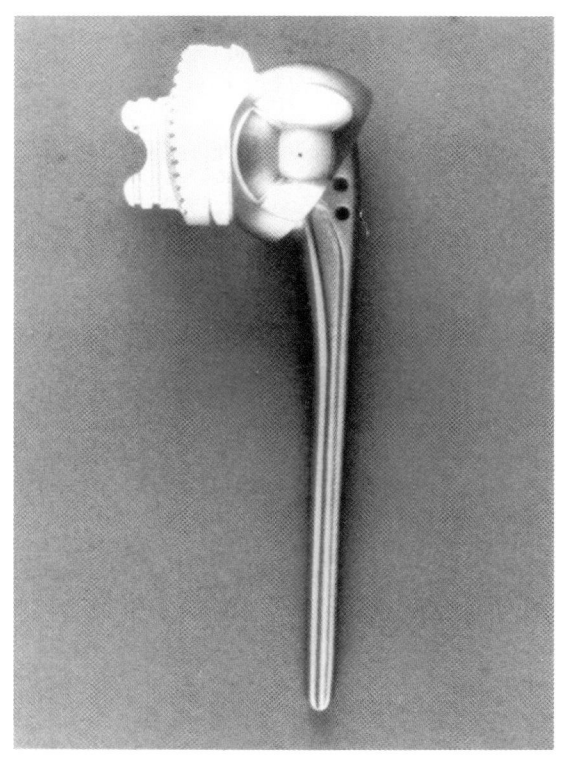

Figure 1–37. Monospherical prostheses designed by Gristina. An example of the semiconstrained devices of the late 1970s. (Reproduced with permission from Gristina et al.[59])

with different-sized humeral components. It was composed of cobalt chrome with a taper and antirotation flange designed for use with methylmethacrylate. New instrumentation included a cutting guide for the humeral head and a glenoid retractor. Between 1976 and 1984, 83 arthroplasties using DANA shoulder prostheses were performed, and 56 patients were available for long-term follow-up. A new shoulder rating scale was also introduced. A radiolucent line had developed at the bone-cement interface of the glenoid component in 53 shoulders. However, only two glenoid components had been revised for loosening. While pain relief and function improved in patients with a hooded glenoid component, range of motion did not.

Another design that emerged in the late 1970s and early 1980s was the monospherical prosthesis by Gristina[84] (Figure 1–37). This shoulder had two glenoids with an over-hemispherical articulating surface and a radius of curvature of either 40 or 44 mm. The humeral stem was recessed with rounded edges to minimize stress and came in two stem sizes. The glenoid was pear-shaped with a bilobate keel configuration, closely approximating the cancellous recesses of the scapula. Two glenoids were designed, one a simple resurfacing prosthesis and the other with an extended hoodlike bearing surface superiorly. One hundred monospherical total shoulder replacements were reviewed in 1987, with 90% of patients experiencing minimal or no postoperative pain. Abduction in the plane of the scapula increased an average of 75 degrees. Radiographic follow-up revealed evidence of glenoid component loosening in three patients. There were no humeral radiolucencies, but radiolucencies less than 1 mm thick at the glenoid bone-cement interface occurred in two-thirds of the patients. It was hoped that metal backing of the glenoid would lower the loosening rate.

A bipolar shoulder prosthesis was designed in 1975 by Swanson (Figure 1–38).[85–87] The large-head humeral implant concept was felt to have the following theoretic advantages: (1) provide smooth concentric total contact for the entire shoulder joint cavity, which includes both the glenoid cavity and coracoacromial arch; (2) decrease the force concentrated at any one contact point, thereby decreasing the coefficient of friction; (3) lengthen the moment arm between the fulcrum and muscle insertion, thereby increasing the efficiency of muscular action; and (4) prevent impingement of the greater tuberosity against the acromion (Figure 1–39).

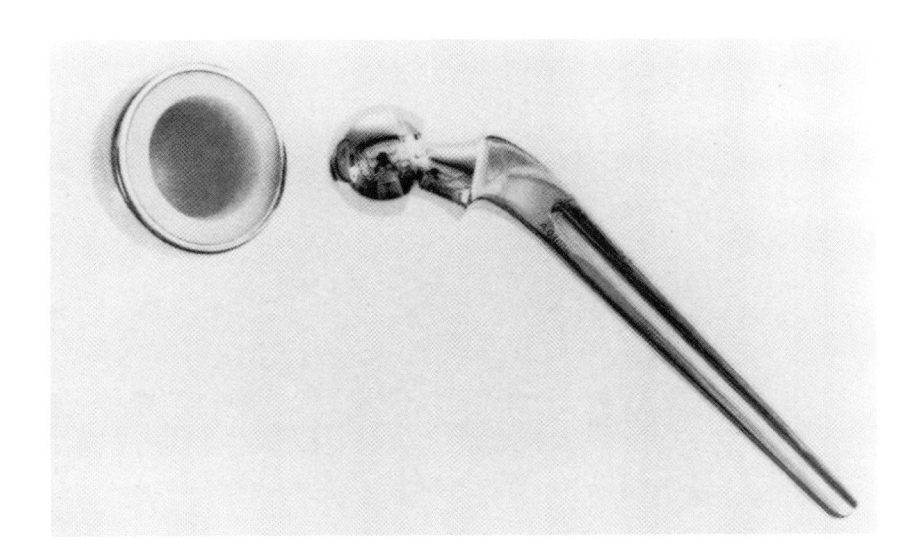

Figure 1–38. Bipolar prostheses of Swanson. (Reproduced with permission from Swanson et al.[87])

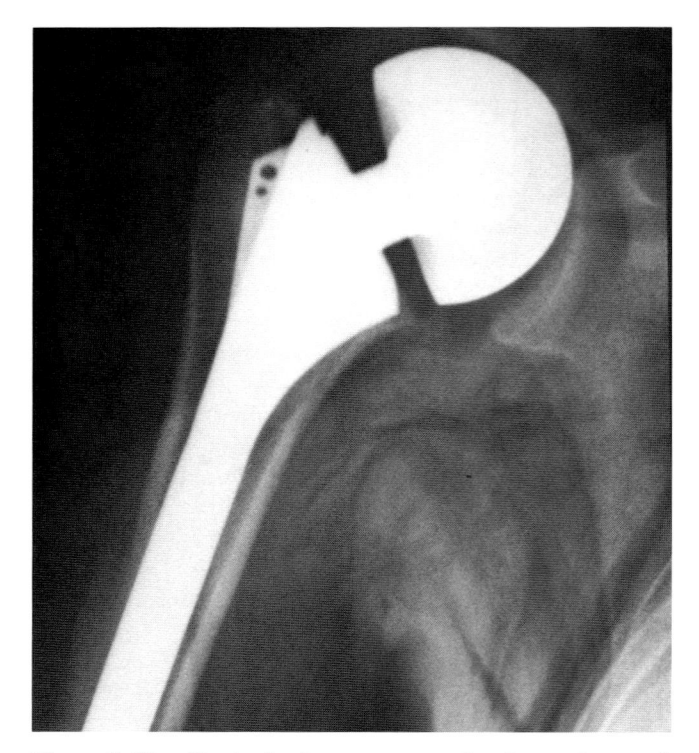

Figure 1–39. Bipolar implant on a cementless humeral stem of the author's design showing the principles of a large-head humeral implant with articulation in the glenoid as well as the coracoacromial arch.

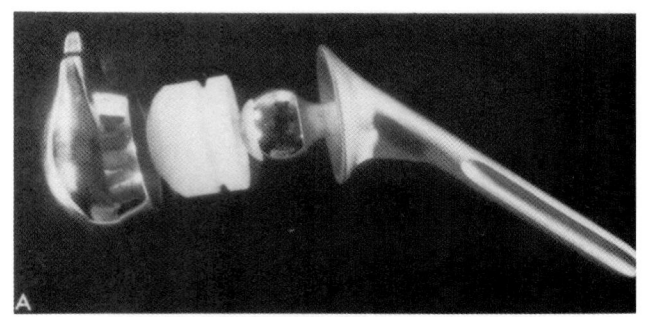

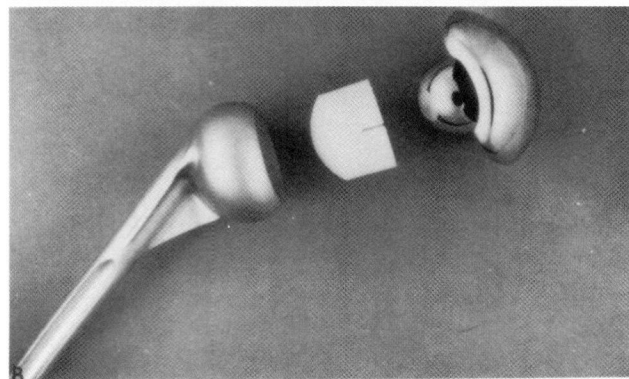

Figure 1–40. Bipolar-type designs by Bateman. **A.** Single-assembly total shoulder. **B.** "Collar button," modification of single-assembly total shoulder. (Reproduced with permission from Bateman.[72])

Commenting on the one-piece silicone on metal large-head implants, Swanson reported the results as good for pain relief but inadequate for motion and durability. Bipolar implant arthroplasty was hoped to be a more durable and efficient method of replacing the shoulder. Fifteen shoulders were operated on between November 1976 and July 1981, and follow-up averaged 41 months. There was no loosening of the stem and no evidence of erosive changes in the glenoid or superior coracoacromial arch. A single dislocation was the only complication. The results did not deteriorate with time and no erosive changes developed in the coracoacromial arch over a longer period of follow-up.[88]

Bateman[72] developed two bipolar designs, one a single-assembly total shoulder prosthesis (Figure 1–40A) and the other a "collar button," modification. Both have a polyethylene inner bearing and are implanted without secure scapular fixation. In the second modification, a reverse ball-and-socket joint was utilized (Figure 1–40B).

At the other end of the spectrum from constrained, semiconstrained, and bipolar designs are the more simplified surface replacements. Bateman[72] developed such a design as well (Figure 1–41). This extremely conservative model replaces only the articular surface of the humeral head. A curved fin that is fenestrated and transfixes the cortex substitutes for an intramedullary stem.

Along the same lines of Bateman's simple resurfacing procedure was the cup arthroplasty described by Jonsson for

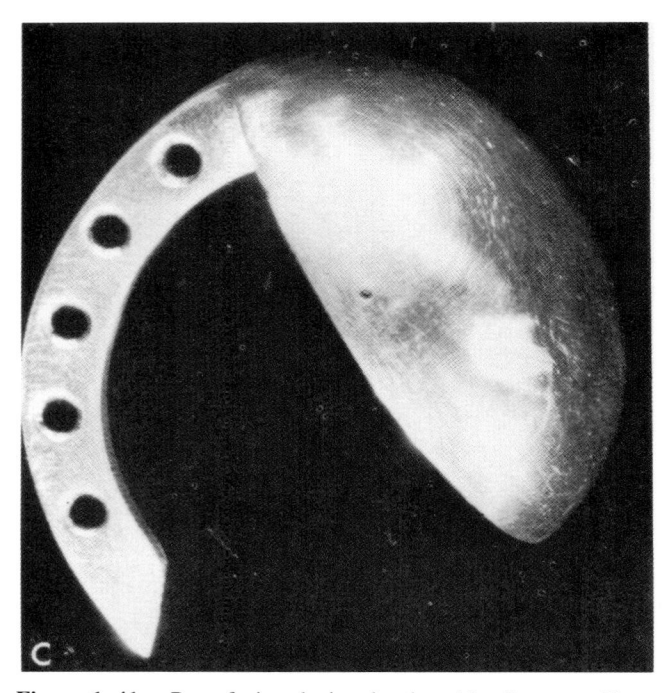

Figure 1–41. Resurfacing device developed by Bateman. Note the fenestrated curved stem designed to transfix the cortex. (Reproduced with permission from Bateman.[72])

rheumatoid patients in Scandinavia (Figure 1–42).[88–90] The Indiana conservative hip has also been utilized in a similar manner. Other conservative stem designs include those of Figgie[91] and Copeland.[92]

In 1982, Neer, Watson, and Stanton presented the largest series to date on total shoulder arthroplasties.[93] The glenoid components utilized in this series are pictured in Figure 1–43. A metal-backed glenoid was added in the late 1970s, coinciding with finite element analysis data that metal backing of the acetabular component decreased the stress at the bone-cement interface. It has been assumed by many that the metal-backed glenoid was introduced for the same reason, but in actuality, it was introduced to avoid breakage of the polyethylene glenoid component, which had occurred in two cases. Subsequently, it was discovered that the glenoid components fractured because they were supported by cement and not bone, and when the cement failed, toggling and fracture of the polyethylene occurred.

The humeral component (Figure 1–44) was designed to match the radius of curvature of the glenoid, with the edges rounded off to avoid abrasion of the polyethylene from a sharp edge on the humeral component. The triflange mechanism was modified and only two holes were left for suturing the tuberosities laterally. Flutes were added for cement egress, as this prosthesis was originally designed for use with methylmethacrylate.

McElwain and English,[55] Cofield,[94] Copeland,[92] and Roper et al.[95] reported results on cementless fixation of total shoulder implants, which are presented in Chapter 23.

Fenlin (personal communication) investigated modular humeral replacement using metal glenoids articulating with polyethylene humeral heads. Design changes led to the development of the Fenlin total shoulder (Figure 1–45). This modular humeral system, designed to be used with cement, has a standard Morse taper on the humeral component for articulation with cobalt chrome heads. The glenoid is a preassembled, metal-backed, finned device that requires cement fixation.

Several other modular designs appeared in the late 1980s. These include the Biomodular developed by Warren and Dines, the Select Shoulder-System by Burkhead, and the Biangular by Werlin. The Biomodular design (Figure 1–46) incorporates a unique reverse Morse taper design which makes revision of a loose glenoid and painful hemiarthroplasty easier. However, a number of head dissociations have occurred with this design. It is unclear whether this is related to debris or fluid within the reverse Morse taper, prohibiting full seating and engagement of the taper, or the longer lever arm and increased stress at the taper junction inherent in this design.

A less constrained glenoid replacement was introduced by the author in 1987 (Figure 1–47). The glenoid is flat-backed

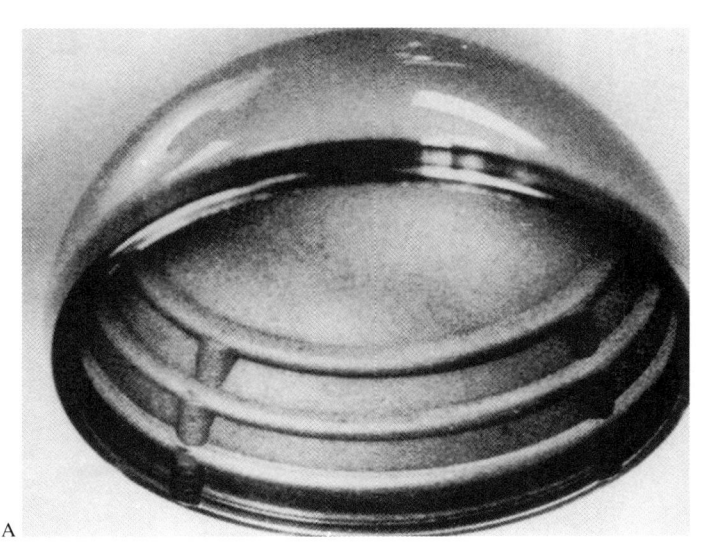

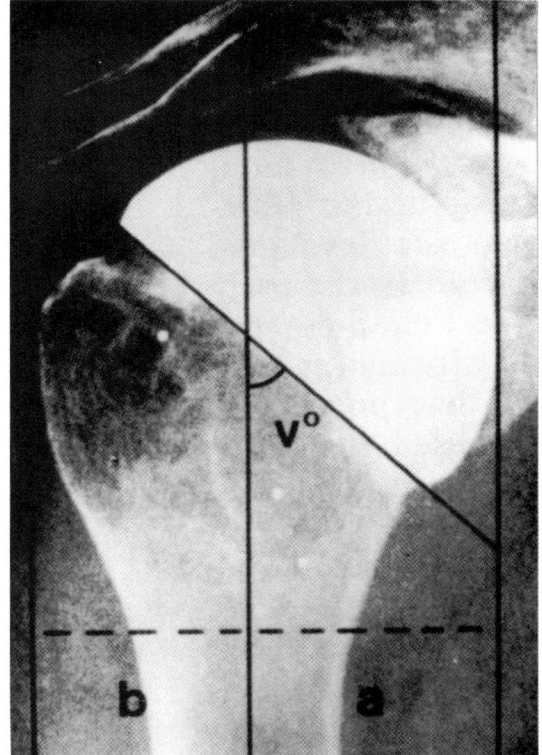

Figure 1–42. A and B. Cup arthroplasty described for Scandinavians by Jonsson. This conservative resurfacing device gave improved function when compared to arthrodesis in rheumatoid patients. (Reproduced with permission from Jonsson et al.[90])

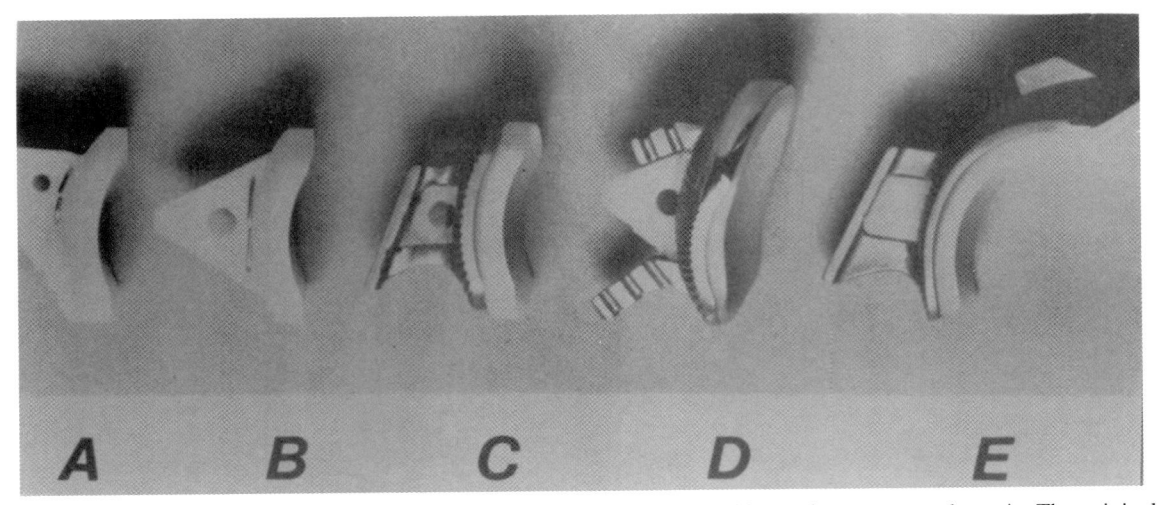

Figure 1–43. Glenoid component utilized in the largest series of shoulder replacements to date. **A.** The original polyethylene component used in 1973 by Neer. **B.** The standard polyethylene glenoid component used since 1974. **C.** Metal-backed standard-size glenoid component. **D.** Metal-backed glenoid component, 200% larger than the standard size, which does allow reattachment of the supraspinatus. **E.** Metal-backed glenoid component, 600% larger than standard size, designed to be used with the long head humeral component, precluding reattachment of the supraspinatus. (Reproduced with permission from Neer et al.[94])

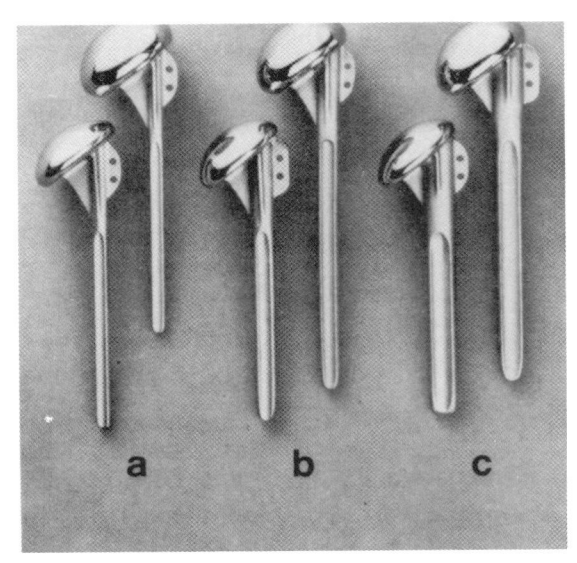

Figure 1–44. Humeral stems available for the Neer II system including stems for juvenile rheumatoid arthritis and long stems for fracture and tumor surgery. Two head sizes, 15 and 22 mm, are available with the same radius of curvature. The 10 humeral components used in the largest series of shoulder replacement to date. **a, b,** and **c.** The standard lengths of stem, each with three stem diameters and two head lengths (thickness of head). The long head was felt to provide better leverage. The short head simplifies repair of large defects of the rotator cuff and is used in small patients. (Reproduced with permission from Neer et al.[93])

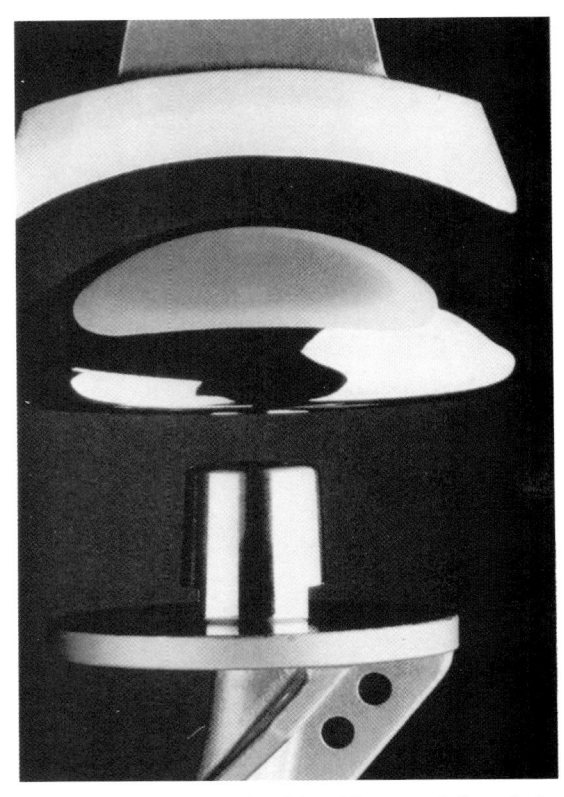

Figure 1–45. Fenlin total shoulder. Note metal-finned glenoid bonded to the polyethylene, decreasing the overall thickness of the glenoid component. Conventional Morse taper on the humeral side.

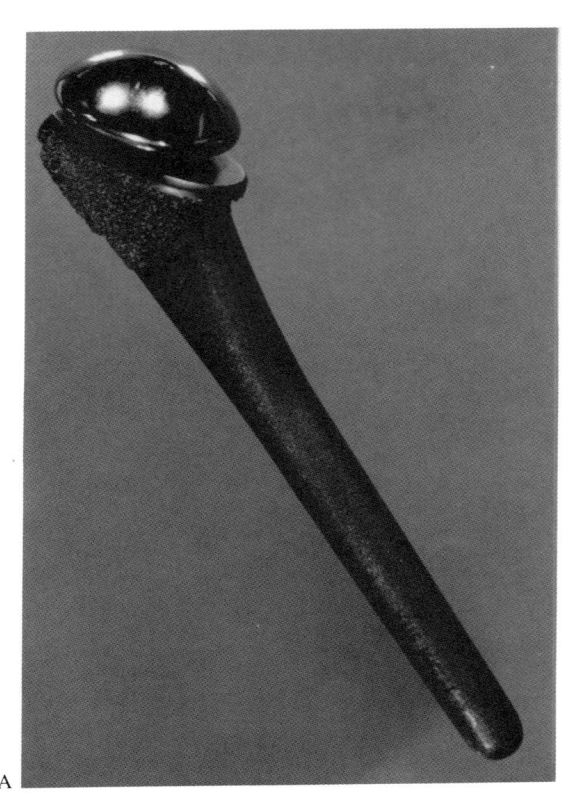

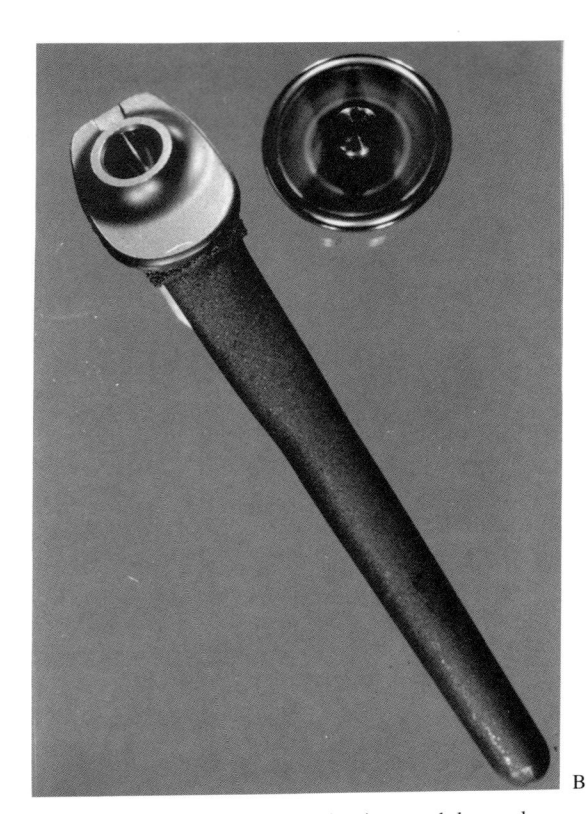

Figure 1–46. Biomodular total shoulder. **A.** Biomodular prosthesis assembled. When implanting modular replacements, it is important to select a head size that covers the collar so that the collar does not impinge against the glenoid. **B.** Biomodular prosthesis disassembled. Note the reverse Morse taper design. Note that the stem of taper is on the humeral component.

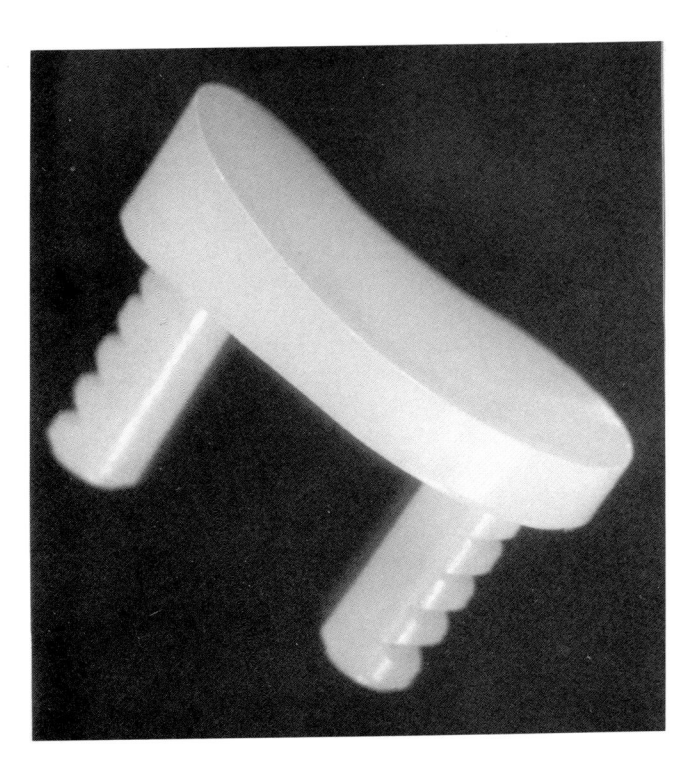

Figure 1–47. Glenoid component of the author's design, a polyethylene component utilized with cement, showing a flat back to avoid the rocking-horse effect, dual-peg fixation, allowing preservation of subchondral bone, pressurization of cement, and a less-constrained bearing surface allowing up to 10 mm of translation.

to avoid the rocking-horse effect, and has two pegs rather than a keel for fixation. The bearing surface allows humeral translation up to 10 mm, which has been described by Wallace[96] as the normal amount of translation seen in young patients during glenohumeral abduction, thereby recreating normal glenohumeral biomechanics.

The Biangular glenoid (Figure 1–48) has two pegs and a fin on the glenoid component placed at a 45-degree angle to the surface. Gagey and Mazas[97] reported on the use of a glenoid component with screw fixation into both the acromion and the glenoid (Figure 1–49). A recent design, the Global Shoulder, designed by Rockwood and Matsen, incorporates a reverse Morse taper similar to the Biomodular on the humeral side and a less constrained glenoid with pegs on the glenoid side.

Alternative materials to cobalt chrome, stainless steel, and titanium have been described. A bioceramic endoprosthesis for replacement of the proximal part of the humerus was reported in 1979; an aluminum oxide, three-component endoprosthesis was implanted without cement for tumor resection.[98] The polyacetal component of Mathys has been used widely in Europe.[99,100] Twelve-year clinical results of the treatment of fractures utilizing the prosthesis have been reported by Burri[101] (Figure 1–50). The prosthesis, which was stabilized with a single screw without cement in 50 cases, had favorable subjective results in more than 80% of the cases. A ceramic head for a shoulder prosthesis has been developed by Fukuda et al.[102,103]

Neer's 1982 series was updated in 1990 to include 776 glenohumeral arthroplasties, with 615 using nonconstrained total shoulder prostheses. Of 408 total shoulder arthroplasties in multiple diagnostic categories, excellent results were obtained in 242 shoulders. The prosthesis as well as his techniques have stood the test of time. Other authors have confirmed the efficacy of his shoulder arthroplasty technique.[19,58,67,72,73,76,78,82,88,94,97,104–117] Clearly, the Neer II prosthesis, with its large clinical experience, is the gold standard upon which all newer modifications must be judged.

Matsen in 1990 said that Neer brought us 90% of the way in glenohumeral replacement. Clearly, he did not do it alone, as there were others struggling in the arena upon whose successes and failures we have all learned and benefited from. The last 10% will come hard, of that fact there is no doubt. Refined techniques, newer biomaterials, and a greater understanding of the complex biomechanics of the replaced shoulder, combined with cooperation, healthy competition, and most importantly, honesty, will help push the boundaries of shoulder replacement surgery.

Codman[118] said, "Give me something different for there's a chance it might be better." To those who dare to improve upon the work of the past, good luck!

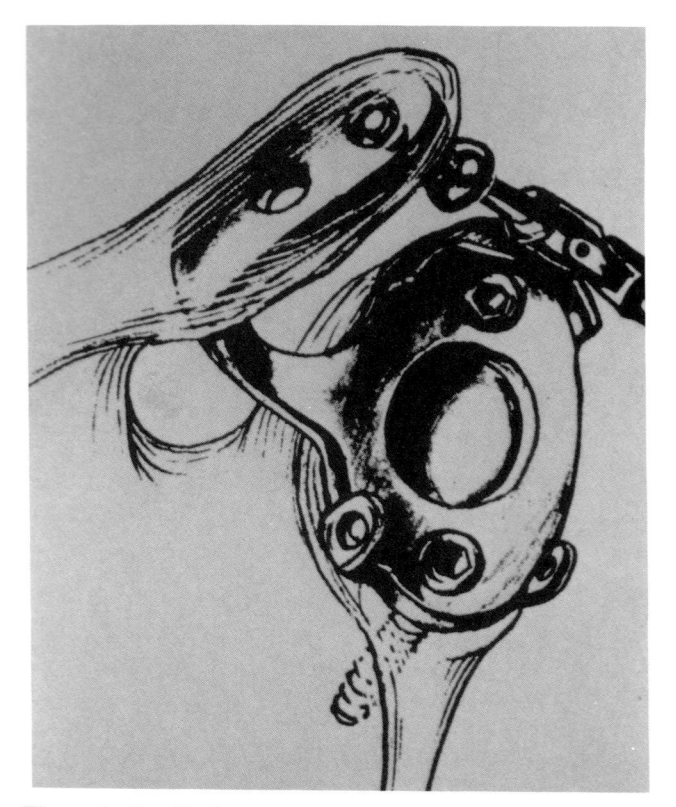

Figure 1–49. Design by Gagey and Mazas. Baseplate showing screw fixation, in both the glenoid and the acromion with a bar linking these two. The authors state that the rotator cuff can be repaired with a bar in place in the interval between the infraspinatus and supraspinatus. (Reproduced with permission from Gagey and Mazas.[97])

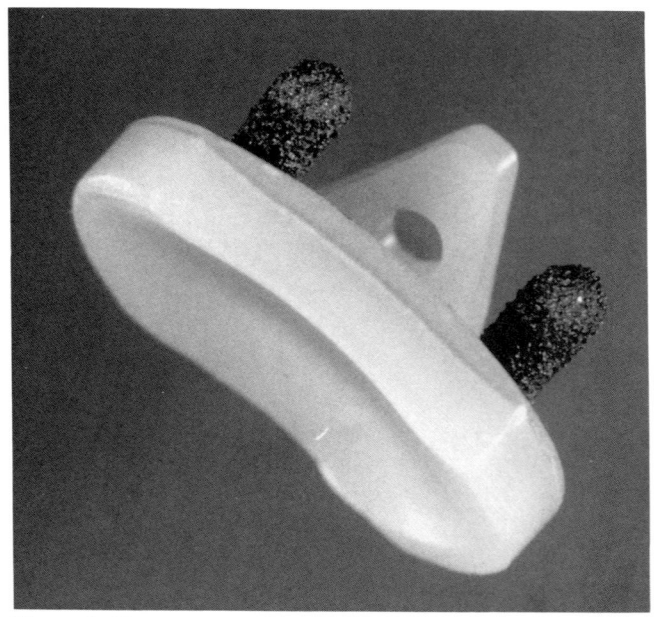

Figure 1–48. Biangular glenoid component combines peg and fin fixation of the glenoid component. The pegs and fin form a 45-degree angle with the back of the prosthesis.

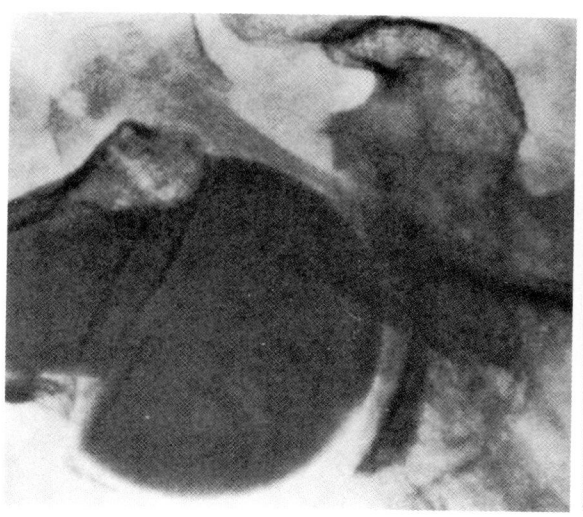

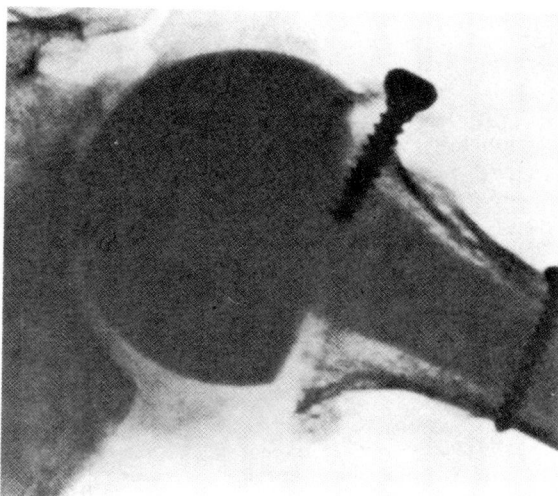

Figure 1-50. Polyacetal component of Mathys. Note the screw fixation for stability. (Reproduced with permission from Burri.[101])

REFERENCES

1. Pean JE. Des moyens prosthetiques destines a obtenir la reparation de parties ossueses. *Gaz Hop Paris* 1894;67:291.
2. Cofield RH. Status of total shoulder arthroplasty. *Arch Surg* 1977;112:1088–1091.
3. Souter WA. The surgical treatment of the rheumatoid shoulder. *Ann Acad Med* 1983;12:243–255.
4. Pean JE, Bick EM, trans. The classic on prosthetic methods intended to repair bone fragments. *Clin Orthop* 1973;94:4–7.
5. Lugli T. Artificial shoulder joint by Pean (1893). The facts of an exceptional intervention and the prosthetic method. *Clin Orthop* 1978;133:215–218.
6. Murphy JB. Fracture and luxation of the neck of the humerus. *Surg Clin Chicago* 1913;II:137–148.
7. Rovsing T. Ein Fall von frieir Knochentransplantation zum Ersatz der zwei oberen Drittel des Oberarmes mit Hilfe der Fibula des Patienten. *Zentralbl Chir* 1910;37:870.
8. Albee FH. *Bone Graft Surgery*. Philadelphia: WB Saunders, 1915:268.
9. Albee FH. Restoration of shoulder function in cases of loss of head and upper portion of humerus. *Surg Gynecol Obstet* 1921;32:1–19.
10. Hammond R. Transplantation of the fibula to replace a bony defect in the shoulder. *J Bone Joint Surg* 1926;8:627–635.
11. Groves EWH. Methods and results of transplantation of bone in the repair of defects caused by injury or disease. *Br J Surg* 1917;5:185.
12. Behrend M. Transplantation of the head and shaft of the fibula to the humerus. *Surg Gynecol Obstet* 1930;51:717.
13. Morison R. Excision of the upper end of the humerus for chondrosarcoma. *Br J Surg* 1914;1:383.
14. Schauffler RM. Transplant of the upper extremity of the fibula to replace the upper extremity of the humerus. *J Bone Joint Surg* 1926;8:723.
15. Skillern PG. Sarcoma of humerus. Resection of upper shaft with transplantation of upper third of fibula to humerus stump. *Int Clin* 1920;1:41.
16. Clark K. A case of replacement of the upper end of the humerus by a fibular graft reviewed after 29 years. *J Bone Joint Surg [Br]* 1959;41:365–368.
17. Konig F. Uber die Implantation von Elfen Hein Zum Eustatz von Knochen und Gelenkenden Brums Beitr. *Klin Chir* 1914;85:613.
18. Jones L. Reconstructive operation for nonreducible fractures of the head of the humerus. *Ann Surg* 1933;97:217–225.
19. Jones L. The shoulder joint—Observations on the anatomy and physiology with an analysis of a reconstructive operation following extensive injury. *Surg Gynecol Obstet* 1942;75:433–444.
20. Smith-Peterson MN, Aufranc OE, Larson CB. Useful surgical procedures for rheumatoid arthritis involving joints of the upper extremity. *Arch Surg* 1943;46:764–770.
21. Baron R, Senn L. Acrylic prosthesis for the shoulder. *Presse Med* 1951;59:1480.
22. Richard A, Judet R, Rene L. Acrylic prosthetic reconstruction of the upper end of the humerus for fracture-luxations. *J Chir* 1952;68:537–547.
23. Lynn TA, Alexakis PG, Bechtol CO. Stem prosthesis to replace lost proximal humerus. *Clin Orthop* 1965;43:245–247.
24. de Anquin CA, de Anquin CE. Prosthetic replacement in the treatment of serious fractures of the proximal humerus. In: Bayley I, Kessel L, eds. *Shoulder Surgery*. New York: Springer-Verlag, 1982:207–215.
25. Monteleone M: L'Endoprotesi sostitutiva mella terapia delle fratture-lussazioni dell'estremità superiore dell'omero. *Chir Organi Mov* 1969;57:404.
26. Krueger FJ. A vitallium replica arthroplasty on the shoulder: A case report of aseptic necrosis of the proximal end of the humerus. *Surgery* 1951;30:1005–1011.
27. Neer CS II, Brown TH Jr, McLaughlin HL. Fracture of the neck of the humerus with dislocation of the head fragment. *Am J Surg* 1953;85:252–258.
28. Neer CS II. Articular replacement for the humeral head. *J Bone Joint Surg [Am]* 1955;37:215–228.
29. Neer CS II. Followup notes on articles previously published in the journal. Articular replacement for the humeral head. *J Bone Joint Surg [Am]* 1964;46:1607–1610.
30. Neer CS II. Replacement arthroplasty for glenohumeral osteoarthritis. *J Bone Joint Surg [Am]* 1974;56:1–13.
31. Neer CS II. *Shoulder Reconstruction*. Philadelphia: WB Saunders, 1990.
32. Engelbrecht E, Stellbrink G. Totale Schulterendoprosthese Modell "St. Georg." *Chirurgie* 1976;47:525–530.

33. Engelbrecht E. Ten years of experience with unconstrained shoulder replacement. In: Bateman JE, Welsh RP, eds. *Surgery of the Shoulder*. St. Louis: CV Mosby, 1984:121–124.
34. Engelbrecht E, Heinert K. More than ten years' experience with unconstrained shoulder replacement. In: Kolbel R, Helbig B, Blauth W, eds. *Shoulder Replacement*. Berlin: Springer-Verlag, 1987:234–239.
35. Kenmore PI, MacCartee C, Vitek B. A simple shoulder replacement. *J Biomed Mater Res* 1974;8:329–330.
36. Cofield RH, Stauffer RN. The Bickel glenohumeral arthroplasty. In: *Joint Replacement in the Upper Limb*. Institution of Mechanical Engineers Conference Publications 1977-5. London: Mechanical Publications Limited for the Institution of Mechanical Engineers, 1977:15–19.
37. Lettin AWF, Scales JT: Total replacement of the shoulder joint (two cases). *Proc R Soc Med* 1972;65:373–374.
38. Lettin AWF, Scales JT. Total replacement arthroplasty of the shoulder in rheumatoid arthritis. *J Bone Joint Surg [Br]* 1973;55:217.
39. Lettin AWF, Copeland SA, Scales JT. The Stanmore total shoulder replacement. *J Bone Joint Surg [Br]* 1982;64:47–51.
40. Post M, Jablon M, Miller H, Singh M. Constrained total shoulder joint replacement: A critical review. *Clin Orthop* 1979;144:135–150.
41. Post M, Haskell SS, Jablon M. Total shoulder replacement with a constrained prosthesis. *J Bone Joint Surg [Am]* 1980;62:327–335.
42. Post M. Constrained arthroplasty of the shoulder. *Orthop Clin North Am* 1987;18:455–462.
43. Post M. Shoulder arthroplasty and total shoulder replacement. In: Post M, ed. *The Shoulder*. Philadelphia: Lea & Febiger, 1988:221–273.
44. Reeves B, Jobbins B, Dowson D, Wright V. A total shoulder endoprosthesis. *Eng Med* 1974;1:64–67.
45. Kessel L, Bayley JL. The Kessel total shoulder replacement. In: Bayley JL, Kessel L, eds. *Shoulder Surgery*. New York: Springer-Verlag, 1982:160–164.
46. Kolbel R, Freidebold G. Moglichkeiten der Alloarthroplastik an der Schulter. *Arch Orthop Unfallchir* 1972;76:31–39.
47. Kolbel R, Boenick U. Biomechanische Probleme der Implantatchirurgie. *Orthopade* 1974;3:153–163.
48. Kolbel R, Friedebold G. Schultergelenksersatz. *Z Orthop* 1975;113:452–454.
49. Kolbel R, Rohlmann A, Bergmann C. Biomechanical considerations in the design of a semi-constrained total shoulder replacement. In: Bayley I, Kessel L, eds. *Shoulder Surgery*. New York: Springer-Verlag, 1982;144–152.
50. Kolbel R. Stabilization of shoulders with bone and muscle defects using joint replacement implants. In: Bateman JE, Welsh RP, eds. *Surgery of the Shoulder*. St. Louis: CV Mosby, 1984.
51. Gerard Y, LeBlanc JP, Rousseau B. Une Prothese Totale D'Epaule. *Chirurgie* 1973;99:655–663.
52. Mazas F, de la Caffiniere JY. Une Prosthese Totale d'epaule non Retentive. A Propos de 38 cas. *Rev Chir Orthop* 1982;68:161–170.
53. Amstutz HC, Thomas BJ, Kabo M, Jinnah Rh, Dorey FJ. The DANA total shoulder arthroplasty. *J Bone Joint Surg [Am]* 1988;70:1174–1182.
54. Amstutz HC, Hoy AL, Clarke IC. UCLA anatomic total shoulder arthroplasty. *Clin Orthop* 1981;155:7–20.
55. McElwain JP, English E. The early results of porous-coated total shoulder arthroplasty. *Clin Orthop* 1987;218:217–224.
56. Fenlin JM Jr. Total glenohumeral joint replacement. *Orthop Clin North Am* 1975;6:565–583.
57. Beddow FH, Elloy MA. Clinical experience with the Liverpool shoulder replacement. In: Bayley I, Kessel L, eds. *Shoulder Surgery*. New York: Springer-Verlag, 1982:164–167.
58. Buechel FF, Pappas MJ, DePalma AF. "Floating-socket" total shoulder replacement: Anatomical, biomechanical, and surgical rationale. *J Biomed Mater Res* 1978;12:89–114.
59. Gristina AG, Romano RL, Kammir GC, Webb LX. Total shoulder replacement. *Orthop Clin North Am* 1987;18:445–453.
60. Wheble VH, Skorecki J. The design of a metal-to-metal total shoulder joint prosthesis. In: *Joint Replacement in the Upper Limb*. Institution of Mechanical Engineers Conference Publications 1977-5. Conference Sponsored by the Medical Engineering Section of the Institution of Mechanical Engineers and the British Orthopaedic Association, London, 1977:7–13.
61. Fenlin JM Jr. Semi-constrained prosthesis for the rotator cuff deficient patient. *Orthop Trans* 1985;9:55.
62. Gristina AG, Webb LX. The trispherical total shoulder replacement. In: Bayley I, Kessel L, eds. *Shoulder Surgery*. New York: Springer-Verlag, 1982;153–157.
63. Zippel J. Arthroplastik des Schultergelenkes. *Orthopade* 1973;2:107–109.
64. Zippel J. Luxationssichere Schulterendoprothese Modell BME. *Z Orthop* 1975;113:454–457.
65. Zippel J. Der Endoprotetische Ersatz des Schultergelenikes. *Therapiewoche* 1975;27:70–79.
66. Zippel J. Luxationssichere Schulterendoprosthese Modell BME. In: Burri C, Ruter A, Hrsg. *Aktuelle Probleme in Chirurgie und Orthopadie*, Bd 1, Teil I. Bern: Huber, 1977.
67. Benjamin A, Hirschowiz D, Arden GP, Blackburn N. Double osteotomy of the shoulder. In: Bayley I, Kessel L, eds. *Shoulder Surgery*. New York: Springer-Verlag, 1982:170–175.
68. Kay SP, Amstutz HC. Shoulder arthroplasty at UCLA. *Clin Orthop* 1988;228:42–48.
69. Tillmann K, Braatz D. Results of resection arthroplasty and the Benjamin double osteotomy. In: Kolbel R, Helbig B, Blauth W, eds. *Shoulder Replacement*. Berlin: Springer-Verlag, 1987;47–50.
70. Gariepy R. Glenoidectomy in the repair of the rheumatoid shoulder. *J Bone Joint Surg [Br]* 1977;59:122.
71. Wainwright D. Glenoidectomy—A method of treating the painful shoulder in severe rheumatoid arthritis. *Ann Rheum Dis* 1974;33:110.
72. Bateman JE. Arthritis of the glenohumeral joint. In: *The Shoulder and Neck*. Philadelphia: WB Saunders, 1978:343–362.
73. Swanson AB. Implant resection arthroplasty of shoulder joint. In: Swanson AB, ed. *Flexible Resection Arthroplasty in the Hand and Extremities*. St. Louis: CV Mosby, 1973:287–295.
74. Varian JPW. Interposition Silastic cup arthroplasty of the shoulder. *J Bone Joint Surg [Br]* 1980;62:116–117.
75. Spencer R, Skirving AP. Silastic interposition arthroplasty of the shoulder. *J Bone Joint Surg [Br]* 1986;68:375–377.
76. Sledge CB, Kozinn SC, Thornhill TS. Total shoulder arthroplasty in rheumatoid arthritis. In: Lettin AWF, Petersson C, eds. *Rheumatoid Arthritis. Surgery of the Shoulder*. New York: S. Karger, 1989;95–102.
77. Clayton ML, Ferlic DC, Jeffers PD. Prosthetic arthroplasty of the shoulder. *Clin Orthop* 1982;164:184.
78. Clayton ML, Ferlic DC. Surgery of the shoulder in rheumatoid arthritis. *Clin Orthop* 1974;106:166.
79. Ferlic DC. *Subacromial Spacer. Orthopaedic Consultation*, discussed by Neer CS II. New York: HP Publishing, 1981:3.

80. Grammont PM. The Acropole prosthesis. In: Bateman JE, Welsh RP, eds. *Surgery of the Shoulder*. St. Louis: Mosby-Year Book, 1984:200–201.
81. Ellman H, Jinnah R, Amstutz HC. Experience with the DANA hooded component for cuff deficient shoulder arthroplasty. *Orthop Trans* 1986;10:217.
82. Brownlee RC, Cofield RH. Shoulder replacement for rotator cuff arthropathy. *Orthop Trans* 1986;10:230.
83. Maki S, Gruen TAW. Anthropometric studies of the glenohumeral joint. *Trans Orthop Res Soc* 1976;1:162.
84. Gristina AG, Webb LX, Carter RE. The monospherical total shoulder. *Orthop Trans* 1985;9:54.
85. Swanson AE. Bipolar implant shoulder arthroplasty. In: Bateman JE, Welsh RP, eds. *Surgery of the Shoulder*. St. Louis: CV Mosby, 1984:211–223.
86. Swanson AB, Swanson GdeG, Sattel AB, Cendo RD, Hynes D, Jar-Ning W. Bipolar implant shoulder arthroplasty. *Orthopedics* 1986;9:343–351.
87. Swanson AB, Swanson GdeG, Sattel AB, Cendo RD, Hynes D, Jar-Ning W. Bipolar implant shoulder arthroplasty: Long-term results. *Clin Orthop* 1989;249:227–247.
88. Jonsson E, Kelly N. Cup arthroplasty of the rheumatoid shoulder. *Acta Orthop Scand* 1986;57:542–546.
89. Jonsson E. *Surgery of the Rheumatoid Shoulder with Special Reference to Cup Hemiarthroplasty and Arthrodesis*. The University Department of Orthopaedics, Lund, Sweden. Malmo, Sweden: Infotryck, 1988.
90. Jonsson E, Brattstrom M, Lidgren L. Evaluation of the rheumatoid shoulder function after hemiarthroplasty and arthrodesis. *Scand J Rheumatol* 1988;17:17–26.
91. Figgie MP, Inglis AE, Figgie H, Solbel M, Burstein A. Custom total shoulder arthroplasty for inflammatory arthritis. In: Post M, Morrey BF, Hawkins RJ, eds. *Surgery of the Shoulder*. St. Louis: Mosby-Year Book, 1990:285–288.
92. Copeland S. Cementless total shoulder replacement. In: Post M, Morrey BF, Hawkins RJ, eds. *Surgery of the Shoulder*. St. Louis: Mosby-Year Book, 1990:289–293.
93. Neer CS II, Watson KC, Stanton FJ. Recent experience in total shoulder replacement. *J Bone Joint Surg [Am]* 1982;64:319–337.
94. Cofield RH. Preliminary experience with bone ingrowth fixation. In: Kolbel R, Helbig B, Blauth W, eds. *Shoulder Replacement*. Berlin: Springer-Verlag, 1987:209–212.
95. Roper BA, Paterson JMH, Day WH. The Roper-Day total shoulder replacement. *J Bone Joint Surg [Br]* 1990;72:694–697.
96. Wallace WA. The dynamic study of shoulder movement. In: Bayley J, Kessel L, eds. *Shoulder Surgery*. New York: Springer-Verlag, 1982.
97. Gagey O, Mazas F. A new total shoulder prosthesis with acromial fixation. In: Post M, Morrey BF, Hawkins RJ, eds. *Surgery of the Shoulder*. St. Louis: Mosby-Year Book, 1990:282–284.
98. Salzer M, Knahr HL, Stark N, Matejovsky Z, Plenk H Jr, Punzet G, Zweymuller K. A bioceramic endoprosthesis for the replacement of the proximal humerus. *Arch Orthop Trauma Surg* 1979;93:169–184.
99. Mathys R. Stand der Verwedung von Kunststoffen fur Kunstliche Gelenke. *Aktuel Traumatol* 1973;3:253.
100. Mathys R, Mathys R Jr. Isoelastische Prothesen des Schultergelenkes. Werkstoffe—Instrumentarium—Prosthesenmodelle. In: Burri C, Ruter A, Hrsg. *Aktuelle Probleme in Chirurgie und Orthopadie*, Bd 1, Teil I. Bern: Huber, 1977.
101. Burri C. Polyacetal resin shoulder prostheses for posttraumatic conditions and osteoarthritis. In: Kolbel R, Helbig B, Blauth W, eds. *Shoulder Replacement*. Berlin: Springer-Verlag, 1987:149–155.
102. Fukuda H. Ceramic glenohumeral prosthesis. Presented at the Annual Meeting of Japanese Shoulder Society; 1984.
103. Ishibashi T, Mikasa M, Fukuda H. A new humeral prosthesis for the Japanese. In: Post M, Morrey BF, Hawkins RJ, eds. *Surgery of the Shoulder*. St. Louis: Mosby-Year Book, 1990:273–276.
104. Brenner BC, Ferlic DC, Clayton ML, Dennis D. Survivorship of unconstrained total shoulder arthroplasty. In: Post M, Morrey BF, Hawkins RJ, eds. *Surgery of the Shoulder*. St. Louis: Mosby-Year Book, 1990:294–297.
105. Cofield RH. Total shoulder arthroplasty: Associated disease of the rotator cuff, results, and complications. In: Bateman JE, Welsh RP, eds. *Surgery of the Shoulder*. St. Louis: CV Mosby, 1984:229–233.
106. Bodey WN, Yeoman PM. Prosthetic arthroplasty of the shoulder. *Acta Orthop Scand* 1983;54:900–903.
107. Bell SN, Gschwend N. Clinical experience with total arthroplasty and hemiarthroplasty of the shoulder using the Neer prosthesis. *Int Orthop* 1986;10:217–222.
108. Cofield RH. Unconstrained total shoulder prostheses. *Clin Orthop* 1983;173:97–108.
109. Cofield RH. Total shoulder arthroplasty with the Neer prosthesis. *J Bone Joint Surg [Am]* 1984;66:899–906.
110. Friedman RJ, Ewald FC. Arthroplasty of the ipsilateral shoulder and elbow in patients who have rheumatoid arthritis. *J Bone Joint Surg [Am]* 1987;69:661–666.
111. Hawkins RJ, Bell RH, Jallay B. Experience with the Neer total shoulder arthroplasty: A review of 70 cases. *Orthop Trans* 1986;10:232.
112. Huten D, Duparc J, Lajoie D, Garcon P. Arthroplasty for shoulder injuries. *Orthop Trans* 1988;12:206.
113. Neer CS II, Morrison DS. Glenoid bone-grafting in total shoulder arthroplasty. *J Bone Joint Surg [Am]* 1988;70:1154–1162.
114. Samilson RL, Prieto V. Dislocation arthropathy of the shoulder. *J Bone Joint Surg [Am]* 1983;65:456–460.
115. Wilde AH, Borden LS, Brems JJ. Experience with the Neer total shoulder replacement. In: Bateman JE, Welsh RP, eds. *Surgery of the Shoulder*. St. Louis: CV Mosby, 1984:224–228.
116. Kelly IG, Foster RS, Fisher WD. Neer total shoulder replacement in rheumatoid arthritis. *J Bone Joint Surg [Br]* 1987;69:723–726.
117. Kelly IG. Shoulder replacement in rheumatoid arthritis. In: Post M, Morrey BF, Hawkins RJ, eds. *Surgery of the Shoulder*. St. Louis: Mosby-Year Book, 1990:305–307.
118. Codman EA. *The Shoulder* Malabar, Fla. Robert E. Krieger, 1934.

ADDITIONAL REFERENCES

Burrows AJ. Replacement of bone by internal prostheses. *J Bone Joint Surg [Br]* 1954;36:694.

Cofield RH. Arthrodesis and resection arthroplasty of the shoulder. In: McCollister EC, ed. *Surgery of the Musculoskeletal System*. New York: Churchill-Livingstone, 1983:109–124.

Coughlin MJ, Morris JM, West WF. The semiconstrained total shoulder arthroplasty. *J Bone Joint Surg [Am]* 1979;61:574–581.

Egund N, Jonsson E, Lidgren L, Kelly I, Pettersson H. Computed tomography of humeral head cup arthroplasties: A preliminary report. *Acta Radiol* 1987;28:71–73.

Marmor L. Hemiarthroplasty for the rheumatoid shoulder. *Clin Orthop* 1977;122:201–203.

Neer CS II. The rheumatoid shoulder. In: Cruess RR, Mitchell HS, eds. *Surgery of Rheumatoid Arthritis*. Philadelphia: JB Lippincott, 1971:117–125.

Neer CS II. Reconstructive surgery and rehabilitation of the shoulder. In: Kelley WN, Harris ED Jr, Ruddy S, Sledge CB, eds. *Textbook of Rheumatology*. Philadelphia: WB Saunders, 1981:1944–1959.

Neer CS II. *Surgical Protocol. Neer II Proximal Humerus. Arthroplasty of the Shoulder: Neer Technique*. St. Paul, MN: Minnesota Mining and Manufacturing Company, 1982.

Neer CS II, Kirby RM. Revision of humeral head and total shoulder arthroplasties. *Clin Orthop* 1982;170:189–195.

Oveson J, Nielsen S. Prosthesis position in shoulder arthroplasty. *Acta Orthop Scand* 1985;56:330.

Ovesen J, Sojbjerg JO, Sneppen O. A humeral head cutting guide: Instrument to secure correct humeral component retroversion in shoulder joint arthroplasty. *Clin Orthop* 1987;216:193–194.

Pahle JA, Kvarnes L. Shoulder synovectomy. *Ann Chir Gynaecol* 1985;74:198, p. 37–39.

Poppen NK, Walker PS. Normal and abnormal motion of the shoulder. *J Bone Joint Surg [Am]* 1976;58:195–201.

Wolff R, Kolbel R. The history of shoulder joint replacement. In: Kolbel R, Helbig B, Blauth W, eds. *Shoulder Replacement*. Berlin: Springer-Verlag, 1987:3–13.

SECTION II

Basic Principles

2 Biomechanics and Design of Shoulder Arthroplasties

Richard J. Friedman, M.D., F.R.C.S.(C)

The shoulder joint, which comprises four different articulations, is one of the most complex in the body. The glenohumeral, sternoclavicular, acromioclavicular, and scapulothoracic joints all work in concert to produce many different and often nonrepetitive movements. Most of the motion occurs in the glenohumeral and scapulothoracic joints, with the others participating at the extremes of motion. This allows for 180 degrees of elevation, combined internal and external rotation of up to 150 degrees, and horizontal flexion of approximately 170 degrees, thus making the shoulder joint the most mobile in the human body.[1]

When considering the function and design of a total shoulder arthroplasty, the biomechanics of the glenohumeral joint are most relevant. Normal anatomic and biomechanical principles concerning stability, forces, and motion of the glenohumeral joint are described and related to the biomechanical and design considerations of a total shoulder arthroplasty. This is followed by a careful examination of various prosthetic designs, and their success or failure based on these principles.

The development of a successful shoulder arthroplasty has lagged behind that of the hip and knee replacements for many reasons. The biomechanics of the normal and abnormal shoulder joint have been studied for many years, yet great controversy has existed, in part due to the complexity of this anatomic region. The incidence of the various arthritic and traumatic conditions that may require treatment with a shoulder arthroplasty is less than that in other joints. Also, affected patients are initially able to compensate somewhat with scapulothoracic motion.[2] The hip and knee have no such compensatory motion. Until recently, therefore, less research time and effort were spent on understanding the biomechanics and arthroplasty design compared to the other major joints, and as a result, progress has been slow.

ANATOMY

One of the main criteria for a successful shoulder arthroplasty is the recreation of normal anatomy and anatomic relationships between the humeral head and glenoid fossa. Many difficult anatomic considerations must be dealt with in the design of a successful shoulder arthroplasty, including the small volume of bone that the components must be fixed to and the large circumference of motion allowed by the surrounding soft-tissue envelope.

The scapula, and therefore the plane of the glenoid articular surface, lies on the posterior chest wall inclined approximately 30 to 40 degrees anterior to the coronal plane of the body when viewed in the transverse plane.[3,4] The humeral head and its articular surface are retroverted a corresponding amount, so that the articular surfaces of the glenoid and humeral head line up[5] (Figure 2–1).

The articular surface of the glenoid cavity subtends an arc of enclosure of 76 degrees in the coronal plane, and somewhat less (62 degrees) in the transverse plane (Figure 2–2).[6] This means that the glenoid cavity is flatter in the transverse plane and therefore has a larger radius of curvature, compared to the coronal plane. With the arm at the side, the scapula angles downward approximately 5 degrees. However, the relationship of the articular surface to the body of the scapula is highly variable and difficult to define precisely. Others have found that the glenoid faces 3 to 5 degrees superiorly.[7] In the transverse plane, the glenoid fossa in normal individuals lies in a slightly anteverted position (2 degrees) relative to the long axis of the scapula in normal individuals, while others have reported a slightly retroverted position.[8]

The articular surface of the humeral head, defined by the anatomic neck, encloses an arc of 155 degrees and is oriented upward 47 degrees.[6] The axis of the humeral shaft lies 2.5 degrees off the vertical in a resting position. The relationship between the two articular surfaces allows for 79 degrees of glenohumeral elevation in the scapular plane, and combined with 41 degrees of scapulothoracic motion, the arm can elevate 120 degrees before the greater tuberosity impinges on the acromion. At this point, the humerus externally rotates to expose more of the humeral articular surface to the glenoid fossa for further elevation to 180 degrees to occur.

In any given anatomic position, the contact area between the two articulating surfaces is small, and the glenoid fossa only covers 25 to 30% of the humeral head.[1,9] Consequently, the articular surfaces provide little inherent bony stability to the joint.[10]

In order for any arthroplasty to be successful, these anatomic features should be restored as much as possible, so that the soft tissues and surrounding musculotendinous cuff are properly balanced and the normal kinematics of the glenohumeral joint are restored.

The conformity between the humeral head and glenoid cavity in the transverse plane has only recently been exam-

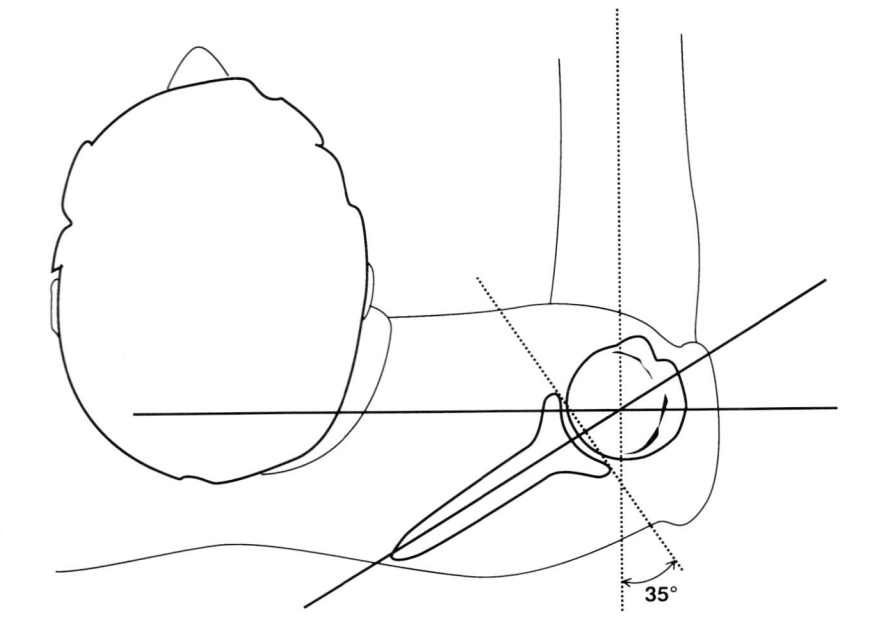

Figure 2–1. Transverse view of the right shoulder from above, demonstrating the relationship of the humeral head and glenoid to the body. With the shoulder in neutral rotation, the humeral head is retroverted 35 degrees, while the face of the glenoid cavity lies off the coronal plane of the body a similar amount, so that the two articular surfaces line up.

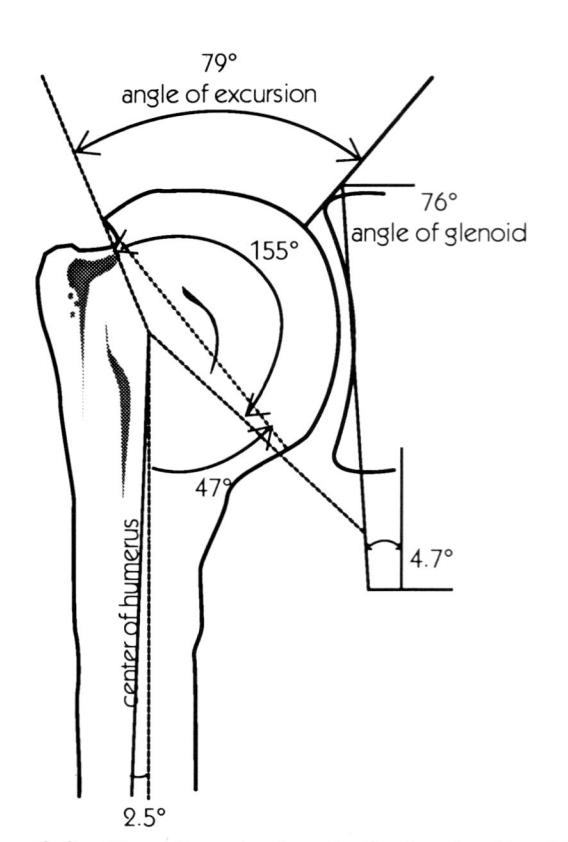

Figure 2–2. Mean dimensional angles for the glenoid and humerus with the arm at the side. The humeral head articular surface subtends an angle of 155 degrees, and with the glenoid arc of enclosure measuring 76 degrees, leaves only 79 degrees for glenohumeral elevation before the humeral head must externally rotate to clear the greater tuberosity from the undersurface of the acromion.

ined.[5,11–13] Three possible situations can exist. In type A, the radius of curvature of the humeral head is less than that of the corresponding glenoid, so that the glenoid is flatter and the humeral head rounder. Type B has equal radii of curvature between the two surfaces, and they conform exactly to each other. In type C, the radius of curvature of the humeral head is greater than that of the glenoid, and therefore it appears flatter compared to a more rounded glenoid (Figure 2–3).

Type B would theoretically have 100% contact between the two surfaces, with the joint forces evenly distributed. Type C would have the humeral head contacting and loading the glenoid peripherally on its rim, without any central contact. Type A would allow the humeral head to contact the middle portion of the glenoid, with the forces concentrated over a smaller area. Anteroposterior translation could also occur with this configuration. This dimensional relationship can be quantified as the glenohumeral or conformity index, defined as the radius humeral head/radius glenoid ratio, for both the anteroposterior and lateral planes. These ratios have been reported as 0.75 in the anteroposterior plane and 0.6 in the lateral plane by Saha,[5] and 0.86 and 0.58, respectively, by Maki and Gruen.[12]

A more recent study utilizing a highly accurate, reproducible computer analysis technique defined these values as 0.67 and 0.39, respectively.[13] Only 9% had radii that matched (type B). The vast majority had a more curved humeral head and flatter glenoid (type A), with less conformity in the lateral versus the anteroposterior plane. A constraint index, defined as the arc of enclosure/360, had a value of 0.18 in the anteroposterior plane and 0.10 in the lateral plane, meaning that there was more curve to the glenoid in the anteroposterior versus the lateral plane. These anatomic features help to

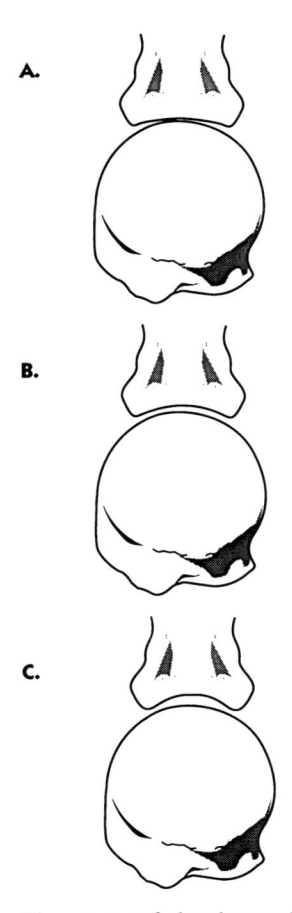

Figure 2–3. A–C. Three types of glenohumeral configurations.

keep the humeral head from translating in a superior-inferior direction, but allow translation in an anteroposterior direction.

The relationship between the contact area and the radius of curvature was recently examined (Friedman RJ, An Y, Kessler L, unpublished data, 1992). Ninety-three percent of the shoulders studied were type A, where the rounder humeral head articulated with a flatter glenoid surface, and resulted in a mean contact area of 30%. It is over this area that the forces across the glenohumeral joint are transmitted. The contact area was found to decrease in certain positions, such as abduction and external rotation, resulting in a greater force per unit area across the joint. These anatomic features may contribute to wear patterns and impingement, and should be considered in the design of a total shoulder arthroplasty.

STABILITY

The shoulder joint is the developmental equivalent of the hip joint in the upper extremity. The hip joint is a true ball-and-socket design, with a great deal of bony stability between two conforming surfaces and very little stability contributed by the surrounding soft tissues. As a result, motion is limited in this joint. The glenohumeral joint, on the other hand, has very little inherent bony stability.[5] A soft-tissue socket provides the necessary stability to the joint, thus allowing for a wide range of motion. This soft-tissue socket includes (1) the capsular-ligamentous complex, consisting of the superior, middle, and inferior portions, and the coracohumeral ligament, all of which are static stabilizers[14]; and (2) the rotator cuff and the surrounding shoulder muscles, which are dynamic stabilizers.[15]

Studies of the capsular-ligamentous complex show the inferior glenohumeral ligament to be the major static stabilizer of the shoulder joint.[16,17] However, the capsule itself is often thin and redundant, which may represent a congenital variation in normal individuals or be secondary to an underlying disease process such as inflammatory arthritis.[18] The static elements contributing to the stability of a total shoulder arthroplasty are, therefore, minimal.[19] On the other hand, if the disease process results in scarring and contracture of the capsule, this may well interfere with the postoperative motion and stability of a total shoulder arthroplasty.

The dynamic stabilizers of the shoulder can be grouped anatomically into three categories: scapulohumeral, axioscapular, and axiohumeral. The latter two groups include the trapezius, rhomboids, serratus anterior, and levator scapulae muscles (axioscapular), and the latissimus dorsi and pectoralis major muscles (axiohumeral). These muscle groups are important for their contributions towards motion and the forces generated about the glenohumeral joint.

The scapulohumeral muscle group, consisting of the supraspinatus, infraspinatus, subscapularis, teres major and minor, and deltoid muscles, is thought to play the significant role in dynamic stabilization of the glenohumeral joint.[20] Electromyographic studies have shown that the supraspinatus functions both as a humeral head compressor and as an arm abductor.[21,22] The subscapularis and infraspinatus, in addition to being internal and external rotators, respectively, both act as compressors of the humeral head when abduction, or elevation, is initiated. The deltoid muscle appears to function strictly as an abductor, or elevator, of the upper extremity. In general, the stability of a total shoulder arthroplasty as well as its mobility, is maintained by a well-functioning scapulohumeral musculature. The necessity of a properly functioning rotator cuff to the clinical success of an arthroplasty has been recognized since the early development of a total shoulder arthroplasty.[23]

FORCES

The forces across the glenohumeral joint are complex, varying not only with the load applied, but also with the position of the arm.[6,24,25] While the glenohumeral joint is often referred to as "non–weight-bearing," significant forces are transmitted across the joint.

With simple arm elevation to 90 degrees, a force of one times the body weight is generated. Lifting an object weighing only 5 kg held in the laterally extended hand generates a force approximately 2.5 times the body weight across the joint, similar to loads that act across the hip joint.[25] However, this load is transmitted across a significantly smaller articular surface area in the shoulder compared to the hip, meaning that the magnitude of mechanical stresses the glenohumeral joint or prosthetic components are subjected to is substantial.

The forces to consider around the glenohumeral joint include the weight of the extremity and any external forces, the abducting muscles (deltoid and supraspinatus), the muscles pulling in a downward direction (subscapularis, infraspinatus, teres minor), and the resultant vector of the compression and shear forces of the humeral head on the glenoid.[26] Studies have shown that the deltoid muscle itself can generate a maximum force of six times the limb weight; the supraspinatus, two and one-half times the limb weight; the rotators, five times the limb weight; and a joint reaction force, seven times the limb weight (Figure 2–4).[24,27]

When abduction of the arm is initiated, compressive forces are generated by the rotator cuff muscles to hold the humeral head against the glenoid fossa and counter the shear forces up the face of the glenoid being created by the abducting muscle forces. This allows the extremity to abduct efficiently and prevents the humeral head from simply sliding up the face of the glenoid. The combination of compressive forces and shear forces gives the resultant force. Up to 60 degrees, the compression and shear forces are roughly equal. After this, the shear force decreases as abduction increases. The compressive force continues to increase to a maximum at 90 degrees of abduction, and then decreases as abduction continues to increase (Figure 2–5).[28] The resultant force also peaks at 90 degrees of abduction, and then decreases at the same rate it increased as abduction increases. For example, considering the weight of the arm as the only load, the resultant force is 0.4 times the body weight at both 30 and 150 degrees of abduction, and 0.6 times the body weight at 60 and 120 degrees of abduction. At 90 degrees of abduction, the joint force is approximately one times the body weight.

In addition to the magnitude, the direction of the resultant force vector is also important. For the humeral head to remain in the glenoid cavity with abduction, the resultant

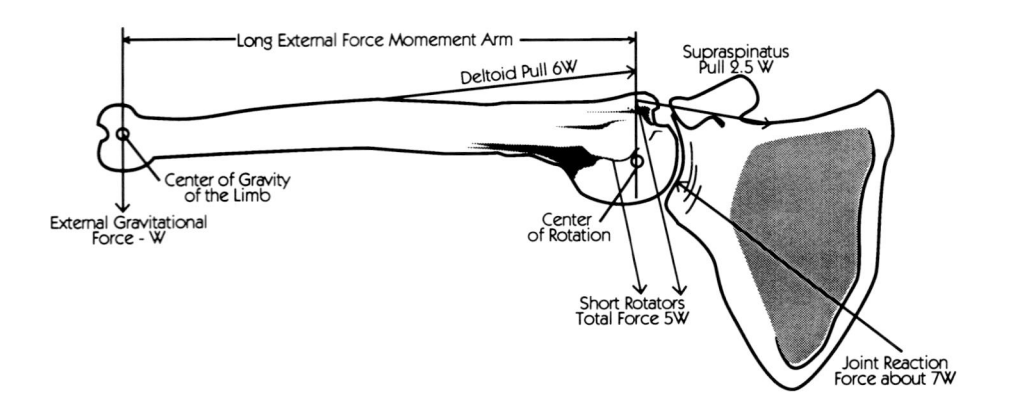

Figure 2–4. Forces generated across the glenohumeral joint with the arm elevated 90 degrees.

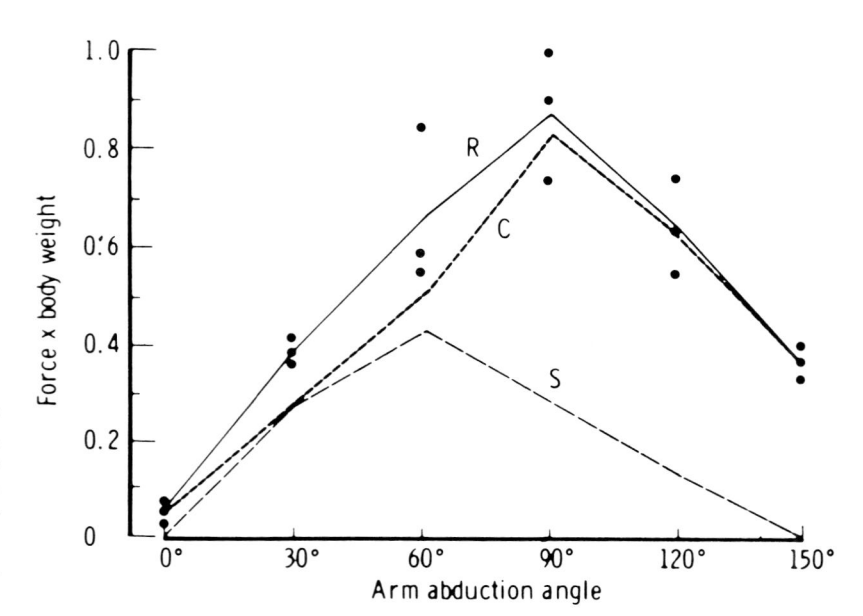

Figure 2–5. The resultant force (R) of the glenohumeral joint is a combination of the compressive component (C) perpendicular to the face of the glenoid and the shear force (S) up the face of the glenoid. (Reproduced with permission from Poppen and Walker.[28])

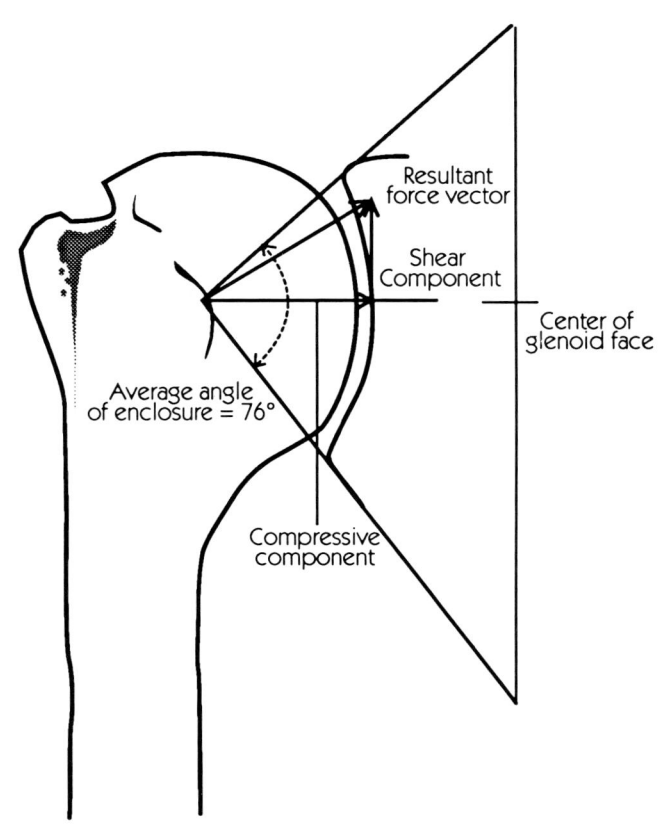

Figure 2-6. The compressive and shear forces comprise the resultant force vector, which must fall within the glenoid angle of enclosure for elevation to occur.

force vector must lie within the angle, or arc of safety, of the glenoid (Figure 2–6).[28] During abduction of the arm in the scapular plane with neutral rotation, the initial force is directed downward and contained within the inferior border of the glenoid. As the arm abducts to 30 and 60 degrees, the force moves to the superior edge of the glenoid, consistent with the high shear forces generated, and then moves back towards the center of the glenoid as abduction continues to increase (Figure 2–7).[29]

Similar calculations with the arm in internal and external rotation show that muscle efficiency and stability are superior in external compared to internal rotation.[28] Forces in external rotation are similar to those in neutral rotation, but the resultant force vector is directed more centrally into the glenoid cavity, due to the deltoid muscle increasing its contribution to compressive forces and decreasing the shear component.

The force vector for internal rotation is larger than in neutral or external rotation, and directed more superiorly, due to an increased shear force. The resultant joint forces in internal rotation are twice those in external rotation at 90 degrees of abduction. This is easily demonstrated by an individual abducting both arms to 90 degrees, with one in maximum internal and the other in maximum external rotation. The arm in internal rotation will fatigue and become painful much more quickly than the arm in external rotation.

In neutral rotation with abduction to 60 degrees, the resultant force vector of the humeral head is contained just within the arc of enclosure of the glenoid. The loss of a functioning rotator cuff mechanism, particularly the supraspinatus, causes a decrease in the compressive forces and an increase in the shear forces, shifting the resultant force vector superiorly out of the arc of enclosure of the glenoid (Figure 2–8). The resulting instability is seen clinically with superior subluxation of the humeral head on the glenoid (Figure 2–9).

The significant forces across the glenohumeral joint mentioned above are transferred to the prosthetic interface in a total shoulder arthroplasty. While the humeral component has a large surface area and a canal-filling stem over which the forces can be distributed, the fixation of the glenoid

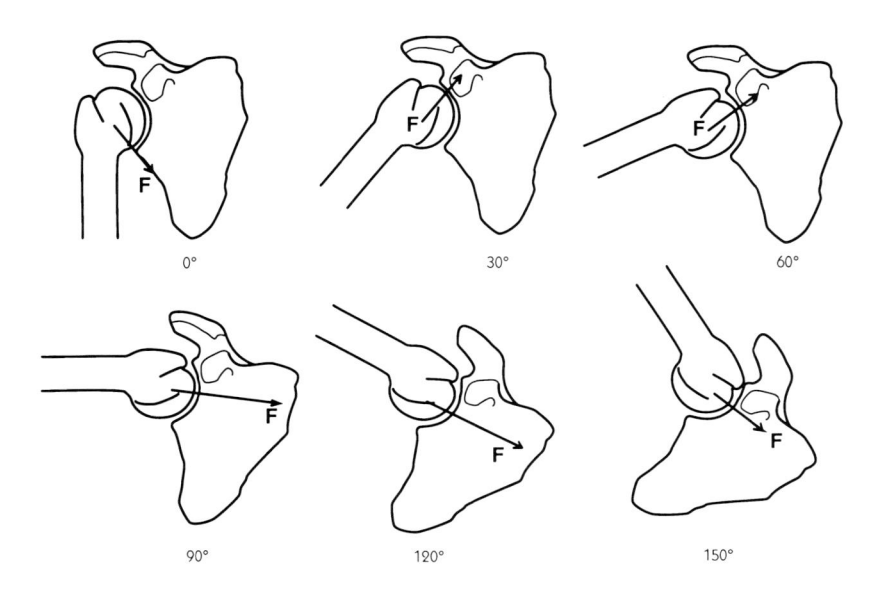

Figure 2–7. The resultant force vectors change with relation to their direction in the glenoid cavity as the arm is abducted. Stability increases with abduction.

Figure 2–8. With the rotator cuff intact, the resultant force vector lies within the arc of enclosure and the humeral head remains centered as the arm is elevated (left). When a large rotator cuff tear is present, the resultant vector lies outside the glenoid articular surface, causing the humeral head to sublux superiorly when the deltoid muscle initiates elevation (right).

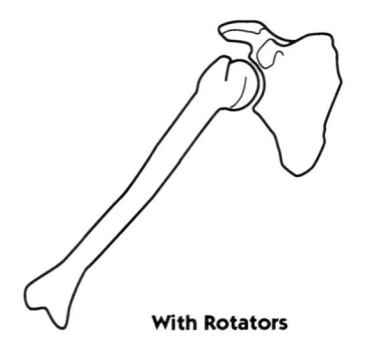

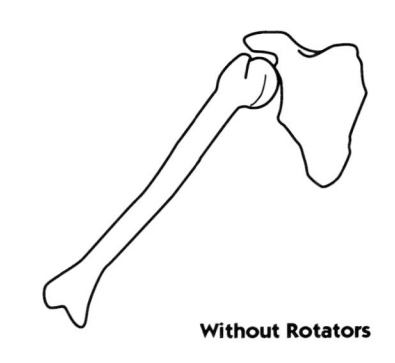

component is much more tenuous. Forces greater than one times the body weight are transmitted across a small surface area, so that the load per unit area is high, possibly surpassing that of the fixation and leading to failure.

Understanding the mechanism for superior migration of the humeral head in the rotator cuff–deficient shoulder helps to explain some cases of glenoid loosening seen after total shoulder arthroplasty.[30] Elevating the glenohumeral joint to 60 degrees loads the glenoid component with high shear forces, and causes the humeral head component to migrate in a superior direction. This eccentrically loads the superior portion of the glenoid component, exerting a downward tilting force, the so-called rocking-horse effect, which can lead to glenoid component loosening.[31] Thus, caution should be exercised in the use of a glenoid component for the rotator cuff–deficient shoulder.

In the everyday use of a total shoulder arthroplasty, significant forces are transmitted across the glenoid component. The available glenoid bone stock is limited, and therefore the fixation technique, whether cemented or uncemented with a porous or ceramic coating, is critical to the long-term success. Appropriate design parameters and glenoid fixation must be optimized as much as possible to take advantage of the anatomy and resist the applied forces.

MOTION

Elevation of the arm, one of the most important functions of the shoulder joint, results from a combination of glenohumeral and scapulothoracic motion. This has been studied extensively in normal individuals, initially examining the question referable to the coronal plane, but more recently referencing the scapular plane.[9,24,32–34] Many authors have stressed the importance of using the scapular rather than the coronal plane, since the true plane of the glenohumeral joint is 30 to 40 degrees anterior to the coronal plane.[3,4] The plane of scapular abduction where maximum glenohumeral elevation occurs has recently been defined as 23 degrees anterior to the plane of the scapula.[35] However, neither reference system is ideal, since scapular rotation is not taken into account.[36]

Early studies defined the relative contributions of glenohumeral and scapulothoracic motion to shoulder abduction in the coronal plane as being a 2:1 ratio throughout.[9,24] In other words, for every 2 degrees of glenohumeral motion, there is 1 degree of scapulothoracic motion contributing to shoulder abduction. In abducting the arm to 120 degrees, 80 degrees would come from the glenohumeral joint and 40 degrees from the scapulothoracic joint. Following external rotation of the humeral head to clear the greater tuberosity from the undersurface of the acromion and expose more articular surface to the glenoid, abduction proceeds to 180 degrees, resulting from 120 degrees of glenohumeral motion and 60 degrees of scapulothoracic motion.[6]

More recent studies of abduction in the scapular plane

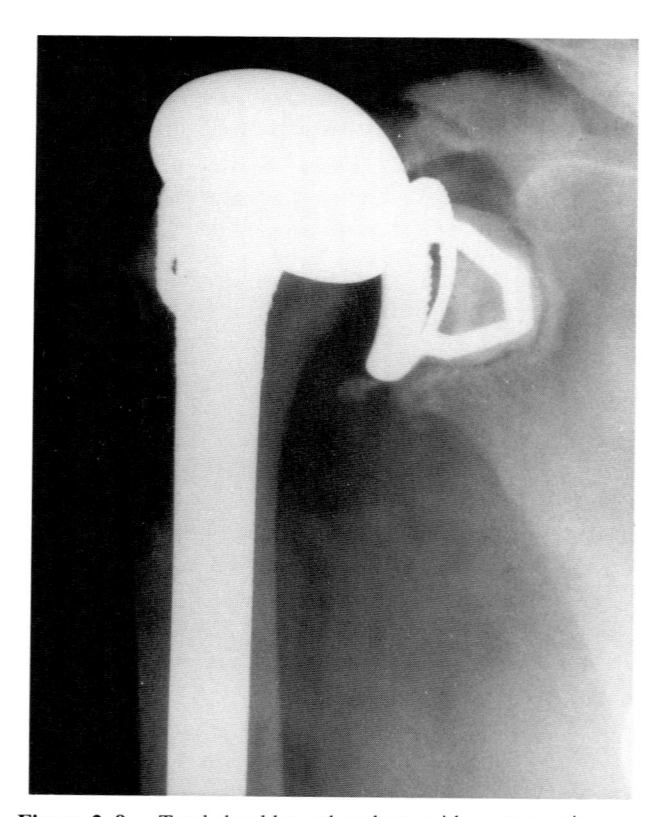

Figure 2–9. Total shoulder arthroplasty with postoperative rotator cuff tear in a patient with a cadaveric renal transplant who was on high-dose corticosteroids, demonstrating superior subluxation of the humeral component against the glenoid prosthesis and a continuous radiolucent line around the glenoid prosthesis.

Figure 2–10. Based on various studies, the relationship of glenohumeral to scapulothoracic motion with increasing elevation of the arm. In general, the ratio of glenohumeral to scapulothoracic motion is 2:1 in the normal shoulder. (Reproduced with permission from Bergmann.[25])

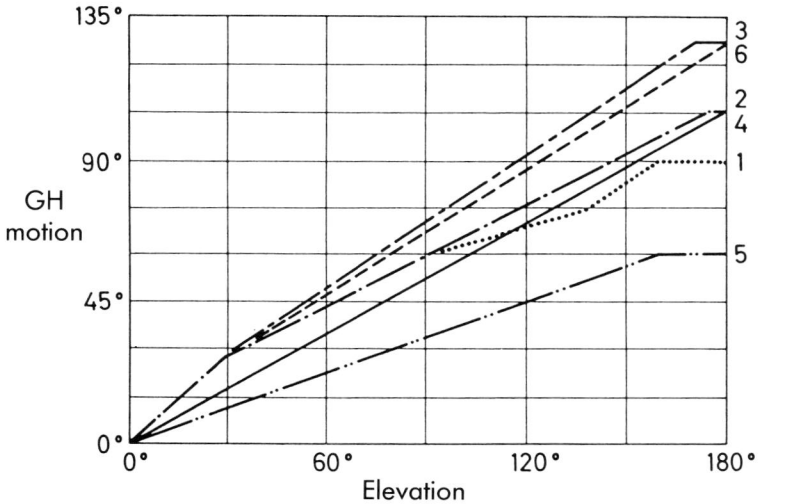

1 Nobuhara et. al. 1977
2 Poppen u. Walker 1976
3 Inman et. al. 1944
4 Freedman u. Munro 1966
5 Wallace 1982
6 Reeves 1972

have confirmed this ratio throughout the full range of motion, but it appears to vary during the first 25 to 30 degrees of abduction.[32–34] Findings from these and other studies are summarized in Figure 2–10. Greater motion occurs at the glenohumeral joint during the first 30 degrees of elevation. An equal contribution of glenohumeral and scapulothoracic motion occurs in the last 60 degrees of elevation, but the overall ratio remains approximately 2:1 throughout the entire arc of elevation.

The relative contributions of glenohumeral and scapulothoracic motion differ in patients with shoulder pathology, such as rotator cuff tears and instabilities.[32] To examine the effects of the disease process, surgical technique, and postoperative rehabilitation on glenohumeral motion, the relative contributions of glenohumeral and scapulothoracic motion have been studied in detail in patients undergoing a nonconstrained total shoulder arthroplasty for severe arthritis without rotator cuff tears.[2,37] Various parameters were defined to determine the biomechanics of the glenohumeral and scapulothoracic joints following total shoulder arthroplasty in 15 patients (Figure 2–11). In this group, the glenohumeral to scapulothoracic ratio from 0 to 90 degrees of elevation in the scapular plane was 1:2, indicating that for every 1 degree of glenohumeral motion, 2 degrees of scapulothoracic motion occurred.[37] This means that less motion occurs between the prosthetic components compared to a normal joint, but that scapulothoracic motion is essentially unchanged. The patients all had statistically significant improvements in pain, motion, and function and what would be considered successful clinical results.

In order to determine whether these abnormal biomechanics were a function of the total shoulder arthroplasty or the underlying disease process, and if these abnormal biomechanics could be altered, 9 patients were prospectively studied. Preoperatively, the glenohumeral to scapulothoracic ratio was found to be 1:2, and all patients had significant pain, decreased motion, and therefore decreased function.[2] This alteration in the glenohumeral to scapulothoracic ratio likely represents the patients' attempt to immobilize the glenohumeral joint for pain relief, and at the same time maximize shoulder motion through the scapulothoracic joint.

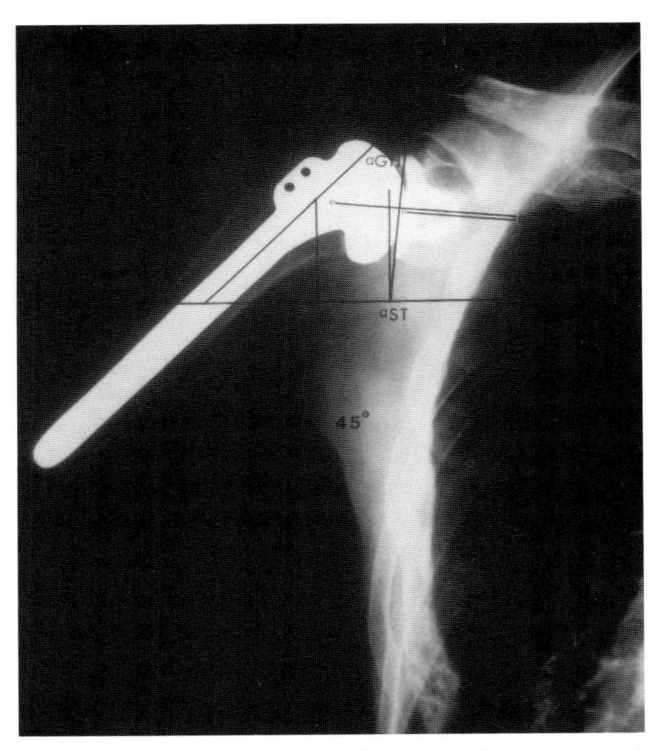

Figure 2–11. Anteroposterior radiograph of the glenohumeral joint following total shoulder arthroplasty, with the various parameters measured to determine glenohumeral and scapulothoracic motion. The scapulothoracic angle (αST) is between the face of the glenoid and the vertical. The glenohumeral angle (αGH) lies between the humeral and glenoid prostheses. The arm angle (αA) is between the long axis of the humeral component and the vertical.

Postoperatively, the ratio of glenohumeral to scapulothoracic motion was not significantly different, despite a wide surgical release and aggressive physical therapy. Therefore, the amount of elevation that can be achieved is limited, since normal glenohumeral motion is not fully restored. The abnormal biomechanics appear to be a function of the underlying disease process. If greater elevation is to be obtained following total shoulder arthroplasty, different surgical and rehabilitation techniques will have to be developed to increase glenohumeral motion and restore normal shoulder biomechanics.

The instant centers of rotation of the glenohumeral joint have been shown to lie close to each other and to the center of the humeral head itself in normal subjects.[6,32] In contrast, patients with shoulder pathology demonstrated instant centers that deviated considerably from the center of the humeral head. In patients who had undergone a nonconstrained total shoulder arthroplasty, the instant centers lay close to each other and to the center of the prosthetic humeral head.[37] This indicates that the center of rotation of a prosthetic glenohumeral joint is located very near the geometric center of the humeral prosthesis, similar to the normal situation.

A correlation exists between the instant centers of rotation and excursion, or translation, of the humeral head in a superior-inferior direction. A small amount of superior translation averaging 3 mm has been found to occur during the first 30 degrees of elevation.[32] Thereafter, approximately 1 mm of further excursion in an upward or downward direction occurs between positions measured. In patients with rotator cuff tears, significantly more translation occurs.

Following total shoulder arthroplasty, a correlation still existed between the instant centers of rotation and excursion.[37] The mean translation was approximately 2 mm from 0 to 90 degrees of scapular plane abduction. Less excursion occurred throughout the arc of motion in the prosthetic shoulder compared to the normal joint, reflecting the conformity existing between the humeral and glenoid components studied. In summary, it appears that the biomechanics of a total shoulder arthroplasty differ significantly from the normal shoulder with respect to excursion and the relative contributions of glenohumeral and scapulothoracic motion, but the prosthetic components appear to rotate on a fixed center, similar to the normal joint.

The above discussion deals with motion in the coronal plane. Differences exist when studying motion of the glenohumeral joint in the transverse plane. With less conformity in the transverse compared to the coronal plane, a variety of motions—rotation, translation, and rolling—are possible.[38] During rotation, the humeral head rotates and the contact point on the glenoid does not change (Figure 2–12). With translation, the contact point of the humeral head does not change, but the glenoid has a constantly changing contact point. Rolling occurs when the contact points between the two surfaces change continuously by an equal amount and is a combination of rotation and translation.

Surface motion of the normal glenohumeral joint is pri-

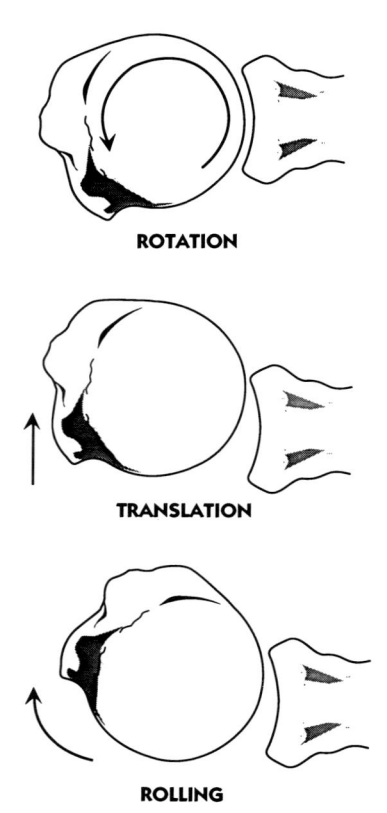

Figure 2–12. Three types of motion—rotation, translation, and rolling—occur at the glenohumeral joint.

marily rotation in the transverse plane, with very little translation occurring. A study of 20 normal individuals demonstrated that the humeral head remained centered in the glenoid cavity throughout the range of horizontal flexion, except in a position of maximum extension and external rotation, when 4 mm of posterior translation occurred.[39] In patients with anterior instability, translation of the humeral head on the glenoid occurred, indicating a significant disruption of the structures responsible for anterior stability.

Recent studies have suggested that anteroposterior translation can occur in normal, asymptomatic shoulders.[40,41] While the amount of translation varied between individuals, all exhibited some degree of glenohumeral translation in the anteroposterior direction during clinical testing for instability. The translation was also found to be reproducible in each subject. None of the normal subjects studied had any symptoms consistent with shoulder instability.

As discussed, cadaveric studies examining the glenohumeral joint have shown that the glenoid and humeral head do not have equal radii of curvature, but in the majority of cases, the radius of curvature of the normal glenoid is larger than that of the corresponding humeral head.[13] With the glenoid flatter and the humeral head more rounded, there is little inherent bony stability, and this anatomic relationship allows translation in the anteroposterior direction to occur. In contrast, many of the total shoulder arthroplasty components available today have an equal radius of curvature between the glenoid and humeral components. This is done to distribute the forces more evenly over a larger contact area, thereby decreasing the stresses across the interface and theoretically improving the long-term fixation. However, this design does not allow anteroposterior translation to occur during normal shoulder motion. The question arises that if normal shoulder biomechanics allow some anteroposterior translation to occur, does the constraint inherent in a system with equal radii of curvature prevent this from happening?

Retrieval studies of failed glenoid components provide some answers to this question.[42] The polyethylene is often worn away asymmetrically at the anterior or posterior edges (Figure 2–13). This creates polyethylene wear debris, which can contribute to osteolysis and loosening. In order for this asymmetric wear to occur, the humeral prosthesis must be moving in an anteroposterior direction relative to the glenoid component.

To answer this more completely, 13 patients were studied following a nonconstrained total shoulder arthroplasty to define the amount and direction of anteroposterior translation of the glenohumeral joint in the transverse plane. No patients had any clinical evidence of anterior, posterior, or inferior instability. The components had matching radii of curvature, and the mean total translation was 4 mm, ranging from 0 to 12 mm.[43] At -30 degrees, the humeral head was centered in the glenoid component. Most translation occurs between -30 and 30 degrees, mainly in a posterior direction.

For this anteroposterior translation to occur between humeral and glenoid components with equal radii of curvature, the prosthetic humeral head must ride up and over the polyethylene rim of the glenoid component. This subjects the glenoid component to repeated eccentric loading, resulting in a rocking-horse effect and thereby increasing the potential for loosening. Asymmetric polyethylene wear and debris formation can also occur and are known to induce osteolysis and subsequent component loosening in total hip and knee arthroplasty. Thus, anteroposterior translation can potentially lead to loosening through two different mechanisms.

While total shoulder arthroplasty components of the design used in this study are referred to as nonconstrained, this is really a misnomer. It is true that no mechanical linkage exists between the components, as was seen in earlier total shoulder arthroplasty designs. However, total shoulder arthroplasty components with conforming surfaces and equal radii of curvature have an inherent constraint that does not allow free movement or translation between them. When the humeral and glenoid components are properly lined up, there is 100% contact between them, with an equal distribution of the stresses over the entire contact area. If displacement of only 1 to 2 mm occurs between the components, then the contact area decreases significantly, thereby increasing the load per unit area on the polyethylene of the glenoid component and the stress distribution across the interface. The end result, as mentioned above, could be loosening through both polyethylene wear and eccentric loading.

The inherent conformity and constraint between the components of this design are not sufficient to prevent anteroposterior translation from occurring. A glenoid component with a greater radius of curvature (a flatter glenoid) would not only recreate the normal anatomy, but also allow translation to occur between the components without eccentric loading and polyethylene wear. However, if the glenoid component is too flat, then the area of contact between the humeral and glenoid components would be minimal, increasing the stress concentration to an unacceptable level. The exact amount of mismatch between a more curved humeral implant and a flatter glenoid component that would allow translation to occur and at the same time optimize the stress transfer and limit the stress concentration has yet to be determined. In the future, total shoulder arthroplasty systems could be designed with less conformity and constraint between the glenoid and humeral components, allowing anteroposterior translation to occur without eccentric loading and polyethylene wear and thus recreating normal shoulder anatomy and biomechanics.

PROSTHESIS DESIGN

In the design of a total shoulder arthroplasty system, one should attempt to recreate both the normal anatomy and the biomechanics of the shoulder joint as much as possible. Theoretically, by restoring normal anatomy and biomechanics, the total shoulder arthroplasty would provide better function and decrease the frequency of component loosening. Certain criteria with regards to design, biomechanics,

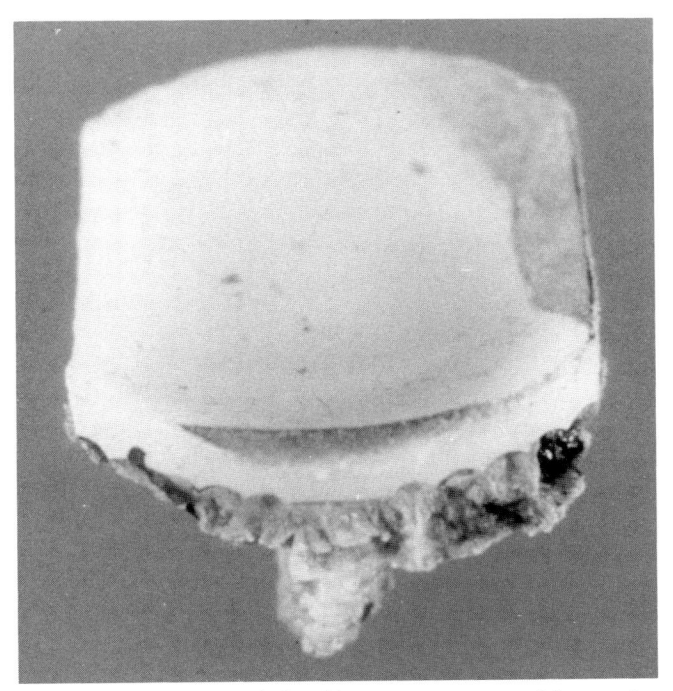

Figure 2–13. Cemented glenoid component removed for aseptic loosening. Note the asymmetric wear of the polyethylene. (Photograph courtesy of Dr. W. Z. Burkhead.)

and surgery must be kept in mind for a successful outcome.[26] The design criteria include reproducing normal anatomy, restoring normal anatomic relationships, and providing functional stability. From a biomechanic point of view, impingement must be avoided, the prosthesis should be able to withstand the expected loads, the materials should provide wear resistance, stress transfer at the bone-cement or cement-prosthesis interfaces must be minimized, and there should be simplicity in the design and manufacturing.

For a total shoulder arthroplasty to be successful, several technical criteria must be accomplished at the time of surgery. The subchondral bone should be preserved by removing only a minimal amount of bone, and the rotator cuff maintained or repaired. The arthroplasty components should be relatively easy to implant, which would minimize technical errors, and should utilize proven fixation methods and biocompatible materials. The ability to start early range of motion postoperatively is essential to a satisfactory outcome. While rarely considered in designs of the past, all prostheses will eventually fail, and therefore revision surgery must be planned to minimize potential complications.[42] Revision criteria include allowing removal of the prosthesis with minimal damage to the soft tissues, maintaining sufficient bone stock to allow for reimplantation or fusion, and allowing for replacement of component parts subject to wear.

Constrained

Historically, the earliest total shoulder arthroplasty designs failed to take many of these criteria into account and were not very successful. The first generation of total shoulder arthroplasty components were of the constrained variety, with the humeral and glenoid components mechanically coupled around a fixed center of rotation. They were indicated for use in patients with severe rotator cuff deficiencies and designed to prevent superior migration of the humeral component on the glenoid prosthesis.

Constrained implants were generally of a ball-and-socket design and required greater resection of bone for implantation. A sphere with a small radius of curvature was seated in a congruous deep socket with or without a locking ring to minimize or prevent subluxations or dislocations. This resulted in a compromise between stability and mobility. While stability was greatly increased, most would not allow abduction past 90 degrees.

In addition to limited motion, these prostheses produced many stress-related mechanical problems. Large forces ended up being borne by the prosthesis, or the bone-prosthesis interface, without the surrounding soft-tissue envelope transmitting much of the load. Fracture of the components, breakage of the linkage, or high loosening rates eventually occurred.[44,45] Little indication exists today for a constrained total shoulder arthroplasty.

One of the earliest designs was the Stanmore prosthesis, developed by Lettin and Scales in 1969 (see Figure 1–23). It had metal humeral and glenoid components articulating, with a high-density polyethylene retention ring designed to capture and hold the humeral head in place.[46–48] Abduction to only 90 degrees was possible.

The Michael Reese total shoulder was developed by Post and Haskell a few years later in 1973.[44,49–51] The basic principle was similar to that of the Stanmore prosthesis, but the system had a metal-to-plastic rather than a metal-to-metal capture. The small spherical metal head is captured in the metal-backed polyethylene glenoid component by a slightly smaller peripheral lip (Figure 2–14). This permits controlled subluxation when the humeral component is forced beyond its maximum range of motion with excessive torque, and theoretically dissipates the forces and reduces the stresses at the bone-cement interface of the glenoid component.

In an attempt to improve motion and decrease the incidence of loosening and dislocation, several designs of a reverse ball-and-socket prosthesis were developed. A larger radius of curvature is possible with the hemispherical

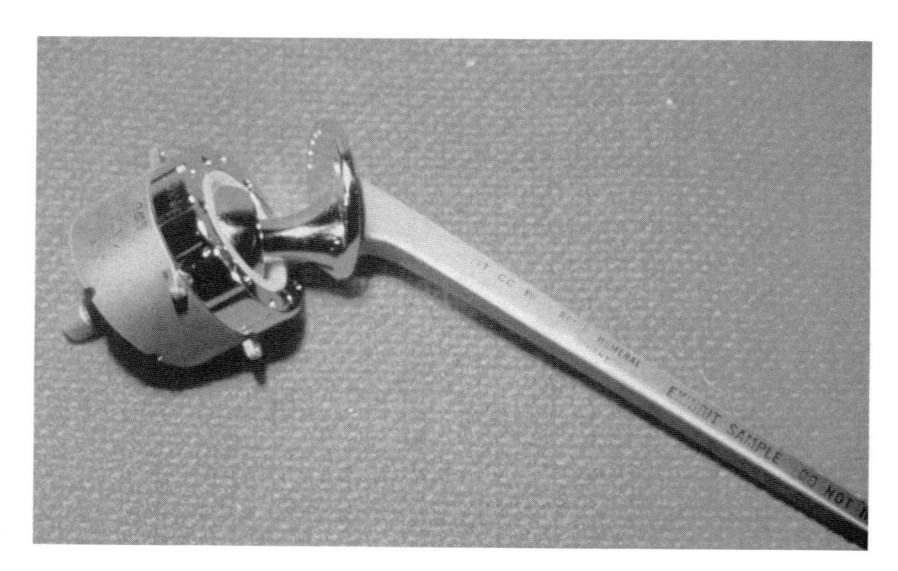

Figure 2–14. Michael Reese constrained total shoulder arthroplasty.

head fixed to the glenoid and the socket on the humeral side, resulting in a greater range of motion before the head impinges on the socket rim. The Jefferson prosthesis, designed by Fenlin, had a large plastic ball attached to the glenoid encased in a thin, metal housing on top of the humeral component.[45] The screw joining the ball to the glenoid component was a weak link and fractured under the loads transmitted (see Figure 1–29).

To try and minimize the stress-induced mechanical problems that were occurring with constrained prostheses, a double ball-and-socket design was developed. The trispherical, developed by Gristina, contained two joints with a free-moving central element (Figure 2–15). This was thought to allow for increased motion between the humeral and glenoid components, but the motion achieved clinically was not as expected.[52,53] This was most likely due to the fact that active motion under a load can only occur when one of the joints is being impinged.

Nonconstrained

A nonconstrained total shoulder arthroplasty has no physical link between the humeral and glenoid components. It resurfaces the glenohumeral joint in a situation analogous to a total hip arthroplasty and relies on the surrounding musculotendinous cuff for stability. Little constraint is built into the system. In this regard, this system is the most anatomic of shoulder prosthesis designs, whereby an attempt is made to recreate normal anatomy. This theoretically allows for unrestricted motion. The spherical humeral components have a large radius of curvature approaching the normal humeral head. The glenoid component generally conforms to the humeral head, and its design preserves bone stock.

The most successful nonconstrained design to date has been the Neer II, which evolved from the original Neer I hemiarthroplasty.[54,55] Many of the previously outlined criteria have been taken into account.[56] Minimal bone resection is required, and the surrounding soft tissues are preserved and repaired if necessary. The components attempt to recreate normal anatomy and anatomic relationships, thereby permitting a maximum range of motion. No mechanical linkage or blockage to motion exists, minimizing the stresses at the interface. Immediate and secure fixation is achieved, allowing for early rehabilitation of the soft tissues.

The humeral component, modified from the original endoprosthetic design, has smooth rounded contours added to the head to prevent impingement on the glenoid component (see Figure 1–44).[57] The humeral head is spherical with a 44-mm radius, matching that of the average humeral head. The stem permits a press-fit if the bone quality is satisfactory, and the stem allows the forces to be dissipated throughout the proximal part of the humerus. The glenoid component is curved to match that of the normal bone and has a 44-mm radius that conforms exactly to the humeral component

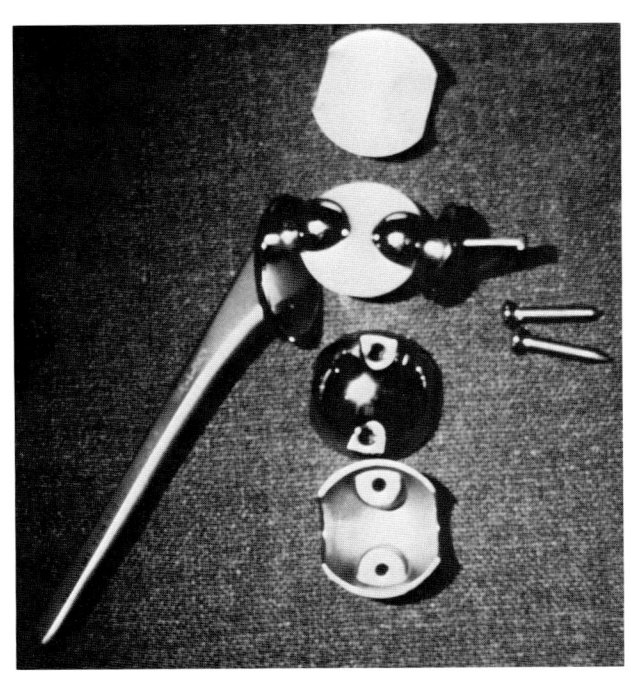

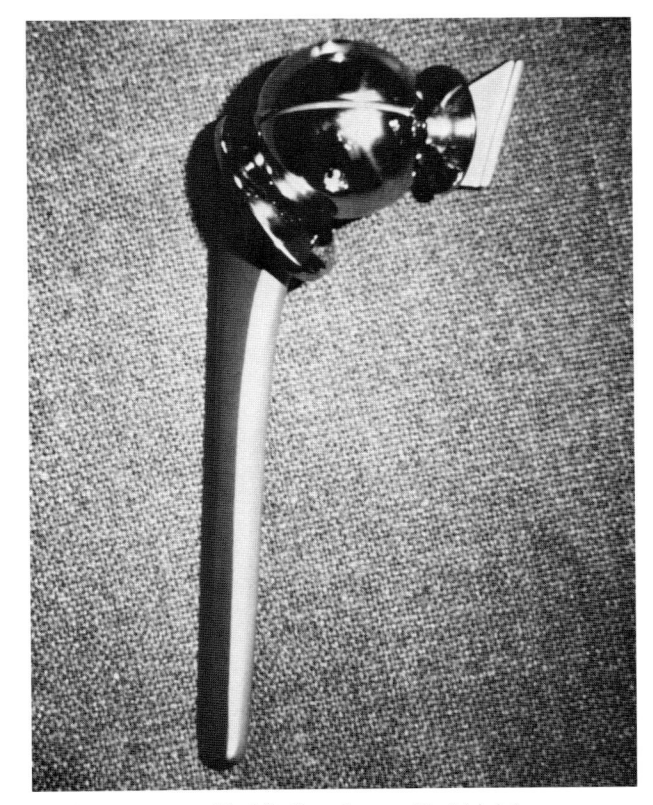

Figure 2–15. Trispherical constrained total shoulder arthroplasty, shown unassembled (left) and assembled (right).

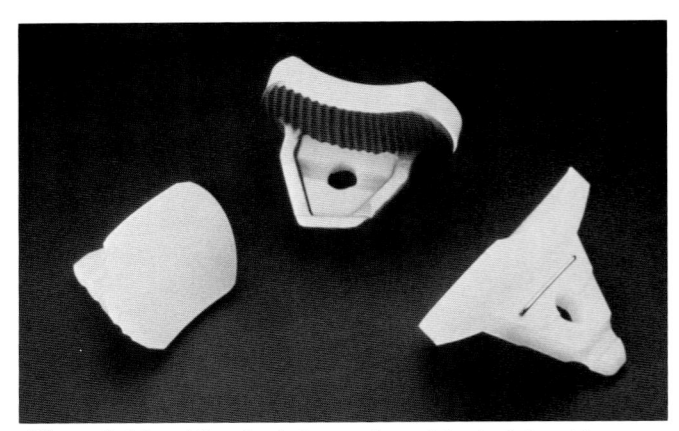

Figure 2–16. All-polyethylene and metal-backed glenoid components for the Neer II total shoulder arthroplasty.

(Figure 2–16). The dimensions match that of the average glenoid, but it is not anatomic in shape. There is no inferior extension, thereby avoiding impingement, or superior buttress that if present might limit abduction.

The original all-polyethylene design, which is still widely used, has been modified to a metal-backed component. Theoretic advantages, based on finite element studies of the acetabulum, included a more even distribution of the stresses at the interface and a decrease in polyethylene deformation and cold flow. However, recent finite element studies have suggested that an all-polyethylene glenoid component provides a more physiologic stress distribution in the surrounding bone.[58,59]

Surgical technique is critical to the success of a nonconstrained total shoulder arthroplasty. Proper tensioning of the capsuloligamentous and musculotendinous structures is essential for stability and function. If the abduction lever arm is not fully restored, weakness of the deltoid and supraspinatous muscles can result in poor function.[60] Conversely, if the components are put in with the center of rotation lateralized, then the soft-tissue structures will be overtightened and the range of motion limited.

Recent advances in the nonconstrained design are aimed at improving long-term fixation, particularly of the glenoid component. These changes include a more anatomic design, a variety of sizes, modularity, the use of pegs and screws, porous coating, and ceramic coatings, among others. Long-term follow-up is necessary to determine what will be most beneficial.

A variation of the nonconstrained total shoulder arthroplasty, the bipolar shoulder arthroplasty, was introduced by Swanson and Bateman separately in the mid-1970s.[61] Motion occurs at two interfaces, between the humeral head and the glenoid cup, and the cup and bony glenoid. Indications for its use have expanded recently, and clinical trials are currently underway, evaluating the use of a bipolar arthroplasty for the treatment of cuff tear arthropathies. The bipolar cup articulates with the undersurface of the acromion in addition to the glenoid fossa, providing stability and improving the abduction lever arm.

Semiconstrained

Semiconstrained prostheses are similar to the nonconstrained variety previously mentioned, except that the glenoid component has a superior extension designed to prevent superior migration of the humeral component. One of the first developed, the McNab-English prosthesis, was made of chrome cobalt with a porous coating over the entire humeral and glenoid component surfaces (Figure 2–17). A cranial curva-

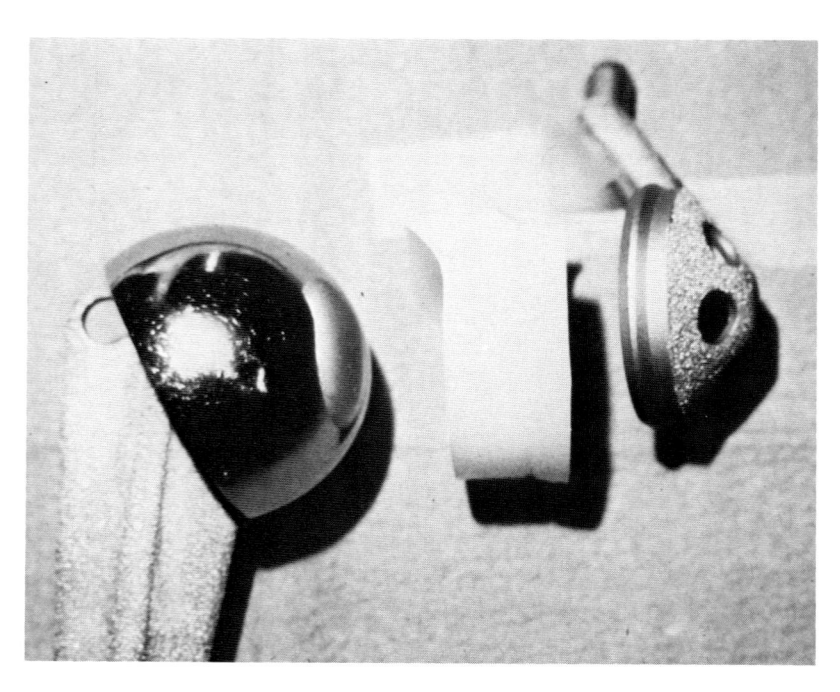

Figure 2–17. McNab-English semiconstrained total shoulder arthroplasty.

ture to the glenoid is designed to increase stability and maintain mobility, but abduction is restricted to some degree.[62,63]

SUMMARY

To design a successful total shoulder prosthesis and properly perform the surgical implantation, it is essential to understand the normal anatomy and biomechanics of the shoulder joint. Currently, nonconstrained prostheses offer the most consistent and durable long-term results, allowing for the restoration of normal anatomy and motion close to that of the normal shoulder joint. Despite the successes to date, improvements on the current state of the art are still needed and will result from increasing our understanding of the complex biomechanics of the shoulder joint.

REFERENCES

1. Seindler A. *Kinesiology of the Human Body under Normal and Pathological Conditions*. Springfield, IL: Charles C Thomas, 1955.
2. Friedman R. Total shoulder biomechanics before and after total joint arthroplasty. In: *Proceedings of the 17th SICOT Meeting*. 1990:350.
3. Johnston T. The movements of the shoulder joint. A plea for the use of the 'plane of the scapula' as the plane of reference for movements occurring at the humero-scapular joint. *Br J Surg* 1937;25:252–260.
4. Saha A. Mechanism of shoulder movements and a plea for the recognition of "zero position" of glenohumeral joint. *Indian J Surg* 1950;12:153–165.
5. Saha A. Dynamic stability of the glenohumeral joint. *Acta Orthop Scand* 1971;42:491–505.
6. Walker P. *Human Joints and Their Artificial Replacements*. Springfield, IL: Charles C Thomas, 1977.
7. Basmajian J, Bazan F. Factors preventing downward dislocation of the adducted shoulder. *J Bone Joint Surg [Am]* 1959;41:1182.
8. Friedman R, Hawthorne K, Genez B. Evaluation of glenoid bone loss with computerized tomography. *J Bone Joint Surg [Am]* 1992;74:1032–1037.
9. Codman E. *The Shoulder*. Boston: Thomas Todd, 1934.
10. Sarrafian S. Gross and functional anatomy of the shoulder. *Clin Orthop* 1983;173:11–19.
11. Saha A. Mechanics of elevation of glenohumeral joint. Its application in rehabilitation of flail shoulder in upper brachial plexus injuries and poliomyelitis. *Acta Orthop Scand* 1973;44:668–678.
12. Maki S, Gruen T. Anthropometric study of the glenohumeral joint. *Trans Orthop Res Soc* 1976;1:173.
13. McPherson E, Friedman R, Dooley R. Anatomic basis of total shoulder design. *J Shoulder Elbow Surg* 1993;2:528.
14. Black J, Dumbleton J. *Clinical Biomechanics*. 2nd ed. New York: Churchill-Livingstone, 1988.
15. Lucas D. Biomechanics of the shoulder joint. *Arch Surg* 1973;107:425–432.
16. Turkel S, Panio M, Marshall J, Girgis F. Stabilizing mechanisms preventing anterior dislocation of the glenohumeral joint. *J Bone Joint Surg [Am]* 1981;63:1208–1217.
17. Ovesen J, Nielsen S. Anterior and posterior shoulder instability. *Acta Orthop Scand* 1986;57:324.
18. Uhthoff H, Piscopo M. Anterior capsular redundancy of the shoulder: Congenital or traumatic? *J Bone Joint Surg [Br]* 1985;67:363–366.
19. An K, Morrey B. Biomechanics. In: Morrey B, eds. *Joint Replacement Arthroplasty*. New York: Churchill-Livingstone, 1990:397–405.
20. Spiegelmann J, Woo S-Y. A rigid-body method for finding centers of rotation and angular displacements of planar joint motion. *J Biomech* 1987;20:715.
21. Celli L, Balli A, de Luise G, Rovesta C. Some new aspects of the functional anatomy of the shoulder. *Ital J Orthop Traumatol* 1985;11:83–91.
22. Ito N. Electromyographic study of shoulder joint. *J Jpn Orthop Assoc* 1980;54:53–64.
23. Reeves B, Jobbin B, Flowers M. Biomechanical problems in the development of a total shoulder endoprosthesis. *J Bone Joint Surg [Br]* 1972;54:193.
24. Inman V, Saunders M, Abbot L. Observations on the function of the shoulder joint. *J Bone Joint Surg [Am]* 1944;26:1–30.
25. Bergmann G. Biomechanics and pathomechanics of the shoulder joint with reference to prosthetic joint replacement. In: Kobel R, Helbig B, Blauth W, eds. *Shoulder Replacement*. Berlin: Springer-Verlag, 1987:33.
26. Buechel F, Pappas M, DePalma A. "Floating socket" total shoulder replacement: Anatomical, biomechanical, and surgical rationale. *J Biomed Mater Res* 1977;12:89–114.
27. de Luca C, Forrest W. Force analysis of individual muscles acting simultaneously on the shoulder joint during isometric abduction. *J Biomech* 1973;6:385–393.
28. Poppen N, Walker P. Forces at the glenohumeral joint in abduction. *Clin Orthop* 1978;135:165–170.
29. Walker P, Poppen N. Biomechanics of the shoulder joint during abduction in the plane of the scapula. *Bull Hosp J Dis Orthop Inst* 1977;38(2):107–111.
30. Morrey B, An K. Biomechanics of the shoulder. In: Rockwood C, Matsen F, eds. *The Shoulder*. Philadelphia: WB Saunders, 1990:208–245.
31. Franklin J, Barrett W, Jackins S, Matsen F. Glenoid loosening in total shoulder arthroplasty. *J Arthroplasty* 1988;3:39–46.
32. Poppen N, Walker P. Normal and abnormal motion of the shoulder. *J Bone Joint Surg [Am]* 1976;58:195–201.
33. Doody S, Freedman L, Waterland J. Shoulder movements during abduction in the scapular plane. *Arch Phys Med Rehabil* 1970;51:595–604.
34. Freedman L, Munro R. Abduction of the arm in the scapular plane: Scapular and glenohumeral movements. *J Bone Joint Surg [Am]* 1966;48:1503–1510.
35. Browne A, Hoffmeyer P, Tanaka S, An K, Morrey B. Glenohumeral elevation studied in three dimensions. *J Bone Joint Surg [Br]* 1990;72:843–845.
36. Laumann U. Kinesiology of the shoulder joint. In: Kobel R, Helbig B, Blauth W, eds. *Shoulder Replacement*. Berlin: Springer-Verlag, 1987:23–31.
37. Friedman R. Biomechanics of the shoulder following total shoulder replacement. In: Post M, Morrey B, Hawkins R, eds. *Surgery of the Shoulder*. St. Louis: Mosby-Year Book, 1990:263–266.
38. Zuckerman J, Matsen FA. Biomechanics of the shoulder. In: Goldberg V, Nordin M, eds. *Biomechanics* 1990:225–247.
39. Howell S, Galinat B, Renzi A, Marone P. Normal and abnormal mechanics of the glenohumeral joint in the horizontal plane. *J Bone Joint Surg [Am]* 1988;70:227–232.
40. Sidles J, Harryman D, Harris S, Matsen FA. In vivo quantification of glenohumeral stability. *Trans Orthop Res Soc* 1991;16:646.

41. Harryman D, Sidles J, Clark J, McQuade K, Gibb T, Matsen F. Translation of the humeral head on the glenoid with passive glenohumeral motion. *J Bone Joint Surg [Am]* 1990;72:1334–1343.
42. Cofield R, Edgerton B. Total shoulder arthroplasty: Complications and revision surgery. *Instr Course Lect* 1990;39:449–462.
43. Friedman R. Glenohumeral translation following total shoulder arthroplasty. *J Shoulder Elbow Surg* 1992;1:312–316.
44. Post M, Jablon M, Miller H, Singh M. Constrained total shoulder joint replacement: A critical review. *Clin Orthop* 1979;144:135–150.
45. Fenlin J. Total glenohumeral joint replacement. *Orthop Clin North Am* 1975;6:565–583.
46. Copeland S, Lettin A, Scales J. The Stanmore total shoulder replacement: A critical review. *J Bone Joint Surg [Br]* 1978;60:144.
47. Lettin A, Scales J. Total replacement of the shoulder joint (two cases). *Proc R Soc Med* 1972;65:373–374.
48. Lettin A, Copeland S, Scales J. The Stanmore total shoulder replacement. *J Bone Joint Surg [Br]* 1982;64:47.
49. Post M, Jablon M. Constrained total shoulder arthroplasty. Long-term follow-up observations. *Clin Orthop* 1983;173:109–116.
50. Post M. Constrained total shoulder replacement. *Instr Course Lect* 1985;34(287):287–294.
51. Post M, Haskell S, Jablon M. Total shoulder replacement with a constrained prosthesis. *J Bone Joint Surg[Am]* 1980;62:327–335.
52. Gristina A, CW. The trispherical total shoulder replacement. In: Bayley J, Kessel L, eds. *Shoulder Surgery*. New York: Springer-Verlag, 1982:xx–xx.
53. Gristina A, Romano R, Kammire G, Webb L. Total shoulder replacement. *Orthop Clin North Am* 1987;18:445–453.
54. Neer C. Articular replacement of the humeral head. *J Bone Joint Surg [Am]* 1964;46:7.
55. Neer C. Articular replacement of the humeral head. *J Bone Joint Surg [Am]* 1955;37:215.
56. Neer C. Unconstrained total shoulder arthroplasty. *Instruct Course Lect* 1985;34:278.
57. Neer C II, Watson K, Stanton F. Recent experience in total shoulder replacement. *J Bone Joint Surg [Am]* 1982;64:319–337.
58. Friedman R, LaBerge M, Dooley R, O'Hara A. Finite element modeling of the glenoid component: Effect of design parameters on stress distribution. *J Shoulder Elbow Surg* 1992;1:261–270.
59. Friedman R, Brookings G, Dooley R. Finite element analysis of glenoid component design. *Orthop Trans* 1990;14:253.
60. Rietveld A, Daanen H, Rozing P, Obermann W. The lever arm in glenohumeral abduction after hemiarthroplasty. *J Bone Joint Surg [Br]* 1988;70:561–565.
61. Swanson A. Bipolar implant shoulder arthroplasty. In: Bateman J, Welsh R, eds. *Surgery of the Shoulder*. St. Louis: CV Mosby, 1984:211–223.
62. McElwain E, English E. The early results of porous coated total shoulder arthroplasty. *Clin Orthop* 1987;218:217–224.
63. Faludi D, Weiland A. Cementless total shoulder arthroplasty: Preliminary experience with 13 cases. *Orthopedics* 1983;6:431.

3 Preoperative Clinical Evaluation

Melvin Post, M.D., and Enrique Grinblat, M.D.

Successful treatment of the arthritic shoulder may require an arthroplasty in order to relieve pain and improve function. A thorough preoperative evaluation of the patient should include an accurate history and physical examination, adequate imaging studies, and pertinent laboratory tests. Planning of the operation, including the surgical approach, selection of a specific device, and consideration of the quality and function of the bone and soft tissues, is an essential part of the preoperative evaluation. The more information that is at hand assists the surgeon in performing the correct operation and achieving the desired result. Other parameters must also be considered, including patient goals and their understanding of the procedure and the possible complications that can result. The surgeon must also consider other treatment options and have the patient be a part of the decision-making process.

HISTORY

An accurate history must be obtained to help determine how the physician proceeds with the medical evaluation and how the patient will be treated. All necessary information may not be gathered in a single interview so that a second or third examination may be needed. The surgeon should not rush ahead and render treatment without being certain of the diagnosis. An effort should be made to place a priority on the patient's answers, and only when all the facts related to the symptoms are obtained and fully understood in a correct sequence should the physical examination be undertaken. It is primarily the history that will permit an early working differential diagnosis of the disease state.

The surgeon should attempt to classify various conditions into categories such as acquired or congenital, and then further divide disease states into the various systems such as hematologic, infectious, metabolic, traumatic, and endocrine that may affect the shoulder. The examining surgeon must obtain a complete history reviewing all the medical systems before the interview is complete, because shoulder symptoms and findings may relate to these in addition to the musculoskeletal system. For example, rheumatoid arthritis often affects other joints and the surrounding soft tissues, and this can influence the sequence of different joint operations. If the knees are severely involved with rheumatoid arthritis and need replacement, it may be best to treat the lower extremities before the shoulders. Treatment of lupus erythematosus with oral steroids may cause osteonecrosis in the proximal part of the humerus, while a history of diabetes causing a polyneuropathy and associated pain in the shoulder girdle may affect the decision to operate. A Charcot neuropathy affecting the shoulder can cause pain and is a relative contraindication to arthroplasty. Electromyography studies may be helpful in the diagnosis. The age of the patient, occupation and specific job requirements, handedness, and educational level are important factors to consider. It is far better to overinterview than to accept an inadequate history.

If the patient's complaints are few and localized, and there are no other significant considerations, such as with a traumatic four-part fracture of the proximal end of the humerus, the surgeon may then elect to perform a hemiarthroplasty as the best treatment for that patient. In contrast, a chief complaint of pain may cross many lines of specialization. The surgeon should recognize a disturbance in form and function regardless of the involved system, as well as understand the pathogenesis of a disease process. Once the surgeon has considered the patient's whole problem, he or she should explain it to the patient so that both can make an intelligent choice regarding treatment.

When a patient complains of pain, attention should be placed on its location, character, frequency, duration, variation, aggravation, distribution or radiation, intensity, and course.[1] Was the pain caused by trauma or was trauma superimposed on a preexisting condition? If so, what was the kind and degree of trauma? Was the pain increased or relieved by specific motions, stress, or activity? How has medication affected the pain? Varying kinds of pain may relate to a neurologic condition or peripheral nerve, muscle, or joint. As this part of the history is obtained, the surgeon should attempt to correlate the symptoms with shoulder anatomy and physiology.

The general history must include a history of previous operations, allergies, and medications as well as emotional stresses that can affect the postoperative rehabilitation and outcome.

PHYSICAL EXAMINATION

Physical examination requires inspection, palpation, percussion, smell, and auscultation. In addition, one must test muscle strength, examine the range of motion for all the joints in both upper extremities, assess joint stability, perform complete neurologic and vascular examinations as well as a general physical examination, and carry out any special tests that may be indicated.

During the general examination, any deviations from the norm are recorded so that a data base is created for later comparison. A general examination must include a description of the skin, including texture, scars, elasticity and pigmentation, and palpation of the subcutaneous tissues. The color of the extremities, especially in the hands, and any evidence of edema should be recorded. For example, does the patient have a vascular shunt in the involved extremity for renal dialysis to the extent that the entire venous system is dilated? Examination of the cervical spine in a patient with rheumatoid arthritis may demonstrate limited extension that can interfere with endotracheal intubation, thereby requiring fiberoptic intubation.

Muscle Examination

A standardized numerical system for grading muscles and muscle groups is recommended.[1] Using this method allows any changes from the initial examination to be recognized. A numerical muscle grade of 5 represents normal power while a decreasing grade indicates the power of a muscle is decreasing. The surgeon should not rely solely on this, but also examine the muscle fully, since a grade of 5 is consistent with a significant amount of muscle atrophy. This is especially true in patients who are well developed and for whom a false numerical rating is obtained because of residual strength of the muscles. In older patients and those recently operated upon, care should be exercised during muscle testing, for fear of causing iatrogenic injury to the soft tissues and bone.

Muscles should be tested with and without gravity eliminated, and a determination made as to whether or not a muscle contraction is present. Endurance of the muscles and dexterity of the glenohumeral joint should be noted. Is the muscle tender, of normal contour, or in spasm? Is the muscle prevented from fully contracting due to pain rather than to any intrinsic weakness within the muscle? A comparison of active and passive motion during muscle testing is needed, since active motion requires muscle strength with a grade of at least 3. The examiner must also know whether or not there is nerve paralysis causing weakness. Is there injury to the brachial plexus that could affect an arthroplasty procedure? Even the muscles of the scapula must be tested, since it is important to know whether or not the fulcrum of the scapula against the chest wall can be fixed, especially if another procedure such as a glenohumeral arthrodesis is being considered.

DATA FORM FOR BASIC SHOULDER EVALUATION (SHEXAM)
American Shoulder and Elbow Surgeons

Name ____________ Shoulder: R / L

Date of Examination ____________ Hospital # ____________

(Mark line)
I. PAIN: |________________|

No Pain (5) Completely disabling pain (0)

II. MOTION:
A. Patient sitting (enter motion or NA if not measured):

1. Active total elevation of arm: ______ degrees
2. Passive internal rotation:
(Circle segment of posterior anatomy reached by thumb
Enter "NA" if reach restricted by limited elbow flexion.)

1=Less than trochanter	8=L2	15=T7
2=Trochanter	9=L1	16=T6
3=Gluteal	10=T12	17=T5
4=Sacrum	11=T11	18=T4
5=L5	12=T10	19=T3
6=L4	13=T9	20=T2
7=L3	14=T8	21=T1

3. Active external rotation with arm at side: ______ degrees
4. Passive external rotation at 90° abduction: ______ degrees
(enter "NA" if patient cannot acheive 90° of abduction)
5. Assisted horizontal cross body adduction: ______ cm
(measure from antecubital fossa to anterior tip of acromion)

B. Patient supine:

1. Passive total elevation of arm: ______ degrees*
2. Passive external rotation with arm at side: ______ degrees

*Total elevation of the arm is measured by viewing the patient from the side and using a goniometer to determine the angle between the arm and the thorax.

III. STRENGTH (5=normal, 4=good, 3=fair, 2=poor, 1=trace, 0=paralysis, NA=not available) [enter numbers below]

A. Anterior deltoid ______
B. Middle deltoid ______
C. External rotation ______
D. Internal rotation ______

IV. DYNAMOMETER EXAM: (Isometric contraction against resistance, arm in neutral position)

	Left	Right
A. Forward flexion	______kg	______kg
B. Abduction	______kg	______kg
C. Extension	______kg	______kg
D. External rotation	______kg	______kg
E. Internal rotation	______kg	______kg

V. STABILITY (5=normal, 4=apprehension, 3=rare subluxation, 2=recurrent subluxation, 1=recurrent dislocation, 0=fixed dislocation, NA=not available) [enter numbers below]

A. Anterior ______
B. Posterior ______
C. Inferior ______

VI. FUNCTION (4=normal, 3=mild compromise, 2=with difficulty, 0=unable, NA=not available) [enter numbers below]

A. Use back pocket? ______
B. Perineal care? ______
C. Wash opposite axilla? ______
D. Eat with utensil? ______
E. Comb hair? ______
F. Use hand with arm at shoulder level? ______
G. Carry 10-15 lbs. with arm at side? ______
H. Dress? ______
I. Sleep on affected side? ______
J. Pulling? ______
K. Use hand overhead? ______
L. Throwing? ______
M. Lifting? ______

VII. ECONOMICS (yes, no, NA, X)
A. Do usual work? ______
B. Working light duty? ______
C. Do usual sport? ______
D. Earning power same as before injury? ______
E. Vocational rehab in progress? ______
F. Receiving physical therapy? ______
G. Receiving home help? ______
H. Legal claim settled? ______

VIII. PATIENT RESPONSE: (Mark line below)

Much better (3) Same (1) Much worse (0)
|________________|________________|

Completed by: ____________. Date____________.
SHEXAM (revised 3-14-89)

Figure 3–1. American Shoulder and Elbow Surgeons form for evaluating shoulder pain and function.

Joint Motion

The accepted method for testing joint motion is based upon the principle of a neural zero first described by Cave and Roberts, which allows for standardization of motion testing.[1,2] A practical basic shoulder evaluation form approved by the American Shoulder and Elbow Surgeons for evaluating pain and function is recommended for serial examinations (Figure 3–1). It is important to note if the shoulder complex moves as an integrated unit.

Rotator Cuff

Since the rotator cuff is so important in providing synchronous motion of the glenohumeral joint, and a prosthetic device is highly dependent upon the integrity of the rotator cuff for its active function, it is essential to know as much as possible about the rotator cuff. This information is especially important when a nonconstrained device is used. It is unwise to repair a tear of the rotator cuff alone in the presence of significant glenohumeral arthritis.[2-5] Evidence of impingement and symptomatic disease of the acromioclavicular joint must be considered in the total treatment of a patient having an arthroplasty procedure.

Preoperative evaluation of the soft tissues and capsule must be considered. Is the joint capsule enlarged or redundant, especially at the inferior recess (Figure 3–2)? If there are anterior contractures, they must be differentiated from a mechanical block to joint motion. A contracture may require lengthening the anterior soft-tissue structures, including the subscapularis.[2,6-8] If the rotator cuff is torn, is it a partial or full-thickness tear? In osteoarthritis, for instance, rotator cuff tears are found in only about 5% of cases.[9,10] If there is degeneration or scarring, especially of the subscapularis, it must be dealt with. Are loose bodies embedded in the soft tissues or within the joint or subscapularis bursa? If other contractures exist, they must be released and the proper tension obtained in the entire rotator cuff mechanism so as to achieve maximum function with a prosthetic device.[2] Is there thinning, stretching, or tearing of the capsule (Figure 3–3)? Is the synovial lining inflamed or hypertrophied? If significant synovitis is present, it must be treated intraoperatively.

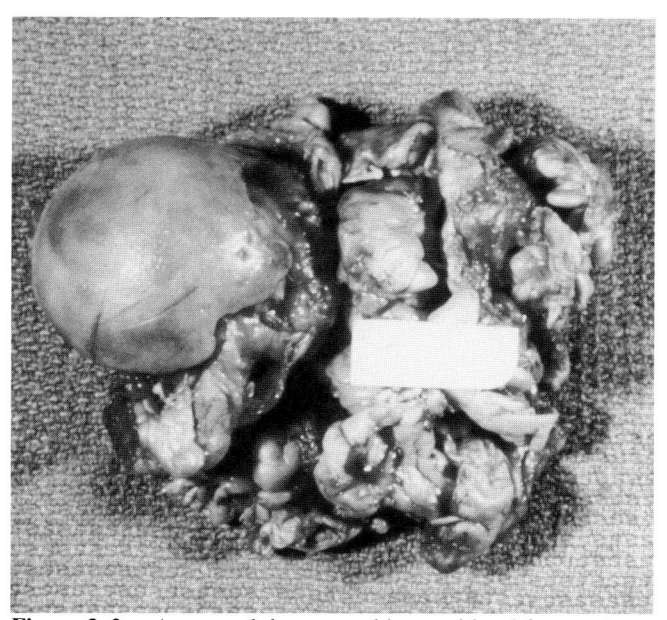

Figure 3–2. A resected degenerated humeral head from a rheumatoid patient is shown. Note the exuberant synovium and its granulation tissue. The rotator cuff was completely nonfunctional and the humeral head was unstable and dislocated from its joint. In this case a constrained prosthesis was required to stabilize the humeral shaft with good results.

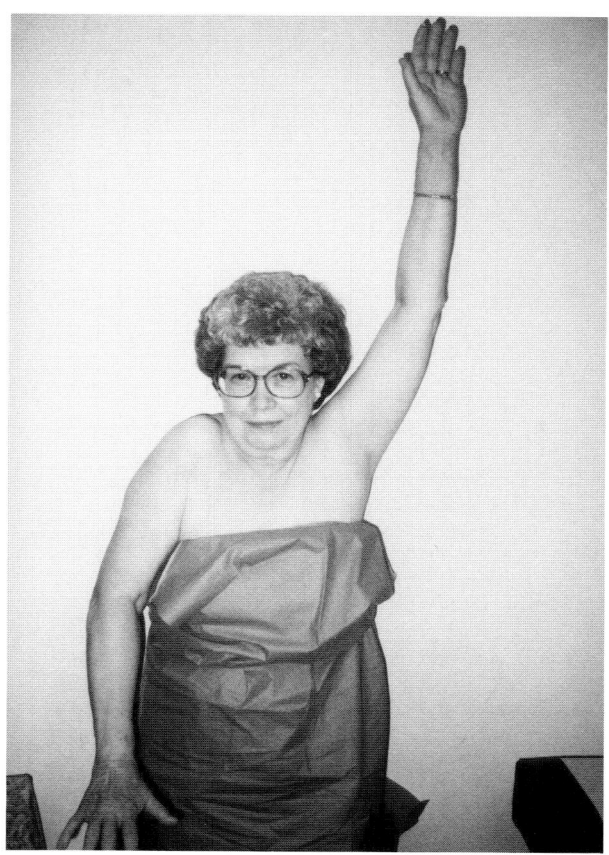

Figure 3–3. An adult woman had an attempted repair of a severely torn rotator cuff. The shoulder was nonfunctional. The glenohumeral joint was arthritic. In this case the patient had a severe cuff arthropathy and required not only a rotator cuff repair but also an arthroplasty as well.

Instability

Instability of the joint must be studied in relation to the underlying process. The condition of the humeral head upon the glenoid is important to know in advance. Whether it is central or posteriorly subluxated, for example, must be known and taken into account during the operation (Figures 3–4 and 3–5).

It is important to know whether or not there was any history of glenohumeral instability due to such factors as

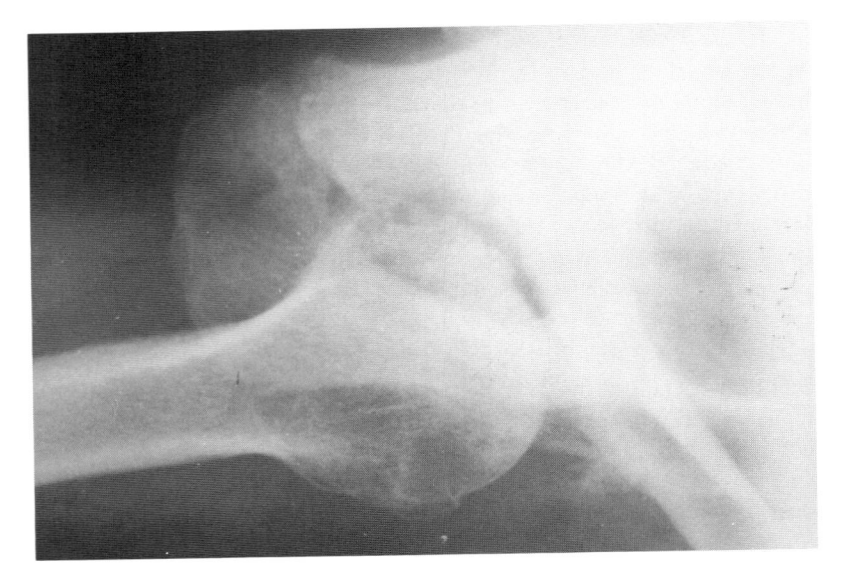

Figure 3–4. An elderly man complained of pain in his shoulder following an inability to actively elevate his arm. Following a thorough evaluation it was discovered that the patient had Charcot disease and a chronic posterior dislocation of his shoulder. Arthroplasty often will not relieve pain and improve function in Charcot disease and is not recommended.

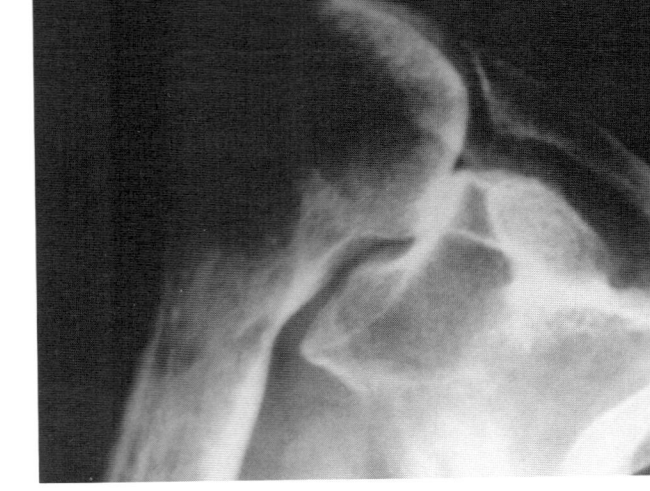

Figure 3–5. An elderly woman had severe rheumatoid arthritis. The shoulder was nonfunctional. Pain was severe. Note the severe erosion of the upper half of the glenoid and undersurface of the acromion. In this case a decision had to be made whether or not a nonconstrained arthroplasty would suffice or whether a constrained joint would be needed to fix the fulcrum of the humeral head. In the vast majority of patients, nonconstrained arthroplasty can be successfully used.

congenital deficiencies, trauma, and arthritis. This must be dealt with intraoperatively, and having this information preoperatively helps in planning the procedure. Previous operations for instability can cause contractures which have to be dealt with, by lengthening the subscapularis or achieving length in the supraspinatus or other structures. Proper circumferential tension within the rotator cuff structures and its underlying capsule is needed in order to obtain optimum function and avoid postoperative subluxation or instability.

IMAGING STUDIES

Plain films, including axillary and anteroposterior views of the glenohumeral joint in internal and external rotation, are needed. In order to achieve a true profile of the glenohumeral joint, the anteroposterior views can be taken with the patient standing and the scapula flush against the x-ray cassette, which results in the torso rotated 30 to 40 degrees, thereby showing the glenohumeral space and its adjacent bony structures.

The humeral head should be studied to determine if it is flattened, sclerotic, or eroded. Large subchondral cysts must be identified and managed intraoperatively with methylmethacrylate or bone grafting.[2,11] Peripheral osteophytes are most often observed inferiorly. The amount and location of cartilage loss should be assessed. The quality of the bone must be considered. These questions are important in the preoperative planning.

Superior subluxation of the humeral head often indicates a severe rotator cuff tear or disease.[12,13] Arthrography is still the gold standard for determining full-thickness rotator cuff tears.[14] It is considered more useful than a routine magnetic resonance imaging scan in most cases.

On the glenoid side, the amount of cartilage loss and sclerosis should be observed, and whether it is central or posterior should be noted.[2] Peripheral osteophytes sometimes may interfere with function of the prosthetic head or placement of the glenoid component. The degree of erosion, whether central, posterior, or anterior, with flattening and narrowing of the glenoid vault will help determine whether or not a glenoid prosthesis can or should be inserted.

The position and size of osteophytes, anterior glenoid rim erosions and fractures, depth of the glenoid vault, posterior glenoid erosions, malunion of any fractured tuberosities, and osteonecrosis of the humeral head are important features to note preoperatively. Erosions of the undersurface of the acromion indicate severe rotator cuff disease (Figure 3–5). Computerized tomographic scanning is especially useful in defining these abnormalities.

If the glenoid is seriously eroded, it may require bone grafting.[2,11] This should be determined preoperatively so that adequate preoperative planning can be carried out. Often, the bone graft can be taken directly from the resected humeral head, making sure to incorporate some of the subchondral bone in the graft, as well as cancellous bone.

Radiographic examination of the humeral shaft in two planes will help to determine the quality of bone, thickness of the cortices, and diameter of the intramedullary canal. Preoperative templating allows the surgeon to plan for the correct stem size.

OTHER CONSIDERATIONS

In considering a patient for shoulder arthroplasty, the surgeon should determine if the procedure will achieve the desired result of relieving pain and restoring function. The surgeon must understand the biomechanics and physiology of the shoulder, and also take into account limitations of the prosthetic device to minimize the risk of failure.[12,13,15,16] If the rotator cuff is extensively torn, severely attenuated, or completely ineffective, a nonconstrained shoulder arthroplasty may not provide the desired results in terms of pain relief and improved function.[17,18] In unusual circumstances, a constrained device or shoulder arthrodesis may need to be considered.[16,19–23]

The rotator cuff tissues are often of better quality and function in osteoarthritis than in rheumatoid arthritis.[10,24] Moreover, multiple operations done on the shoulder produce a less desirable result than a well-done initial operation.

Gratifying results can be obtained with a shoulder arthroplasty if patients are carefully selected, the correct prosthesis is chosen, the operation is performed well, and a careful postoperative rehabilitation program is carried out. The rehabilitation program is very different for nonconstrained versus constrained devices.

Shoulder arthroplasty prostheses are of three types: constrained, semiconstrained, and nonconstrained.[25] Nonconstrained arthroplasty devices can be used to manage the vast majority of patients with glenohumeral arthritis. However, they are highly dependent upon an effective rotator cuff to obtain maximum function. Constrained devices are seldom indicated, except in certain instances when the entire rotator cuff mechanism is lost. A constrained arthroplasty prosthesis should be considered only when there is no hope of restoring the rotator cuff or it is completely absent. This type of device provides an artificial fulcrum between the prosthesis and bone.[2] It is not nearly as durable as a nonconstrained device, and often fails in the short term. Even a semiconstrained arthroplasty prosthesis still relies on the musculotendinous complex for stability.[26]

If glenohumeral tension exceeds the compression force, a nonconstrained arthroplasty will fail. Every effort should be made to restore rotator cuff function, release contractures, and achieve proper tension of the soft tissues surrounding the prosthetic device so that residual muscle power can maximize muscle contraction for function. Active function depends upon the quality of the rotator cuff, its muscle strength, and adequacy of the operation.

When a glenoid component is needed, excessive removal of cancellous bone in the glenoid vault should be avoided since this will only lead to early loosening.[2,8,16,17] The authors recommend glenoid components only when there is severe glenoid erosion, large glenoid bone cysts, or an incongruous glenoid.[27] When good subchondral bone is present with an adequate volume in the glenoid vault, a glenoid component is not routinely used. An incongruous nonconstrained glenoid component is recommended in selected cases since it permits some translation of a metal humeral head against the glenoid component.[28]

INDICATIONS

The indications for shoulder arthroplasty include osteoarthritis,[10] rheumatoid arthritis,[25] fracture,[29,30] posttraumatic arthritis, osteonecrosis, old sepsis, rotator cuff disease associated with severe glenohumeral arthritis,[31–33] and revision surgery.

Osteoarthritis

In osteoarthritis the joint space is narrowed, peripheral osteophytes of varying sizes are noted, subchondral sclerosis is present, and cystic changes in the subchondral metaphyseal area of the humeral head are often observed. The rotator cuff is intact in more than 90% of the cases. Glenoid erosions, both central and peripheral, may be severe in the most advanced cases.

Osteophytes may be present at the glenoid rim or along the inferomedial aspect of the humeral head. Often, the joint may contain osteochondral loose bodies that may not be evident on plain radiographs. The subscapularis bursa can be enlarged, communicate with the joint, and contain loose bodies. If contractures of the anterior capsule and subscapularis are present, lengthening of these anterior soft-tissue structures may become necessary.

Rheumatoid Arthritis

In rheumatoid arthritis all the tissues are affected. In this disease process, the soft tissues, especially the rotator cuff mechanism, are affected much more frequently than in osteoarthritis. The rotator cuff is often torn, attenuated, and scarred. Rheumatoid granulation tissue can be found in and about the joint in a patient with active disease.[1] Both soft-tissue and bone loss can be severe, leading to joint instability. Erosions may be severe, along with osteopenia. Synovial hypertrophy can be extensive (see Figure 3–2). Cysts are often found within the glenoid and humeral head. In the most advanced cases, cartilage loss may be complete. The capsule can become stretched and thinned, leading to great instability. Neer et al.[5,7] described three forms of the rheumatoid process: dry, wet, and resorptive. In the dry form, the joint space may be lost, particularly with periarticular sclerosis. Bone cysts and stiffness may result. In the wet form, the synovial lining may be exuberant with marked erosions at the margins of the bone, and the humeral head may displace within the glenoid. Marked bone resorption is present in the resorptive form.

Other inflammatory conditions that may cause arthritis of the glenohumeral joint include hemophiliac arthritis, chondrocalcinosis, Lyme arthritis, pigmented villonodular synovitis, and psoriasis. Steroid therapy may cause osteonecrosis of the humeral head.

Posttraumatic Arthritis

Posttraumatic arthritis resulting from fracture of the proximal part of the humerus or fracture-dislocation is often associated with a malunion of the tuberosities causing impingement, and the rotator cuff may be severely torn. The humeral head can be deformed and malunited, with nonunions present in some cases.[3,29,34,35] In other cases, single and multiple episodes of dislocation may present with radiographic evidence of glenohumeral arthritis.

Arthritis can result from previous surgery involving the use of internal fixation devices.[11,36] Patients who have had previous operations for recurrent shoulder dislocations often show degenerative changes of the glenohumeral joint (Figure 3–6). In some cases, posttraumatic osteonecrosis may develop. Shoulder arthroplasty following old trauma is very difficult surgery, and complications occur more frequently because of scarring, malunion, nonunion, bone loss, humeral shortening, and muscle and soft-tissue contractures.

Osteonecrosis

Osteonecrosis due to injury or oral corticosteroid usage for systemic disease results in varying degrees of collapse of the humeral head. The glenoid articular surface is often intact. The rotator cuff is rarely torn. In this event, hemiarthroplasty is often successful.

Rotator Cuff Disease Associated with Severe Glenohumeral Arthritis

A form of rotator cuff disease associated with severe glenohumeral arthritis, known as the "Milwaukee shoulder," was described by McCarty et al. in 1981.[31] In this condition the synovial fluid was found to have aggregates of hydroxyapatite crystals, active collagenase, and proteases.[32] It was assumed that active enzymes within the synovium resulted in damage to the joint surfaces and surrounding soft tissues.[37,38] Later, basic calcium phosphate (BCP) was identified as the crystal that formed in the synovial fluid. The synovial lining absorbs these crystals, secretes collagenase that further damages the tissues, and causes the release of additional crystals.

Neer et al.[5] described another form, called "cuff tear arthropathy," whose features included massive rotator cuff tearing, glenohumeral instability, loss of articular cartilage with humeral head collapse, and bone loss (Figure 3–7). The condition was not related to osteoarthritis. It is not clear how Neer's description of cuff tear arthropathy is related to the "Milwaukee shoulder." Due to the marked instability, it is possible that a rocker-bottom effect can result in glenoid component loosening[15] (Figure 3–8).

Acute Fractures

In surgical neck fractures, the tuberosities are often fractured, comminuted, and superiorly displaced, with the rotator cuff being extensively torn. When a four-part surgical neck fracture or fracture-dislocation occurs, the blood supply to the humeral head is lost.[39] Older patients can be treated with a hemiarthroplasty, while in younger individuals open reduction and internal fixation may be indicated if secure fixation and early motion are possible. Otherwise, a hemiarthroplasty may be performed.

Infection

Septic arthritis of the shoulder is uncommon, and often signifies an underlying systemic illness.[40] It can be debilitating and painful, leading to destruction of the articular cartilage. Associated shoulder diseases and systemic illnesses must be recognized in order to treat the condition adequately and prevent reinfection. A precise diagnosis is needed before treatment is rendered. Elevated white blood cell counts and sedimentation rates along with joint aspiration for bacteriologic testing can supply the information needed for a correct diagnosis. Specific imaging studies may be helpful in difficult cases (Figure 3–9). When a prosthetic joint infection is present, the components may loosen. The rotator cuff may be attenuated, the long head of the biceps may be torn or dislocated, and joint stability may be poor.

Failed Surgery

In a failed shoulder arthroplasty the rotator cuff is often scarred and torn, with the muscles being of poor quality and even fibrotic. Stability may be poor, and infection may be

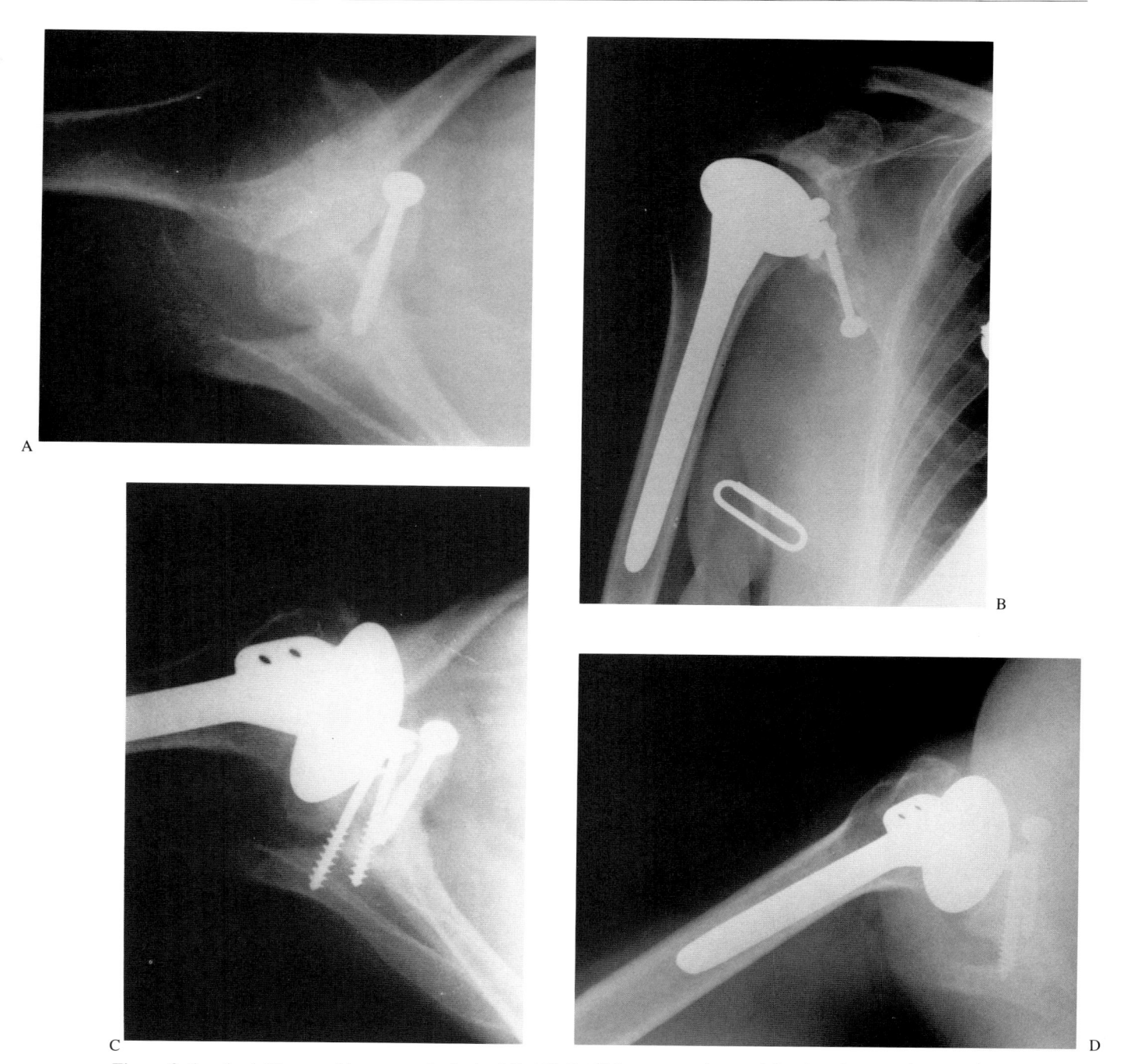

Figure 3–6. **A.** A 55-year-old woman who had a failed Helfet-Bristow procedure and developed severe degeneration and recurring dislocation of the proximal part of the humerus. At surgery, the coracoid and its screw were left alone. The anterior glenoid was absent and eroded. **B** through **D.** Anteroposterior, true axillary, and modified axillary views of the glenohumeral joint show a Neer hemiarthroplasty. The entire front half of the glenoid vault, with a new face, was reconstructed from a bone graft made from the excised humeral head and held with two screws. The screw from the previous coracoid graft in the initial operation was left alone. (Figure continued on next page.)

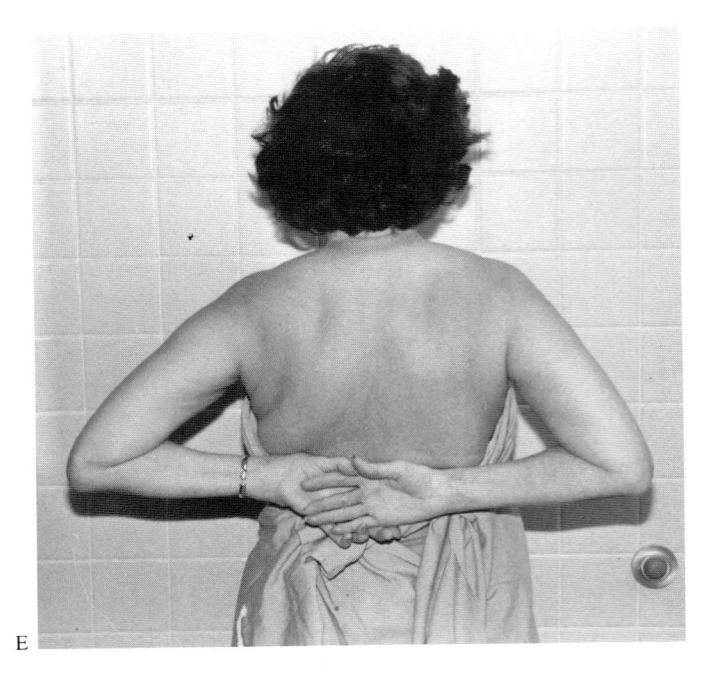

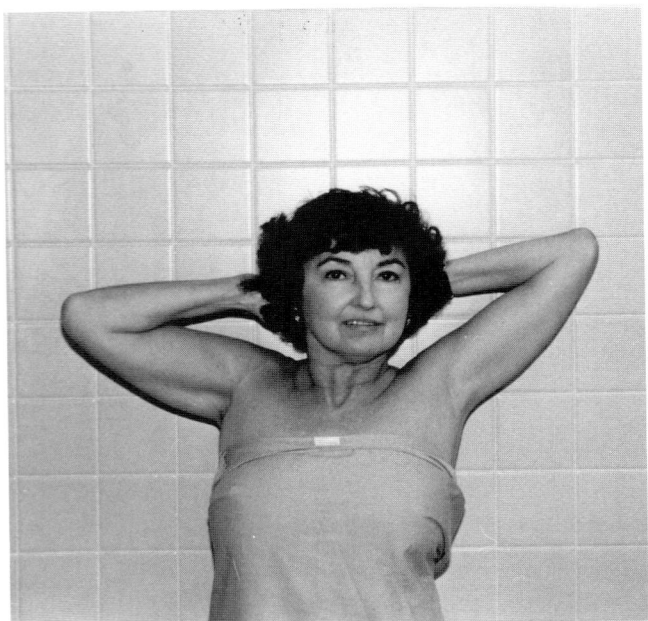

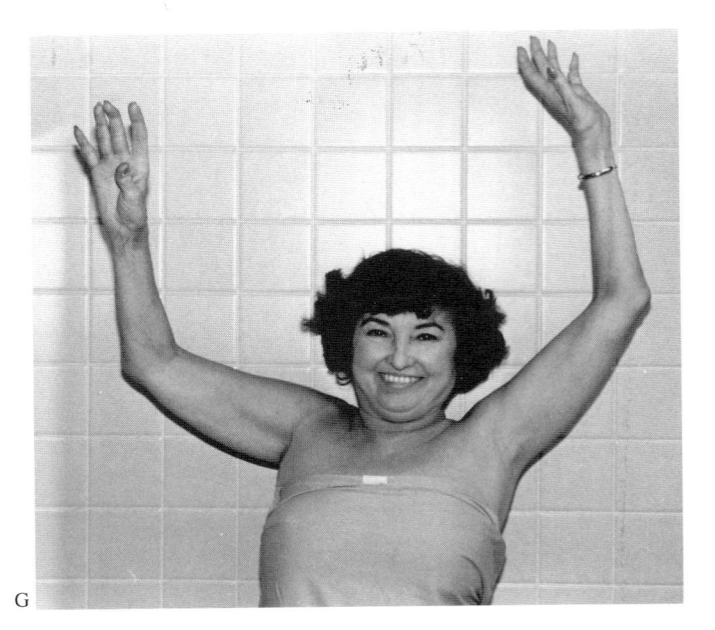

Figure 3–6. (Continued) E through G. Note the active motions several years later. Deltoid weakness and poor endurance of the muscles about the shoulder persisted. Nevertheless, the result was excellent. Pain was relieved. (Reproduced with permission from Post.[2])

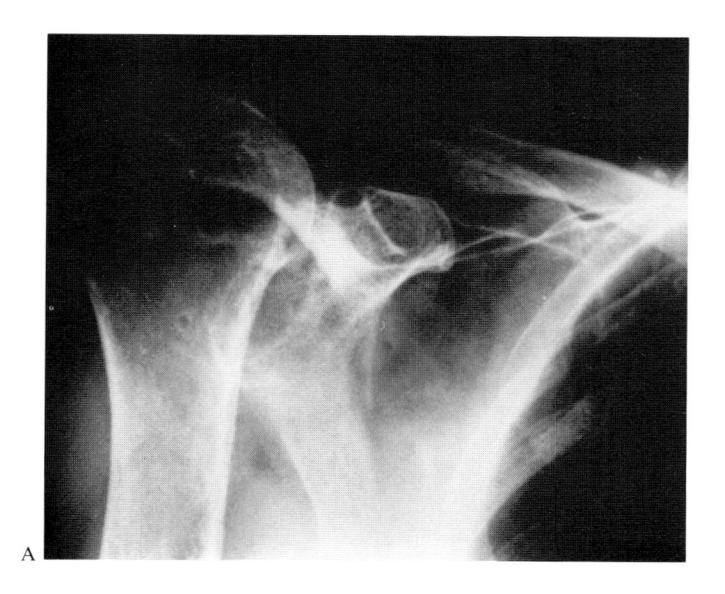

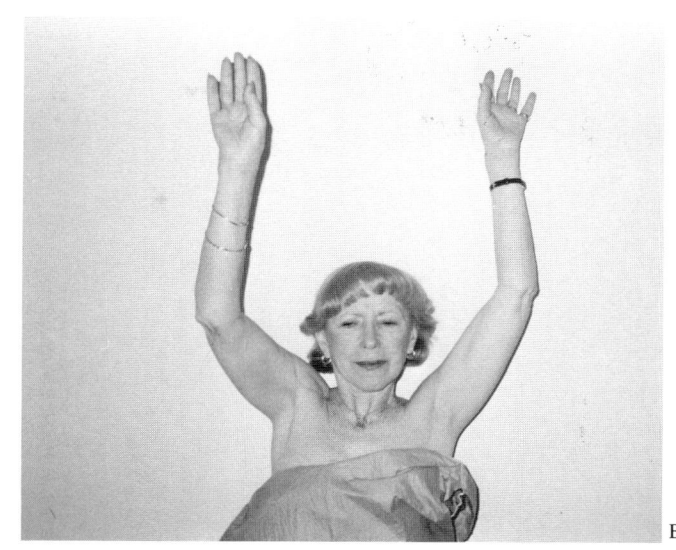

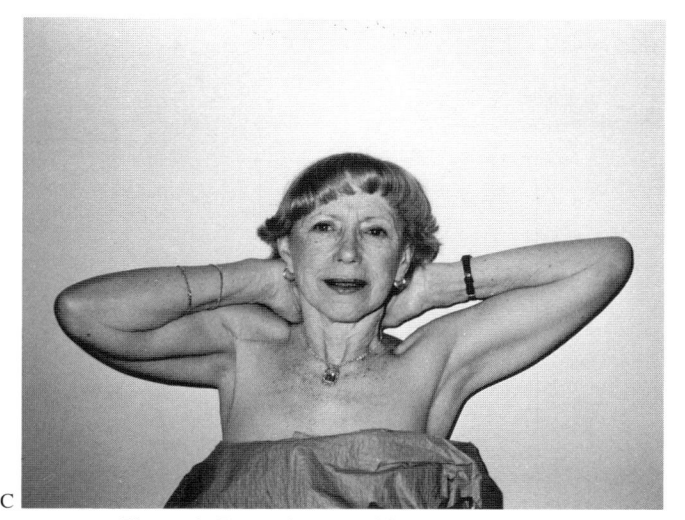

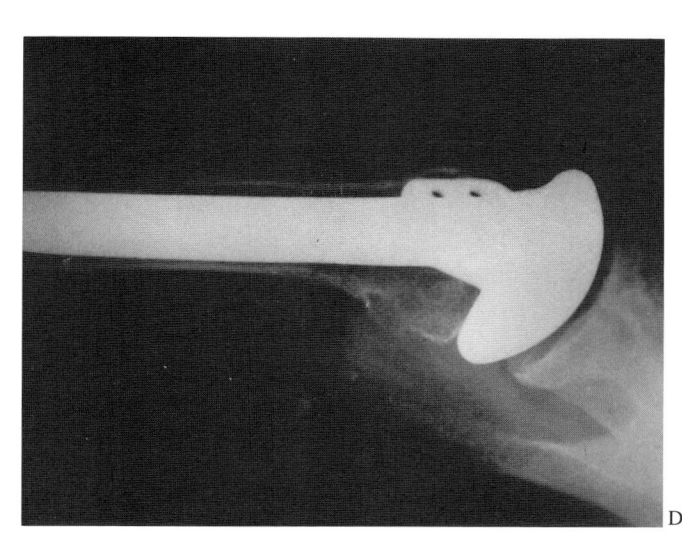

Figure 3–7. A 67-year-old woman had severe rotator cuff tear arthropathy. **A.** An anteroposterior radiograph is shown. Note the severe superior subluxation, degeneration of the humeral head, and degenerative arthritis. **B** and **C.** A Neer II hemiarthroplasty was performed. There was good active motion in the right shoulder but the endurance was poor since the muscles had been severely weakened and endurance diminished. **D.** An axillary view of the shoulder shows the hemiarthroplasty prosthesis with preservation of the joint space several years later. (Reproduced with permission from Post.[2])

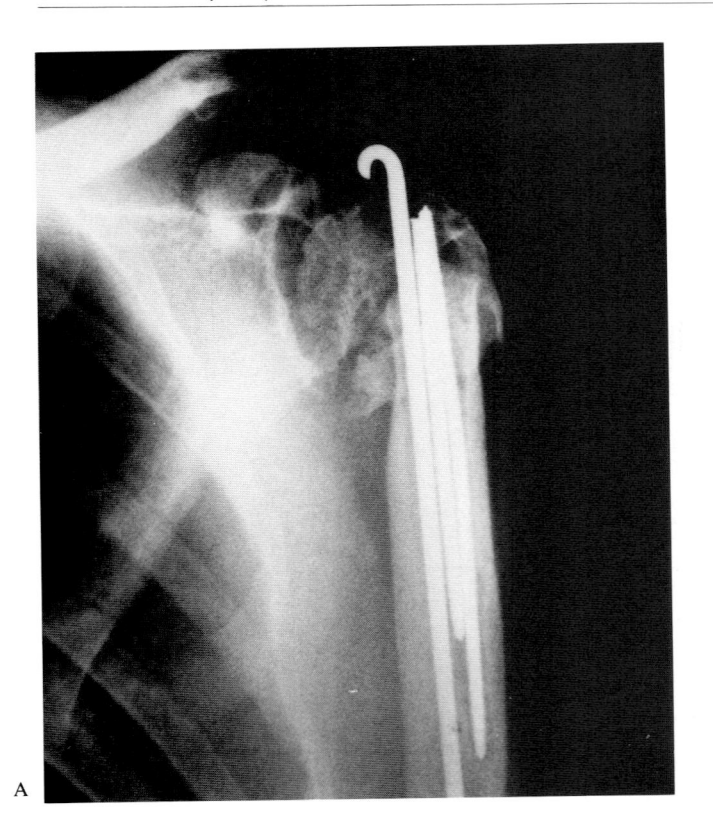

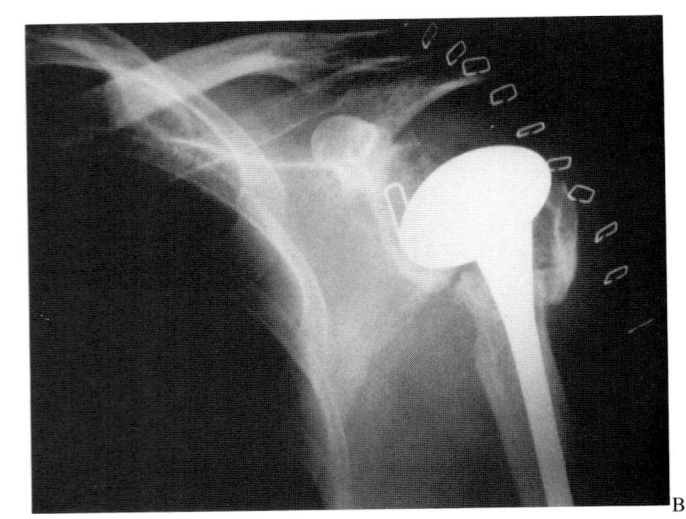

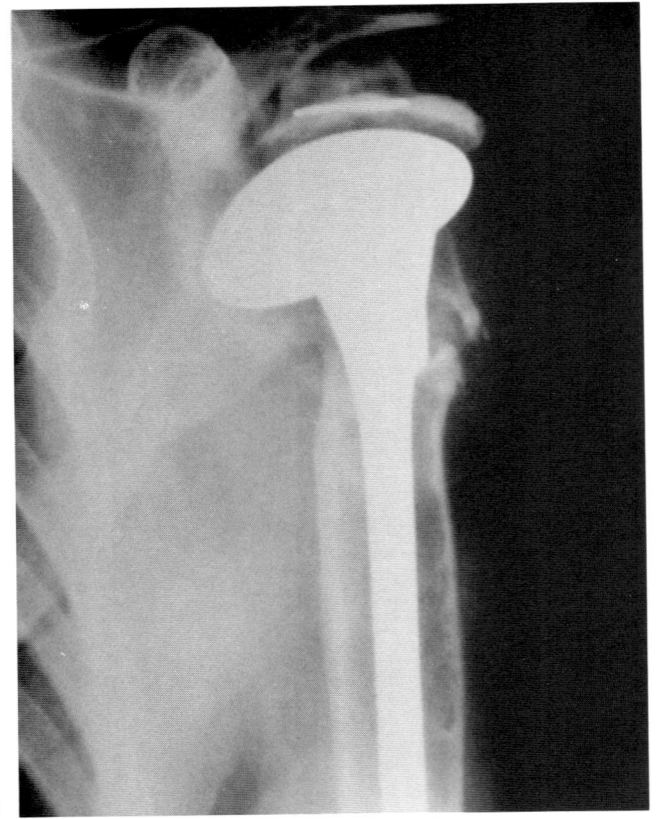

Figure 3–8. **A.** An elderly woman had an open reduction and internal fixation of a surgical neck fracture. The humeral head became necrotic and the shoulder markedly painful. Note the rush rod and threaded pins through the head and into the shaft. The joint showed severe evidence of posttraumatic arthritis. **B.** A total shoulder arthroplasty was performed because the joint was severely degenerated. The rotator cuff showed extensive tearing and attenuation of the tissues, indicating a severe rotator cuff tear arthropathy. The remaining portion of the greater tuberosity was grafted to the shaft. **C.** One year later, note the superior dislocation of the glenoid prosthetic component, most likely due to a rocker-bottom effect. Eventually, the components were removed, with relief of pain. The shoulder was flail.

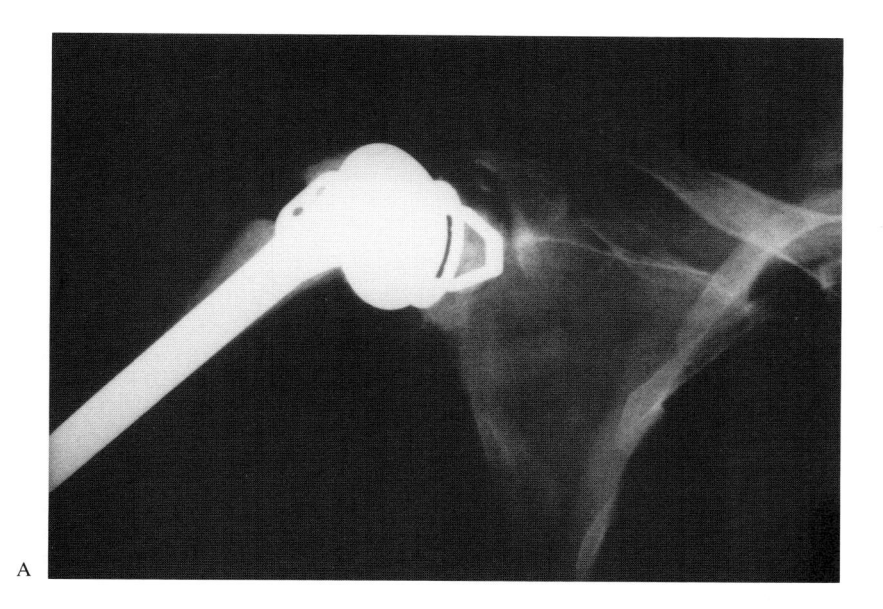

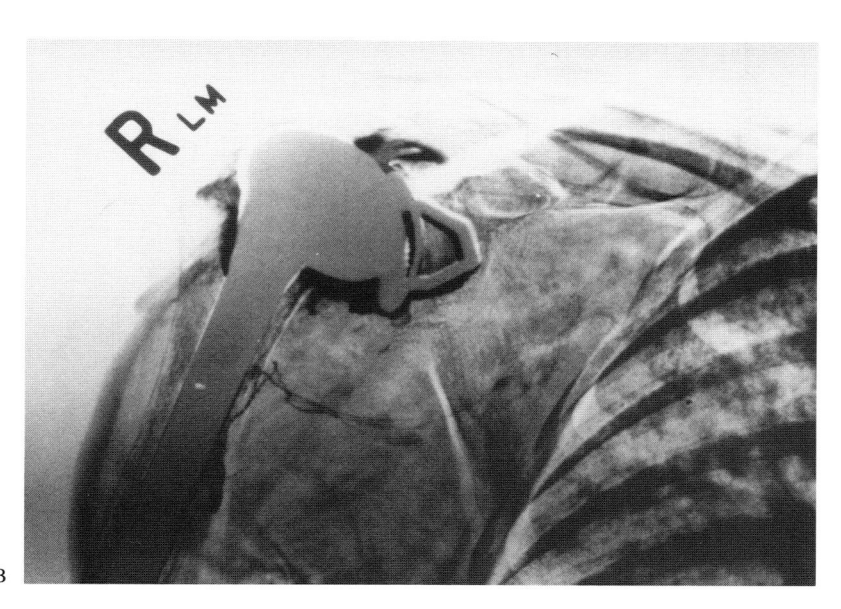

Figure 3–9. A. Aged adult was referred because of persistent severe pain in the shoulder that had a Neer II prosthesis. A computerized tomographic scan and plain films of the right shoulder showed no abnormalities. **B.** Negative subtraction studies showed loose prosthetic components with movement of the glenoid that was infected. The components were removed and the pain and infection subsided.

present. Complications of shoulder arthroplasty surgery leading to failure can be avoided with proper patient selection, good surgical technique, and the correct choice of prosthetic devices. Instability may be avoided if proper tension is placed on the rotator cuff tissues and contractures are released. Rotator cuff tears must be repaired if possible. However, it should be recognized that later degeneration of the rotator cuff can occur, especially in one that is already diseased. Tuberosity nonunions and malunions must be corrected. If nerve injury is present, optimum function may not be achieved. Infection must be eradicated and avoided. Postoperative follow-up examinations are necessary on a regular basis to follow the patient's progress.

REFERENCES

1. Post M. Physical examination of the shoulder girdle. In: Post M, ed. *Physical Examination of the Musculoskeletal System*. Philadelphia: Lea & Febiger, 1987:13–55.
2. Post M. Shoulder arthroplasty and total shoulder replacement. In: Post M, ed. *The Shoulder*. Philadelphia: Lea & Febiger, 1988:221–278.
3. Cofield RH, Briggs BT. Glenohumeral arthritis. *J Bone Joint Surg [Am]* 1979;61:668–677.
4. Halverson PB, Cheung HS, McCarty DJ. Enzymatic release of microspheroids containing hydroxyapatite crystals from synovium and of calcium pyrophosphate dihydrate crystals from cartilage. *Ann Rheum Dis* 1982;41:527–531.

5. Neer CS II, Craig EV, Fukuda H. Cuff-tear arthropathy. *J Bone Joint Surg [Am]* 1983;65:1232–1244.
6. Neer CS II, Kirby RM. Revision of the humeral head and total shoulder arthroplasties. *Clin Orthop* 1982;170:189–195.
7. Neer CS II, Watson KC, Stanton FJ. Recent experience in total shoulder replacement. *J Bone Joint Surg [Am]* 1982;64:319–337.
8. Post M. Constrained arthroplasty of the shoulder. *Orthop Clin North Am* 1987;18:455–462.
9. Cofield RH. Total shoulder arthroplasty with the Neer prosthesis. *J Bone Joint Surg [Am]* 1984;66:899–906.
10. Neer CS II. Replacement arthroplasty for glenohumeral osteoarthritis. *J Bone Joint Surg [Am]* 1974;56:1–13.
11. Neer CS, Morrison DS. Glenoid bone-grafting in total shoulder arthroplasty. *J Bone Joint Surg [Am]* 1988;70:1154–1162.
12. Post M, Jablon M, Miller H, Singh M. Constrained total shoulder joint replacement: A critical review. *Clin Orthop* 1979;144:135–150.
13. Post M. Forces in the shoulder (letter of reply to the editor). *Clin Orthop* 1988;231:308–310.
14. Cofield RH. Total shoulder arthroplasty: Associated disease of the rotator cuff, results and complications. In: Bateman JE, Welsh RP, eds. *Surgery of the Shoulder.* St. Louis: CV Mosby, 1984:229–233.
15. Franklin JL, Barrett WP, Jackins SE, Matsen FA III. Glenoid loosening in total shoulder arthroplasty. *J Arthroplasty* 1988;3:39–46.
16. Post M, Haskell SS, Jablon M. Total shoulder replacement with a constrained prosthesis. *J Bone Joint Surg [Am]* 1980;62:327–335.
17. Bayley JIL, Kessel L. The Kessel total shoulder replacement. In: Bayley I, Kessel L, eds. *Shoulder Surgery.* New York: Springer-Verlag, 1982:160–164.
18. Coughlin JH, Morris MH, West WF. The semiconstrained total shoulder arthroplasty. *J Bone Joint Surg [Am]* 1979;61:574–581.
19. Cofield RH. Status of total shoulder arthroplasty. *Arch Surg* 1977;112:1088–1091.
20. Fenlin JM Jr. Total glenohumeral joint replacement. *Orthop Clin North Am* 1975;6:565–583.
21. Gristina AG, Webb LX. The trispherical total shoulder replacement. In: Bayley I, Kessel L, eds. *Shoulder Surgery.* New York: Springer-Verlag, 1982:153–157.
22. Gristina AG, Webb LX, Carter RE. The monospherical total shoulder. *Orthop Trans* 1985;9:54.
23. Kölbel R, Friedeboldl G. Schultergelenkersatz. *Z Orthop* 1975;113:452–454.
24. Neer CS II. Articular replacement for the humeral head. *J Bone Joint Surg [Am]* 1955;37:215–228.
26. Lettin AWF, Copeland SA, Scales JT. The Stanmore total shoulder replacement. *J Bone Joint Surg [Br]* 1982;64:47–51.
25. Cofield RH. Unconstrained total shoulder prosthesis. *Clin Orthop* 1983;173:97–108.
27. Barrett WP, Franklin JL, Jackins SE, et al.: Total shoulder arthroplasty. *J Bone Joint Surg [Am]* 1987;69:865–872.
28. Friedman RJ. Glenohumeral translation following total shoulder arthroplasty. *J Shoulder Elbow Surg* 1992;1:312–316.
29. Neer CS, Brown TH Jr, McLaughlin HL. Fracture of the neck of the humerus with dislocation of the head fragment. *Am J Surg* 1955;85:252–258.
30. Neer CS II. Followup notes on articles previously published in the journal. Articular replacement for the humeral head. *J Bone Joint Surg [Am]* 1964;46:1607–1610.
31. McCarty DJ, Halverson PB, Carrera GF, et al. "Milwaukee shoulder"—Association of microspheroids containing hydroxyapatite crystals, active collagenase, and neutral protease with rotator cuff defects. I. Clinical aspects. *Arthritis Rheum* 1981;24:464–473.
32. McCarty D. Crystals, joints, and consternation. *Ann Rheum Dis* 1983;42:243–253.
33. Samilson RL, Prieto V. Dislocation arthropathy of the shoulder. *J Bone Joint Surg [Am]* 1983;65:456–460.
34. Huston KA, Nelson AM, Hunder GG. Shoulder swelling in the rheumatoid arthritis secondary to subacromial bursitis. *Arthritis Rheum* 1978;21:145–147.
35. Zuckerman JD, Matsen FA III. Complications about the glenohumeral joint related to the use of screws and staples. *J Bone Joint Surg [Am]* 1984;66:175–180.
36. Figgie HE III, Inglis AE, Goldberg VM, et al: An analysis of factors affecting the long-term results of total shoulder arthroplasty in inflammatory arthritis. *J Arthroplasty* 1988;3:123–130.
37. Halverson PB, Cheung HS, McCarty DJ, et al. "Milwaukee shoulder"—Association of microspheroids containing hydroxyapatite crystals, active collagenase, and neutral protease with rotator cuff defects. II. Synovial fluid studies. *Arthritis Rheum* 1981;24:474–483.
38. Halverson PB, Garancis MC, McCarty DJ. Histopathological and ultrastructural studies of synovium in Milwaukee shoulder syndrome—A basic calcium phosphate crystal arthropathy. *Ann Rheum Dis* 1984;43:734–741.
39. Tanner MW, Cofield RH. Prosthetic arthroplasty for fractures and fracture-dislocations of the proximal humerus. *Clin Orthop* 1983;179:116–128.
40. Leslie BM, Harris JM, Driscoll D. Septic arthritis of the shoulder in adults. *J Bone Joint Surg [Am]* 1989;71:1516–1522.

4 Radiology of Total Shoulder Arthroplasty

Piran Aliabadi, M.D., and Barbara N. Weissman, M.D.

PREOPERATIVE PLANNING

Normal Examinations

RADIOGRAPHS AND COMPUTERIZED TOMOGRAPHY

Routine preoperative evaluation should consist of an anteroposterior (AP) view of the shoulder with the arm in internal rotation, and a 40-degree posterior oblique AP view with the humerus externally rotated.[1] An additional axillary view may be obtained for evaluation of bone stock but computerized tomography (CT) is often superior for this purpose[2] (Figure 4–1).

Radiographs obtained with the humerus in internal rotation show the rounded contour of the humeral head, whereas external rotation views show the greater tuberosity in profile. While a true AP view of the shoulder does not show the glenohumeral joint in profile, the posterior oblique view does, allowing the width of the cartilage space to be optimally studied. The normal appearances on the axillary view are shown in Figure 4–1.

CT scanning is helpful in the preoperative assessment of the shoulder, particularly for the evaluation of bone stock. The technique has the advantage of allowing imaging in the axial plane and providing excellent spatial resolution and soft-tissue contrast. Cortical outlines are better shown on CT scans than on magnetic resonance (MR) scans. A normal-appearing CT scan of the shoulder is shown in Figure 4–2.

Anatomic Relationships—Humeral Retroversion. Saha emphasized that in humans, the head, neck, and upper part of the humeral shaft are deviated posteromedially on the humeral axis (torsion).[3] Axial views of the shoulder that include the distal part of the humerus (the method of Mukherjee-Sivaya) allow measurement of this inclination (Figure 4–3).[3] Saha noted this angle to average 30 degrees of retroversion.

Glenohumeral anatomy is well demonstrated in the axial plane on CT. Humeral torsion can be assessed by relating the axis of the humeral head on proximal CT sections to the axis of the humeral articular surface on distal sections. The exact methods of obtaining these measurements vary. Hill et al.[4] obtained three to six axial sections through the glenohumeral joint at 5- to 10-mm intervals and several sections through the capitellum and trochlea. The axis of the humeral articular surface was determined by drawing a concentric circle around the radius of the humeral head. Two points were marked on this circle at 90 degrees to the articular margin. A line drawn between these two points and a perpendicular line to this indicated the humeral head axis (Figure 4–4). The difference between this axis and a line parallel to the distal articular surface represents the degree of humeral torsion. Normal individuals displayed retroversion averaging 30 degrees. Similar values were found on CT study by Randelli and Gambrioli.[5]

Anatomic Relationships—Glenoid Tilt. The glenoid tilt in both AP and superior-inferior planes can be assessed on radiographs or on CT scans (Figure 4–5). AP tilt may be evaluated on the axillary radiograph. The plane of the glenoid (drawn from the most anterior to the most posterior points of the glenoid) and the axis of the scapula (drawn from the midpoint of the glenoid line to the junction of the base of the spine) and the vertebral border are constructed.[3] The angle is read on the acromial side of the scapular axis. Nomenclature is confusing, although retroversion angles are usually referred to as negative and anteversion angles as positive. Saha[3] noted the angle of glenoid tilt to average 7.4 degrees of retroversion in almost three-fourths of subjects while slightly more than one-fourth had anterior tilt of 2 to 10 degrees. Similarly, specimen axillary radiography has shown the tilt of the glenoid (glenoid version) to range from +7 (anteversion) to −12 degrees (retroversion), with an average measurement of −2 degrees.[6]

Similarly, the angular tilt of the glenoid may be measured from axial CT scans. A line is constructed from the medial border of the scapula, distal to the intersection of the spine and the body, to the midpoint of the glenoid (Figure 4–5). The angle between a parallel to the glenoid surface and this scapular baseline indicates the tilt of the glenoid. Glenoid tilt on CT scans has been found to vary from superior to inferior,[5] displaying greater retroversion superiorly (superior retroversion averaging 14 degrees, inferior retroversion averaging 1 degree).[4] Mallon et al.[6] found the angle between the scapular blade and the glenoid fossa on pneumoarthrograms to average −6 degrees of retroversion (range, +2 to −13 degrees).

MAGNETIC RESONANCE IMAGING OF THE SHOULDER

Evaluation of the rotator cuff is done by the authors, when necessary, with MR imaging, less often with arthrography, and least often with ultrasonography.[7–15] MR imaging has the advantages of evaluation without ionizing radiation, imaging in any plane, high-spatial resolution, and excellent depiction of soft-tissue structures. Usually, imaging of the

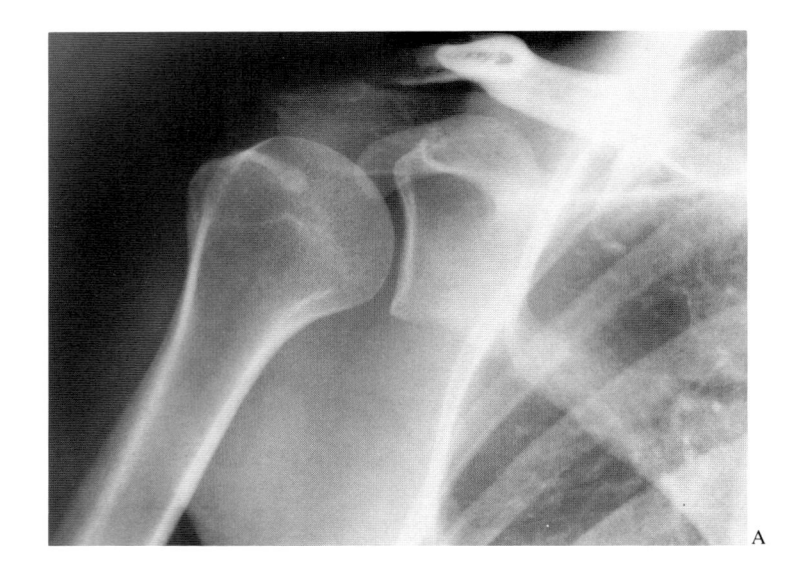

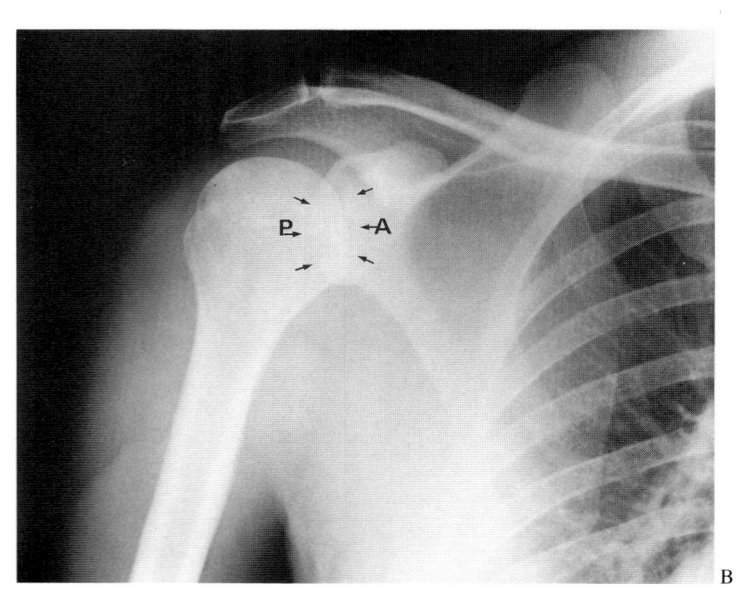

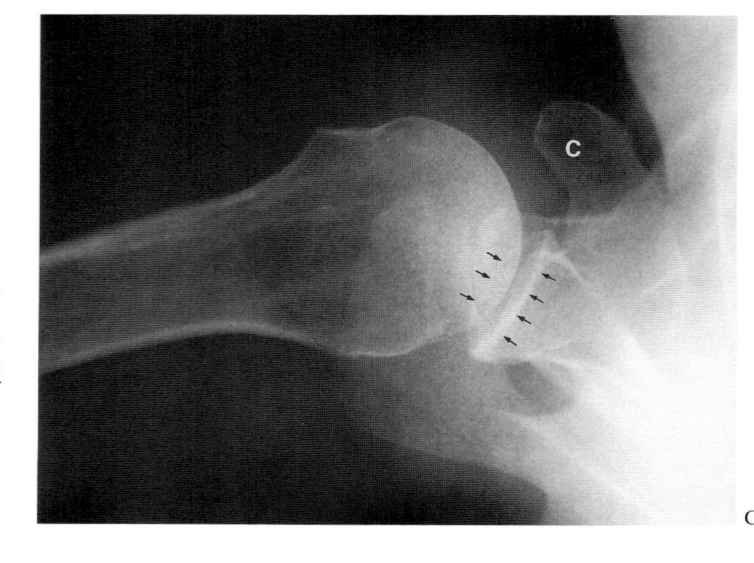

Figure 4–1. Normal radiographic appearance. **A.** The posterior oblique, external rotation view shows the thickness of the glenohumeral cartilage space. The greater tuberosity is seen in profile. The density in the humeral head is a bone island. **B.** The internal rotation view shows the round contour of the humeral head. It is wise to usually include the apex of the lung in this view for evaluation. The anterior (A) and posterior (P) glenoid rims are shown. **C.** The normal axillary view. The arrows indicate the glenoid. C = coracoid.

become very bright on T2-weighted images. The findings are thought to reflect edema and inflammation within the tendon.[7] Partial-thickness tears may be difficult or impossible to distinguish from tendinitis.

IMAGING FOLLOWING TOTAL SHOULDER ARTHROPLASTY

Normal Radiographic Appearances

Three general types of total shoulder arthroplasties are available, constrained, semiconstrained, and nonconstrained[21-23,25-35] (Figure 4-11). Posterior oblique AP radiographs of the shoulder with the humerus externally rotated usually provide a profile view of both components and the joint space and are often the most helpful postoperative radiographs. An internal rotation view usually completes the evaluation. An axillary view provides additional information about the humeral and glenoid components. Radiographs are performed immediately postoperatively, before discharge from the hospital, at 3 weeks, at 6 months, and then annually.[25]

Evaluation of the nonconstrained Neer prosthesis[25] in the posterior oblique projection usually shows the inferior edge of the humeral component to be aligned with the inferior margin of the glenoid. The inferior surface of the head of the prosthesis parallels the cut surface of the neck and the lateral keel is seated in cancellous bone. The superior margin of the prosthetic humeral head should be higher than the greater tuberosity.[35]

MEASURING POSITION

Facing Angle. The facing angle of the glenoid component (Figure 4-12) is the angle between the longitudinal axis of the glenoid and the medial border of the scapula. Closed angles, with the glenoid tilted downward, have been thought to lessen upward subluxation.[23]

Retroversion. Twenty to 40 degrees of humeral component retroversion is usually recommended.[36,37] Ovesen and Nielsen[36] found that in a cadaver model, retroversion of less than 35 degrees was accompanied by limitation of external rotation. Humeral component retroversion explains the observation that radiographs taken with the humerus externally rotated often show the humeral component in profile. The retroversion of the humeral component can be measured directly on the Mukherjee-Sivaya view[3,36] (see Figure 4-3).

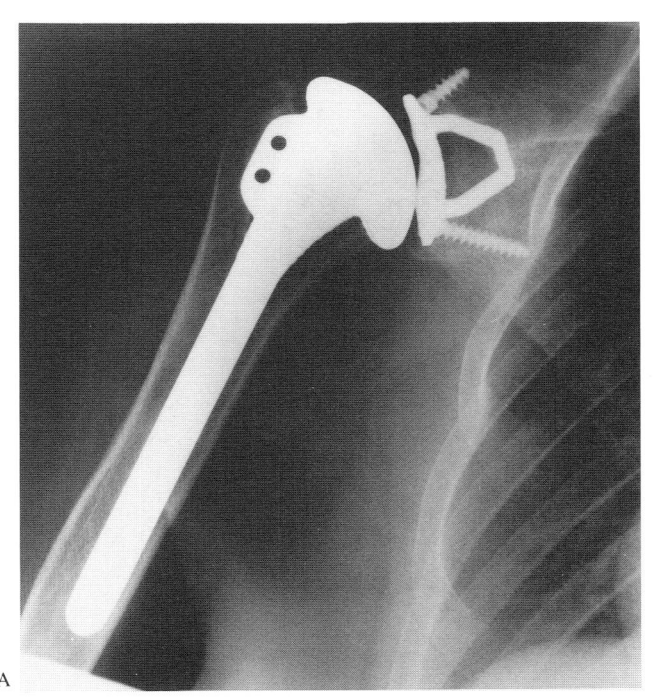

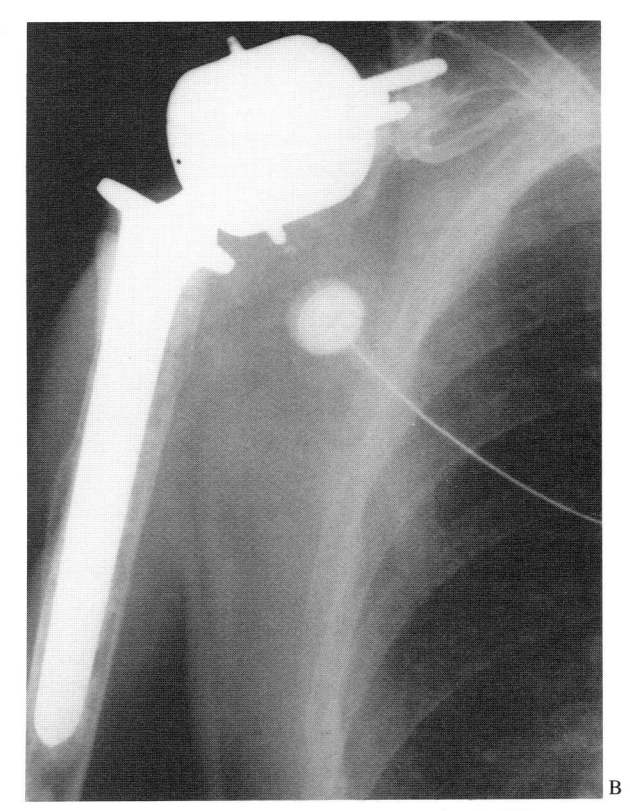

Figure 4-11. Normal radiographic appearances. **A.** Uncomplicated bone-ingrowth nonconstrained prosthesis. The posterior oblique, external rotation view of the shoulder shows the glenohumeral joint nearly in profile and the humeral component in profile. There are no lucencies along the prosthesis-bone interface. The inferior aspect of the humeral component is roughly aligned to the inferior aspect of the glenoid component. **B.** Uncomplicated cemented constrained prosthesis.

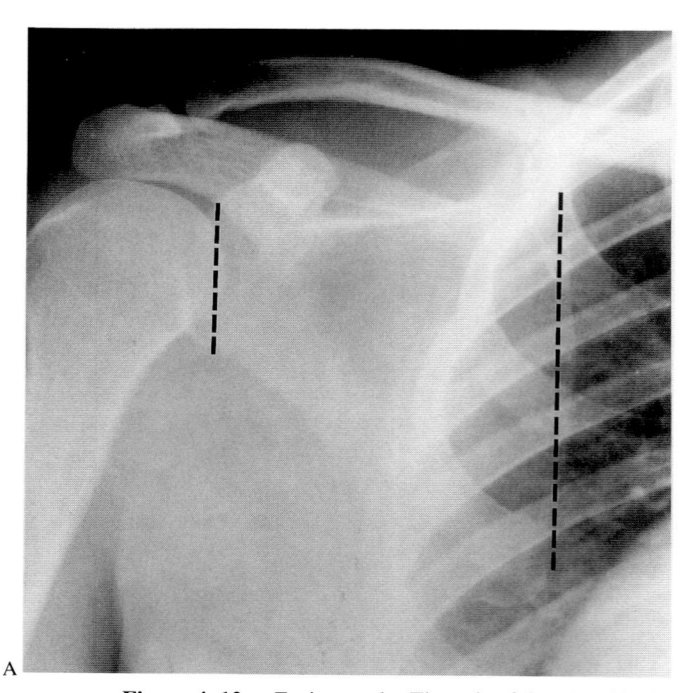

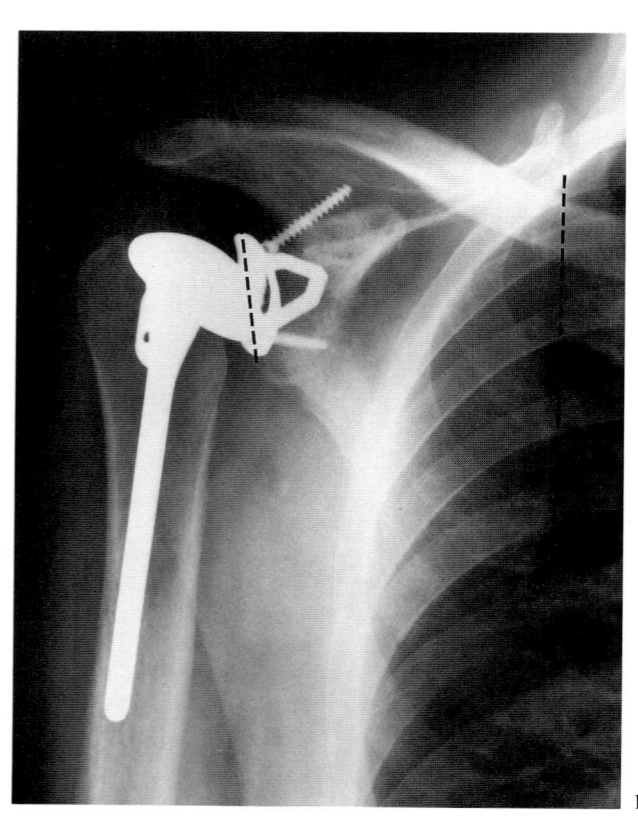

Figure 4–12. Facing angle. The axis of the glenoid with relation to the medial part of the scapula is shown in a normal shoulder (**A**) and a prosthetic shoulder (**B**).

Since this view is not usually available, Frich and Moller[38] determined retroversion from the AP projection of the shoulder obtained with the forearm in 35 degrees of internal rotation (Figure 4–13). In this view, retroversion of the prosthetic humeral head can be determined by the formula $d = \cos^{-1}(tg\ p/tg\ a)$, where d is the true angle of retroversion, a the apparent retroversion angle on the internal rotation view, and p the angle between the head and stem of the prosthesis (50 degrees for the Neer prosthesis). For simplification, the measurement may be compared to a prepared table of calculated values. In addition, an estimation of the retroversion angle can be done by subtracting 40 degrees from the measured angle (a) on the 35-degree internal rotation radiograph. For all but extreme measurements, the error of this estimation is, at most, 5 degrees.

BONE-CEMENT INTERFACE

When both components are cemented, bone-cement lucencies more commonly develop on the glenoid than on the humeral side of the joint. Glenoid bone-cement lucencies are frequent even when nonconstrained prostheses are used. Cofield,[22] for example, found some lucency at the bone-cement interface of the glenoid component in 52 of 65 Neer prostheses that were not loose. Eight additional glenoid components were loose. As in total hip arthroplasty the lucent zone usually measures less than 2 mm in thickness in

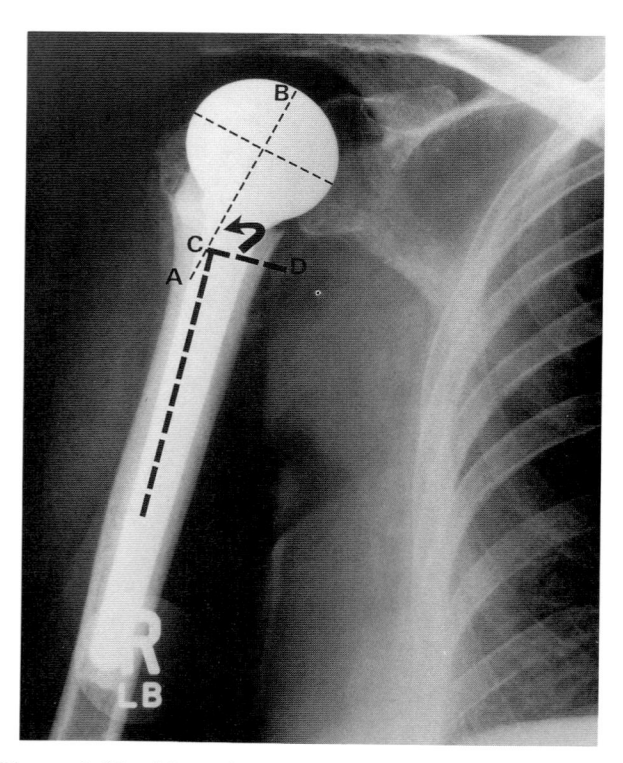

Figure 4–13. Measuring retroversion from 35-degree internal oblique view. The angle between a perpendicular to the humeral head ellipse (AB) and a perpendicular to the humeral shaft axis (CD) is measured and compared to values in a standard table.

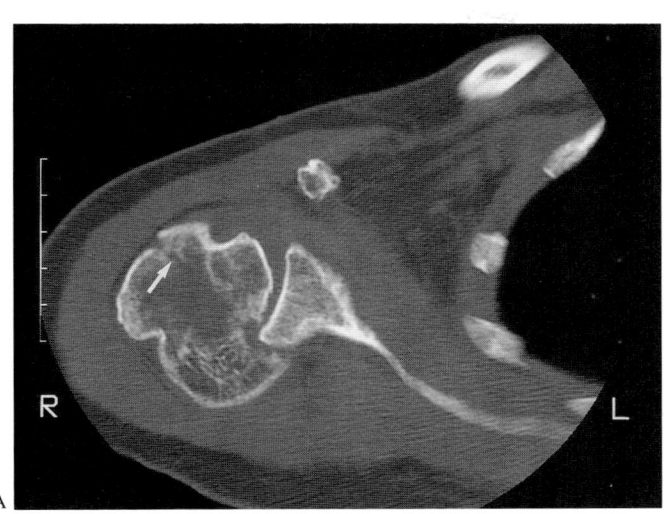

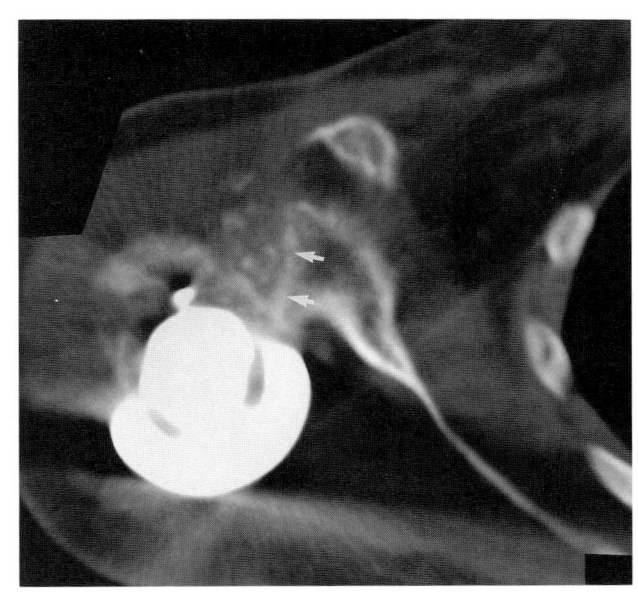

Figure 4–14. Posterior dislocation. **A.** Computerized tomographic scan through the shoulder shows posterior dislocation of the humeral head with impingement on the posterior lip of the glenoid. The fracture line extends to the greater tuberosity (arrow). **B.** Subsequent computerized tomographic scan through the head of the prosthesis confirms posterior dislocation of the humeral component with impingement on the posterior lip of the glenoid (arrows). Small bony fragments are noted in the region.

uncomplicated cases and is made apparent by a thin adjacent zone of sclerosis.

UNCEMENTED COMPONENTS

Remodeling may occur around bone-ingrowth components reflecting altered stress. Bone resorption reflects areas of decreased stress, and new bone production reflects areas of increased stress. McElwain and English[30] noted resorption of the proximal humeral cortex (9 patients), cancellous new bone formation (7 patients), and proximal humeral remodeling (5 patients) in a series of 13 arthroplasties using bone-ingrowth semiconstrained total shoulder prostheses.

Computerized Tomography

Beam-hardening artifact from metal prostheses may interfere with bone and soft-tissue details. Usually, however, the examination suffices for determination of alignment (Figure 4–14) and often for more detailed study. Egund et al.,[39] for example, have used CT (with reconstruction of the obtained information and the high-frequency filter) to evaluate the bone-cement interface inside humeral head cup arthroplasties. This region could not be demonstrated on standard radiographic examination.

Complications

SUBLUXATION/DISLOCATION

Dislocation may occur early or late in the postoperative course. Six cases of dislocation occurred in one series of 98 arthroplasties using nonconstrained total shoulder prostheses: three anterior, one posterior, and two superior.[25] Four occurred within the first 4 months postoperatively (Figures 4–14, 4–15, and 4–16).

Proximal migration of the humerus after total shoulder arthroplasty has been associated with rotator cuff tear, inadequate or failed cuff repair, impingement syndrome, painful shoulder, and a poor result.[27] The abnormally high humeral position has been thought to lead to abnormal motion and glenoid loosening. Boyd et al.,[27] however, found no significant relationship between the presence of proximal

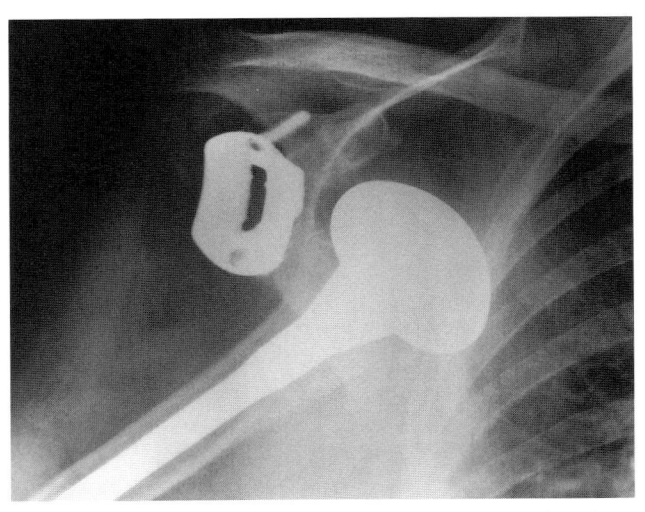

Figure 4–15. Anterior dislocation. The frontal projection shows medial (and anterior) dislocation of the humeral component with relation to the glenoid.

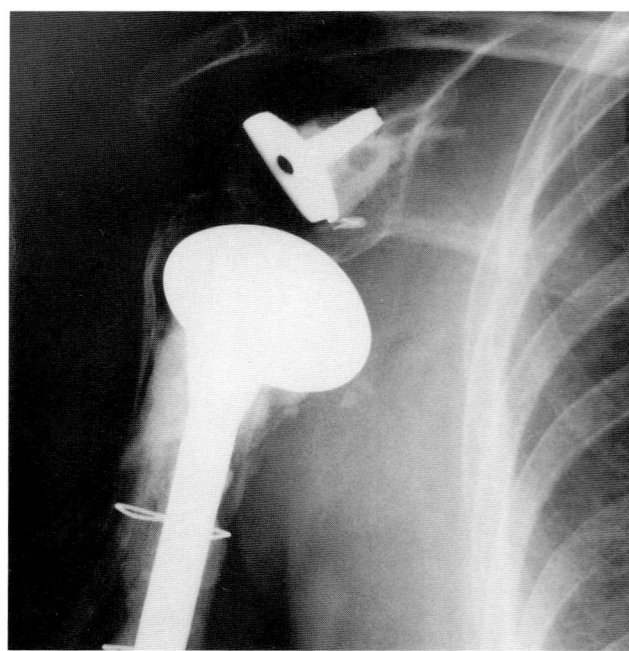

Figure 4-16. Inferior humeral subluxation. This revised total shoulder arthroplasty demonstrates inferior displacement of the humeral component. The glenoid component is tilted inferiorly. Humeral length was decreased.

humeral migration and the presence of major rotator cuff tears, pain relief, or glenoid loosening. Thornhill et al.[23] found proximal subluxation to be more frequent when the postoperative glenoid facing angle significantly exceeded neutral abduction.

While there are no exact measurements used to determine the presence of proximal migration, serial evaluation of the relationship of the inferior edge of the humeral component to that of the glenoid component or evaluation of the decreasing distance between the undersurface of the acromion and the humeral component on AP radiographs usually allows adequate assessment. Boyd et al.[27] recorded proximal migration as present when the humeral head was superior to the center of rotation of the glenoid (Figures 4-17 and 4-18). In that series, 29 (22%) of 131 Neer total shoulder replacements exhibited this finding.

LOOSENING

Loosening requiring revision is more common on the glenoid than the humeral side. For example, Boyd et al.[27] reviewed 131 Neer total shoulder arthroplasties and found radiographic evidence of loosening in 12% of cemented glenoid components and 4% of uncemented humeral components. Similarly, Cofield[22] followed 73 Neer total shoulder arthroplasties and found loosening of the glenoid component in 8 cases (documented in 7 by a change in component position); no loosening of humeral components was identified. Neer et al.,[21] however, found radiologic evidence of humeral loosening in 2 of 194 shoulders and no glenoid components were clinically or radiologically loose.

Theoretically, constrained prostheses place greater stress on the adjacent bone than do nonconstrained prostheses and, hence, are more likely to develop loosening. In a series of 100 constrained prostheses, radiolucencies of 1 to 2 mm developed around 50% of the stems, and 30% of the screws and central posts displayed 1-mm lucencies.[33] Only six posttraumatic cases of loosening occurred in the same series. Twenty-four– to 53-month follow-up of 16 semiconstrained Stanmore prostheses documented loosening of only 1 glenoid component.[28]

Radiographic Evidence of Loosening—Cemented Components. Lucent zones of 2 mm or more along the entire bone-cement interface or any lucent zone at the prosthesis-cement interface suggest loosening. These findings may or may not be associated with symptoms (Figure 4-19). Thus, of a series of 132 patients with nonconstrained prostheses or hemiarthroplasty, 6 patients developed lucencies that increased to greater than 2 mm in width along portions of the glenoid component, but only 3 required revision during the 6- to 73-month follow-up period.[29]

Changes in component position indicate loosening (Figure 4-20). A loose glenoid component may become displaced into the joint (Figure 4-21). Sinking of the humeral component into the humeral shaft has been noted to occur in 5% of uncemented, press-fit Neer humeral components.[27] This assessment may be difficult but is facilitated in the Neer system by noting the relative positions of the proximal lateral keel of the prosthesis to the greater tuberosity on serial radiographs (see Figure 4-18).

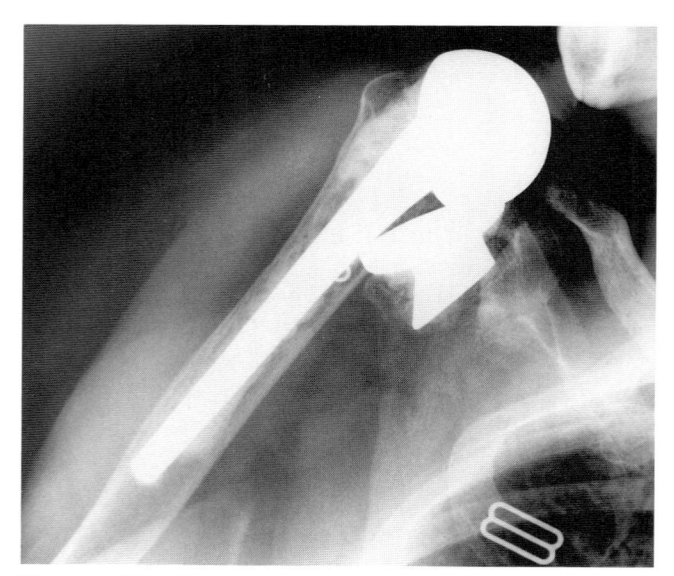

Figure 4-17. Severe upward subluxation of a nonconstrained prosthesis. There is marked elevation of the humeral component of this monospherical cemented prosthesis.

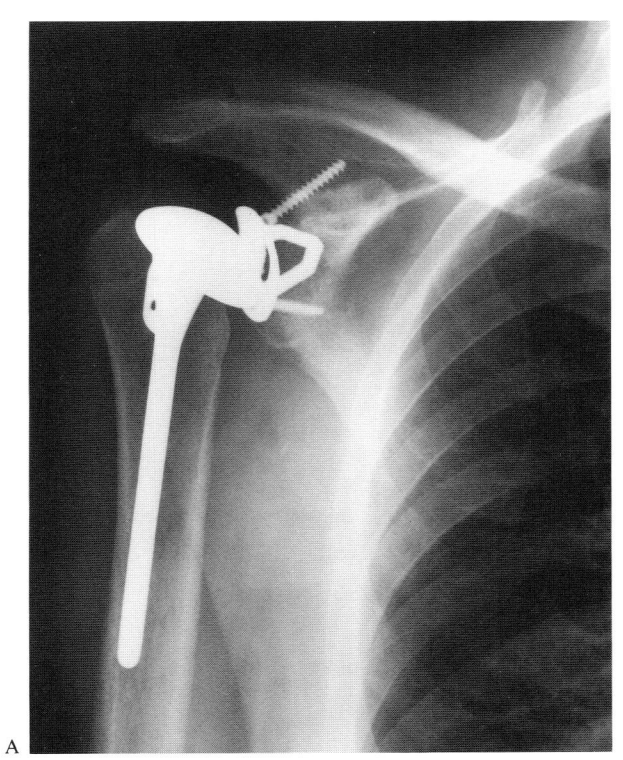

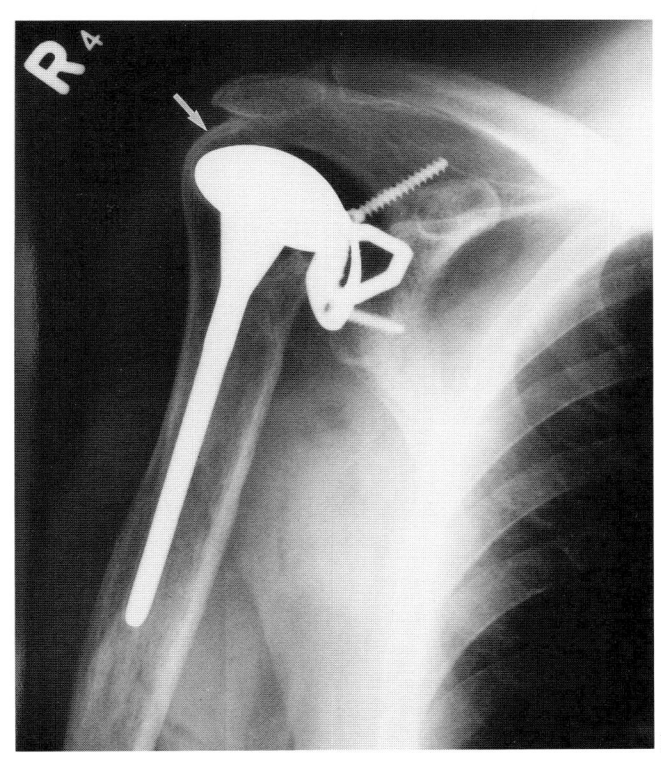

Figure 4–18. Upward subluxation and humeral component subsidence. **A.** Bone-ingrowth glenoid and press-fit humeral components are present without subluxation. **B.** Subsidence of the humeral component into the humerus as indicated by the remodeling of the greater tuberosity (arrow). Upward subluxation of the humeral component with relation to the glenoid is also noted.

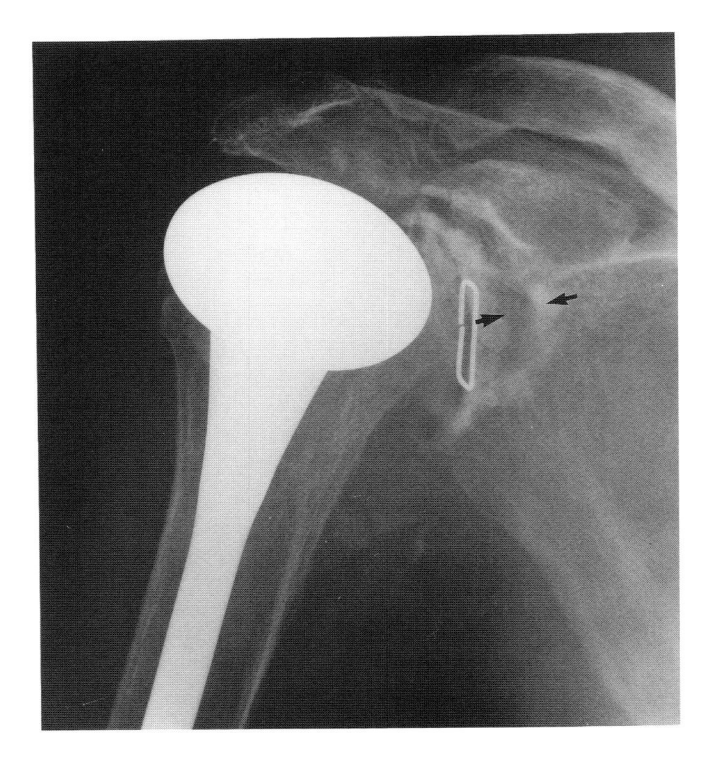

Figure 4–19. Glenoid component loosening. The internal rotation anteroposterior view shows a wide cement-bone interface with the glenoid component (arrows). This finding is indicative of component loosening.

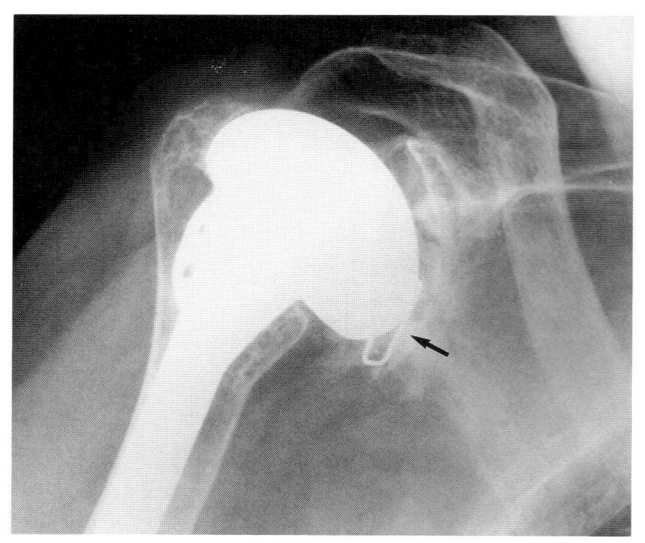

Figure 4–20. Glenoid displacement. The anteroposterior external rotation radiograph shows the low position of the glenoid (arrow). This had changed from postoperative examinations.

Radiographic Evidence of Loosening—Bone-Ingrowth Prostheses. If the findings in total shoulder prostheses are analogous to those of total hip prostheses, then loosening is suggested by a 2-mm or wider lucent zone between the prosthesis and the bone, particularly if this is progressive.[40–42] This lucency is delimited by a thin line of sclerosis. Thin lucencies that do not progress after 2 years suggest the formation of a stable fibrous tissue interface.[43]

Progressive or marked subsidence of components indicates loosening[41] and provided the best correlation with clinical outcome in a series of porous coated hip prostheses followed for an average of 32 months. Increasing numbers of displaced beads from the bone-ingrowth surface indicate component motion.[41] Changes in component position or lucencies of 2 mm or more along the prosthesis-bone interface indicate loosening[42] (Figure 4–22). Although arthrography is often used for the evaluation of loosening of a total hip replacement, the technique is rarely used for the assessment of total shoulder arthroplasty.

INFECTION

Infection following total shoulder arthroplasty is rare and in one series of 98 shoulders with nonconstrained prostheses, no cases of infection were reported.[25] Infection is suggested radiographically by the presence of poorly defined areas of bone destruction, periosteal reaction, or wide bone-cement or prosthesis-bone lucent zones. Lucent zones usually display an adjacent sclerotic line, but when infection is present, this line may be eroded. Infection may, however, be present without any abnormal radiographic findings. Scintigraphy has been used for the evaluation of loosening of and infection around total hip and total knee prostheses but is seldom utilized for the evaluation of total shoulder prostheses.

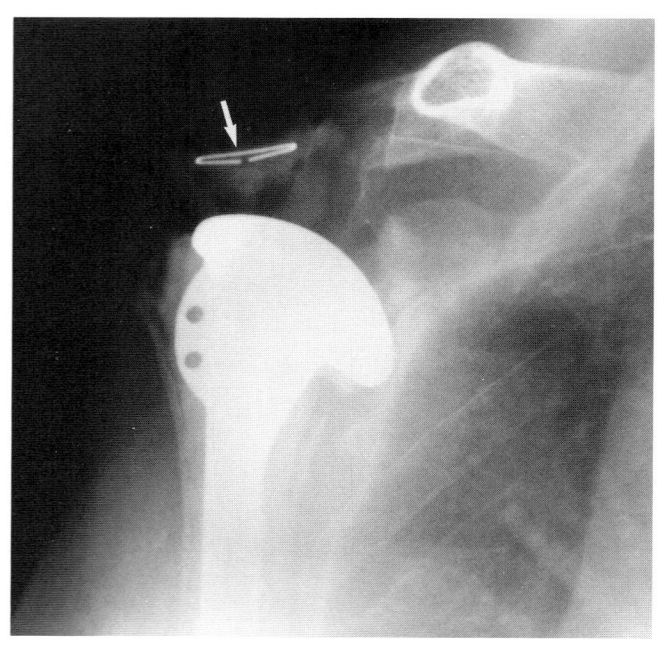

Figure 4–21. Displaced glenoid component. The anteroposterior projection shows displacement of the glenoid component (arrow) from the glenoid.

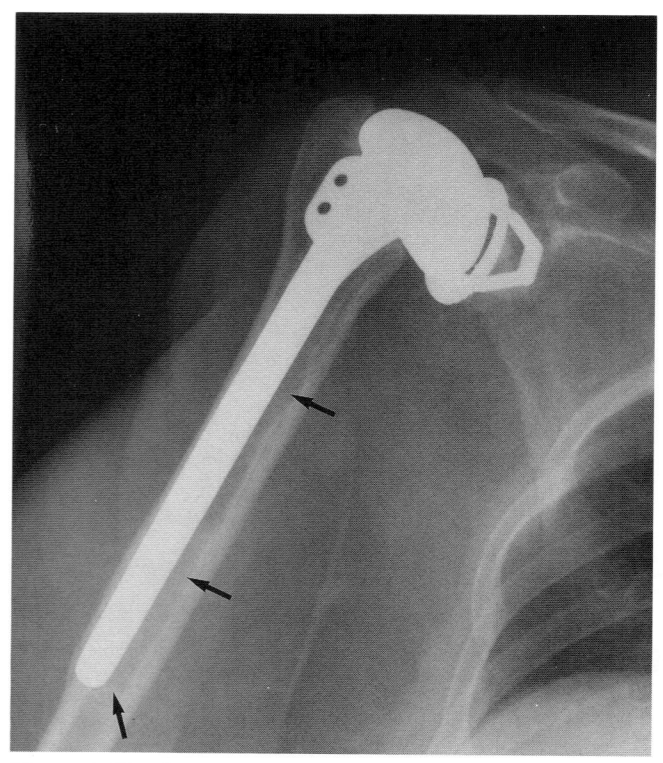

Figure 4–22. Loose uncemented humeral component. There is a wide lucency about the humeral stem and remodeling of the lateral humeral cortex, indicative of humeral component loosening (arrows). Only a thin lucency is present about the glenoid cement.

COMPONENT FRACTURE

Bending or breaking of prostheses has been reported and is more frequent in constrained prostheses.[32] Careful scrutiny of the components may be necessary to identify component bending or disruption (Figure 4–23).

DISSOCIATION OF COMPONENTS

Mechanical dissociation of a snap-fit glenoid liner has been reported.[44] The abnormal liner position was seen on radiographs by the change in position of the radiopaque glenoid marker. The lucency of the liner can often be seen if care is taken to obtain optimal radiographs for the purpose (Figure 4–23) or if arthrography is performed. Dissociation of modular humeral heads has also been reported and is usually evident on plain radiographs.

FRACTURE

Fractures may occur intraoperatively or postoperatively (Figure 4–24). Barrett et al.[45] reported one humeral shaft and one greater tuberosity fracture intraoperatively. A review by Thornhill and Barrett[35] revealed a 1.1% incidence of intraoperative or postoperative fractures in 540 shoulders that underwent Neer total shoulder arthroplasties.

HETEROTOPIC NEW BONE FORMATION

Six (6%) of 98 total shoulder prostheses in one series demonstrated heterotopic bone formation.[25] The clinical outcome was unaffected (Figure 4–25).

SUMMARY

Radiographic evaluation is an integral part of the preoperative workup and postoperative assessment of patients undergoing total shoulder arthroplasty. Utilization of newer imaging methods for postoperative evaluation is in its infancy. Analysis of standard radiographic studies with bone-ingrowth components and long-term series of cemented and press-fit components will help in understanding the roles of various imaging techniques.

Acknowledgment. The authors sincerely thank Mrs. Roberta Otis for her careful manuscript preparation and Mr. Robert Littlefield for his photographic expertise.

REFERENCES

1. Silvka J, Resnick D. An improved radiographic view of the glenohumeral joint. *J Can Assoc Radiol* 1979;30:83–85.

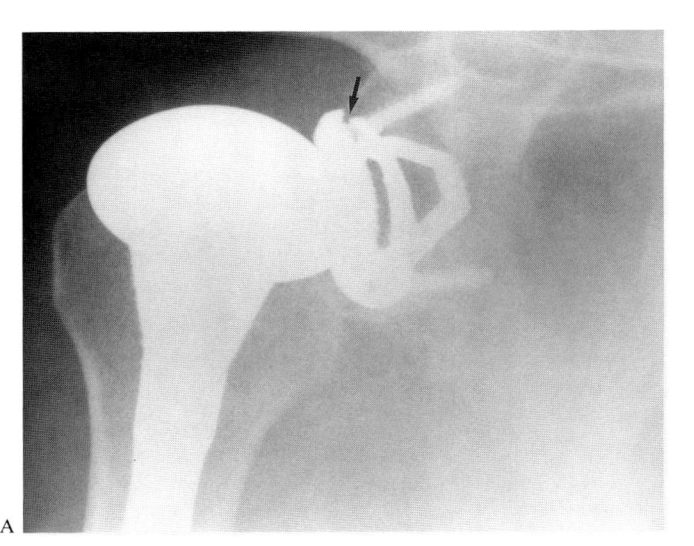

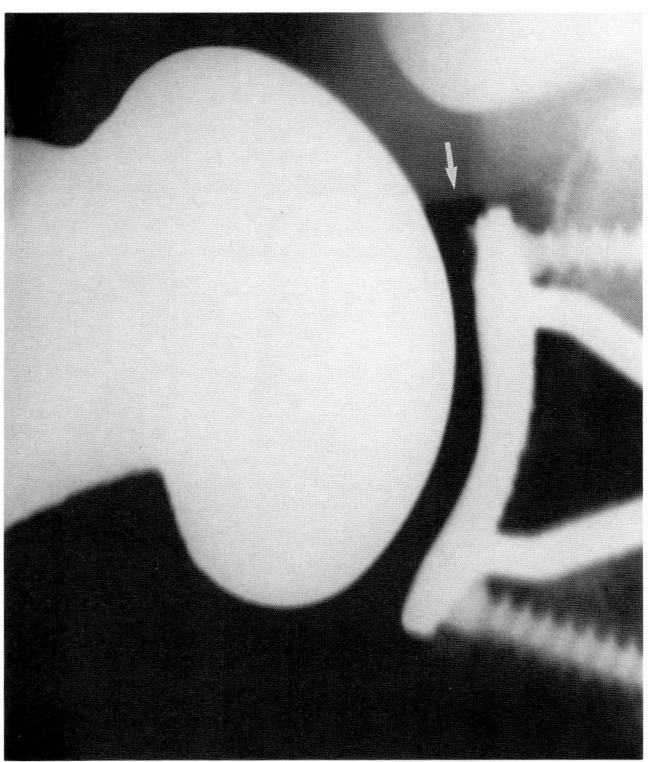

Figure 4–23. Glenoid component fracture. **A.** The anteroposterior, internal rotation view of a bone-ingrowth prosthesis shows disruption of the metal backing of the glenoid component in the region of the uppermost screw (arrow). **B.** A fluoroscopic spot film shows the low density of the polyethylene liner, which appears to be in position. The patient was asymptomatic.

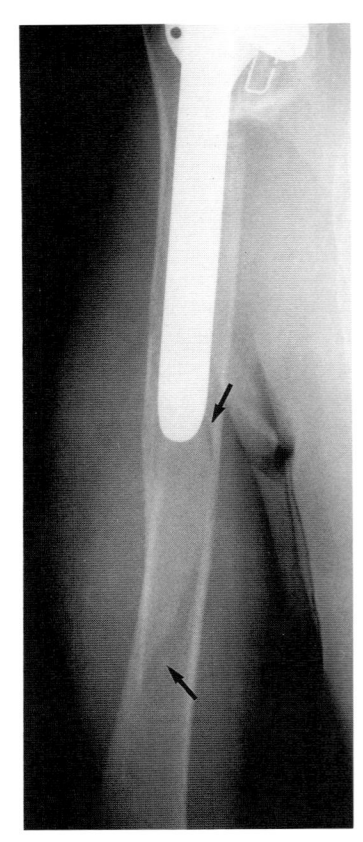

Figure 4–24. Humeral fracture. The anteroposterior, external rotation view shows a spiral fracture (arrows) beginning at the tip of the humeral component.

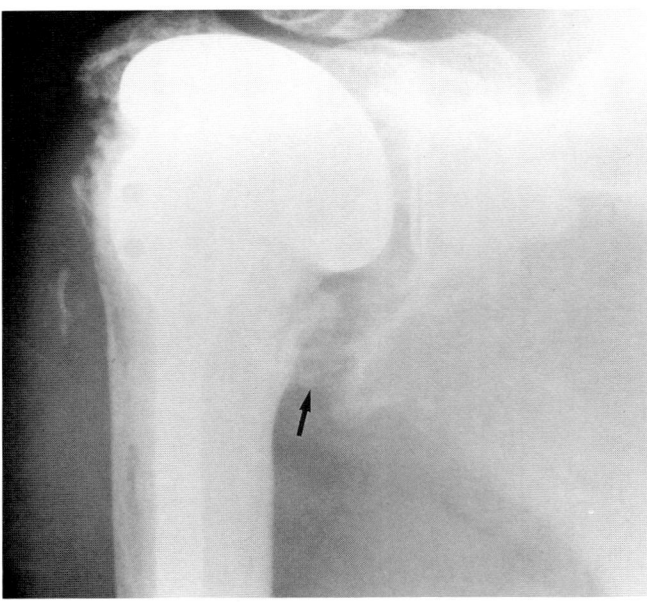

Figure 4–25. Heterotopic bone formation. The anteroposterior, external rotation radiograph shows the glenohumeral joint in profile. New bone (arrow) has developed along the inferior aspect of the joint and appears continuous with the humerus. There is apposition of the humeral head and the acromion, attesting to rotator cuff attrition.

2. DeSmet AA. Axillary projection in radiography of the nontraumatized shoulder. *Am J Radiol* 1980;134:511–514.
3. Saha AK. Dynamic stability of the glenohumeral joint. *Acta Orthop Scand* 1971;42:491–505.
4. Hill JA, Tkach L, Hendrix RW. A study of glenohumeral orientation in patients with anterior recurrent shoulder dislocations using computerized axial tomography. *Orthop Rev* 1989;18:84–91.
5. Randelli M, Gambrioli PL. Glenohumeral osteometry by computed tomography in normal and unstable shoulders. *Clin Orthop* 1986;208:151–156.
6. Mallon WJ, Brown HR, Vogler JB, Martinez S. Radiographic and geometric anatomy of the scapula. *Clin Orthop* 1992;277:142–154.
7. Boorstein JM, Kneeland JB, Dalinka MK, Iannotti JP, Suh JS. Magnetic resonance imaging of the shoulder. *Curr Prob Diagn Radiol* 1992;21:3–27.
8. DeKorvin LB, Ghossein IA, Kadouch R, Duvauferrier R. Value of modern imaging in the radioanatomical study of the shoulder. *Ann Radiol* 1989;32:234–243.
9. Nelson MC, Leather GP, Nirsch RP, Pettrone FA, Freedman MT. Evaluation of the painful shoulder. A prospective comparison of magnetic resonance imaging, computerized tomographic arthrography, ultrasonography, and operative findings. *J Bone Joint Surg [Am]* 1991;73:707–715.
10. Rafii M, Firooznia H, Sherman O, et al. Rotator cuff lesions: Signal patterns at MR imaging. *Radiology* 1990;177:817–823.
11. Zlatkin MB, Iannotti JP, Roberts MC, et al. Rotator cuff tears: Diagnostic performance of MR imaging. *Radiology* 1989;172:223–229.
12. Farin PU, Jaroma H, Harju A, Soimakallio S. Shoulder impingement syndrome: Sonographic evaluation. *Radiology* 1990;176:845–849.
13. Crass JR, Craig EV, Feinberg SB. Ultrasonography of rotator cuff tears: A review of 500 diagnostic studies. *J Clin Ultrasound* 1988;16:313–327.
14. Hodler J, Fretz CJ, Terrier F, Gerber C. Rotator cuff tears: Correlation of sonographic and surgical findings. *Radiology* 1988;169:791–794.
15. Middleton WD, Reinus WR, Melson GL, Totty WG, Murphy WA. Pitfalls of rotator cuff sonography. *AJR* 1986;146:555–560.
16. Kagetsu NJ, Litt AW. Important considerations in measurement of attractive force on metallic implants in MR imagers. *Radiology* 1991;179:505–508.
17. Lackmann RW, Kaufman B, Hans JS, et al. MR imaging in patient with metallic implants. *Radiology* 1985;157:711–714.
18. Shellock FG. MR imaging of metallic implants and materials: A compilation of the literature. *AJR* 1988;151:811–814.
19. Berquist TH. *Magnetic Resonance of the Musculoskeletal System*. New York: Raven Press, 1990.
20. Kerr R, Resnick D, Pineda C, Haghighi P. Osteoarthritis of the glenohumeral joint: A radiologic-pathologic study. *AJR* 1985;144:967–972.
21. Neer CS, Watson KC, Stanton FJ. Recent experience in total shoulder replacement. *J Bone Joint Surg [Am]* 1982;64:319–336.
22. Cofield RH. Total shoulder arthroplasty with Neer prosthesis. *J Bone Joint Surg [Am]* 1984;66:899–906.
23. Thornhill TS, Karr MJ, Averill RM, Batte NJ, Thomas WH. Total shoulder arthroplasty: The Brigham and Women's experience. *Orthop Trans* 1983;7:497.
24. Bigliani LU, Morrison DS, April EW. The morphology of the acromion and its relationship to rotator cuff tears (abstract). *Orthop Trans* 1986;10:216.
25. Aliabadi P, Weissman BN, Thornhill T, Nikpoor N, Sosman JL. Evaluation of a nonconstrained total shoulder prosthesis. *AJR* 1988;151:1169–1172.

26. Amstutz HC, Sew Hoy AL, Clarke IC. UCLA anatomic total shoulder arthroplasty. *Clin Orthop* 1981;155:7–20.
27. Boyd AD, Aliabadi P, Thornhill TS. Postoperative proximal migration in total shoulder arthroplasty. Incidence and significance. *J Arthroplasty* 1991;6:31–37.
28. Coughlin MJ, Morris JM, West WF. The semiconstrained total shoulder arthroplasty. *J Bone Joint Surg [Am]* 1979;61:574–581.
29. Gristina AG, Romano RL, Kammire GC, Webb LX. Total shoulder replacement. *Orthop Clin North Am* 1987;18:445–453.
30. McElwain JP, English E. The early results of porous-coated total shoulder arthroplasty. *Clin Orthop* 1987;218:217–224.
31. Pahle JA, Kvarnes L. Shoulder replacement arthroplasty. *Ann Chir Gynaecol Suppl* 1985;74:85–89.
32. Post M, Haskel SS, Jablon M. Total shoulder replacement with a constrained prosthesis. *J Bone Joint Surg [Am]* 1980;62:327–335.
33. Post M, Jablon M. Constrained total shoulder arthroplasty. Long-term follow-up observations. *Clin Orthop* 1983;173:109–116.
34. Sledge CB, Kozinn SC, Thornhill TS, Barrett WP. Total shoulder arthroplasty in rheumatoid arthritis. *Rheumatology* 1989;12:95–102.
35. Thornhill TS, Barrett WP. Total shoulder arthroplasty. In: Rowe CR, ed. *The Shoulder*. New York: Churchill-Livingstone, 1988:481–505.
36. Ovesen J, Nielsen S. Prosthesis position in shoulder arthroplasty. *Acta Orthop Scand* 1985;56:330–331.
37. Ovesen J, Sojbjerg J, Sneppen O. A humeral head cutting guide: Instrument to secure correct humeral component retroversion in shoulder joint arthroplasty. *Clin Orthop* 1987;216:193–194.
38. Frich LH, Moller BN. Retroversion of the humeral prosthesis in shoulder arthroplasty. Measurements of angle from standard radiographs. *J Arthroplasty* 1989;4:277–280.
39. Egund N, Jonsson E, Lidgren L, Kelly I, Pettersson H. Computed tomography of humeral head cup arthroplasties. A preliminary report. *Acta Radiol* 1987;28:71–73.
40. Kaplan PA, Montesi SA, Jardon OM, Gregory PR. Bone-ingrowth hip prostheses in asymptomatic patients: Radiographic features. *Radiology* 1988;169:221–227.
41. Kattapuram SV, Lodwick GS, Chandler H, Khurana JS, Ehara S, Rosenthal DI. Porous-coated anatomic total hip prostheses: Radiographic analysis and clinical correlation. *Radiology* 1990;174:861–864.
42. Weissman BN. Current topics in the radiology of joint replacement. *Radiol Clin North Am* 1990;28:1111–1134.
43. Engh CA, Bobyn JD, Glassman AH. Porous coated hip replacement—The factors governing bone ingrowth, stress shielding and clinical results. *J Bone Joint Surg [Br]* 1987;62:45–55.
44. Driessnack RP, Ferlic DC, Wiedel JD. Dissociation of the glenoid component in the Macnab/English total shoulder arthroplasty. *J Arthroplasty* 1990;5:15–18.
45. Barrett WP, Jackins SE, Wyss C, Matsen FA III. Total shoulder arthroplasty: the University of Washington experience. *Orthop Trans* 1986;10:232.

5 Anesthesia for Shoulder Arthroplasty

B. Hugh Dorman, M.D., Ph.D., and Gary R. Haynes, M.D, Ph.D.

REGIONAL ANESTHESIA FOR SHOULDER SURGERY

Regional techniques provide excellent anesthesia for shoulder surgery when utilized appropriately. Properly conducted regional anesthesia has certain advantages not shared by general anesthesia. Selective nerve blockade of the shoulder allows for ideal operative conditions without altering the function of vital organs. This becomes increasingly important in patients with preexisting organ system dysfunction, in whom a disturbance in physiology by a general anesthetic may not be well tolerated. Regional anesthesia for the shoulder can provide excellent postoperative analgesia, thereby reducing narcotic requirement. This potentially eliminates many side effects associated with narcotic administration, including nausea, urinary retention, respiratory depression, and pruritus.[1] A reduced incidence of postoperative pulmonary complications and disorientation may result from regional techniques.[2] Since regional anesthesia abolishes afferent impulses from the operative area, the endocrine, metabolic response to pain and sympathetic responses are greatly attenuated.[3] Regional anesthesia also minimizes the danger of aspiration in patients with full stomachs, provides for early ambulation, and allows patients to stay awake who are fearful of the loss of consciousness necessary with general anesthesia.

The use of regional anesthesia for shoulder surgery also has some potential disadvantages. Regional techniques do not always result in adequate analgesia for surgery. The success rate with nerve blocks is very dependent on the expertise of the anesthesiologist. Other potential drawbacks are related to the injection of local anesthetic solutions in the area of the brachial plexus and include pneumothorax, traumatic injury to neural structures, intravascular or neuraxial administration of local anesthetics, and hematoma formation.[4-6]

Innervation of the Shoulder and Upper Extremity

An understanding of neural anatomy and sensory distribution of the shoulder and upper extremity is essential prior to administering regional anesthesia. The brachial plexus supplies sensation to the shoulder joint and a majority of the upper extremity. The skin over the shoulder is supplied by branches of the cervical plexus, and the posteromedial area of the upper arm to the elbow is supplied by the second intercostal nerve (intercostobrachial branch).

The brachial plexus consists of anterior rami from C5–8 and T1 (Figure 5–1). The respective nerve roots pass through their intervertebral foramina and converge inferiorly to form three trunks beneath the prevertebral fascia, between the scalenus anterior and medius muscles. C5 and C6 unite to become the superior trunk, C7 forms the middle trunk, and C8 and T1 converge to form the inferior trunk. The trunks are stacked in a vertical orientation in the interscalene area. They proceed in an inferior and anterolateral direction toward the superior aspect of the first rib, in close proximity to the subclavian artery. As the trunks and subclavian artery emerge from the interscalane area, they are enclosed by prevertebral fascia (Figure 5–2).

Each trunk splits into an anterior and posterior division at the lateral aspect of the first rib. The divisions continue in a lateral and inferior direction beneath the clavicle and enter the axilla where they unite to form three cords, named according to their relationship with the axillary artery. The posterior cord lies posterior to the axillary artery and is formed from all three posterior divisions. The lateral cord is formed from the anterior divisions of the superior and middle trunks, while the medial cord emerges from the anterior division of the inferior trunk. The prevertebral fascial sheath that initially formed around the subclavian artery and brachial plexus trunks also encloses the brachial plexus and axillary artery through the axilla and into the proximal part of the arm. The three cords branch at the lateral aspect of the pectoralis minor muscle into individual nerves. A branch from the lateral cord joins a branch from the medial cord to form the median nerve. The lateral cord is also the origin of the musculocutaneous nerve, which leaves the axillary sheath in the proximal aspect of the axilla. The medial cord gives rise to the ulnar nerve, which is in a posteromedial position relative to the artery. The medial cutaneous nerve of the arm and forearm is also formed from the medial cord. The posterior cord gives rise to both the radial and axillary nerves.

The cervical plexus is formed from the anterior primary rami of the upper four cervical nerves. Anterior rami of C2–4 nerves are responsible for sensory supply to the skin in the distribution of the anterolateral regions of the neck and shoulder. Four distinct nerves from the cervical plexus emerge at the midpoint of the posterior border of the sternocleidomastoid muscle (Figure 5–3). These include the lesser occipital nerve, the great auricular nerve, the supraclavicular nerve, and the anterior cutaneous nerve of the neck. The supraclavicular nerve is important in regional

Anesthesia for Shoulder Arthroplasty 71

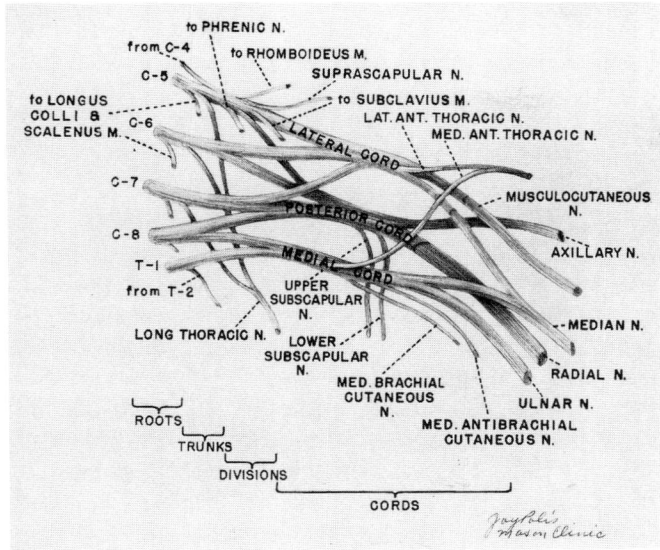

Figure 5–1. Components of the brachial plexus.

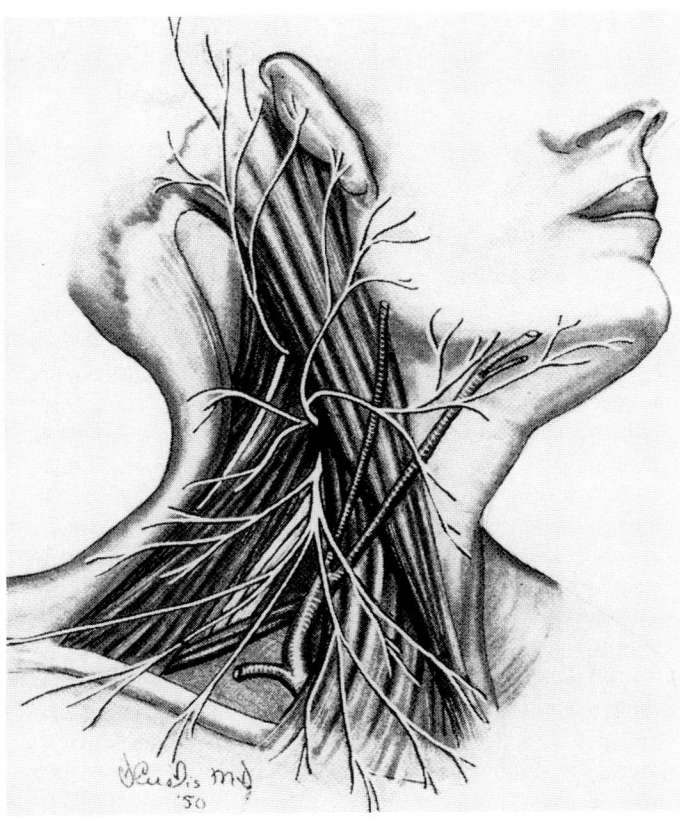

Figure 5–3. The superficial cervical plexus and its relationship to the sternocleidomastoid muscle.

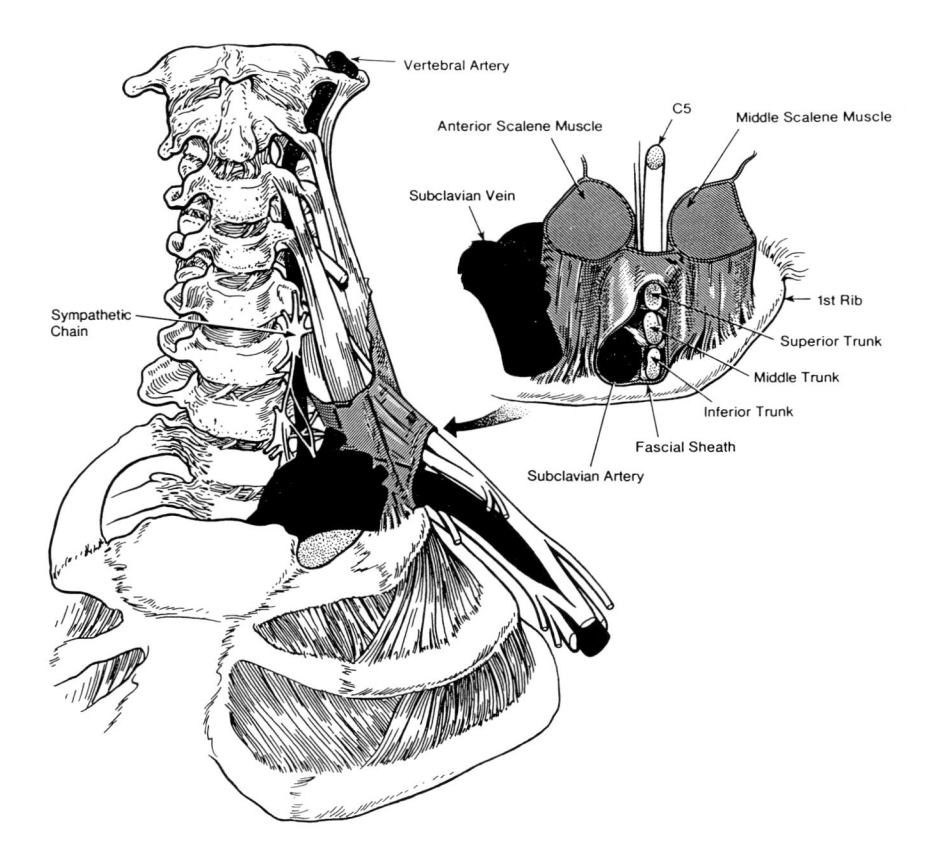

Figure 5–2. Anatomy of the brachial plexus and its relationship to the scalenus anterior and medius muscles, subclavian artery, vertebral artery, and sympathetic chain. The prevertebral fascia forms a sheath around the brachial plexus and subclavian artery upon emergence from the interscalene area.

anesthesia for the shoulder since it supplies the skin over the deltoid muscle. In addition, the supraclavicular nerve supplies sensation posteriorly to the upper aspect of the scapula and anteriorly over the lower portion of the neck and upper chest to the second rib.

Indications

There are no absolute indications for a regional anesthetic technique in shoulder arthroplasty surgery. There are, however, patients who could benefit from avoidance of general anesthesia. Patients with severe pulmonary dysfunction who are at risk for prolonged intubation following surgery are excellent candidates for a regional anesthetic.[7,8] The risk for bronchospasm in a patient with reactive airway disease is avoided with a regional technique. Patients with limited cardiac reserve or in congestive heart failure may be very sensitive to the cardiac depressant effects of many anesthetic agents utilized for general anesthesia.[9] Hemodynamic management of such patients may be facilitated with regional anesthesia. There are many patients who are fearful of the loss of consciousness necessary for general anesthesia, and would prefer to remain awake for surgery. Furthermore, some patients are very susceptible to the side effects associated with general anesthesia. Nausea, vomiting, and disorientation, which can occur following administration of a general anesthetic, may be avoided with a regional technique. Finally, significant postoperative analgesia can be provided following a regional anesthetic, thereby decreasing narcotic requirements in individuals who frequently experience unpleasant opioid-induced side effects.

Contraindications

There are several contraindications to regional anesthesia for shoulder arthroplasty surgery. Patient refusal of a regional technique constitutes one of the most important reasons to perform general anesthesia. Multiple attempts to convince a reluctant patient that regional anesthesia is indicated for shoulder surgery may harm the physician-patient relationship, and place the physician in a difficult medical-legal position at a later date. Furthermore, regional anesthesia performed on a reluctant patient is usually not satisfactory for the patient or sufficient for the surgical procedure. Regional techniques should not be performed on patients with a cutaneous infection, recent burn, or dermatitis in the area of block-needle insertion. Access to administer a regional anesthetic for the shoulder in patients with neck braces or dressings that cannot be temporarily removed is difficult. A preexisting neuropathy of the involved shoulder or ipsilateral upper extremity in the distribution of the brachial or cervical plexus may result in questions of possible nerve damage from the regional technique in the postoperative period. A complete neurologic examination should be performed on every patient who presents with a neuropathy in the distribution of the nerve block, with deficits clearly documented on the patient's chart prior to surgery. Finally, regional anesthesia should not be attempted on patients who are uncooperative or who would not be able to remain still for the nerve block and subsequent surgery.

Preoperative Evaluation

The preoperative visit allows the anesthesiologist to acquire a complete understanding of the patient's physical status and concurrent medical problems that impact on anesthetic management. In addition to the complete history and physical examination that is typically performed on a patient undergoing surgery, there are additional considerations when planning for shoulder surgery using a regional anesthetic. Prior regional anesthetic experiences should be discussed, especially if any were particularly unpleasant. Any history of adverse reactions to local anesthetics should be documented. Furthermore, a detailed examination of the neck and upper chest on the operative side should be performed to confirm the absence of infectious processes, burns, or a recent injury that would preclude use of a nerve block.

Preoperative discussions with patients should include a complete outline of perioperative events. Premedication, monitoring requirements, intravenous catheter placement, and a detailed outline of the nerve block procedure should be discussed. A description of the progressive loss of motor and sensory function following the injection of local anesthetic should be included. The expected duration of nerve blockade should also be discussed, so that patients are not concerned if motor and sensory functions do not immediately return in the postoperative period. Patients should be assured that sedation will be provided as needed during surgery, and general anesthesia will be induced prior to incision if the nerve block is not complete.

Premedication

The requirement for premedication depends on the physical status and personality of the patient, as well as the nerve block technique. Relatively stoic, relaxed individuals will require minimal preoperative sedation, while anxious patients who are sensitive to any degree of discomfort will need generous sedative medication. Nerve block techniques that involve patient feedback about paresthesias require patients to be only minimally sedated. The use of a nerve stimulator to locate the brachial plexus precludes patient participation, and allows for an increased level of sedation preoperatively.

Narcotics, benzodiazepines, or both usually provide adequate preoperative sedation. Narcotics are useful to attenuate the discomfort associated with needle insertion during nerve blockade. Morphine, 0.10 to 0.15 mg/kg intramuscularly; methadone, 0.10 to 0.15 mg/kg orally; and controlled-release morphine, 30 mg orally, are all effective.[10] Benzodiazepines such as diazepam, 0.15 mg/kg orally, and lorazepam, 2 to 4 mg orally, provide anxiolysis and sedation without significant side effects.[11] They offer the additional benefit of increasing the seizure threshold; this may be especially advantageous when large doses of local anesthetics are administered.[12] Other potential benefits of benzodiazepines include the development of anterograde amnesia and the oral route of administration.[13]

Premedication should not be administered to patients with severely compromised cardiopulmonary function. In this subset of individuals, significant doses of sedative or hypnotic agents should only be administered when constant patient monitoring is in effect. Intravenous fentanyl and/or midazolam can be titrated to effect slowly such patients just prior to surgery.[14] Ketamine, 0.25 mg/kg intravenously, is another useful drug that can be administered just prior to block-needle insertion or incision to increase patient cooperation. Concurrent or prior administration of a benzodiazepine is recommended in order to reduce ketamine-related side effects.[15] A combination of intravenous droperidol and fentanyl titrated to take effect just prior to the surgical procedure also results in a relaxed, cooperative patient. Large doses of droperidol should be avoided, however, since there is an increased incidence of hypotension and extrapyramidal dyskinesis.[16,17] Anticholinergic medications should not be routinely included in the premedication regimen, since the antisialagogue effect can be uncomfortable in the awake patient.

Equipment Requirement

When regional anesthesia is used for shoulder surgery, resuscitative equipment must be present to treat accidental injection of local anesthetic agents intravascularly, or into the central neural axis. Equipment for airway management and positive-pressure ventilation must be immediately available, including an Ambu bag, mask, laryngoscope, endotracheal tubes, succinylcholine, suction, oral airways, and a supply of oxygen. Vasopressors, lidocaine, intravenous fluid, and atropine are required to manage hemodynamic instability or arrhythmias. Barbiturates or benzodiazepines are also necessary to treat local anesthetic-induced convulsions. An anesthesia machine should be available to provide positive-pressure ventilation and administer general anesthesia if the regional anesthetic is not sufficient for surgery. Whenever local anesthetics are injected, aspiration tests should be performed to rule out intravascular or intradural needle placement. Furthermore, a 3-mL test dose of the local anesthetic containing epinephrine (5 μg/mL) should be administered prior to injecting a large volume of solution.[18] Unless injected into an artery perfusing the brain, the small test dose does not contain sufficient local anesthetic to cause systemic toxicity. The 15 μg of epinephrine, however, will typically cause an increase in heart rate if administered intravascularly.

Paresthesias Versus Nerve Stimulators

There are two main techniques utilized to locate the brachial plexus, elicitation of paresthesias and electrically stimulating motor components of the plexus. For the paresthesia method, the block needle is inserted toward the nerve until contact is made, and the patient reports a paresthesia in the peripheral distribution of the brachial plexus. A blunt point needle is recommended when performing nerve blocks, since the risk of neural trauma is decreased relative to techniques using a needle with a sharp taper.[19] A blunt needle is especially important when using the paresthesia method, since this technique has been shown to result in a decreased incidence of neural lesions following blockade of the brachial plexus.[20] Additional disadvantages of the paresthesia technique include patient discomfort and the inability of some patients to cooperate or provide reliable information.

Motor nerve stimulation, using a pulse-generated electric current with an exploring needle, is probably a more reliable technique to perform brachial plexus nerve blocks. The motor components of the brachial plexus are stimulated by a low-frequency current, providing feedback on location of the nerves. A standard nerve stimulator can be modified to provide an optimal current, consisting of a low-frequency 1-Hz pulse of 1-millisecond duration.[21] Optimal needle position at the brachial plexus results in painless motor response at currents equal to or less than 0.5 mA.[22,23] The use of insulated needles allows for accurate location of the plexus at the tip of the needle, where the injection of local anesthetic occurs.[23] The use of nerve stimulators does not require patient cooperation and therefore is independent of patient reliability. Furthermore, patients can be heavily sedated for the nerve block procedure.

Intraoperative Management

Intraoperative management of the patient with a brachial plexus block for shoulder surgery can be extremely challenging. Patients undergoing regional anesthesia require the same vigilance and care as patients with a general anesthetic. Continuous attention to vital signs will be necessary to ensure patient safety, especially in heavily sedated individuals with unprotected airways. The anesthesiologist must also continuously monitor the patient to prevent spontaneous movements that impede surgical progress.

Positioning of the patient undergoing regional anesthesia is an important consideration. An excellent nerve block of the shoulder can be a difficult management problem if other areas of the patient become uncomfortable due to improper positioning. In patients who require heavy sedation, neural injury can occur secondary to poor positioning.

The level of sedation required intraoperatively is dependent on the patient's anxiety level, the duration and conditions of surgery, the adequacy of neural blockade, and the patient's physical status. The calm, well-informed individual will require minimal sedative supplementation, while the young or anxious patient may need to be totally unaware of the surgical procedure. The patient with a full stomach, difficult airway, or compromised cardiopulmonary status should receive minimal amounts of sedation, titrated slowly to effect. Prolonged surgical procedures usually require increased amounts of sedative medications, since the patient frequently becomes increasingly uncomfortable and impatient. Shoulder surgery performed under regional anesthesia typically requires sedation, since the surgical manipulations that occur in close proximity to the patient's head and neck often cause anxiety. Finally, incomplete nerve blocks will obviously increase the sedation requirements and may necessitate changing to a general anesthetic.

A variety of medications can provide adequate sedation for regional anesthesia. Good patient-physician rapport, with reassurance and distraction, can be an effective tool to allay anxiety.[24] A number of intravenous agents can effectively provide intraoperative sedation. Intravenous benzodiazepines such as diazepam, lorazepam, and midazolam provide amnesia and sedation in the absence of significant cardiovascular or respiratory effect.[25] Midazolam offers advantages relative to other intravenous benzodiazepines, with a shorter half-life, faster clearance and patient recovery, less venous irritation or thrombophlebitis, and no active metabolites.[26,27]

Intravenous narcotics can provide analgesia for patient discomfort and reduce the requirement for benzodiazepines intraoperatively.[28,29] Newer synthetic compounds, such as alfentanil, have a short clinical duration of effect and can be utilized for quick surgical procedures.[30] All intravenous narcotics must be titrated carefully in patients with preexisting pulmonary disease, since respiratory depression is a potential side effect. Short-acting barbiturates, such as propofol and methohexital, can be administered by continuous intravenous drip, and titrated to a desired level of sedation.[31] Such agents can be extremely useful to ablate patient responses when performing a nerve block with the use of a nerve stimulator, when patient cooperation is not necessary. Propofol's short elimination half-life and rapid metabolic clearance results in rapid patient recovery, even following prolonged infusions.[31] Intravenous ketamine administration, after low doses of benzodiazepines, is efficacious for sedation and analgesia and is relatively free of significant side effects.[32] Finally, supplementation with nitrous oxide in concentrations of 25 to 50% can be useful for sedation and appears to result in more rapid recovery after discontinuation, compared to intravenous agents.[33]

Techniques of Brachial Plexus Block

The two primary approaches utilized to block the brachial plexus for shoulder surgery include the interscalene and supraclavicular approaches. In either case, a superficial cervical block may be required to ablate sensation to the skin overlying the deltoid muscle.

INTERSCALENE BLOCK

The interscalene approach to the brachial plexus has been well described.[34,35] In an interscalene block, local anesthetic is targeted to the roots of the brachial plexus, where they reside in a groove between the scalenus anterior and medius muscles, at the level of C6. In order to facilitate the nerve block, the patient is instructed to lie in a supine position, with the head turned away from the involved shoulder. The C6 level can be identified by palpation of the cricoid cartilage. The area or groove between the scalenus anterior and medius muscles is located by first identifying the lateral edge of the sternocleidomastoid muscle's posterior belly. The operator's index and forefingers are drawn back from the sternocleidomastoid muscle over the scalenus anterior muscle until the groove between the scalene muscles is appreciated. When landmarks are difficult to identify, slow deep breaths may allow for improved palpation of the scalene musculature.[36] The external jugular vein frequently overlies the brachial plexus between the scalene muscles and can serve as a useful landmark once the C6 level is appreciated. The nerve block needle is inserted into the interscalene groove at the level of C6. The direction of the needle should be primarily inward, perpendicular to the skin, but with a slightly caudal and posterior inclination (Figure 5–4). Since the cervical transverse processes at this level are directed primarily in a lateral plane, the caudal tilt should help prevent needle insertion into the central neural axis.

The brachial plexus normally resides at a depth of 1.0 to 1.5 cm in patients without excessive adipose tissue. It is important that the needle lies under the prevertebral fascia, to ensure that local anesthetic enters the brachial plexus sheath. When a paresthesia technique is used for plexus location,

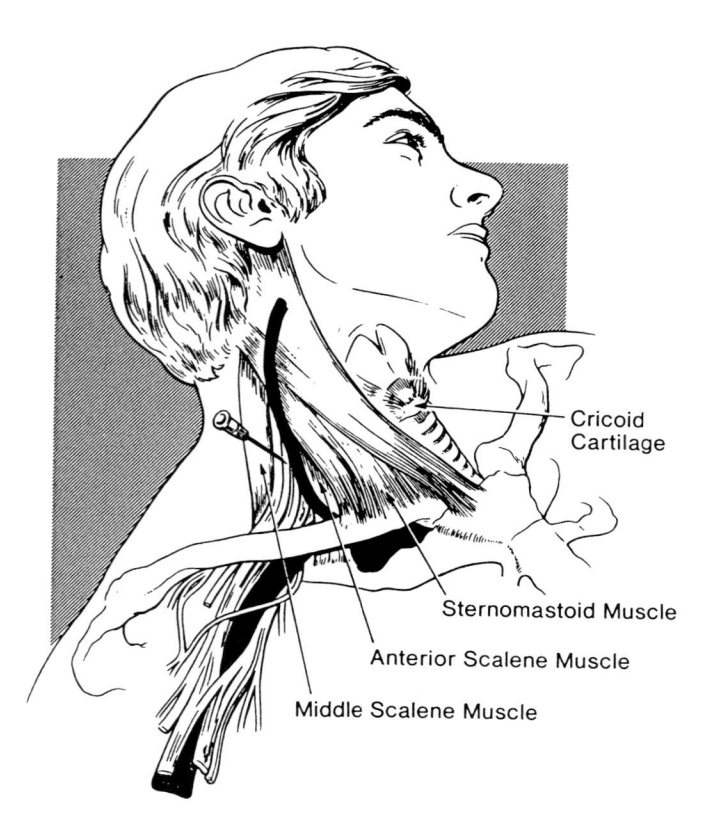

Figure 5–4. Anatomic landmarks and correct needle placement for interscalene block.

confirmation of correct needle placement is provided by induction of paresthesias distal to the elbow, usually involving the thumb or index finger. A stimulating needle is very useful in performing this block; muscle contractions distal to the shoulder reflect the stimulation of nerve roots within the brachial plexus. When correct needle placement is ensured by either technique, 35 to 40 mL of local anesthetic solution is injected following a negative aspiration. This volume of anesthetic fills the sheath to the upper cervical vertebrae and, therefore, can result in anesthesia of both the cervical and brachial plexuses.[37] Stabilization of the needle during injection can be facilitated by the use of a flexible conduit from syringe to needle.[38] This is particularly important for the interscalene block, since the brachial plexus is relatively superficial at this location.

Nerve blockade progresses from C5 distally to T1, with loss of biceps function appearing first; small muscle function of the hand typically disappears last. Sensory loss evolves down the preaxial aspect of the arm to the thumb, across the fingers, and up the postaxial distribution of the upper extremity towards the axilla. Blockade in the ulnar nerve distribution may be delayed or absent with reduced local anesthetic volumes.[34]

There are distinct advantages of the interscalene block for shoulder surgery. Arm position does not affect the ability to perform the block, and the incidence of pneumothorax is minimal. Furthermore, landmarks are usually not obscured by obesity, and the block can be safely completed in patients with infection or trauma of the upper chest, arm, or shoulder.

Several disadvantages and potential complications are associated with the interscalene approach to the brachial plexus. Since sensory function of the postaxial aspect of the arm can be spared with even large volumes of local anesthetic, shoulder surgery that must extend into this area may require additional anesthesia. The vertebral artery lies in close proximity to the brachial plexus; accidental intravascular injection of local anesthetic into the artery can occur with the interscalene approach, and result in significant concentrations of local anesthetic in the brain, with subsequent convulsions.[39] Subarachnoid or epidural injection of large volumes of local anesthetic is also possible due to horizontal or cephalad needle direction and can cause total spinal anesthesia.[5,40] Pneumothorax can occur with improper caudal placement of the nerve block needle. Hoarseness and Horner's syndrome are not rare following interscalene block, but usually are not clinically significant.[41] Finally, transient ipsilateral hemidiaphragmatic paresis has been shown to occur in 100% of patients following interscalene block, and may have clinical significance in patients with preexisting respiratory disease.[42]

SUPRACLAVICULAR BLOCK

In the supraclavicular approach to the brachial plexus, the trunks of the plexus are blocked as they cross over the first rib. The nerve block is most easily performed with the patient supine, with the head slightly turned away from the involved shoulder. The correct position for block-needle placement is a point 1 to 2 cm behind the midpoint of the clavicle. Several landmarks can be useful in confirming a midclavicular position. The lateral border of the scalenus anterior muscle, where the brachial plexus exits the neck, usually lies over the midpoint of the clavicle. The midclavicular region also consistently lies 1.5 to 2.0 cm lateral to the posterior border of the clavicular head of the sternocleidomastoid muscle. The straight portion of the external jugular vein, if continued in a caudal direction, typically intersects the clavicle at the midpoint. Finally, the subclavian artery lies in close proximity to the brachial plexus and frequently can be palpated in the subclavian fossa behind the clavicle.

The nerve block needle is inserted down towards the first rib with a slight medial and posterior inclination. Paresthesias distal to the elbow are usually obtained prior to contacting the first rib. If the rib is located with the needle and a paresthesia has not been obtained, the needle should be walked along the surface of the rib in an anterior or posterior direction, until a paresthesia is elicited. Since the subclavian artery lies just anterior and medial to the plexus at the first rib, aspiration of arterial blood should result in redirection of the needle to a more posterior and lateral position. A stimulating needle can also be utilized to locate the nerve trunks and causes peripheral motor activity at low output in the distribution of the brachial plexus when properly placed. Following a negative aspiration, 30 to 35 mL of local anesthetic solution is injected.

There are several distinct advantages of the supraclavicular approach to brachial plexus block for shoulder surgery. The volume of local anesthetic required for nerve blockade is reduced relative to the interscalene approach, since the brachial plexus is most compactly arranged over the first rib. Less local anesthetic translates into decreased serum levels from vascular absorption. The supraclavicular block typically is quick in onset, and arm or shoulder position does not affect the ability to perform the block.

There are several potential complications associated with the supraclavicular approach. One of the most frequent and potentially serious complications is pneumothorax. The incidence of clinically significant pneumothorax can approach 6%, but usually occurs 1% of the time in experienced hands.[43] The risk of pneumothorax is increased by medial needle inclination towards the dome of the pleura. A high degree of suspicion for pneumothorax is required following a supraclavicular block; a chest x-ray film should be obtained immediately with any suggestive symptoms such as cough, pleuritic pain, or dyspnea. In the absence of symptoms a routine x-ray film is not warranted, especially since most pneumothoraces only become evident 24 hours after the procedure.[44] The risk of pneumothorax strongly suggests that supraclavicular brachial plexus block should never be performed bilaterally.

Other complications of the supraclavicular block include Horner's syndrome, which can appear in up to 70% of patients when large volumes of local anesthetics are administered.[44] Phrenic nerve block is present with a 40 to 60% incidence, but should be well tolerated unless severe preexisting lung disease is present. Toxic reactions from elevated serum concentrations of local anesthetic agents can occur from inadvertent intravascular injection. Aspiration tests for blood with the supraclavicular block are mandatory prior to injection of local anesthetic, since the subclavian artery is in such close proximity to the brachial plexus at the first rib. Finally, nerve damage from needle trauma or ischemia secondary to vasoconstrictor drugs is a potential concern. Nerve damage, however, can also occur from surgical trauma and faulty position of the extremity. Immediate neurologic consultation is necessary to establish the extent of any neurologic dysfunction and to prescribe appropriate treatment.

Superficial Cervical Plexus Block

The skin over the shoulder is supplied by descending branches of the cervical plexus. Typically, 40 mL of local anesthetic solution, administered via the interscalene approach, will block the cervical and brachial plexuses. Occasionally, ineffective cranial spread of local anesthetic results in an absence of cervical plexus blockade. It is, therefore, necessary to test sensation of the skin overlying the deltoid muscle to ensure a block prior to surgery. If the cervical plexus has been spared, then a superficial cervical plexus block is indicated.

The sensory component of the cervical plexus originates in the anterior primary rami of C2–4, and emerges as four nerves behind the lateral edge of the sternocleidomastoid muscle. The superficial cervical plexus block is most easily performed after the brachial plexus block, with the patient supine. The patient's head is turned away from the involved shoulder, and the posterior border of the clavicular head of the sternocleidomastoid muscle is identified. Five milliliters of local anesthetic solution is deposited at the midpoint and lateral edge of the sternocleidomastoid muscle, with an additional 5 mL deposited along the lateral edge of the posterior belly of the sternocleidomastoid muscle, 2 cm from the midpoint, in both a cranial and caudal direction. This superficial infiltration of local anesthetic along the middle third of the posterior border of the muscle ensures a successful block.

Local Anesthetic Agents

Any local anesthetic that is suitable for peripheral nerve block can be utilized in a brachial plexus block for shoulder surgery. The choice of agent depends primarily on the duration of surgery and the requirement for postoperative analgesia. The addition of 5 μg/mL of epinephrine to the local anesthetic is recommended to reduce systemic absorption of anesthetic solution and to prolong the duration of nerve blockade.

There are four local anesthetics that have been extensively utilized for brachial plexus block. Shoulder procedures of relatively short duration (less than 2 hours) that do not result in a significant degree of postoperative discomfort can be effectively performed with either 1.0 to 1.5% lidocaine or 1.0 to 1.5% mepivacaine. Both agents have a rapid onset and reduced toxicity compared to more potent, longer-acting agents.[45–48] For shoulder surgery of prolonged duration, or procedures in which a significant amount of postoperative pain is expected, 0.75 to 1.00% etidocaine or 0.375 to 0.500% bupivacaine is recommended. In addition to providing anesthesia for the surgical procedure, these agents can deliver prolonged analgesia in the postoperative period while the local anesthetic effect is waning.[49] The local anesthetic-induced analgesia can decrease the narcotic requirement in the postoperative period, and thereby reduce narcotic-related side effects. The longer-acting agents, however, are more toxic, especially in cardiac tissue.[50,51] Furthermore, cardiac resuscitation is difficult following bupivacaine-induced cardiac collapse. These observations highlight the need for aspiration tests and slow administration of local anesthetic to prevent increased serum levels.

Postoperative Management

Protection of the anesthetized upper extremity is the primary concern in the postoperative period. Padding for the elbow should be provided for ulnar nerve protection. The limb should not be displaced posteriorly or abducted more than 90 degrees to avoid stretching the brachial plexus.[52] Ideally, the limb should be stabilized postoperatively to help avoid trauma or improper positioning.

GENERAL ANESTHESIA FOR SHOULDER SURGERY

Shoulder surgery encompasses a variety of surgical procedures, ranging from simple manipulation under anesthesia to total shoulder arthroplasty.[53–56] General anesthesia is probably the most commonly used anesthetic technique for shoulder surgery today. The long duration of many shoulder procedures, unfamiliarity with interscalene and supraclavicular blocks, the time required for placing a regional block, and patient anxiety contribute to choosing general anesthesia. General anesthesia and endotracheal intubation, however, may be difficult in many patients who require this operation.

Perioperative Anesthetic Considerations

Several considerations are important for shoulder surgery under general anesthesia. Concurrent diseases such as rheumatoid arthritis present problems in a number of organ systems. The patient for shoulder arthroplasty surgery is usually placed in a "beach chair" position. This elevates the head and trunk and places the legs in a dependent position, creating a good operative field for surgery but resulting in blood pooling and venous stasis of the lower extremities. The head must be supported to prevent sudden flexion or extension, and there must be adequate knee flexion to avoid sciatic nerve injuries. All changes in position should be done slowly, since moving an anesthetized patient from the supine to sitting position may precipitate orthostatic hypotension. This can be treated by reducing the concentration of inhalational agent, administering intravenous fluid or vasopressors, and applying elastic leg stockings. Elderly and arthritic patients usually have atrophic skin which is sensitive to pressure necrosis. Careful padding over all pressure points is an absolute requirement. Whenever the surgical field is above the level of the right atrium, the potential exists for venous air embolism. The risk is small in shoulder surgery, but should be considered in any patient who suddenly becomes hemodynamically unstable.

Coexisting Disease

The most common diseases that necessitate shoulder arthroplasty include rheumatoid arthritis, systemic lupus erythematosus, osteoarthritis, and posttraumatic arthritis.[57] Two-thirds of patients with rheumatoid arthritis complain of shoulder pain and 90% of hospitalized patients with rheumatoid arthritis have arthritic changes in the shoulder.[58,59] These associated diseases can result in a number of problems that must be addressed to facilitate optimal anesthetic management. Furthermore, patients presenting for shoulder arthroplasty surgery are typically older, with an average age of 63 years.[57]

CONCURRENT MEDICATIONS

Patients typically present for shoulder arthroplasty surgery with a long history of using aspirin and/or nonsteroidal anti-inflammatory drugs to reduce inflammation and pain. Aspirin results in a significant degree of platelet dysfunction and can also cause liver damage. Tinnitus and hearing loss have been associated with toxic aspirin levels.[60] It is desirable to discontinue aspirin therapy at least 1 week before surgery so that platelet function can recover. Nonsteroidal anti-inflammatory drugs also impair platelet function and irritate the gastric mucosa, resulting in an increased incidence of gastrointestinal bleeding, gastritis, and peptic ulcer formation.[60] In addition, nonsteroidal anti-inflammatory drugs bind to plasma proteins, and doses of many drugs must often be reduced due to displacement from albumin.[61]

Rheumatoid arthritis and systemic lupus erythematosus patients are also frequently treated with corticosteroids and cytotoxic agents. Problems associated with steroid therapy include poor wound healing, osteoporosis, decreased immune response, mineralocorticoid effect, and gastrointestinal bleeding. Parenteral gold therapy produces remissions in many rheumatoid arthritis patients but can result in pancytopenia and glomerulonephritis. Bone marrow suppression and renal dysfunction are complications of D-penicillamine, another drug utilized in the treatment of rheumatoid arthritis.

ASSOCIATED JOINT AND INFLAMMATORY DISEASE

Patients with rheumatoid arthritis frequently present with inflammatory changes in the head and neck that need to be addressed. Rheumatoid nodules and reactive inflammatory changes in the sclera can cause acute glaucoma or scleral thinning with perforation.[62] Sjögren's syndrome occurs in 10% of rheumatoid arthritis patients; the absence of tearing contributes to the friability of ocular tissue and the increased possibility of inadvertent eye injury.

Arthritic disease in temporomandibular, cricoarytenoid, and cervical spine articulations are common in patients with rheumatoid arthritis. Dysphagia, hoarseness, or stridor suggests severe cricoarytenoid arthritis. Reductions in cricoarytenoid joint mobility may cause marked narrowing of the glottic opening. Indirect laryngoscopy is recommended in questionable cases to assess vocal cord mobility and laryngeal anatomy.[63]

The temporomandibular joint and mouth opening must be evaluated. Limited mandibular movement may make intubation difficult, and if a receding chin, small mandible, or short neck are present, intubation may be impossible. Ideally the uvula and soft palate should be easily visible on examination, and the mouth opening at least five centimeters in width. Rheumatoid inflammatory changes can also produce laryngeal deviation or shortening of the neck. The trachea may rotate rightward and be displaced to the left in this condition, and the larynx may tilt forward.

Arthritic changes in the cervical spine occur in as many as 90% of rheumatoid arthritis patients. Neck pain, pain radiating to the occiput, upper extremity radiculopathy, or limited neck mobility implies cervical arthritis. Instability of the cervical spine must be evaluated in any patient with long-standing rheumatoid arthritis; flexion-extension spine films may help define cervical spine changes. Computerized tomography and magnetic resonance imaging are also used to delineate the degree of cervical spine disease.

Three types of cervical spine changes occur in rheumatoid arthritis patients. The most common is atlantoaxial subluxation (C1–2 subluxation), followed by vertebral body subluxation (subluxation of any C2–7 vertebrae) and then odontoid migration.[64] Any clinical or radiologic evidence of such cervical spine involvement requires neck stabilization during intubation. The use of smaller endotracheal tubes and an awake fiberoptic intubation technique are usually helpful.

ASSOCIATED CARDIAC DISEASE

Cardiac disease is common in both rheumatoid arthritis and systemic lupus erythematosus patients due to advanced age and inflammatory changes.[65] Pericarditis and pericardial effusion with thickening can occur with progression to cardiac tamponade. Myocarditis may result in decreased contractility and conduction changes. Cardiac valve fibrosis due to persistent inflammation has also been described. Furthermore, in rheumatoid arthritis patients, coronary arteritis and thrombosis may cause myocardial infarction. The preoperative evaluation should include an electrocardiogram, and an echocardiogram may also be indicated if a murmur is detected or a pericardial effusion is suspected. Invasive monitoring will be necessary for surgery if significant cardiac disease is diagnosed.

ASSOCIATED PULMONARY DISEASE

Diffuse interstitial fibrosis or infiltrates, cough, dyspnea, and hypoxia can occur in association with a systemic inflammatory disease.[66] Inflammatory changes in the lung may result in a restrictive pattern of pulmonary disease. Chest wall deformities, pleural effusion, and costochondral arthritis may contribute to decreases in total pulmonary compliance. Objective evaluation of lung function with a preoperative chest radiograph, spirometry, and an arterial blood gas analysis may be required to define a patient's pulmonary function.

LABORATORY CHANGES

Patients presenting for shoulder arthroplasty surgery are often anemic due to gastrointestinal bleeding associated with aspirin, nonsteroidal anti-inflammatory drugs, or steroid therapy. The anemia is usually a hypochromic, microcytic type that resists correction with supplemental iron. Pancytopenia can result from many of the cytotoxic drugs used to treat concurrent systemic inflammatory diseases. Any reduction in platelet number may also be accompanied by an inhibition of platelet function due to aspirin therapy. Glomerulonephritis with proteinuria may cause dramatic reductions in the serum level of albumin. Steroid therapy with a potential mineralocorticoid effect can cause a hypokalemic, hypochloremic metabolic alkalosis. Finally, renal failure with elevations in blood urea nitrogen and creatinine can occur secondary to inflammatory disease and must be evaluated preoperatively.

REFERENCES

1. Cousins MJ, Mather LE. Intrathecal and epidural administration of opioids. *Anesthesiology* 1984;61:276–310.
2. Widlund L. Regional blockade vs. analgesic therapy. *Acta Anaesthesiol Scand* 1982;S74:169–172.
3. Kehlet H. The endocrine-metabolic response to postoperative pain. *Acta Anaesthesiol Scand* 1982;S74:173–175.
4. Edde RR, Deutsch S. Cardiac arrest after interscalene brachial-plexus block. *Anesth Analg* 1977;56:446–447.
5. Ross S, Scarborough CD. Total spinal anaesthesia following brachial plexus block. *Anesthesiology* 1973;39:458.
6. Tuominen MK, Pere P, Rosenberg PH. Unintentional arterial catheterization and bupivacaine toxicity associated with continuous interscalene brachial plexus block. *Anesthesiology* 1991;75:356–358.
7. Stein M, Cassara EL. Preoperative pulmonary evaluation and therapy for surgery patients. *JAMA* 1970;211:878–890.
8. Tarhan S, Moffitt EA, Sessler AD, Douglas WW, Taylor WF. Risk of anaesthesia and surgery in patients with chronic bronchitis and chronic obstructive pulmonary disease. *Surgery* 1973;74:220–226.
9. Kemmotsu O, Hashimoto Y, Shimosato S. The effects of fluroxene and enflurane on contractile performance of isolated papillary muscles from failing hearts. *Anesthesiology* 1974;40:252–260.
10. Kay B, Healey TEJ. Premedication by controlled release morphine. *Anaesthesia* 1984;39:587–593.
11. Magbagbeola JAO. A comparison of lorazepam and diazepam as oral premedicants for surgery under regional anaesthesia. *Br J Anaesth* 1974;46:449–451.
12. deJong RH, Heavner JE. Local anaesthetic seizure prevention: Diazepam versus pentobarbital. *Anesthesiology* 1972;36:449–457.
13. McKay AC, Dundee JW. Effect of oral benzodiazepines on memory. *Br J Anaesth* 1980;52:1247–1256.
14. Dundee JW, Wilson DB. Amnesic action of midazolam. *Anaesthesia* 1980;35:459–461.
15. White PF, Way WL, Trevor AJ. Ketamine. Its pharmacology and therapeutic uses. *Anesthesiology* 1982;56:119–136.
16. Patton CM. Rapid induction of acute dyskinesia by droperidol. *Anesthesiology* 1975;43:126–127.
17. Whitwam JG, Russel WJ. The acute cardiovascular changes and adrenergic blockade by droperidol in man. *Br J Anaesth* 1971;43:581–591.
18. Moore DC, Batra MS. The components of an effective test dose prior to epidural block. *Anesthesiology* 1981;55:693–696.
19. Selander D, Dhuner KG, Lundborg G. Peripheral nerve injury due to injury needles used for regional anaesthesia. *Acta Anaesthesiol Scand* 1977;21:182–188.
20. Selander D, Edshage S, Wolff T. Paraesthesia or no paraesthesia? Nerve lesions after axillary blocks. *Acta Anaesthesiol Scand* 1979;23:27–33.
21. Greenblatt GM, Denson JS. Needle nerve stimulator-locator: Nerve blocks with a new instrument for locating nerves. *Anesth Analg* 1962;41:599–602.
22. Koons RA. The use of the block-aid monitor and plastic intravenous cannulas for nerve blocks. *Anesthesiology* 1969;31:290–291.
23. Ford DJ, Pither C, Raj PP. Comparison of insulated and uninsulated needles for locating peripheral nerves with a peripheral nerve stimulator. *Anesth Analg* 1984;63:925–928.
24. Scott DL. Sedation for local analgesia. *Anaesthesia* 1975;30:471–475.
25. Kanto J, Klotz U. Intravenous benzodiazepines as anaesthetic agents: Pharmacokinetics and clinical consequences. *Acta Anaesthesiol Scand* 1982;26:554–569.
26. Aun C, Flynn PJ, Richards J. A comparison of midazolam and diazepam for intravenous sedation in dentistry. *Anaesthesia* 1984;39:589–593.
27. Allonen H, Siegler G, Klotz U. Midazolam kinetics. *Clin Pharmacol Ther* 1981;30:653–661.
28. Corall IM, Strunin L, Ward ME, Mason SA, Alcalay M. Sedation for outpatient conservative dentistry. *Anaesthesia* 1979;34:855–858.
29. Philip BK. Supplemental medication for ambulatory procedures under regional anaesthesia. *Anesth Analg* 1985;64:1117–1125.
30. Bovill JG, Sebel PS, Blackburn CL, Heykants J. The pharmacokinetics of alfentanil (R39209): A new opioid analgesic. *Anesthesiology* 1982;57:439–443.
31. White PF: Propofol: Pharmacokinetics and pharmacodynamics. *Semin Anaesth* 1988;7:4–20.
32. Austin TR. Low dose ketamine and diazepam during spinal analgesia. *Anaesthesia* 1980;35:391–392.
33. Korttila K, Ghoneim MM, Jacobs L, Mewaldt SP, Petersen RC. Time course of mental and psychomotor effects of 30

percent nitrous oxide during inhalation and recovery. *Anesthesiology* 1981;54:220–226.
34. Winnie AP. Interscalene brachial plexus block. *Anesth Analg* 1970;49:455–466.
35. Ward ME. The interscalene approach to the brachial plexus. *Anaesthesia* 1974;29:147–157.
36. Sharrock NE, Bruce G. An improved technique for locating the interscalene groove. *Anesthesiology* 1976;44:431–433.
37. Winnie AP. Regional anaesthesia of the upper and lower extremities. In: Zauder HL, ed. *Anaesthesia for Orthopedic Surgery*. Philadelphia: FA Davis, 1980:89–106.
38. Winnie AP. An "immobile needle" for nerve blocks. *Anesthesiology* 1969;31:577–578.
39. Kozody R, Ready LB, Barsa JE, Murphy TM. Dose requirement of local anaesthetic to produce grand mal seizure during stellate ganglion block. *Can J Anaesth* 1982;29:489–491.
40. Kumar A, Battit GE, Froese AB, Long MC. Bilateral cervical and thoracic epidural blockade complicating interscalene brachial plexus block: Report of two cases. *Anesthesiology* 1971;35:650–652.
41. Seltzer JL. Hoarseness and Horner's syndrome after interscalene brachial plexus block. *Anesth Analg* 1977;56:585–586.
42. Urmey WF, Talts KH, Sharrock NE. One hundred percent incidence of hemidiaphragmatic paresis associated with interscalene brachial plexus anaesthesia as diagnosed by ultrasonography. *Anesth Analg* 1991;72:498–503.
43. Moore DC. Complications of regional anaesthesia. In: Bonica JJ, ed. *Regional Anaesthesia*. Philadelphia: FA Davis, 1969:233.
44. Bridenbaugh LD. The upper extremity: Somatic blockade. In: Cousins MJ, Bridenbaugh LD, eds. *Neural Blockade in Clinical Anaesthesia and Management of Pain*. 2nd ed. Philadelphia: JB Lippincott, 1988:396–397.
45. Liu PL, Feldman HS, Covino BM, Giasi R, Covino BG. Acute cardiovascular toxicity of intravenous amide local anesthetics in anesthetized ventilated dogs. *Anesth Analg* 1982;61:317–322.
46. Foldes FF, Davidson GM, Duncalf D, Kuwabara S. The intravenous toxicity of local anaesthetic agents in man. *Clin Pharmacol Ther* 1965;6:328–335.
47. Scott DB. Evaluation of the toxicity of local anaesthetic agents in man. *Br J Anaesth* 1975;47:56–61.
48. Scott DB. Toxicity caused by local anaesthetic drugs. *Br J Anaesth* 1981;53:553–554.
49. Richards L, Dorman BH, Conroy JM, Friedman RJ, Duc TA. A comparison of etidocaine versus marcaine for postoperative analgesia following interscalene block for shoulder surgery. *South Med J* 1991;84(9):2S–8.
50. Liu PL, Feldman HS, Giasi R, Patterson MK, Covino BG. Comparative CNS toxicity of lidocaine, etidocaine, bupivacaine and tetracaine in awake dogs following rapid intravenous administration. *Anesth Analg* 1983;62:375–379.
51. Morishima HO, Pederson H, Finster M, Feldman HS, Covino BG. Etidocaine toxicity in the adult, newborn and fetal sheep. *Anesthesiology* 1983;58:342–346.
52. Jackson L, Keats AS. Mechanism of brachial plexus palsy following anaesthesia. *Anesthesiology* 1965;26:190–194.
53. Garland DE, Razza BE, Waters RL. Forceful joint manipulation in head injured adults with heterotopic ossification. *Clin Orthop* 1982;169:133–138.
54. Blassingame WM, Bennett GB, Helm PA, Purdue GF, Hurst JL. Range of motion of the shoulder performed while patient is anesthetized. *J Burn Care Rehabil* 1989;10:539–542.
55. Snyder SJ. Rotator cuff lesions—Acute and chronic. *Clin Sports Med* 1991;10:595–619.
56. Russ SJ, Sonnaben DH, Tonkin M, Tyndall A. A place for surgery in arthritic diseases. *Med J Aust* 1990;152:426–430.
57. Inglis AE. Advances in implant arthroplasty in the upper extremity. *Clin Exp Rheumatol* 1989;7(S3):141–144.
58. Gschwend N. The rheumatoid shoulder. In: Stutgart, ed. *Surgical Treatment of Rheumatoid Arthritis*. New York: Thieme, 1980:35–44.
59. Peterson CJ. Painful shoulders in patients with rheumatoid arthritis. Prevalence, clinical and radiological features. *Scand J Rheumatol* 1986;15:275–279.
60. Flower RJ, Moncada S, Vane JR. Analgesic-antipyretics and anti-inflammatory agents; drugs employed in the treatment of gout. In: Gilman AG, Goodman LS, Gilman A, eds. *The Pharmacologic Basis of Therapeutics*. 6th ed. New York: MacMillan, 1980:682–716.
61. Antiarthritic drugs. In: Bennett DR, ed. *AMA Drug Evaluations*. 5th ed. Chicago: American Medical Association, 1983:107–138.
62. Hollingsworth JW, Saykaly RJ. Systemic complications of rheumatoid arthritis. *Med Clin North Am* 1977;61:217.
63. Funk D, Raymon F. Rheumatoid arthritis of the cricoarytenoid joints: An airway hazard. *Anesth Analg* 1974;54:742–744.
64. Keenan MA, Siles CM, Kaufman RL. Acquired laryngeal deviation associated with cervical spine disease in erosive polyarticular arthritis. *Anesthesiology* 1983;58:441–449.
65. Cathcart ES, Spodick DH. Rheumatoid heart disease: A study of the incidence and nature of cardiac lesions in rheumatoid arthritis. *N Engl J Med* 1962;266:959–961.
66. Lee FI, Bain AT. Chronic diffuse interstitial pulmonary fibrosis and rheumatoid arthritis. *Lancet* 1962;2:693–694.

6 Surgical Anatomy and Technique

Gordon I. Groh, M.D., and Charles A. Rockwood, Jr., M.D.

Although a number of surgical approaches for performing arthroplasty of the shoulder have been described,[1-9] the vast majority of procedures are performed through an anterior approach to the joint. The anterior, long deltopectoral approach without detaching the origin of the deltoid as described by Neer et al.[9,10] is currently the preferred approach for shoulder arthroplasty. Two important principles of this approach include preservation of the deltoid, and protection of the axillary and musculocutaneous nerves.[11]

The anterior portion of the deltoid must be preserved, since there is no effective muscle to compensate for the loss of this powerful shoulder flexor.[12] Weakness of the posterior portion of the deltoid is less disabling, since the latissimus dorsi is a strong synergistic muscle. Detachment of the anterior deltoid is problematic, since secure reattachment of this muscle following shoulder arthroplasty is difficult, and impairs postoperative rehabilitation for the patient.[13] Patients with a detached or denervated anterior deltoid after shoulder arthroplasty have a poor outcome in that they have limited motion, have decreased strength, and are extremely dissatisfied with the procedure.[14]

The relationship of the axillary and musculocutaneous nerves must always be of concern to the surgeon. Although positioning the arm in adduction and external rotation may make anterior approaches to the glenohumeral joint safer,[9,10,15] it is far better to identify the nerves and protect them during the entire surgical procedure. Burkhead et al.[12,16] have described in detail the tremendous variation, from specimen to specimen, in the course and position of these nerves. Laceration of the axillary nerve denervates the entire deltoid muscle. Since all important shoulder function requires elevation in the scapular plane, injury to the axillary nerve is the most catastrophic neurogenic injury that may occur during shoulder arthroplasty. Disastrous consequences await those surgeons who embark on a shoulder arthroplasty without an exact knowledge of the location of the axillary nerve, and fail to protect it.

ANATOMIC LANDMARKS

Three anterior prominences, the clavicle, acromion, and coracoid, are excellent guides to the placement of the incision and are intimately related to important structures in developing the exposure. The clavicle is just superior to the upper portion of the deltopectoral groove. Its position is readily palpable and marks the most superior aspect of the incision.

The acromion serves as a large surface area for attachment of the deltoid, increasing the muscle's efficiency.[5] Should wide reflection of the deltoid become necessary, the deltoid should never be released from the acromion during arthroplasty. Rather, the deltoid insertion can be released instead.[9,10,13] The interval between the acromion and coracoid process is spanned by the tough, wide coracoacromial ligament. It may be necessary to divide and resect a portion of this ligament when the rotator cuff is intact, but it must be left intact when the cuff is deficient, since this ligament serves as a buttress to anterior displacement of the humeral head.

The coracoid serves as a "lighthouse" to the deltopectoral interval.[17] It lies within the deltopectoral groove and its palpation is a landmark for the position of the cephalic vein and the brachial plexus. The cephalic vein is intimately attached to the deltoid and directly overlies the coracoid. The brachial plexus and its terminal divisions lie medial to the base of the coracoid.

NERVES

The axillary nerve is one of the two terminal branches of the posterior cord of the brachial plexus. It arises posterior to the coracoid process and crosses the anterior-inferior and then lateral border of the subscapularis muscle. At this point the nerve joins the posterior humeral circumflex artery, and together they exit posteriorly through the quadrangular space where the axillary nerve sends two branches to supply the capsule. The axillary nerve then splits into two major trunks. The posterior trunk gives off branches to the teres minor and posterior deltoid, terminating as the superior lateral cutaneous nerve. The anterior trunk passes forward around the humerus and supplies first the middle deltoid and then the anterior deltoid.[3,12,18]

The musculocutaneous nerve originates from the lateral cord of the brachial plexus and innervates the coracobrachialis muscle as well as the biceps brachii and brachialis muscles. The coracobrachialis muscle is occasionally innervated directly from the lateral cord of the brachial plexus. Flatow et al.[19] noted that the lateral portion of the musculocutaneous nerve penetrates into the coracobrachialis muscle at a distance of 3.1 to 8.2 cm from the tip of the coracoid. The most common cause of damage to this nerve during shoulder arthroplasty is overzealous retraction. Powerful retraction of the conjoint tendon, made up of the short head of the biceps and the coracobrachialis, may produce a traction injury to the musculocutaneous nerve. Careful attention to retraction should minimize this possibility.

SURGICAL APPROACH

Although a posterior approach for shoulder arthroplasty has been described, Neer et al.[9,10] delineated the disadvantages of this approach for an arthroplasty: (1) Obstruction to exposure is created by the posterior aspect of the acromion. (2) Release of internal rotation contractures by this approach is hazardous. (3) Division and repair of the infraspinatus tendon, which is far more variable in its quality than the subscapularis tendon, is required.

Neer et al.[9,10] described the development of the currently preferred anterior surgical approach. Initially, a short deltopectoral approach with detachment of the anterior portion of the deltoid from the clavicle was used, but this weakened the muscle. During 1976 and 1977, Neer utilized a superior approach with detachment of the middle section of the deltoid; however, this approach was found to weaken the middle part of the deltoid. In September 1977, Neer[9] began to exclusively utilize the long deltopectoral approach, which has become the standard for shoulder arthroplasty because of the greater ease of rehabilitation after surgery, and is the technique described here.

SURGICAL TECHNIQUE

The patient is positioned on the operating room table in the semi-Fowler position with the legs parallel to the floor to avoid dependency (Figure 6–1A). The standard headrest from the operating table is removed and replaced with either a Mayfield or McConnell headrest. This allows the patient to be positioned at the top and edge of the table (Figure 6–1B,C), which is necessary in order to extend the externally rotated arm off the side of the table down towards the floor, enabling the surgeon to ream the intramedullary canal and insert the prosthesis. The patient's head can then be secured

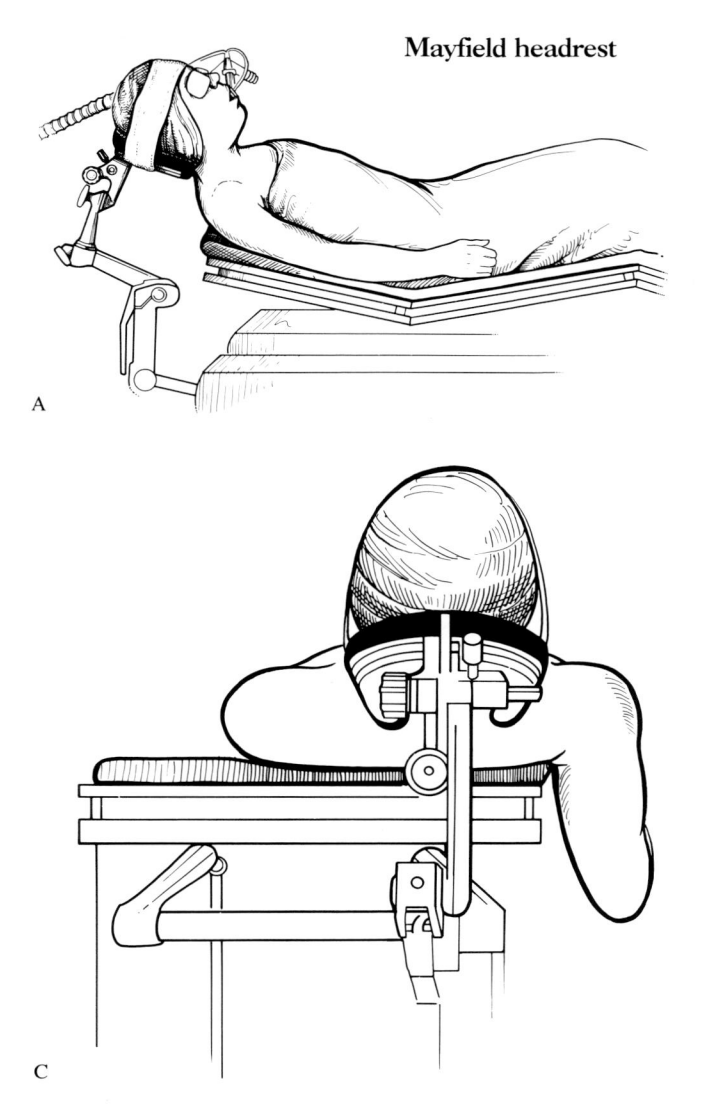

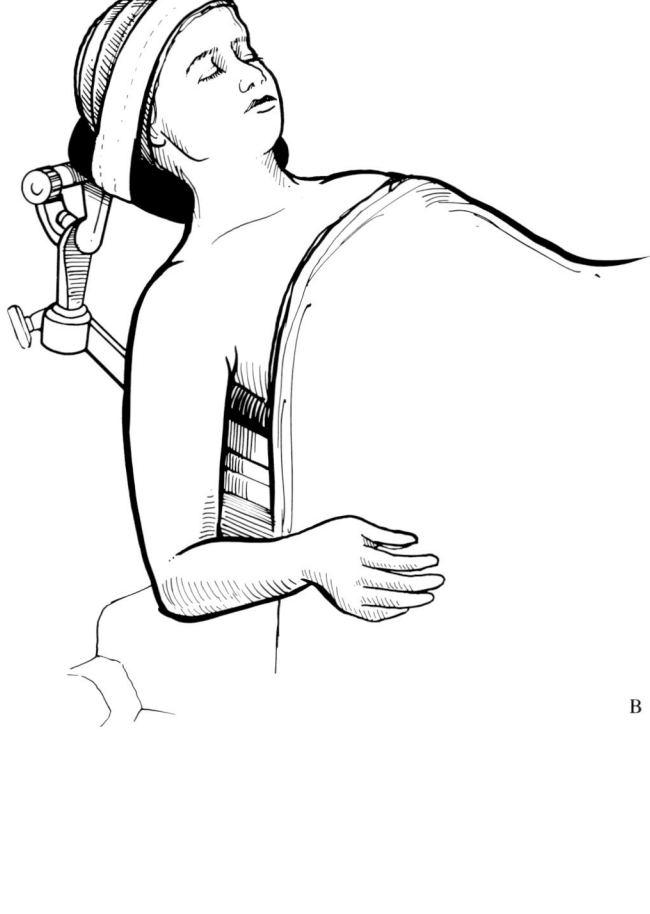

Figure 6–1. A–C. Position of the patient on the operating table with the head supported by a Mayfield or McConnell headrest.

82 Arthroplasty of the Shoulder

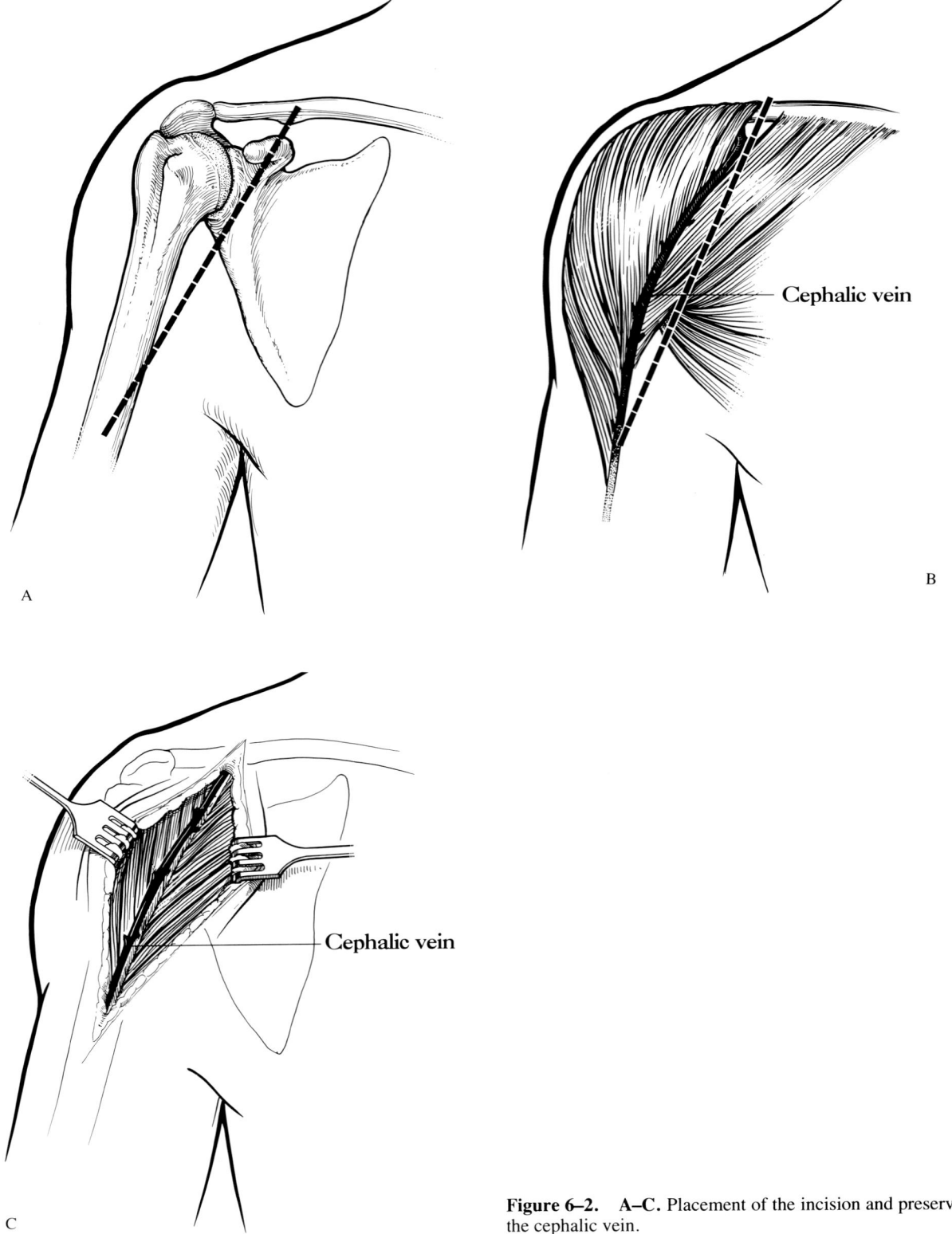

Figure 6–2. **A–C.** Placement of the incision and preservation of the cephalic vein.

to the headrest with tape if the patient is under general anesthesia. Care should be taken to rest the head in a position that avoids hyperextension or tilting of the neck, which may cause compression of the cervical roots.

Plastic towel drapes can be used to block out the area being prepped and to isolate the anesthesia equipment from the operative field. The entire upper extremity is prepped and the arm is draped free. The axilla is separated as much as possible from the sterile surgical field. After the skin incision is marked, the surgical site is covered with adherent plastic drapes.

The skin incision is made in a straight line with the arm held in 30 degrees of abduction (Figure 6–2A,B). The incision should begin from the superior aspect of the clavicle, over the top of the coracoid, and extend down the anterior aspect of the arm. Once the incision has been made, the cephalic vein near the deltopectoral interval should be identified (Figure 6–2C) and saved, since postoperative extremity swelling and pain will be decreased by its preservation. The vein is usually intimately associated with the deltoid, because of the many feeding vessels from the deltoid into the cephalic vein. It is for this reason that the authors recommend the cephalic vein be taken laterally with the deltoid muscle. The feeding vessels coming into the vein from the region of the pectoralis major muscle should be clamped and tied, allowing retraction of the deltoid muscle with the vein laterally. The deep surface of the deltoid is then freed from the underlying tissues using a combination of blunt and sharp dissection all the way from its origin on the clavicle down to its insertion onto the humeral shaft. On occasion, as recommended by Neer,[9,10] it may be necessary to partially free the insertion of the deltoid from the humeral shaft.

When the deep surface of the deltoid has been completely freed, abduct and externally rotate the arm. Protect the exposed surface of the deltoid with a moist sponge and retract the deltoid laterally with two Richardson retractors or a deltoid retractor. Then, retract the conjoined tendon medially with a Richardson retractor. Only in unusual circumstances is it necessary to release a portion of the conjoined tendon or divide the coracoid process for additional exposure.

The tendon of the upper portion of the pectoralis major is identified and the upper portion of the tendon is released with an electrocautery cutting blade to aid in the exposure of the inferior aspect of the joint (Figure 6–3). Care must be taken to avoid injury to the long head of the biceps tendon during this maneuver. If the patient has a marked internal rotation contracture, most of the pectoralis major tendon can be released from its insertion. This tendon release should not be repaired at the completion of the operation.

The anterior humeral circumflex vessels are then identified in the lower one-third of the subscapularis tendon. The vessels are then isolated, clamped, and ligated (Figure 6–4). Due to the extensive anastomoses of blood supply in this area, other sources of bleeding should be expected and controlled with electrocautery during release of the subscapularis tendon.

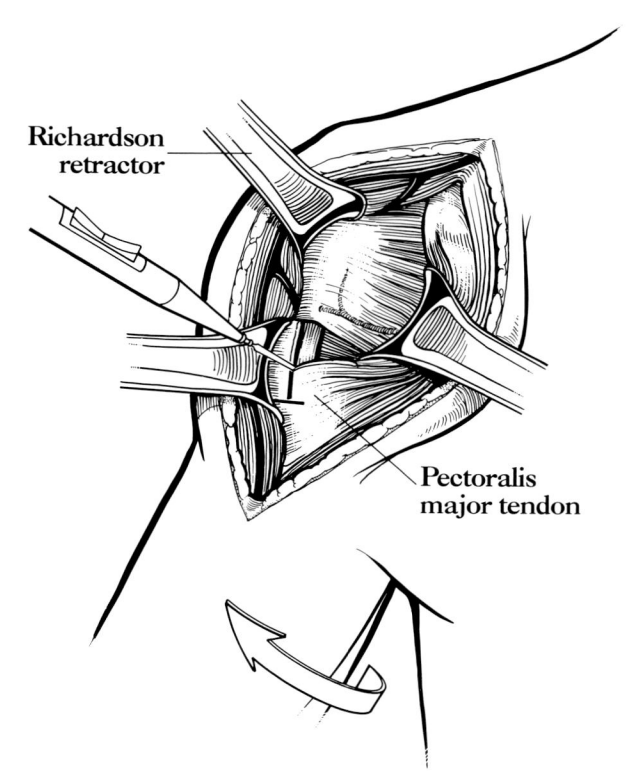

Figure 6–3. Release of the upper portion of the pectoralis major tendon to aid in exposure. The tendon should not be repaired at the completion of the operation.

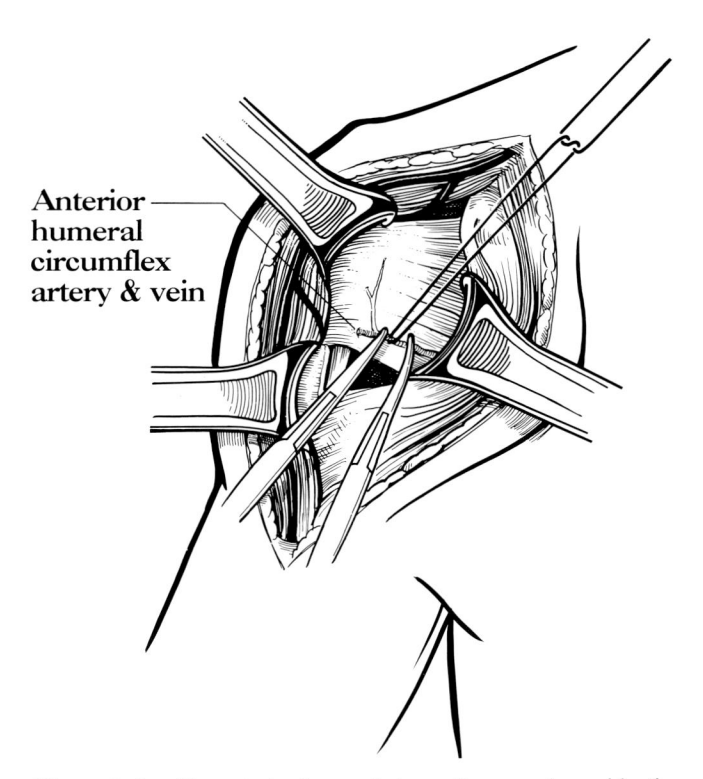

Figure 6–4. The anterior humeral circumflex vessels are identified and ligated.

It is now important to identify the musculocutaneous and axillary nerves. Palpate the musculocutaneous nerve as it comes from the brachial plexus into the medial aspect of the conjoined tendon (Figure 6–5A). The nerve usually penetrates the muscle about 4 to 5 cm inferior to the tip of the coracoid, but in some instances the nerve has a higher penetration into the conjoined muscle-tendon unit.[17,20] The proximity of this nerve must be kept in mind during retraction of the conjoined tendon.

The axillary nerve is then located by passing the volar surface of the index finger down along the anterior surface of the subscapularis muscle (Figure 6–5B). The finger is then rotated and hooked anteriorly to identify the axillary nerve (Figure 6–5C). Scarring and adhesions may result in the nerve being plastered onto the anterior surface of the subscapularis on occasion. This situation makes identification of the nerve difficult. When this occurs, an elevator can be passed along the anterior surface of the subscapularis muscle

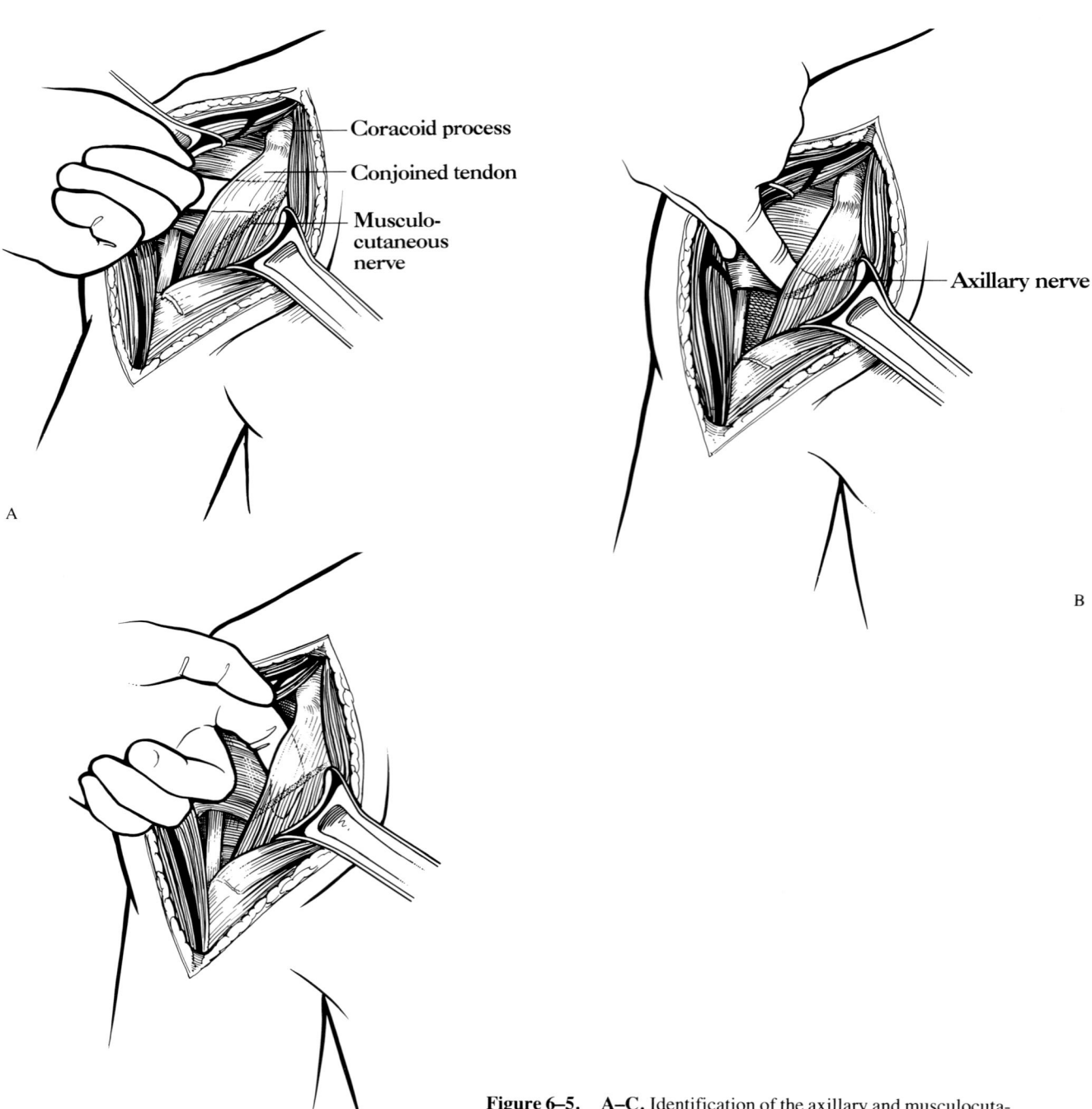

Figure 6–5. A–C. Identification of the axillary and musculocutaneous nerves.

to create an interval between the muscle and the nerve. Always identify the axillary nerve and carefully retract and hold it out of the way, especially during the critical steps of releasing and resecting the anterior-inferior capsule.

The amount of passive external rotation present at this point in the procedure determines the specific technique for subscapularis tendon release. If the shoulder can be externally rotated 35 degrees or more, simply divide the subscapularis tendon 1.5 cm medial to its insertion, after tagging it with stay sutures.

If the patient has only 15 to 20 degrees of external rotation, release the tendon from its insertion into the lesser tuberosity, just medial to the long head of the biceps tendon (Figure 6–6A). At the time of closure, the tendon is repaired to the cut surface of the humerus using a nonabsorbable heavy suture (Figure 6–6B). If the patient's shoulder has less than 15 degrees of external rotation, then lengthen the tendon using a coronal Z-plasty technique (Figure 6–6C,D). Each centimeter of tendon lengthened will equal approximately 20 degrees of additional external rotation. When the coronal Z-plasty procedure is performed, include the capsule on the lateral stump of the tendon for additional strength. At the time of closure, the subscapularis tendon should be repaired with heavy nonabsorbable 1-mm surgical tape.

After the subscapularis tendon has been released, free the tendon of any scarring or adhesions from the back of the coracoid process and the capsule as it attaches onto the anterior glenoid rim, so it once again becomes a dynamic muscle-tendon unit. This process requires that the subscapularis muscle-tendon unit be released 360 degrees around its border. This usually requires a fair amount of soft-tissue dissection along the anterior aspect of the neck of the scapula. During this dissection, it is imperative to identify, protect, and retract the axillary nerve with a Scoffield-type retractor. It is important to have a free, dynamic, and functioning subscapularis muscle-tendon unit at the time of its repair.

On occasion, the capsule is divided or released with the subscapularis tendon. If that occurs, the anterior capsule must be dissected from the posterior surface of the subscapularis so that a free, dynamic subscapularis tendon can be obtained. A Scoffield retractor can be used to retract the previously identified axillary nerve away from the inferior capsule. Externally rotate the arm to place tension on the capsule. The anterior-inferior capsule should be released from the humerus all the way inferiorly to at least the 6 o'clock position, even in the presence of a large inferior osteophyte (Figure 6–7A). Failure to do so will make it very difficult to deliver the head up and out of the glenoid fossa. This can be achieved using a knife or electrocautery blade. Once the capsule has been released, pass a small bone hook around and under the neck of the humerus. With a large Darrach retractor in the joint and a bone hook around the neck of the humerus, the arm is externally rotated, adducted, and

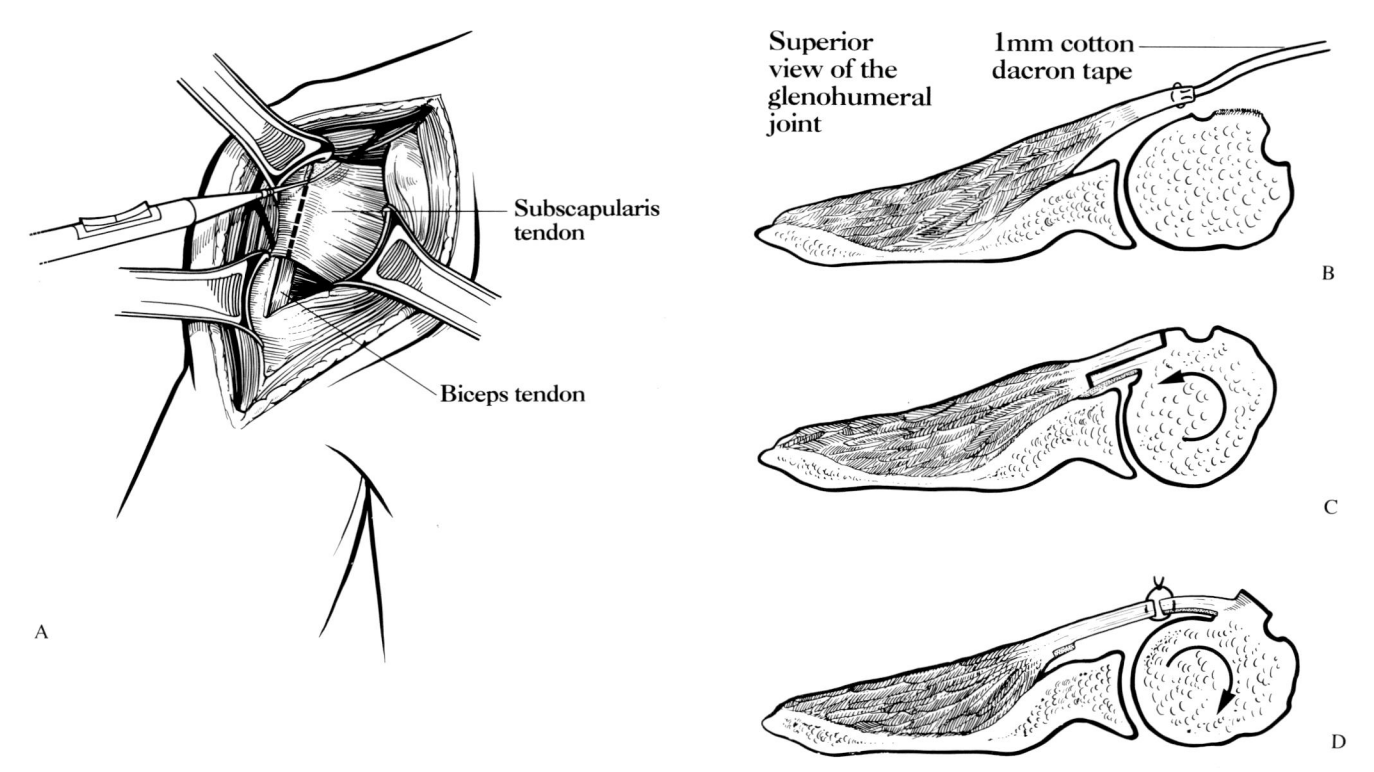

Figure 6–6. **A** and **B.** Release of the subscapularis tendon at its insertion onto the lesser tuberosity and repair to the cut surface of the neck of the humerus using a heavy nonabsorbable suture. **C** and **D.** In cases in which the patient has less than 20 degrees of external rotation, lengthen the subscapularis tendon using a coronal Z-plasty technique.

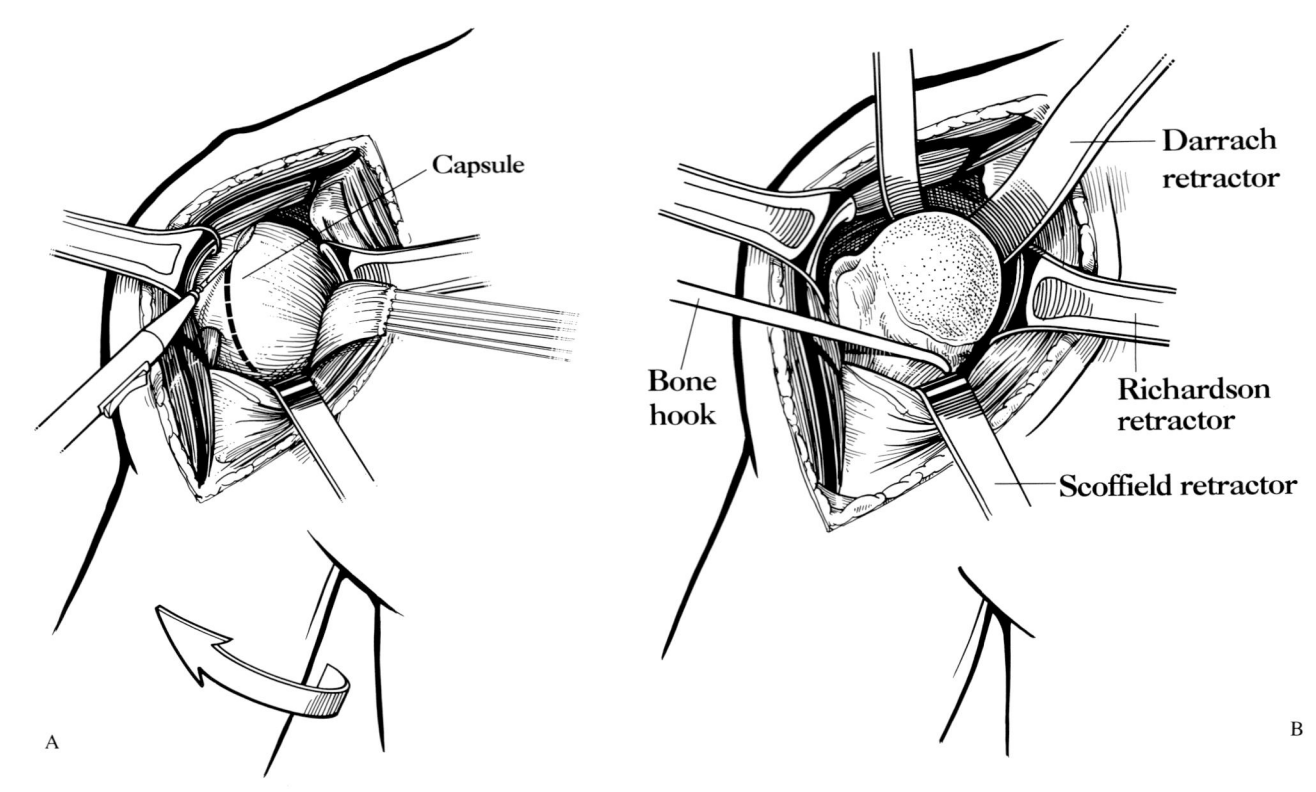

Figure 6–7. A and B. Resection of the anterior-inferior capsule and dislocation of the humeral head.

extended to deliver the head up and out of the glenoid fossa (Figure 6–7B). If the humeral head cannot be delivered in this fashion, the inferior capsule is likely still intact and must be completely released. It is important to obtain this exposure with the arm extended off the side of the table in external rotation before proceeding with humeral head resection.

TECHNIQUE FOR NONCONSTRAINED SHOULDER ARTHROPLASTY

Resection of Humeral Head

Resection of the humeral head is a critical part of the procedure. When there is no posterior glenoid erosion, as exhibited on an axillary lateral radiograph or computerized tomographic scan, the humeral head should be removed with the arm in 30 to 35 degrees of external rotation. This can be accomplished by flexing the elbow 90 degrees and then externally rotating the arm 30 to 35 degrees (Figure 6–8).

The varus-valgus angle of the head to be removed is determined using a humeral osteotomy template. Place the template along the anterior aspect of the arm parallel to the shaft of the humerus, and mark the angle at which the head will be removed with an electrocautery blade (Figure 6–9A). The superior-lateral portion of the mark should be at the junction of the articular surface with the attachment of the rotator cuff on the greater tuberosity. In many instances, the inferior portion of the mark will be medial to the inferior osteophyte of the flattened and deformed humeral head (Figure 6–9B). Using the osteotomy template will ensure that the prosthesis sits properly on the supporting medial neck of the humerus. If the resection is in too much of a varus position, then support for the collar of the prosthesis will be compromised (Figure 6–9C,D).

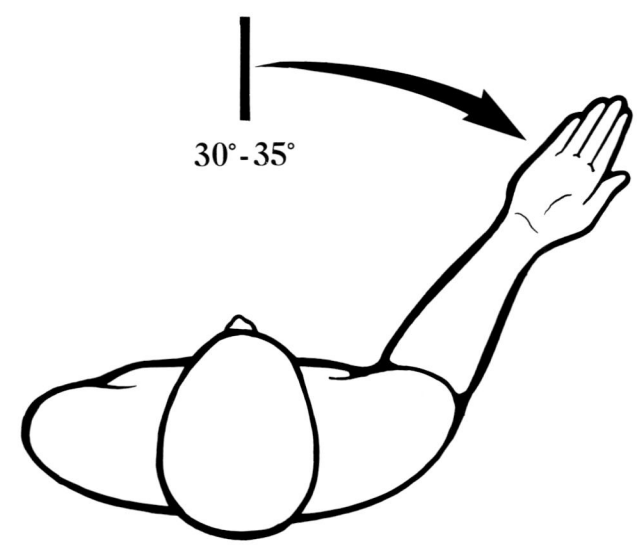

Figure 6–8. Arm position for resection of the humeral head.

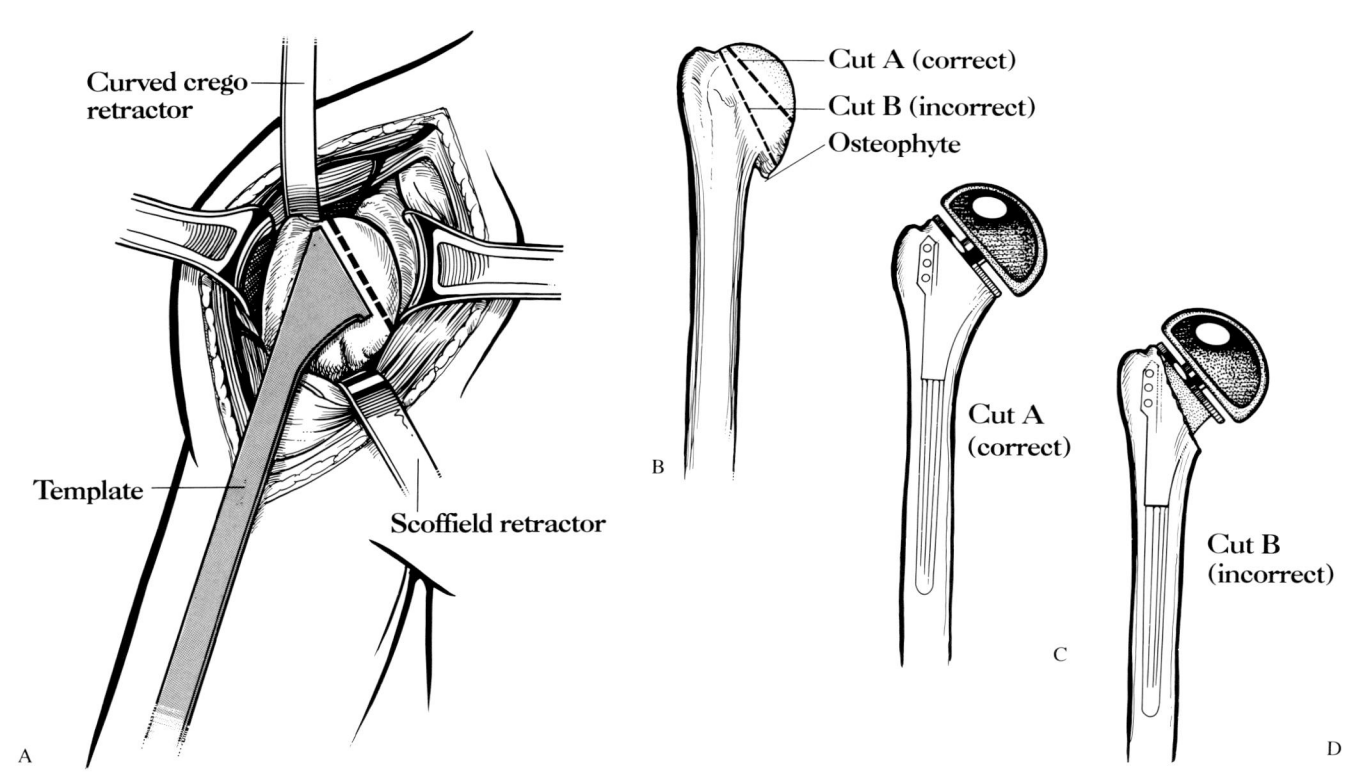

Figure 6–9. Marking the varus-valgus angle for resection of the humeral head using a template (**A**). Excess resection leads to insufficient support for the prosthesis on the neck of the humerus (**B–D**).

If a preoperative axillary lateral radiograph or computerized tomogram has shown posterior glenoid erosion, then several options are available: Remove the anterior half of the glenoid with an air burr or a glenoid reamer, graft bone to the posterior glenoid, or resect the humeral head with the arm in less than 30 to 35 degrees of external rotation. For example, if there is 20 degrees of posterior glenoid erosion, then the head should be resected with the arm externally rotated only 15 to 20 degrees.

Before the oscillating saw or osteotome is used to remove the head, the biceps tendon and insertions of the supraspinatus, infraspinatus, and teres minor into the proximal part of the humerus must be protected. Pass a curved Crego or a small Darrach retractor under the biceps and curl it around to protect these structures during humeral head resection (Figure 6–10). With a large Darrach retractor in the joint, a sagittal power saw or osteotome can be used to remove the humeral head at the predetermined angle.

Once the humeral head has been removed, use a bone hook in combination with extension and external rotation of the arm off the side of the table to deliver the cancellous bone surface of the proximal end of the humerus up and out of the incision (Figure 6–11A). Once again, positioning of the patient on the operating room table is extremely important, since it is exceedingly difficult to insert the medullary canal reamers, as well as the prosthesis, unless the arm can be extended off the side of the table (Figure 6–11B,C).

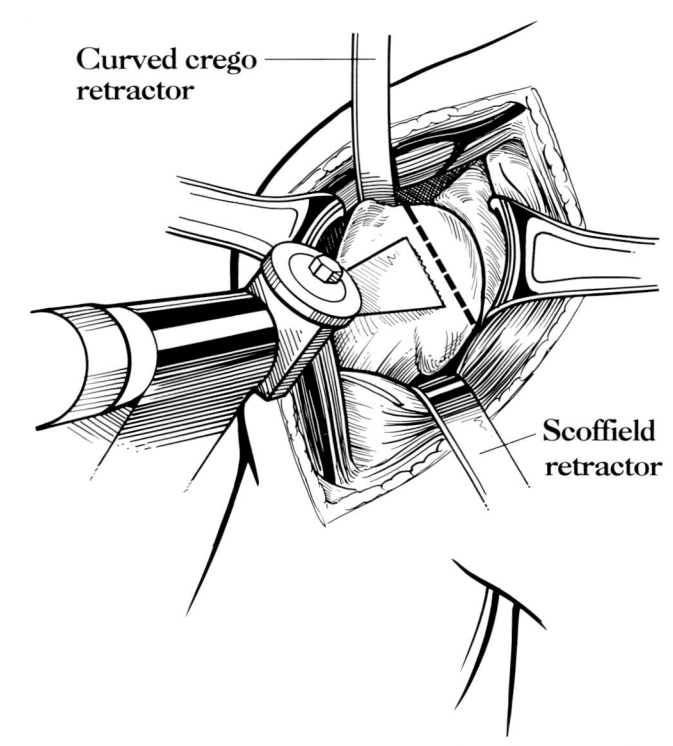

Figure 6–10. The biceps tendon and insertion of the supraspinatus, infraspinatus, and teres minor tendons into the proximal part of the humerus are protected with a Crego retractor prior to humeral head removal.

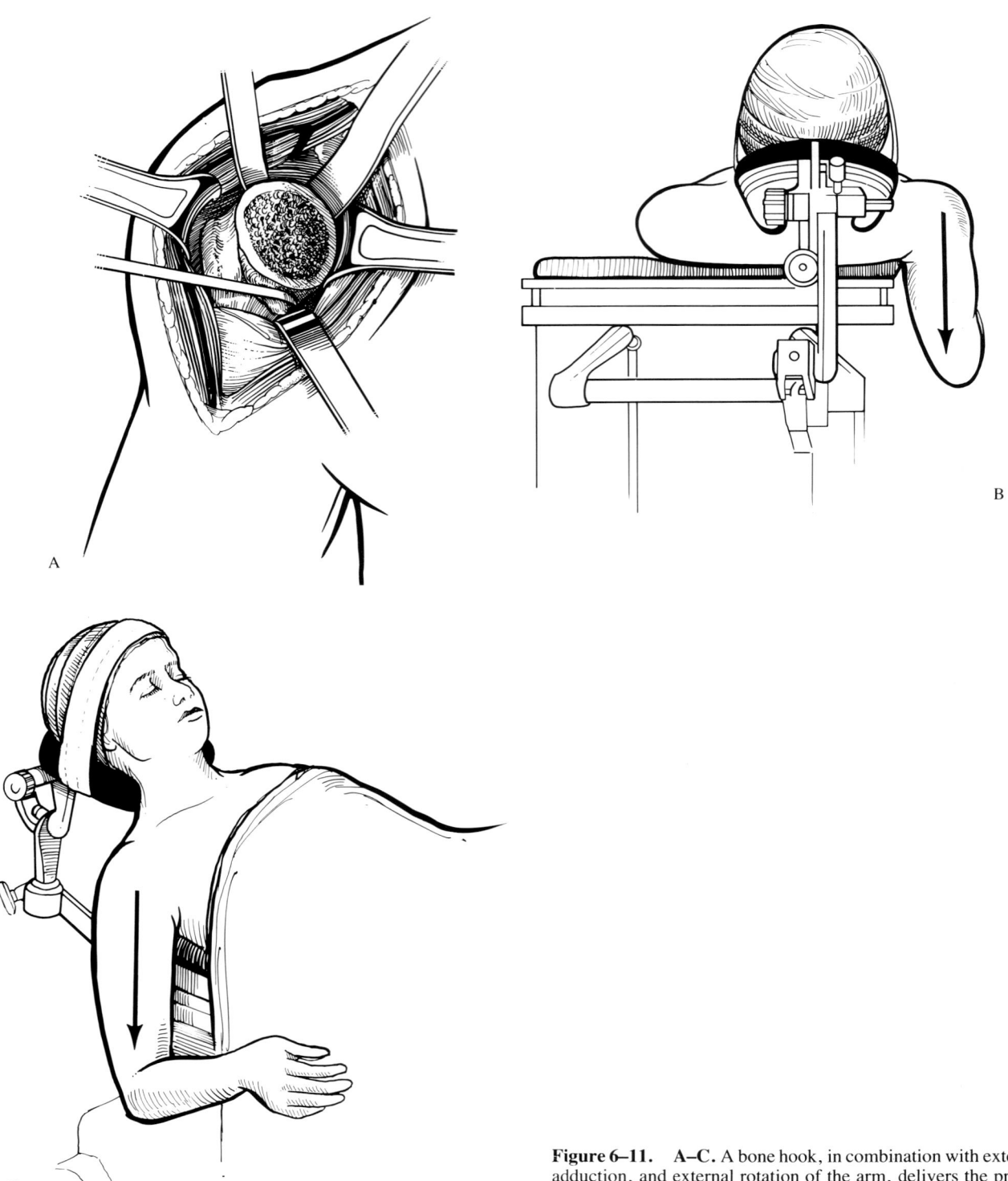

Figure 6–11. **A–C.** A bone hook, in combination with extension, adduction, and external rotation of the arm, delivers the proximal part of the humerus up and out of the incision.

A 6-mm medullary canal reamer is used to start a pilot hole in the superior-lateral cancellous surface of the bone so the reamer will pass directly down the intramedullary canal (Figure 6–12A,B). The humeral reamer is inserted down the humerus until the top flute pattern is at the level of the cut surface of the bone. Once the initial reamer is seated, proceed with the 8-mm, 10-mm, and 12-mm reamers until the reamer begins to bite on the cortical bone of the intramedullary canal. The final reamer size chosen will determine the stem size of the final broach and implant.

The body-sizing osteotome matching the size of the final reamer is selected. If a 12-mm reamer was used, then a 12-mm body-sizing osteotome and 12-mm intramedullary rod would be selected. The rod is then threaded into the osteotome body and inserted down the intramedullary canal (Figure 6–13A). The rod placed down into the reamed canal prevents the sizing osteotome from drifting into a varus position. The collar of the body-sizing osteotome is used to determine proper rotation prior to cutting the bone. When the lateral fin of the osteotome touches the greater tuberosity, slide the collar down the osteotome until it touches the cancellous bone. Then rotate the osteotome until the collar lies flat on the cut-bone surface. Slide the collar up before driving down the osteotome.

Driving the body-sizing osteotome down into the cancellous bone accomplishes three things. First, it cuts out the appropriate amount of bone to receive the lateral fin of the body broach in the area of the greater tuberosity. Second, it creates the anterior, posterior, and inferior fin tracks. Finally, it outlines the amount of cancellous bone that will need to be removed before seating the broach and the prosthesis (Figure 6–13B). The bone can be removed with a rongeur or small osteotome prior to inserting the body broach. If the bone in the proximal part of the humerus is not removed, a fracture of the proximal humerus could occur when the body broaches are driven down into place.

Broaching is done in a sequential manner starting with a smaller broach and gradually increasing to the correct size. The correct stem and body size has already been determined from the intramedullary reaming and size of the body-sizing osteotome used. If, for example, a 12-mm reamer and 12-mm body-sizing osteotome were used, then attach the driver-extractor to the 10/10 broach and lock it into position (Figure 6–14A). Following the fin tracks previously established with the sizing osteotome, seat the 10/10 broach. This broach is then removed, and the 12/12 broach is then seated. Sequential broaching ensures progressive removal of bone to reduce the possibility of fracturing the humeral shaft.

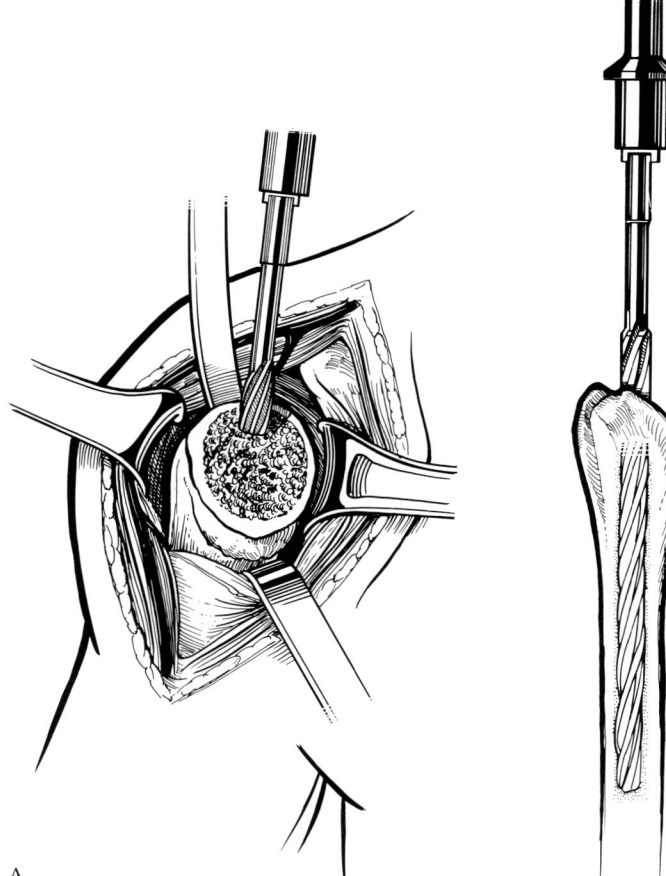

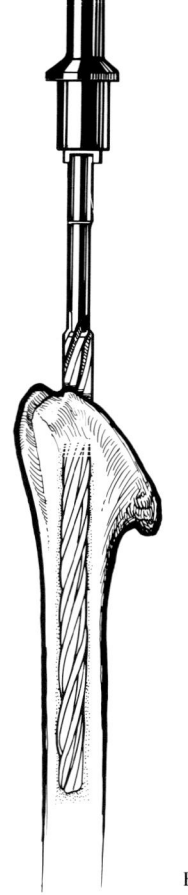

Figure 6–12. **A** and **B.** A 6-mm reamer is placed eccentrically, as superiorly as possible, to enter the medullary canal.

90 Arthroplasty of the Shoulder

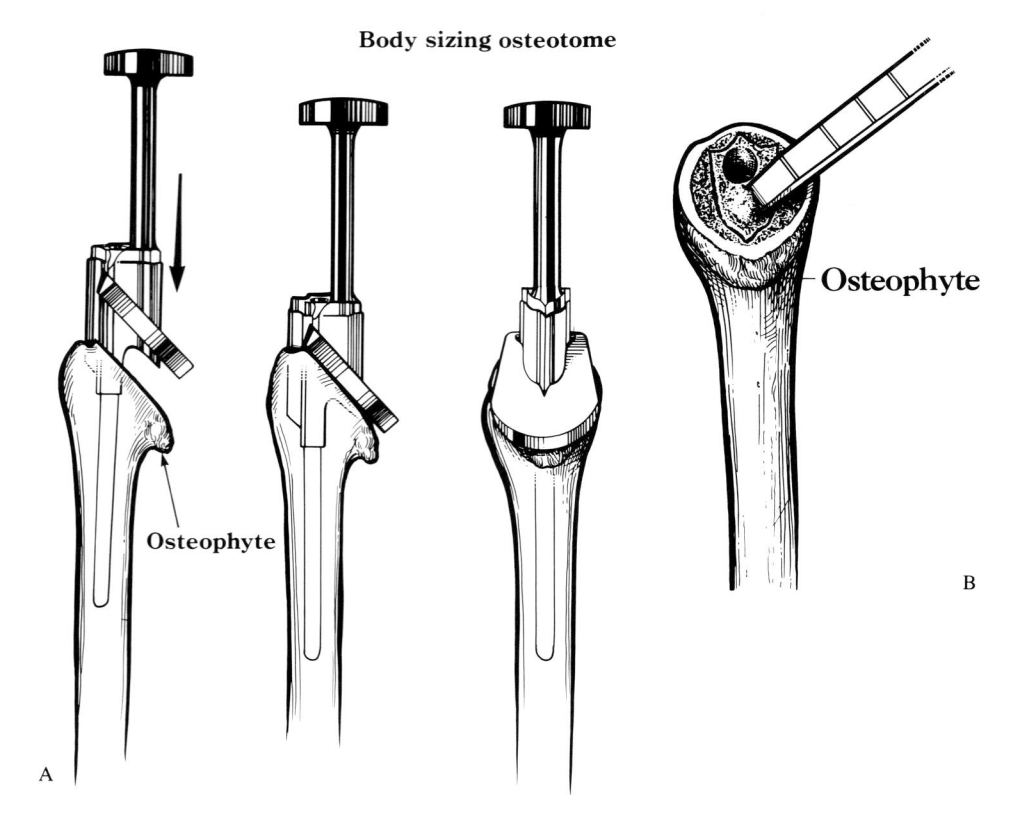

Figure 6–13. **A.** The body-sizing osteotome is inserted down the reamed canal. The body-sizing osteotome collar is used to determine proper rotation prior to cutting the bone. When the collar lies flat along the cut surface of the bone, the proper rotation is ensured. **B.** After removing the body-sizing osteotome, the proper amount of cancellous bone to extract from the proximal end of the humerus is outlined and removed using an osteotome, prior to insertion of the broaches.

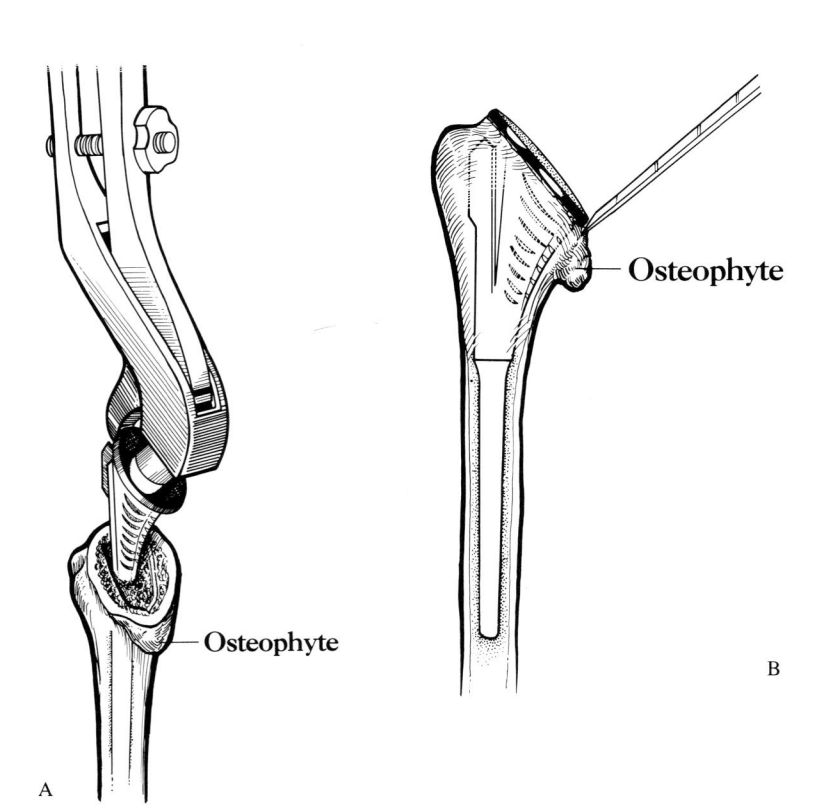

Figure 6–14. **A** and **B.** Insertion of the broach and removal of inferior osteophytes.

While broaching, be sure to maintain proper version of the broach by following the previously cut fin tracks. If the proximal part of the humerus is large in proportion to the intramedullary canal, a mismatched humeral body-stem combination is available. If the intramedullary canal was reamed to 12 mm and the proximal part of the humerus is quite large, then a 14/12 broach and prosthesis could be used. If a larger body size is selected for better fit in the proximal end of the humerus, then the appropriate body-sizing osteotome with rod must be utilized before inserting a larger broach. The humeral prosthesis is approximately 1 mm larger than the corresponding broach size, so a press-fit can be obtained. However, the prosthesis may be easily cemented, if indicated.

With the final broach in place, remove any osteophytes extending inferiorly from the cut surface of the medial humeral neck using an osteotome and/or rongeurs (Figure 6–14B). While the glenoid fossa is being evaluated and prepared, one of the body broaches should be left in place to protect the proximal humerus from compression fractures or deformation by retractors.

With the broach in place, use a humeral head retractor to displace the proximal end of the humerus posteriorly to expose the glenoid fossa (Figure 6–15A). The Scofield retractor should again be utilized to protect the axillary nerve as the labrum and thickened anterior-inferior capsule is removed. The capsule should be dissected and then resected free from the posterior surface of the subscapularis tendon. If the capsule is not excised and left in place to be reattached to the humerus, then it can restrict external rotation postoperatively. Resection of the anterior-inferior capsule will not lead to any instability of the joint.

A variety of glenoid sizer discs are utilized to determine the proper size of the glenoid (Figure 6–15B). Select the one that best fits the size of the glenoid fossa. Since the normal shoulder joint allows anterior-posterior translation of the head in the glenoid fossa,[21] glenoid prostheses have been developed with a radius of curvature 3 mm larger than the corresponding humeral head. If a 52 mm size glenoid is selected, then a short, medium, or long 52-mm humeral head, which allows for a 3-mm mismatch between the prosthetic head and glenoid, should be used.

If the humerus can be sufficiently displaced posteriorly to use motorized glenoid preparation equipment, then create a hole in the center of the glenoid fossa using either a punch or air burr (Figure 6–16). Attach the gold-colored, anodized drill guide to the handle and place it into the glenoid fossa over the centering hole. Insert the gold-colored anodized drill bit into the guide and drill (Figure 6–17A). It is important that the drill bit be perfectly centered in the drill guide and the power engaged before the bit comes into contact with the bone. If the bit is not properly aligned in the guide, the bit will bind in the guide, which can cause damage to the drill and other instruments (Figure 6–17B).

If the joint is so tight that the longer gold-colored, anodized drill bit cannot be inserted, the shorter silver bit

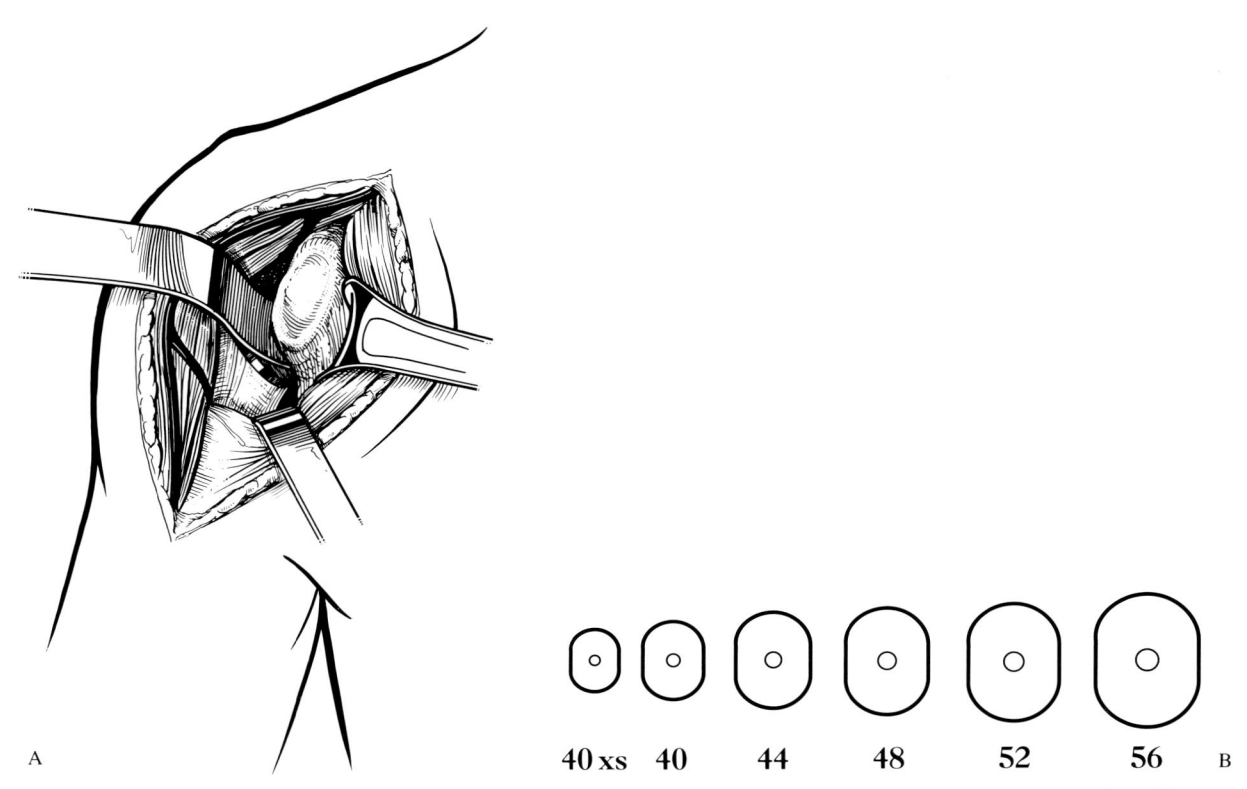

Figure 6–15. A humeral head retractor is used to expose the glenoid fossa (**A**), which is sized using the sizer discs (**B**).

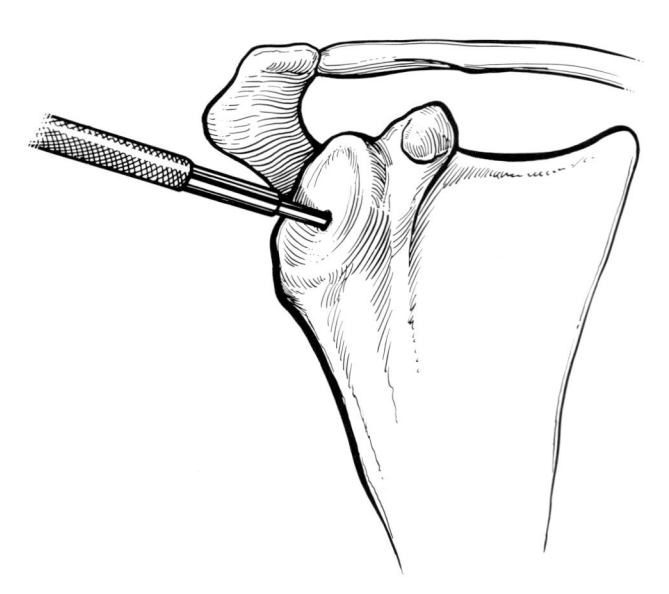

Figure 6–16. A central hole is placed in the glenoid fossa with a punch or air burr in preparation for placement of the pegged glenoid.

may be used to create the central drill hole. After "bottoming out" the silver drill bit, the central drill guide should be removed and the drilling resumed until the silver drill bit bottoms out. The depth of the central drill hole using the silver bit without using the central drill guide will be the same as if the longer gold anodized drill bit with the guide had been used.

Next, attach to the drill the glenoid reamer that best fits the size of the glenoid fossa. Insert the hub of the reamer into the central hole and ream the glenoid until it has a smooth configuration that matches the size of the previously selected glenoid (Figure 6–18A,B). This ensures a perfect fit between the back of the glenoid prosthesis and the face of the glenoid. Again, the power should be engaged to the glenoid reamer while the tip of the reamer is in the pilot hole but before it comes in contact with the bone. If the reamer is held tightly against the glenoid before the power is started, then the reamer may bind and cause damage to the power drill and bone.

The silver-colored peripheral drill guide is now attached to the handle. The central peg on the drill guide slips into the hole previously drilled in the center of the glenoid fossa. Use the silver-colored drill bit, which is shorter than the gold anodized drill bit, to create four peripheral holes in the glenoid fossa (Figure 6–19). Drill the superior hole first, and then place the antirotation peg to prevent any rotation of the guide while the other holes are being drilled. Insert the previously selected, trial pegged glenoid prosthesis and keep it in place during sizing of the trial humeral head (Figure 6–20). The final pegged glenoid prosthesis is slightly smaller than the trial prosthesis, to allow room for cement.

If the proximal end of the humerus cannot be displaced posteriorly enough to use the drill bit because of a tight or

Long gold-anodized drill bit

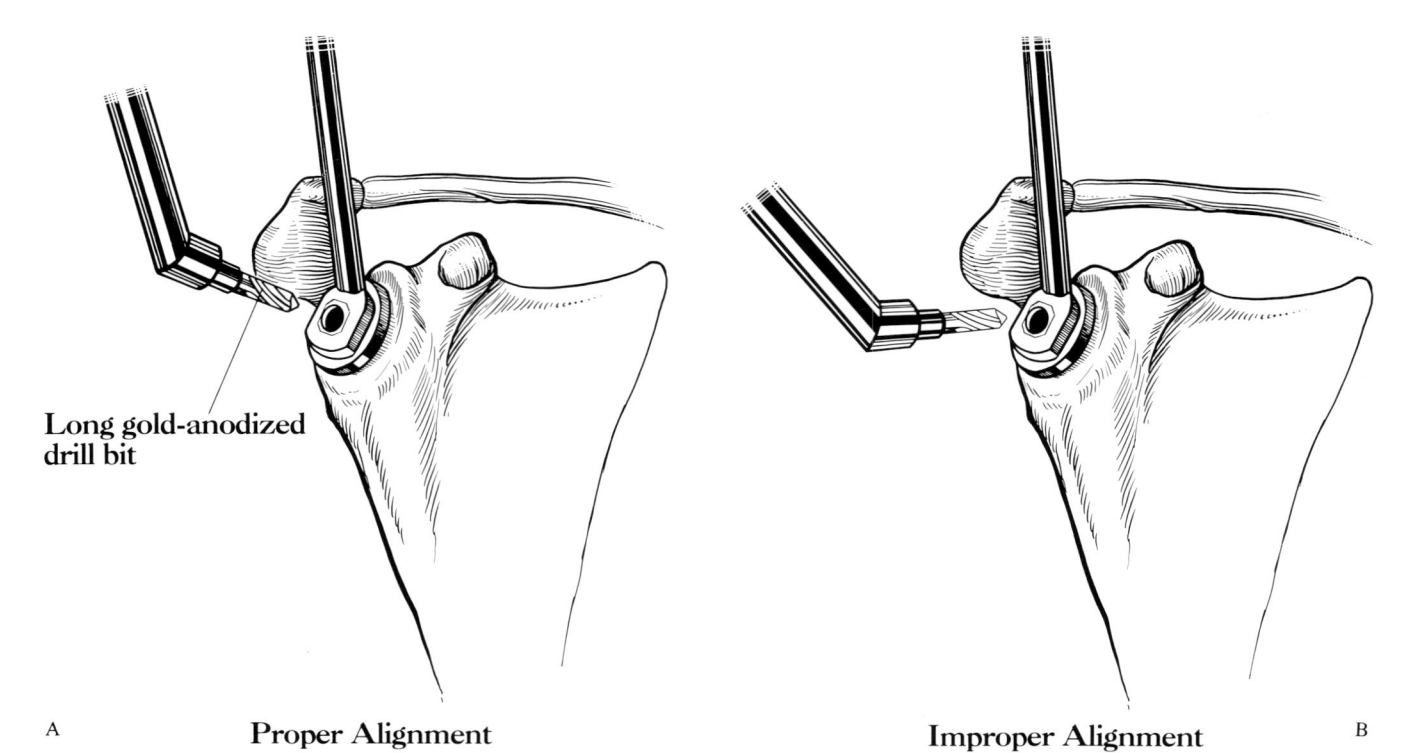

A   **Proper Alignment**   **Improper Alignment**   B

Figure 6–17. **A** and **B.** The gold anodized drill and drill guide are used to drill the central hole. The drill must be placed straight into the drill guide and powered to "drill" before the drill comes into contact with the bone.

Surgical Anatomy and Technique 93

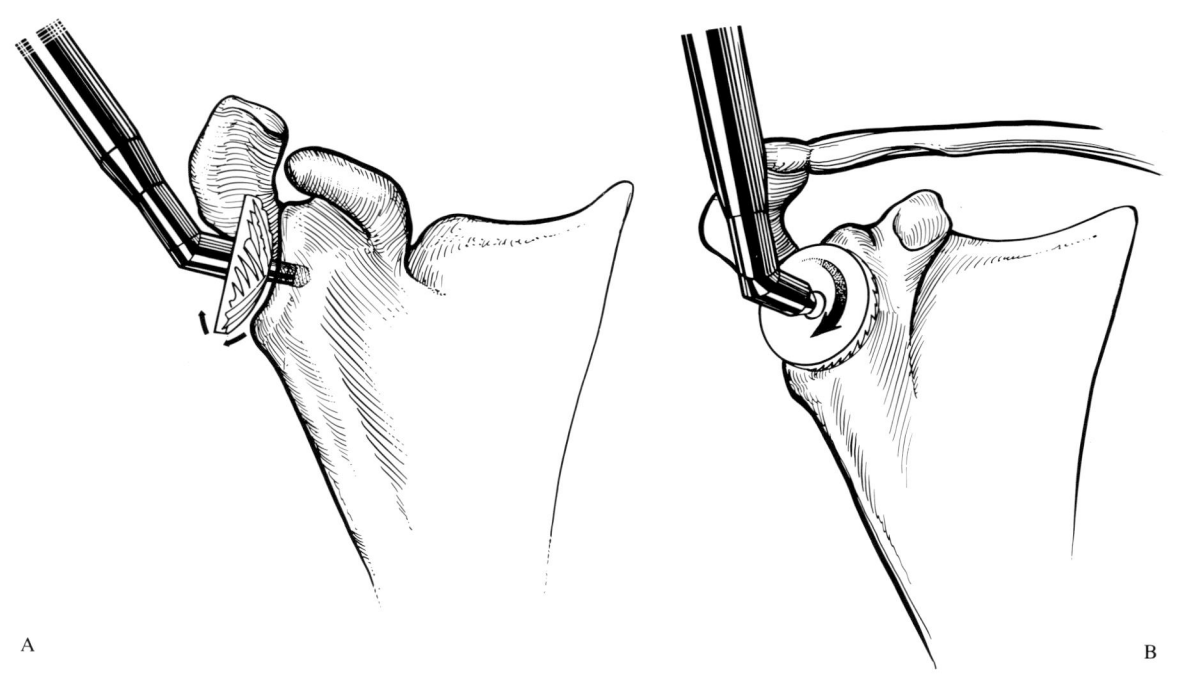

Figure 6–18. A and B. Reaming the glenoid fossa.

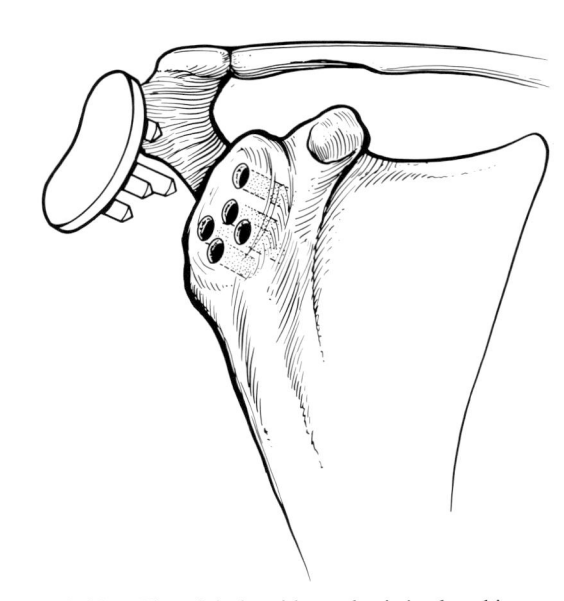

Figure 6–20. The trial glenoid prosthesis is placed into position.

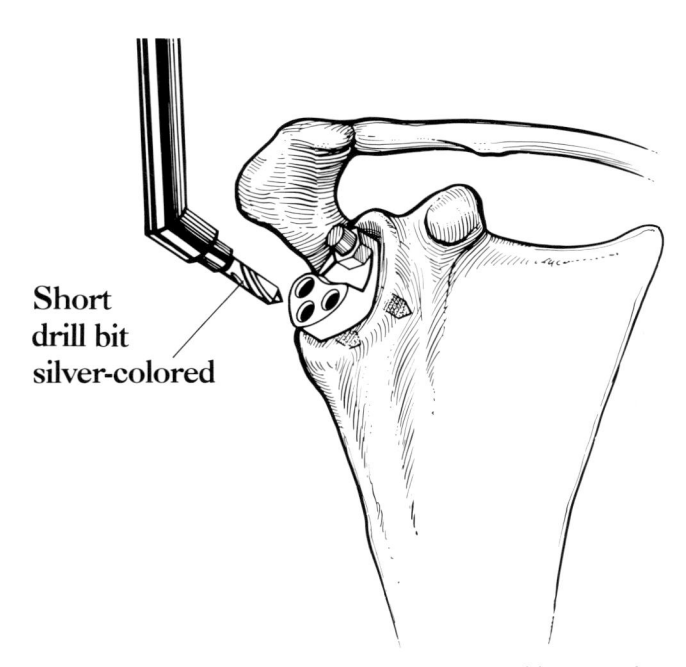

Figure 6–19. The silver-colored drill and drill guide are used to create the four peripheral holes in the glenoid fossa.

heavily muscled shoulder, then the keeled glenoid component should be used. To utilize the keeled component, use an air burr to partially create a slot in the glenoid fossa. Then insert the hub of the appropriate-size glenoid reamer into the slot and ream the glenoid until it has a smooth configuration that matches the size of the previously selected glenoid component. Continue to use the air burr with curettes to remove enough bone to receive the keel (Figure 6–21A). Evacuate cancellous bone in the base of the coracoid and down the lateral border of the scapula to help lock in the keeled prosthesis with cement (Figure 6–21B). The keel of the final prosthesis is slightly smaller than the trial prosthesis, to accommodate cement.

With the trial glenoid prosthesis and appropriately sized humeral broach in place, select a suitable short, medium, or long humeral head (Figure 6–22). The size of the head has been previously determined by the glenoid size selection. Selecting a humeral head of the appropriate length allows the soft tissues to be balanced with proper tension. With the correct head size in place, a stable configuration of the joint without gross anterior or posterior instability should be achieved. In addition, it should be possible to reapproximate the subscapularis tendon back to bone and have at least 30 to 35 degrees of external rotation. With the arm in 90 degrees of abduction, 20 to 30 degrees of internal rotation should be achieved. If the fit of the humeral head is so tight that functional internal or external rotation cannot be obtained, then a shorter head should be used. Similarly, if gross anterior or posterior instability exists, a longer head should be utilized.

With the broach in place and the trial humeral head removed, displace the humerus posteriorly to prepare the

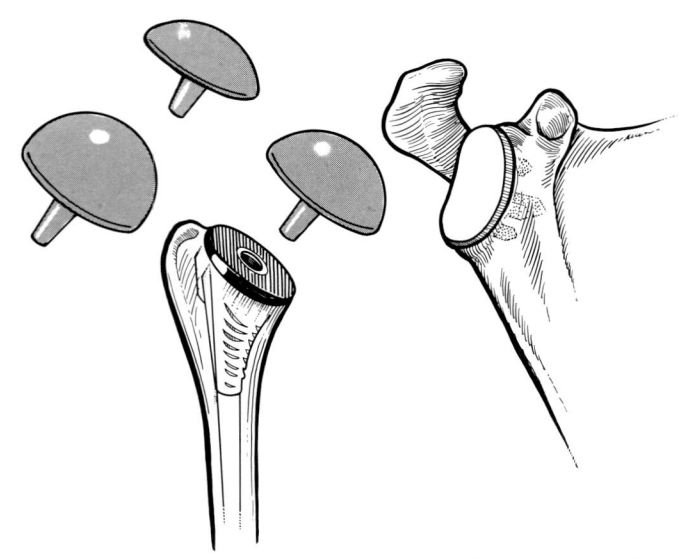

Figure 6–22. With the trial glenoid prosthesis in place and the appropriate-size humeral broach in place, select the appropriate short, medium, or long humeral head.

glenoid fossa for insertion of the glenoid prosthesis. Insert a probe into each of the drilled holes to determine if the holes have exited the anterior or posterior cortex of the glenoid. If exit holes are found, it is important to not put an excessive amount of cement into the holes, where it could extrude out and possibly damage the surrounding soft tissues.

Carefully irrigate and/or use pulsatile lavage to remove any clotted blood from the holes. For hemostasis, spray thrombin and insert a piece of surgical gauze into each of the

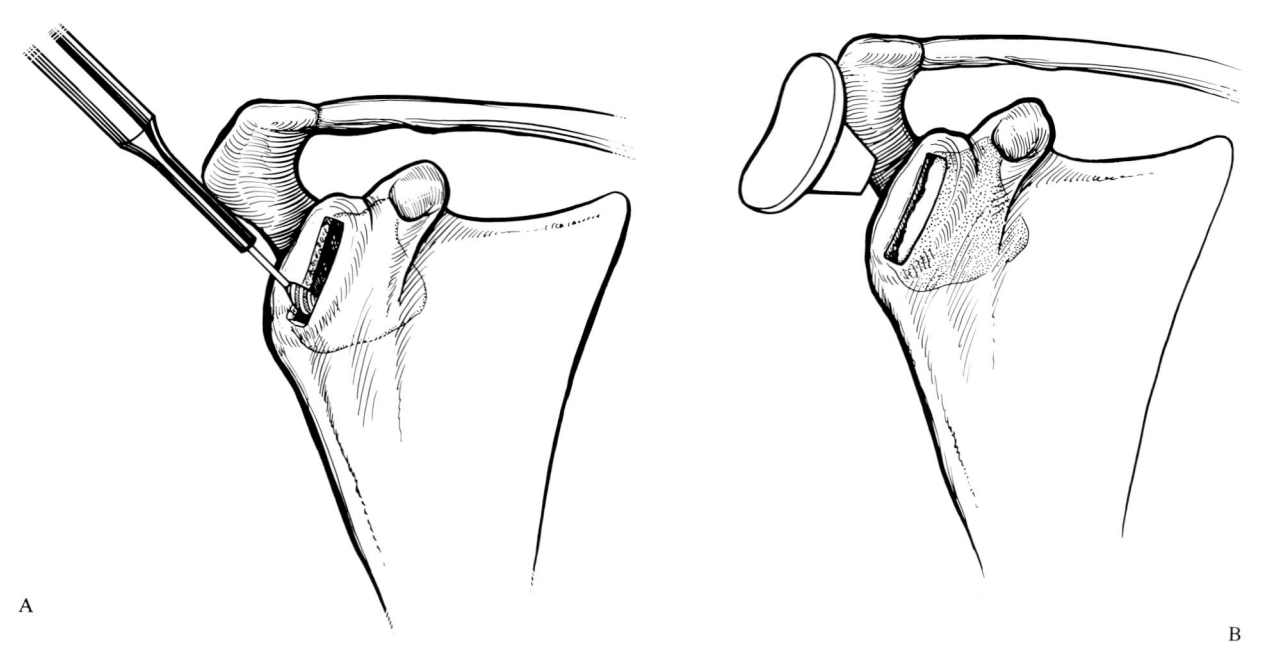

Figure 6–21. **A.** An air burr is utilized to create a slot in the glenoid fossa. **B.** The trial keeled prosthesis (which is a little larger than the final prosthesis) is placed in position.

holes (Figure 6–23A). Mix a half-package of methylmethacrylate, remove the gauze from the holes, and place a small amount of methylmethacrylate into each of the holes using your fingertip (Figure 6–23B). Only a small amount of methylmethacrylate is necessary in each hole to create the proper cement mantle around each peg. Insert the glenoid prosthesis and hold it in position with finger pressure until the cement is cured and the prosthesis is secure (Figure 6–23C).

A disposable syringe that will deliver a precise volume of cement into each hole can be used; it prevents excess cement from being displaced out of the holes and being deposited between the back of the prosthesis and the face of the glenoid. Excessive cement extruding out of the holes and lying between the prosthesis and the glenoid fossa is undesirable for two reasons. First, it will create an uneven seat for the glenoid prosthesis, and second, the cement may become fragmented and loosen in the joint, causing three-body wear of the polyethylene.

If the keeled glenoid prosthesis is to be used, hemostasis in the keel hole must be obtained. The slot should be irrigated to remove any clots, and then sprayed with thrombin, packed with Surgicel and a sponge. When the methylmethacrylate is ready, remove the sponge and the Surgicel and impact the cement into the slot with finger pressure. Firm finger pressure and several small batches of cement will ensure a good cement mantle in the slot to receive and secure the keeled prosthesis. As mentioned, cement between the glenoid fossa and the back of the prosthesis is undesirable. The methylmethacrylate can be pressurized prior to insertion of the prosthesis. This will prevent any excess cement from lying between the face of the glenoid and the back of the prosthesis. Insert the keeled prosthesis and hold it in position with finger pressure until the cement is set and the prosthesis is secure (Figure 6–24).

Before the humeral component is inserted, plan how the subscapularis tendon will be repaired. If the tendon was

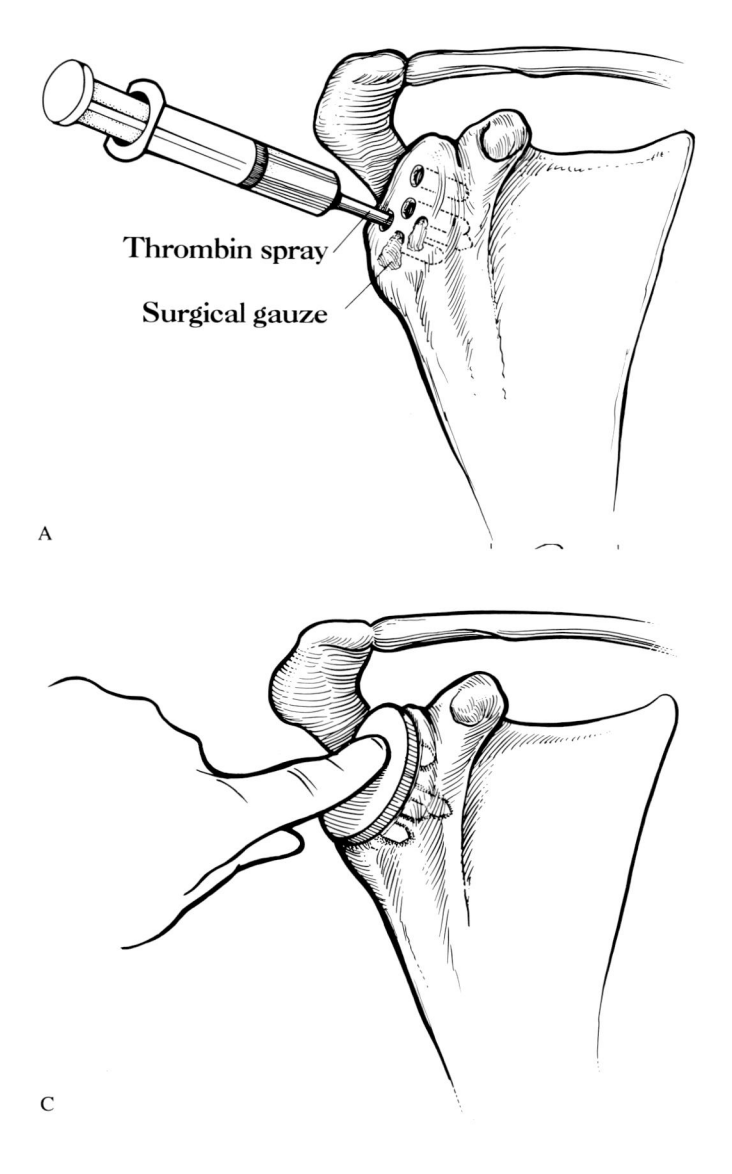

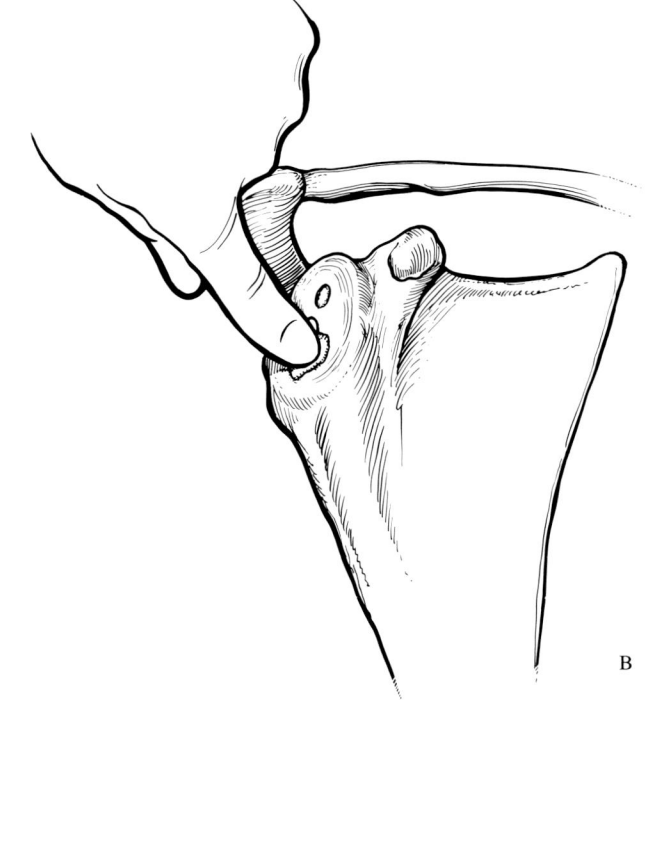

Figure 6–23. **A.** The drill holes are irrigated with thrombin spray and packed with surgical gauze. **B.** A small amount of bone cement is placed into each of the holes using pressure from a fingertip. **C.** The glenoid prosthesis is inserted and held in position with finger pressure until the cement is set.

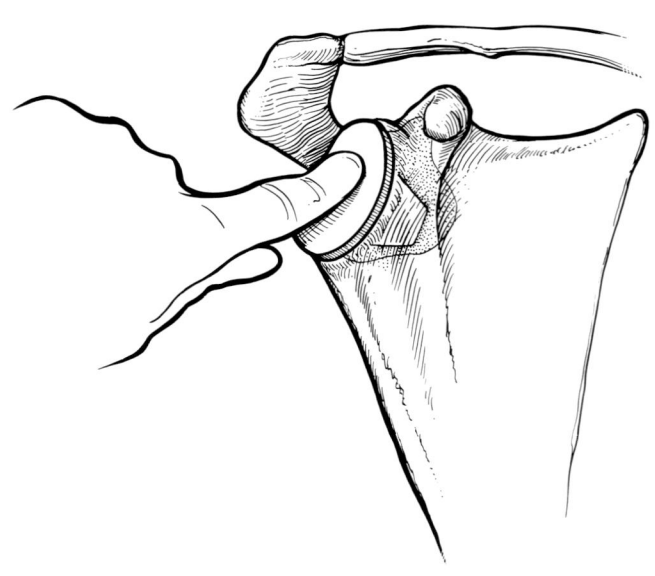

Figure 6–24. The keeled glenoid prosthesis is inserted into position and held there until the cement has set.

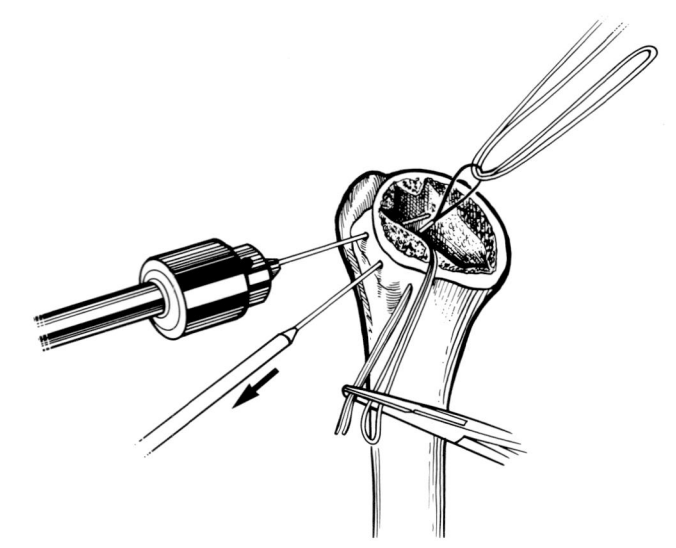

Figure 6–25. If the subscapularis tendon has been released from the bone, then drill three or four holes into the anterior neck of the remaining humerus to reattach the tendon to bone.

simply divided or a coronal Z-plasty lengthening was performed, then insertion of the humeral component may proceed. If the tendon was taken directly off its insertion, then drill three or four holes into the anterior neck of the remaining humerus for reattaching the tendon to bone. Use a suture passer to pull loops of suture through these drill holes to repair the tendon after the prosthesis has been inserted (Figure 6–25).

Attach a humeral prosthesis that is the same size as the final broach size to the driver-extractor and insert the prosthesis down the humeral canal. The fins of the prosthesis must be aligned with the fin tracks previously created by the body broach (Figure 6–26). The prosthesis is 1 mm larger overall than the broach so a press-fit without cement can be obtained. The cancellous bone of the resected head can be used as graft to help fill any defects in the proximal part of the humerus or to ensure a good tight press-fit. The decision to use cement or a press-fit technique is up to the individual surgeon. In some instances, it may be necessary to use methylmethacrylate due to a previous surgical procedure, fractures, osteoporosis, rheumatoid arthritis, or degenerative cysts in the humerus.

Before the final humeral head is inserted, thoroughly clean the Morse taper socket in the humeral prosthesis with a dry sponge and insert the appropriate-size head. Use a plastic-tipped driver to secure the head in place by sharply striking it four to five times with a 2-lb mallet (Figure 6–27). Make sure to impact the head in the direction of the Morse taper. Grasp the head to be sure that it is securely attached to the humeral prosthesis.

With gentle traction, internal rotation, and finger pressure on the humeral prosthesis, reduce the head into the glenoid fossa (Figure 6–28). Following joint irrigation, pass the previously placed stay sutures in the subscapularis tendon into the loop of sutures in the proximal part of the humerus, pull the loops and sutures through the bone, and secure the tendon back to bone (Figure 6–29).

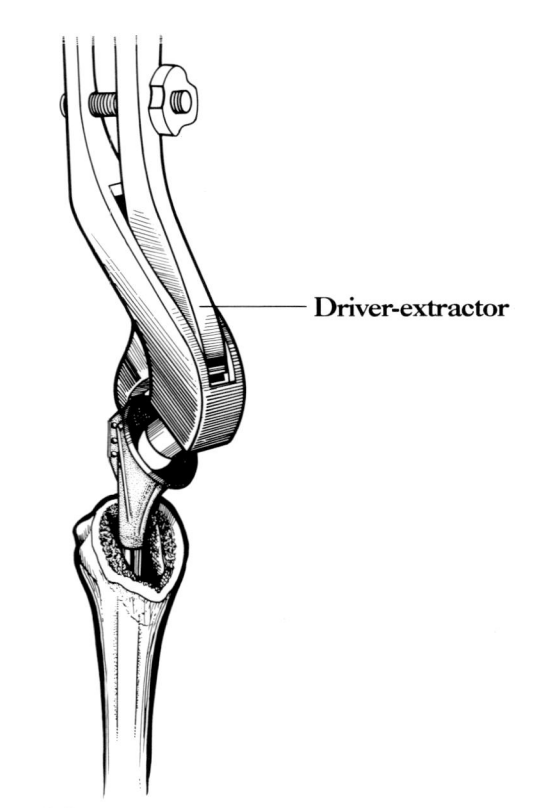

Figure 6–26. The final driver-extractor is utilized to place the prosthesis body into the humeral canal.

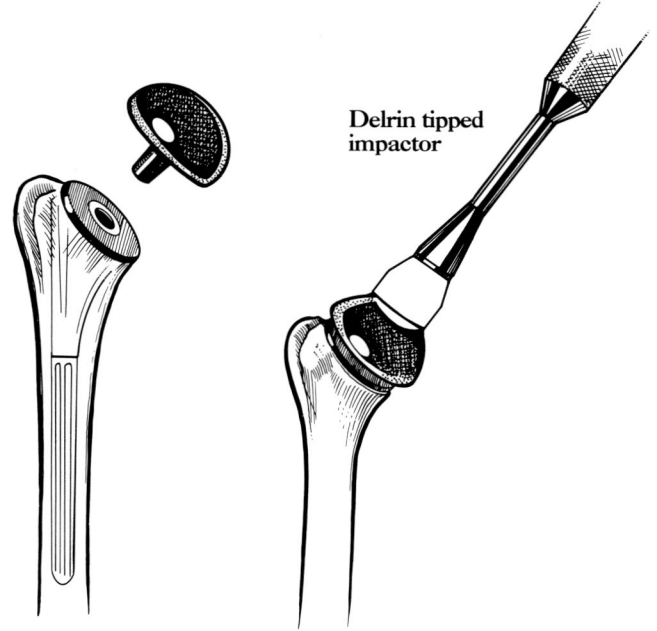

Figure 6-27. Before the final humeral head is inserted, thoroughly clean the reverse Morse taper socket in the humeral prosthesis. The Delrin-tipped driver is used to secure the head in place by sharply striking the head four times with a 2-lb mallet.

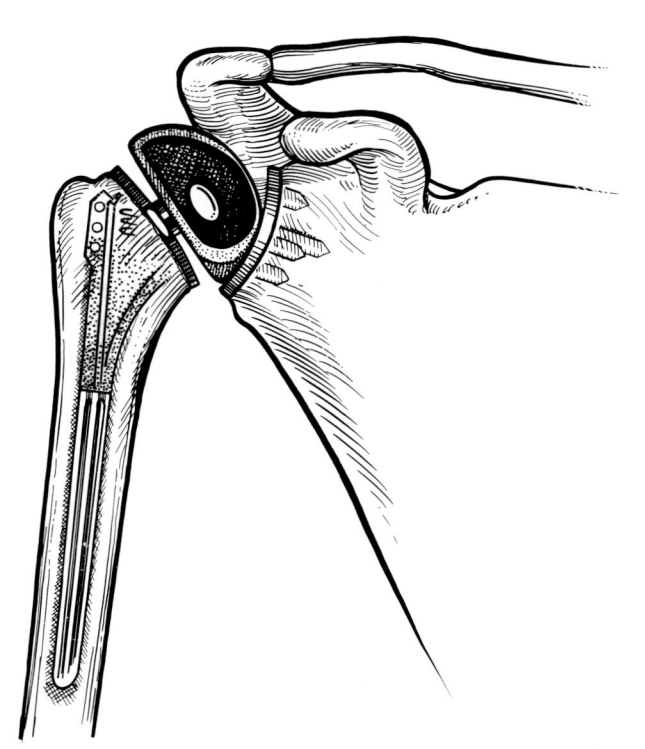

Figure 6-28. The prosthesis is reduced using gentle traction, internal rotation, and finger pressure.

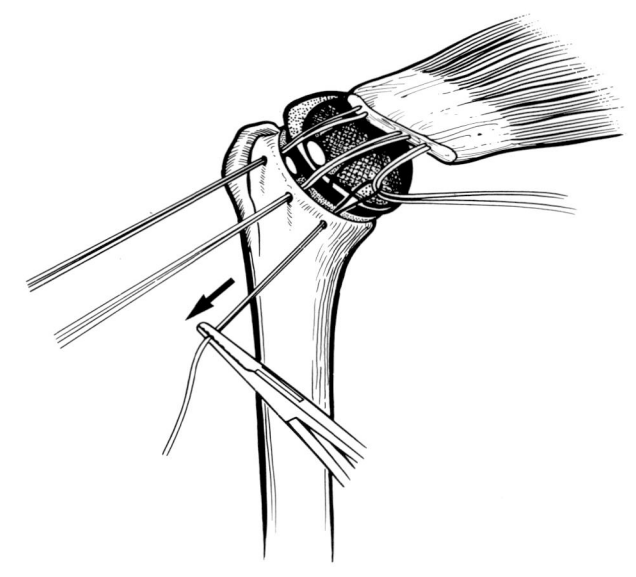

Figure 6-29. The subscapularis is reattached to bone using the previously placed drill holes in the anterior neck of the remaining humerus.

If the tendon was previously divided or was lengthened with a coronal Z-plasty technique, then repair and secure it with heavy nonabsorbable sutures, such as 1-mm Dacron tape. Use of the heavy 1-mm tape sutures allows immediate passive movement beginning the day of surgery without fear of detaching the subscapularis tendon.

Before wound closure, palpate the axillary nerve a final time to be sure that it is in its normal position and intact. Thoroughly irrigate the wound with antibiotic solution. Infiltrate the subcutaneous and muscle tissues with 0.25% bupivacaine solution to ease immediate postoperative pain (Figure 6-30). One or two portable wound evacuation units are used to prevent the formation of a postoperative hematoma.

The wound may be closed according to the surgeon's preference. The deltopectoral fascia can be closed with a running no. 0 absorbable suture, and the deep layer of fat with a no. 0 or 2-0 absorbable suture. The subcuticular fat is closed as a separate layer, and the skin is closed with a running subcuticular nylon suture. Careful attention to wound closure will result in a cosmetically acceptable incision (Figure 6-31).

REFERENCES

1. Henry AK. *Exposure of the Bones and Other Surgical Methods*. New York: William Wood, 1927.
2. Hoppenfeld S, de Boer P. *Surgical Exposures in Orthopaedics*. Philadelphia: WB Saunders, 1990.
3. Abbott LC, Saunders JBM, Hogey H, et al. Surgical approaches to the shoulder joint. *J Bone Joint Surg [Am]* 1949;31:235-244.

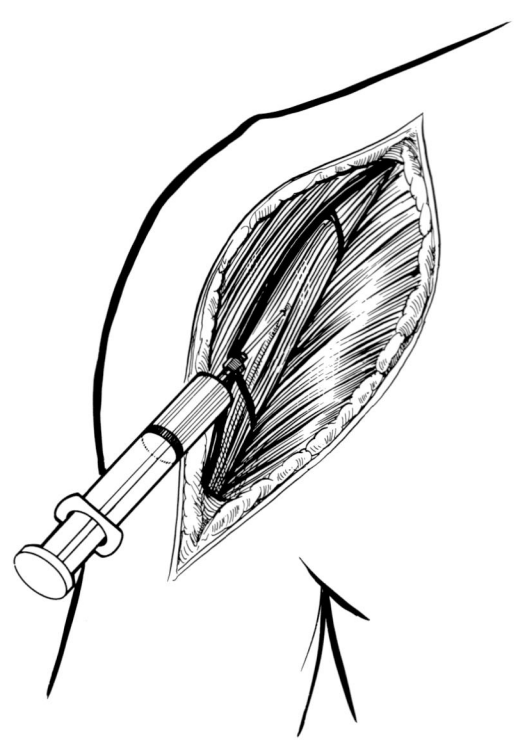

Figure 6–30. The wound is infiltrated with 0.25% bupivacaine prior to closure.

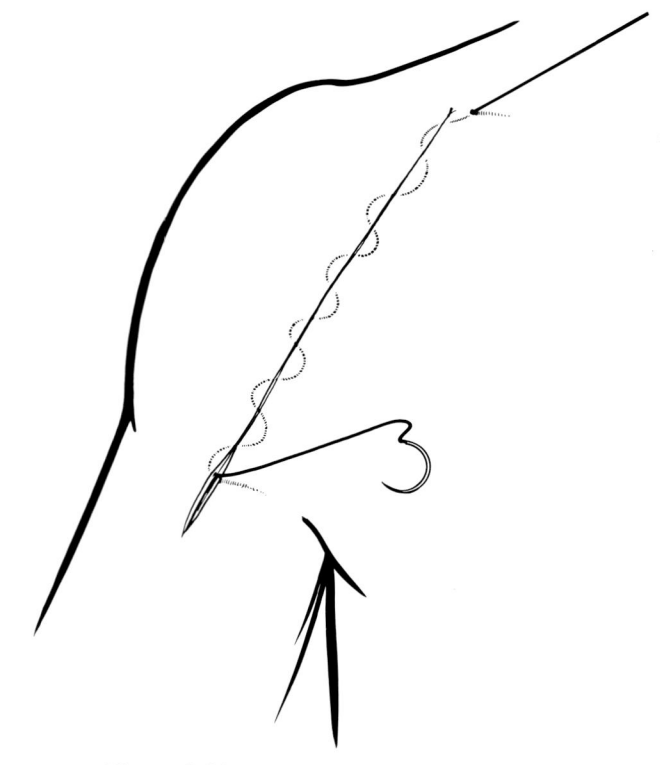

Figure 6–31. Subcuticular nylon skin closure.

4. Banks SW, Laufman H. *Surgical Exposures of the Extremities.* Philadelphia: WB Saunders, 1953.
5. DePalma AF. *Surgery of the Shoulder.* 3rd ed. Philadelphia: JB Lippincott, 1983.
6. Henry AK. *Extensile Exposure Applied to Limb Surgery.* Edinburgh: Livingstone, 1945;15.
7. Hollinshead WH. *Anatomy for Surgeons.* 2nd ed. New York: Harper & Row, 1969.
8. Johnston TB. *Gray's Anatomy.* 27th ed. New York: Longmans, Green, 1988:769–776.
9. Neer CS, Watson KC, Stanton FJ. Recent experience in total shoulder replacement. *J Bone Joint Surg [Am]* 1982;64:319–337.
10. Neer CS. *Shoulder Reconstruction.* Philadelphia: WB Saunders, 1990.
11. Rockwood CA. The technique of total shoulder arthroplasty. *Instr Course Lect* 1990;39:437–447.
12. Burkhead WZ, Scheinberg RR, Box G. Surgical anatomy of the axillary nerve. *J Shoulder Elbow Surg* 1992;1:31–36.
13. Cofield RH. Degenerative arthritis revisions of the glenohumeral joint. In: Rockwood CA, Matsen FA, eds. *The Shoulder.* Philadelphia: WB Saunders, 1990.
14. Groh GI, Rockwood CA. Loss of deltoid following shoulder operations: An operative disaster. Presented at the meeting of the Western Orthopaedic Association; 1992; Monterey, CA. October.
15. Bryan JB, Schouder K, Tullos HS, et al. The axillary nerve and its relationships to common sports medicine shoulder procedure. *Am J Sports Med* 1986;14:113–116.
16. Burkhead WZ. Musculocutaneous and axillary nerve position after coracoid graft transfer. In: Post M, Morrey BF, Hawkins RJ, eds. *Surgery of the Shoulder.* St. Louis: Mosby-Year Book, 1990, pg 152–155.
17. Neer CS II, Rockwood CA. Fractures and dislocations of the shoulder. In: Rockwood CA, Green DP, eds. *Fractures in Adults.* 2nd ed. Philadelphia: JB Lippincott, 1984, pg 675–985.
18. Linell EA. The distribution of nerves in the upper limb with reference to variabilities and their clinical significance. *J Anat* 1921;55:79–112.
19. Flatow EL, Bigliani LU, April EW. An anatomical study of the musculocutaneous nerve and its relationship to the coracoid process. *Clin Orthop* 1989;244:166–171.
20. Helfet AJ. Coracoid transplantation for recurring dislocation of the shoulder. *J Bone Joint Surg [Br]* 1958;40:198–202.
21. Harryman DT, Sidles JA, Clark JM, et al. Translation of the humeral head of the glenoid with passive glenohumeral motion. *J Bone Joint Surg* 1990;72:1334–1343.

7 Rehabilitation Following Shoulder Arthroplasty

John J. Brems, M.D.

Shoulder replacement will fail without adequate rehabilitation . . . only the surgeon can and must direct the rehabilitation program.—Charles S. Neer, II

Total shoulder arthroplasty may be a technical exercise in the operating suite, but a successful outcome requires many hours of faithful attention to a well-designed and well-performed rehabilitation program. This will maximize motion, strength, and ultimately patient satisfaction.

The term "physical therapy" encompasses a broad spectrum of modalities, from hands-on joint stretching to muscle toning and strengthening. Other treatment options, including heat, ice, ultrasound, phonophoresis, and electrical stimulation, are part of the physical therapy regimen and are more fully discussed in physical therapy texts.[1-3] Their use following shoulder arthroplasty rehabilitation should necessarily be minimal.

Proper postarthroplasty rehabilitation must follow a logical sequence allowing for tissue healing, joint mobilization, and finally muscle strengthening. Variance from this logical progression of recovery and rehabilitation frustrates both the patient and physician. The patient must view himself or herself as an active agent in the program, not the passive receiver of another care giver. Although benefits of phonophoresis, ultrasound, deep heat, and myoelectric stimulation are possible, they cannot substitute for the major goals of joint mobility and muscle strengthening.

The main goals of postarthroplasty rehabilitation are joint mobility, maximizing range of motion, and muscle strengthening—in that order. Joint mobilization itself is subdivided into three phases which must progress in a logical fashion. Strengthening is also divided into three phases which must be followed sequentially to allow maximal chance for return of function. When the surgeon realizes that technical expertise is responsible for only a small part of an arthroplasty's success, and that a well-designed and well-executed rehabilitation program, performed by a well-trained and experienced shoulder therapist, is mandatory, then a successful outcome can be realized.

PREOPERATIVE REHABILITATION

The rehabilitation program does not begin after the surgical procedure; rather, it begins at the preoperative visit when the decision has been made to proceed with shoulder arthroplasty. The person designated to be the physical therapist postoperatively should see the patient prior to surgery to discuss and demonstrate the postoperative rehabilitation program. This implies that a relationship needs to be established not just between patient and surgeon, but also between surgeon and physical therapist. Although nearly impossible to statistically quantify, the author's recurring experiences and impressions are that the best rehabilitation results do not just happen, they are caused. Those physical therapists who are experienced in shoulder rehabilitation obtain better results than those physical therapists who are not so specialized.

At the time of the presurgical evaluation, the physical therapist should meet with the patient and ideally the spouse or other family member who will participate in the postsurgical home care. At this time, the same therapist who will manage the postoperative rehabilitation should discuss the rehabilitation program, its intent, purpose, and expectation. The physical therapist should examine the involved shoulder for range of motion and muscle tone, discuss these findings with the patient and surgeon, and then demonstrate the range-of-motion program that will begin after the shoulder arthroplasty. The patient is reassured that pain and stiffness will be both normal and conquerable. Reassurance builds confidence and confidence builds success.

A successful physical therapist is not just a mechanic who puts a joint through motion. One must have empathy and an ability to communicate that empathy to the patient. The best way to judge the quality of a successful relationship with a physical therapist is seeing that the patient looks forward to the interaction, despite the fact that it will result in discomfort and pain.

Of equal importance with the therapist-patient relationship is the surgeon-therapist relationship. Many orthopaedic surgeons have access to physical therapists in their office setting, and even when this is not possible, preoperative communication between these two care givers is most desirable. Even when this surgeon-therapist relationship is not possible, the identified therapist should at least see the patient preoperatively. Since patients may travel a long distance, a physical therapist in the patient's hometown should be identified prior to surgery and spoken to about the postoperative rehabilitation program. Furthermore, it is the surgeon's responsibility to communicate the desired program and modifications that may be necessary to the physical therapist. One cannot expect the patient to communicate the plans and precautions to the physical therapist. Merely completing a standard prescription form with the physical therapy order should be considered inadequate if it is not supplemented with a direct conversation and explanation from the surgeon.

Physical therapy is not just a mechanical exercise program performed on an individual. A successful physical therapist not only is experienced in the exercise mechanics, but also must be empathetic, sympathetic, and interactive with the patient. Laying on of hands is important in rehabilitation, but for success the patient must see the physical therapist as a professional, supporter, and friend who understands the pain and apprehension. This type of necessary relationship is better established preoperatively rather than after surgery when pain is most likely to be very significant. Preoperative discussions with the physical therapist provide an opportunity for the patient and family helper to have the postoperative rehabilitation program demonstrated. This may help diminish questions and misunderstandings that arise after surgery. The preoperative visit provides the opportunity to establish a rapport between patient and therapist that can account for much of the success in postarthroplasty rehabilitation.

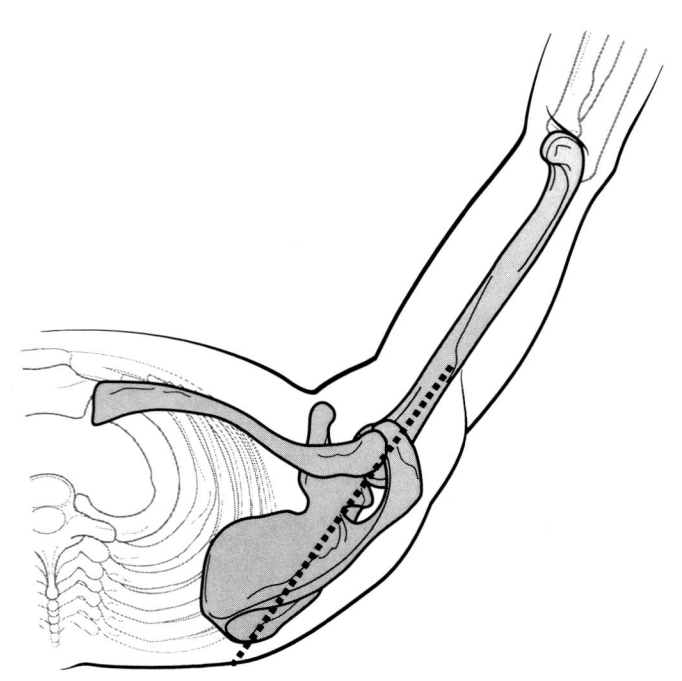

Figure 7–1. Maximal supine elevation of the arm occurs when the long axis of the humerus lies in the plane of the scapula. This plane is approximately 45 degrees from the coronal plane.

EVALUATION OF MOTION

For years attempts have been made to establish a system for measuring and recording shoulder motion. Whereas it is relatively simple to describe the normal motion of a hinge joint such as the proximal interphalangeal joint of the finger, consistent reproducible measurement of shoulder motion is much more difficult. The shoulder complex consists of multiple joints: glenohumeral, scapulothoracic, acromioclavicular, and sternoclavicular. Dysfunction in one joint will affect the others; in some cases compensation may occur, and in others decompensation of other joints may affect total motion.

This discussion focuses on the maximization of three planes of shoulder motion: (1) elevation (total of glenohumeral and scapulothoracic elevation), (2) external rotation, and (3) internal rotation.

Elevation

The American Shoulder and Elbow Surgeons has formed a committee to establish standards for recording shoulder motion. Classic shoulder motion assessment has been based on recording of shoulder abduction and forward flexion, and most contemporary physical therapy texts still refer to shoulder motion in these terms. However, the maximal elevation of the arm occurs when the plane encompassing the long axis of the humerus lies in the same plane as the body of the scapula (Figure 7–1). The plane of the scapula is approximately 45 degrees to the frontal plane of the body. Hence, traditional therapy with stretching and mobilization in the abduction and forward flexion planes not only is unnecessary, but also does not even allow maximum joint motion because of intrinsic anatomic barriers.[4] When glenohumeral motion is maximized in the plane of elevation, scapulothoracic motion automatically allows maximum motion in the forward flexion and abduction planes.

External Rotation

Possibly the most important functional motion of the shoulder complex is external rotation. Loss of external rotation results in a significant functional disability as seen in patients with osteoarthritis. Most people tolerate a 90-degree loss of glenohumeral elevation, but cannot tolerate more than a 45-degree loss of external rotation without significant impairment. Proper technique to maximize external rotation is mandatory to obtain maximal recovery of this motion. Experience shows that patients find this exercise the most painful and hence the most difficult.

To maximize external rotation, one must recognize the capsular and mechanical constraints of the glenohumeral joint. The capsular contribution (glenohumeral ligaments and subscapularis) is dictated by the surgical reconstruction. Most surgical approaches to the glenohumeral joint involve division and reconstruction of the anterior structures. Their repair will then dictate the amount of allowable external rotation. It is important to remember that a patient will never obtain more external rotation than was mechanically permitted at the time of joint closure.

In the normal anatomic situation, the capsular ligaments allow the most external rotation when the long axis of the

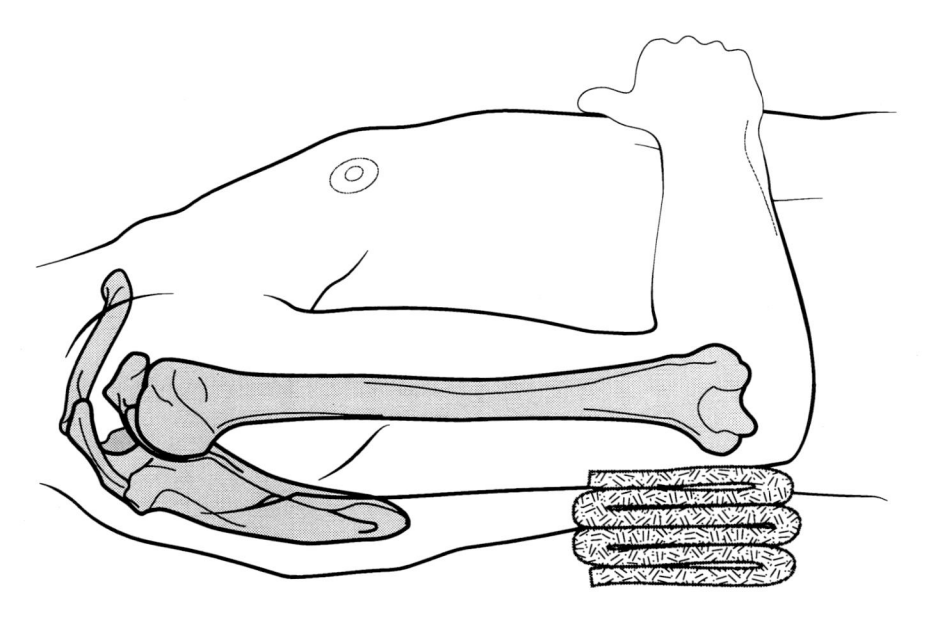

Figure 7-2. The patient lies supine with the elbow held off the table by towels to maintain the long axis of the humerus parallel to the long axis of the spine and body of the scapula for supine external rotation.

humerus is parallel to the body of the scapula (Figure 7–2). To establish this in the supine position, the elbow must be raised off the table so it is parallel to the body of the ipsilateral scapula. Furthermore, these capsular structures are in their most relaxed state when the central axis of the glenoid is perpendicular to the long axis of the humerus (Figure 7–3). The examiner or physical therapist therefore must abduct the arm so that the elbow is approximately 4 to 6 in from the patient's side. This amount will vary from patient to patient depending on body somatotype.

During the measuring, stretching, mobilizing, and recording of total shoulder elevation and external rotation, the patient should be in the supine position on a relatively hard surface without a pillow under the head. In the supine position, one avoids the accessory spinal motion that may contribute to overall apparent shoulder motion.

Internal Rotation

Maximizing internal rotation is particularly important in the postoperative rehabilitation of the shoulder following any surgical procedure. The ability to internally rotate allows women to comfortably fasten their bras behind their backs, and permits the patient to pass belts, zip zippers, tuck in shirts and blouses, and do other activities routinely performed with the hand behind the back. When one realizes that loss of internal rotation occurs early in most pathologic processes affecting the shoulder, it becomes easier to understand why recovery of this motion is characteristically difficult.

At first glance it would appear that internal rotation is merely pulling the arm in across the chest. However, internal rotation of the humerus progressively increases as the thumb is pulled higher up the thoracic spine. The higher the thumb tip reaches up the spine, the more humeral internal rotation occurs (Figure 7–4). By convention, the spinal level to which the tip of the thumb reaches in the midline is recorded as maximal internal rotation. Surface anatomy features help determine the spinal level that the thumb reaches. The superior angle of the scapula is opposite the fourth thoracic vertebra (T4), and the seventh thoracic vertebra (T7) is opposite the inferior angle (Figure 7–5). A Sprengel's deformity or scoliosis may alter these otherwise normal anatomic

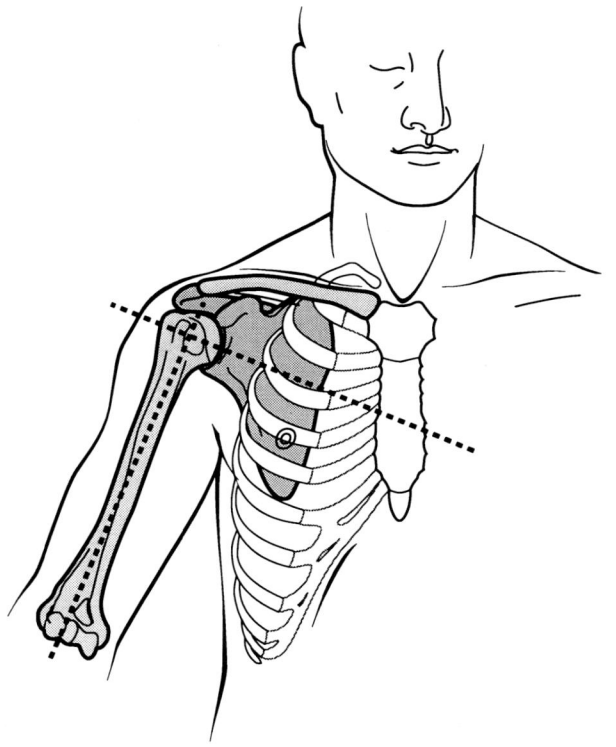

Figure 7-3. The elbow should be brought away from the side to establish perpendicularity between the long axis of the humerus and the central axis of the glenoid. This ensures maximal capsule relaxation, allowing improved external rotation.

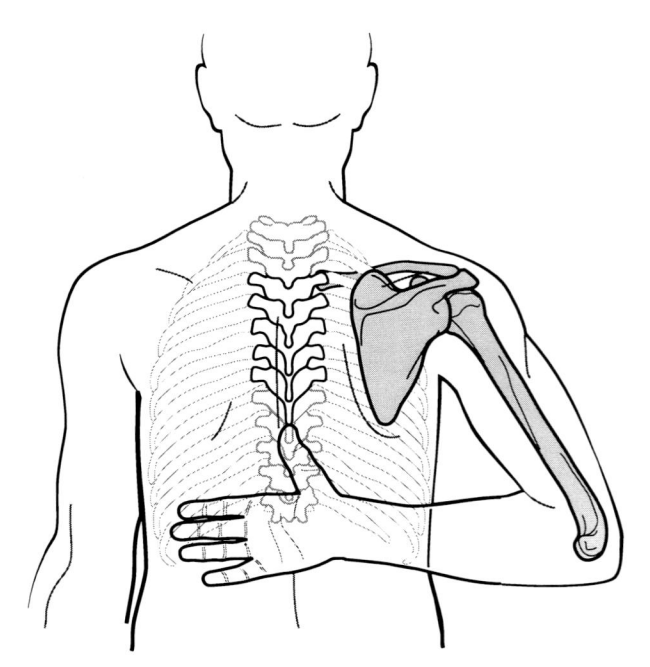

Figure 7–4. Internal rotation is recorded by the maximal extent the tip of the thumb reaches up the dorsal aspect of the spine.

relationships. The iliac crest is opposite the fourth lumbar vertebra (L4) and the sacrum begins at the gluteal crease. If the patient cannot get the arm behind the midline of the side, then their internal rotation would be to the greater trochanter.

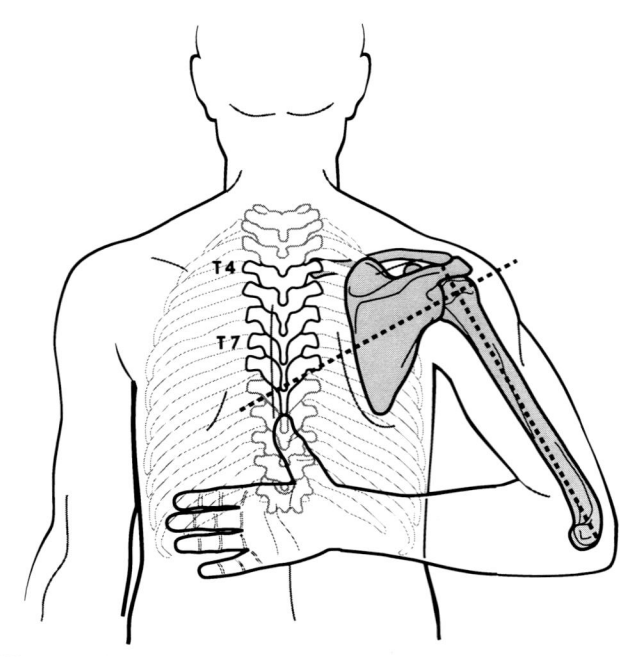

Figure 7–5. In keeping the thumb along the midline, the humerus is abducted to establish perpendicularity between the long axis of the humerus and the central axis of the glenoid. The superior angle of the scapula is opposite the spinous process of T4 and the inferior angle is opposite the spinous process of T7.

POSTOPERATIVE REHABILITATION

As discussed, the rehabilitation program is best initiated prior to surgery, but when does it begin after surgery and how long should it continue for? Several years ago, the postarthroplasty rehabilitation program did not begin for several days after surgery. Much of this delay was necessitated by surgical exposures and procedures that included release of the deltoid muscle origin. To allow sufficient healing of this important muscle, active use of the arm had to be restricted for many weeks. Concern for dislocation of the joint also led to a delay of several days in initiating the rehabilitation program. Many surgeons discharged patients from the hospital with slings or other supportive devices and many continue this practice today.

The more recent trend by experienced shoulder surgeons has been to start the physical therapy program very early. Rockwood begins his rehabilitation program the same day as the surgery, initiating passive movement of the extremity a few hours after the shoulder arthroplasty.[5] Newer techniques of surgery that allow preservation of the deltoid, proper component orientation, proper respect for myofascial sleeve tension, and modification of component design all provide intrinsic joint stability and thus permit safe, early rehabilitation.[6]

There will always be specific concerns and situations that will require modification and delays in certain exercises to protect the soft tissues. For example, anterior capsular lengthening done for a severe long-standing loss of external rotation could require a delay in passive external rotation stretching to allow sufficient healing of the subscapularis capsule construct. This illustrates why the surgeon should and must direct the rehabilitation program. Only the surgeon knows the specific surgical considerations that may alter the otherwise standard protocol.

One intraoperative benefit in using regional anesthesia such as an interscalene block is that at the completion of the procedure, while still in the operating suite and prior to placing the dressing, the surgeon can take the involved shoulder through a range of motion with the patient watching.[7] By viewing their arm and the extent of motion that is allowed by virtue of the anesthesia, patients appear to regain motion more quickly. They are more easily convinced that the pain spasm reflex limits their motion and is not a true mechanical block. In learning to relax in the face of pain, the patient will usually find a dramatic improvement in motion. Unless there are unusual intraoperative problems, the rehabilitation program should begin within days to minimize scarring and adhesions between muscle groups. In the contemporary surgical approach to shoulder arthroplasty, the only muscle divided is the subscapularis, and its motor function as an internal rotator is duplicated by many other muscles.

The author's preference is to initiate the rehabilitation program following shoulder arthroplasty on the first postoperative day. On the evening of surgery, the patients are in a compressive dressing to minimize swelling of the forearm, and are encouraged to use their arm for feeding the following day. In preparation for the therapy session, the patients are given analgesics at least 30 minutes before the program is to begin, allowing time for the analgesic to reach peak effect. In addition, moist heat can be applied to the shoulder for a minimum of 30 minutes prior to the therapy session. Moist heat appears to be subjectively soothing to the patient; it may act as a mild analgesic and seems to diminish the perception of stiffness.

Stretching

There are many published rehabilitation protocols, both in physical therapy texts and in orthopaedic texts.[8-10] The fact that there are so many published protocols is testimony to the fact that there is no best one. The surgeon should understand the principles and develop a program that satisfies patient needs and produces a successful result. These principles include (1) early initiation of the rehabilitation program, (2) allowing early active motion, (3) eliminating or limiting supportive devices such as slings and immobilizers, and (4) maximizing passive joint motion in the cardinal planes (elevation, internal and external rotation) prior to initiation of a strengthening program.

Multiple short periods of stretching exercises are more beneficial than fewer prolonged sessions. Patients should spend no more than 5 minutes per session three or four times per day. None of us looks forward to pain, and prolonged exercise becomes psychologically very debilitating. The stretching or mobilization portion of the rehabilitation program is designed to progressively increase the range of motion available to the shoulder complex. This implies maximizing motion at the glenohumeral, scapulothoracic, acromioclavicular, and sternoclavicular joints.

Mobilization is progressive and proceeds through various phases. The first-phase exercises are designed to initiate elevation and external rotation. Phase I continues until elevation is approximately 140 degrees and external rotation is 40 degrees. The phase II program continues with elevation up to 160 degrees and external rotation to approximately 60 degrees. In addition, the phase II stretching initiates internal rotation and shoulder level adduction. The final phase of stretching is designed to increase the range of all cardinal motions to their anatomic maximum.

PHASE I STRETCHING

Phase I exercises are initiated within 24 to 48 hours of shoulder arthroplasty. One-half hour prior to therapy, both heat and analgesics are given as described.

1. *Pendulum Exercise* (Figure 7–6). The patient bends forward at the waist and supports his or her weight with the nonsurgical arm. Ideally the thoracic spine should be parallel to the floor. The involved arm should circle one way and then the other. In one direction, the hand should be maximally

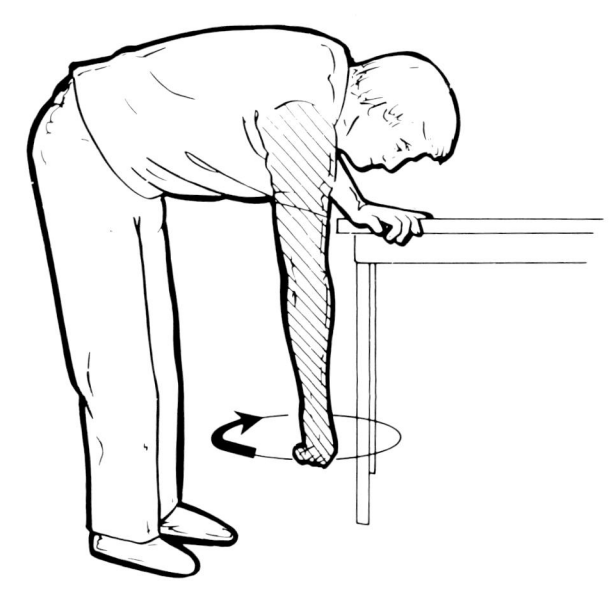

Figure 7–6. For pendulum exercises, the patient bends forward at the waist and rotates the arm clockwise and counterclockwise while keeping the back parallel to the floor.

pronated while circling and then the direction should be reversed with the hand now supinated. Time spent per exercise: 30 to 60 seconds.

2. *Assisted Supine Elevation* (Figure 7–7). The patient should be placed supine without a pillow. A pillow raises the head and may tend to raise the shoulder and scapula off the table, which may adversely affect joint mobility. The physical therapist puts gentle traction on the humerus and gradually elevates in the scapular plane. When the patient begins to experience pain, a gentle firm pressure is applied for only 3 to 5 seconds. Stretching is always by firm gentle continuous pressure and not with pulsating force. The arm is then gently

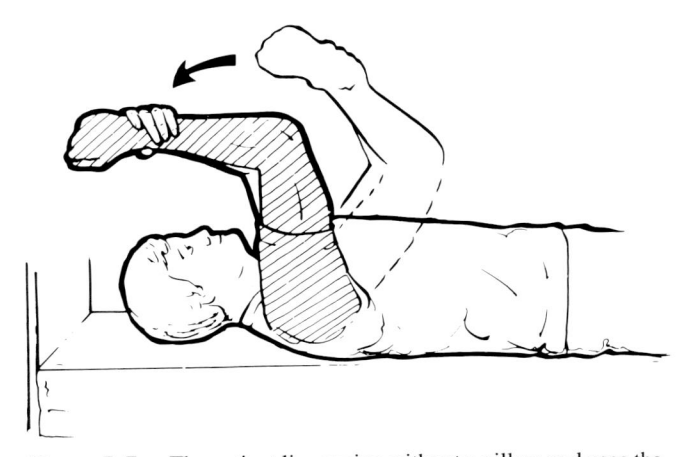

Figure 7–7. The patient lies supine without a pillow and uses the uninvolved arm to passively elevate the involved arm. Gentle longitudinal traction along the axis of the humerus may improve the motion and stretching during this exercise.

Figure 7–8. The patient is positioned supine with a towel underneath the elbow to make the humerus parallel to the floor. The elbow is brought 4 to 6 in away from the side and a stick or dowel is used to passively rotate the involved arm into external rotation. It is important to maintain perpendicularity between the forearm and the upper arm at the elbow.

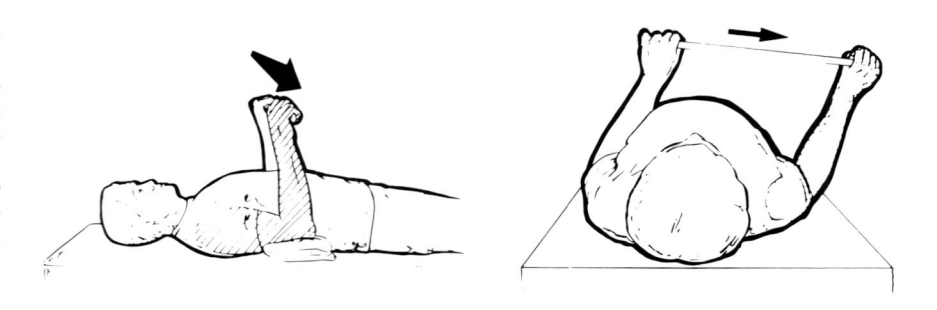

assisted back down to the side. This may be repeated two or three times at each exercise session. Total time spent per exercise: 15 to 30 seconds.

3. *Assisted External Rotation* (Figure 7–8). The patient again is positioned on the back without a pillow. A folded towel is placed under the arm so the long axis of the humerus is parallel to the spine. As discussed previously, the elbow is brought 4 to 6 in away from the side to reestablish the proper glenohumeral axis relationship. The physical therapist instructs the patient in using a dowel or some sort of stick to push the forearm away from the side so as to rotate the humerus itself. Care must be taken to have proper orientation of the stick so it rotates the humerus and does not merely extend the elbow. The stick itself must not be parallel to the waist, but rather is maintained perpendicular to the humerus at all times. The patient, helper, and physical therapist should apply constant firm pressure in external rotation; pulsating force should not be used. Total time for exercise: 30 to 45 seconds.

4 *Assisted Elevation with Pulley* (Figure 7–9). The pulley exercise assists the patient in passive elevation of the arm. Pulley placement is critically important. Ideally, the pulley itself should be at least 1 ft higher than the extended reach of the normal arm. Furthermore, the pulley placement relative to the patient should be directly above the head or possibly even behind it. If the pulley is too far in front of the patient, maximal elevation will be considerably less than ideal. By having the pulley above or slightly behind the patient's head, it will ensure that as the operated arm is raised by the good arm, maximal elevation is occurring.

The patient must be carefully instructed in using the pulley, especially if the physician is concerned about limiting early active motion, such as when a rotator cuff repair was part of the arthroplasty. As the affected arm is descending with the pulley, an undesirable eccentric contraction of the deltoid and supraspinatus may occur.

Occasionally the patient's domiciles do not allow a pulley to be placed at the appropriate height. It is possible to mount a pulley over the top of a door. The patient sits on a chair with the back to the door (Figure 7–10). While doing the pulley exercise, the patient should concentrate on trying to get the arm as high as possible and not worry whether or not he or she is standing on the toes, hiking the shoulder, or arching the back. Each of these secondary motion artifacts will diminish spontaneously as total shoulder elevation improves. Total time spent per exercise: 60 to 90 seconds.

5. *Assisted Abduction* (Figure 7–11). The patient lies supine without a pillow and uses the normal arm to assist elevation of the operated extremity. The fingers are intertwined as in a clasp and the arms are brought up overhead and placed behind the neck. The elbows are then gently brought down by the side with the aid of a physical therapist. The elbows are actively brought together and returned to the side. Total time spent per exercise: 30 to 60 seconds.

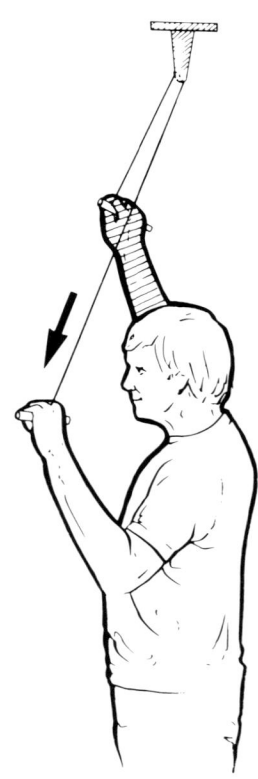

Figure 7–9. The patient stands with a pulley directly over his head. The pulley should be 1 ft higher than the extended reach of the normal arm. The involved arm is passively elevated by pulling the rope through the pulley with the uninvolved shoulder.

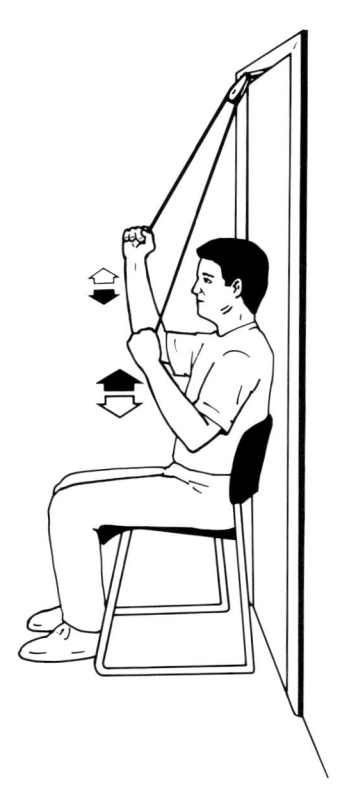

Figure 7–10. If the pulley cannot be placed 1 ft higher than the extended reach of the patient's normal arm, the pulley may be placed over a door, as shown. The patient should sit with the back to the door as the pulley is used in this fashion.

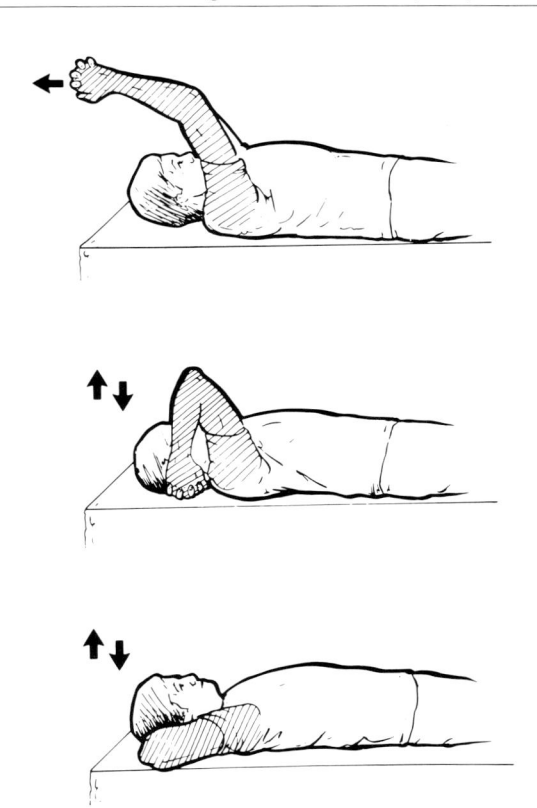

Figure 7–11. The patient is positioned supine and uses the uninvolved arm to stretch the involved shoulder overhead. The fingers are intertwined and placed behind the head and the elbows gently lowered to the side.

PHASE II STRETCHING

This phase of the stretching begins 10 to 14 days after the shoulder arthroplasty, at the time of suture removal. Internal rotation exercises are introduced at this point. The patient continues with stretching in elevation and external rotation using slightly different techniques than those of the phase I program to further assist in maximizing these motions.

1. *Assisted Internal Rotation* (Figure 7–12). Both arms are placed behind the back and the hand of the normal arm grasps the wrist of the operated shoulder. It is first pulled into extension trying to keep the upper arm and forearm in the true sagittal plane and then when maximal extension has been reached, the good arm pulls the wrist up the back as shown. As the elbow is flexed and the thumb comes up the back, internal rotation is increased. The higher the thumb reaches up the spine, the greater the degree of internal rotation.

2. *Assisted Elevation* (Figure 7–13). The patient lays on a bed ideally fitted with a headboard under which the hands can easily fit, as shown in the figure. The patient then lies on the back without a pillow to keep the scapula resting comfortably on the mattress. Using the uninvolved arm, the operated arm is lifted up overhead while arching the back, allowing the hands to reach under the headboard. While still holding on to

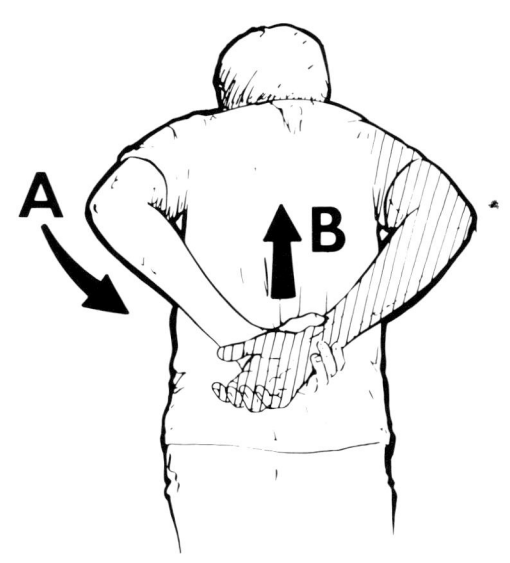

Figure 7–12. **A.** The uninvolved arm initially pulls the operated arm into extension. **B.** The wrist is then pulled up the back, keeping the hand in the midline as shown.

Figure 7–13. The patient lies on a bed with a headboard. The surgical arm is elevated passively using the other arm until the fingers can reach underneath the headboard. This may cause some arching of the back, but as the back is lowered, the arms are further elevated.

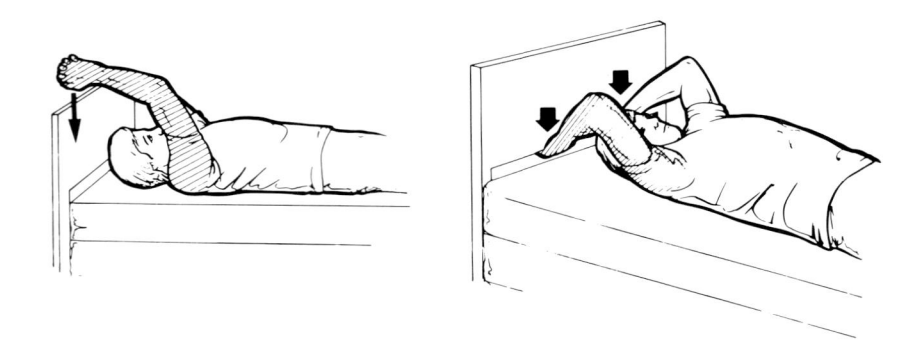

the underside of the headboard, the arch in the back is slowly lowered, effectively increasing elevation of the shoulder.

3. *Assisted External Rotation* (Figure 7–14). The patient stands in a doorway with the elbow placed against the side and flexed to 90 degrees. By keeping the elbow tight up against the side and turning in place, the shoulder is externally rotated. This is most useful in increasing external rotation from 40 to 60 degrees. These phase II exercises require no more than 3 to 4 minutes and should be preceded by the phase I program.

PHASE III STRETCHING

These exercises are designed to help attain the last 20 degrees of shoulder motion in all directions. Like the exercises described above, they should ideally be performed twice daily. The first set is done in the morning upon awakening, preferably immediately following a hot shower. The second set should be performed in the early afternoon.

1. *Assisted Elevation* (Figure 7–15). The patient should stand approximately 12 to 14 inches away from a convex corner. The major concentration should be to keep the elbow straight and apply minimal pressure on the corner with the hand of the affected extremity. The patient slowly leans inwards, forcing the axilla, elbow, and wrist to lie on the corner. The patient keeps steady pressure on the axilla for several seconds as the stretching occurs. It is important to note that pulsing or jerking should not be performed, as this will only tend to further irritate an already sore shoulder.

2. *Assisted External Rotation* (Figure 7–16). The patient stands in a doorway with both forearms flat against the doorjamb, keeping the humeri parallel to the floor. The patient leans forward into the open doorway, which stretches the anterior capsule and assists in external rotation with the elbow in 90 degrees of abduction. The patient should keep pressure on the shoulders for approximately 5 to 10 seconds and should not pulse or jerk the shoulder during the exercise.

3. *Assisted Internal Rotation* (Figure 7–17). The patient may stand, as shown in the figure, with the back up against a table or ledge. The affected arm is placed so that the back of the wrist lies on the table with the thumb along the midline of the spine. As the knees are flexed, the table acts as a platform that will forcefully flex the elbow and increase internal rotation as the thumb is pulled up the back. The further the tip of the thumb rises along the thoracic spine, the more internal rotation is required.

4. *Assisted Adduction* (Figure 7–18). This is a particularly valuable exercise in benefiting the patient who is having difficulty sleeping. The arm is lifted up to shoulder level just below the chin. The unaffected arm pulls the affected arm up

Figure 7–14. **A.** The patient stands holding the elbow of the involved arm tight up against the side of the body. **B.** While the patient keeps the forearm held on the doorjamb and turns in place, the arm is pulled into increasing external rotation.

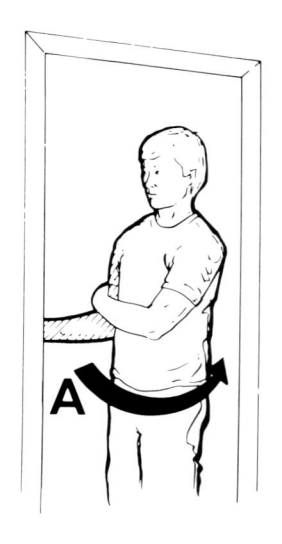

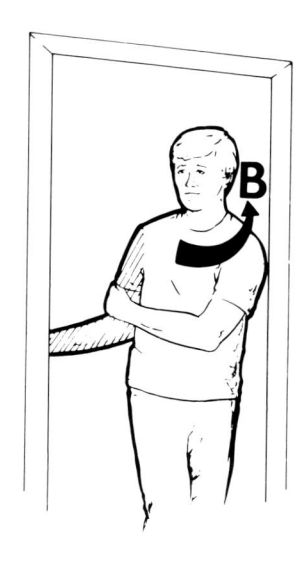

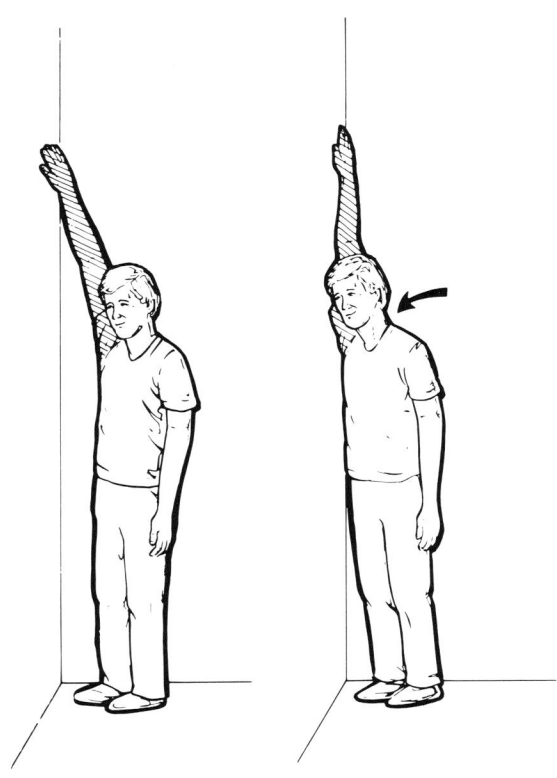

Figure 7–15. The patient stands, as shown, 1 ft away from the corner. The elbow of the involved extremity is kept in full extension. In leaning towards the corner trying to place the axilla on the edge, the arm is forced up into near full elevation.

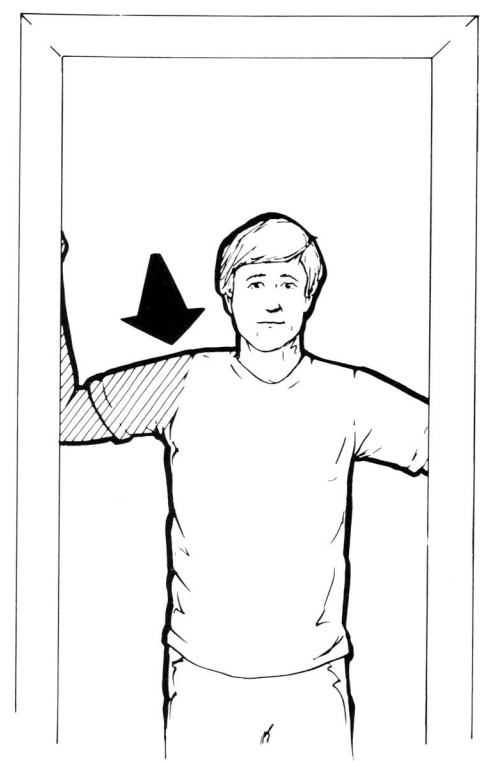

Figure 7–16. The patient stands in a doorway with the upper arms parallel to the floor and the forearms held on the doorjamb. As the patient leans forward, the arms are forced into external rotation and extension.

underneath the chin, stretching the posterior capsule. While sleeping, if the patient rolls over on the affected side, the arm is forced into adduction. Recovery of this adduction motion tends to diminish associated night pain. Patients should continue these four phase III stretching exercises indefinitely. Total time spent on phase III stretching is 3 to 5 minutes.

SUMMARY OF STRETCHING

Virtually all patients begin their postarthroplasty rehabilitation program within 24 to 48 hours, starting with the phase I stretching program. The program is done two to three times daily and should be completed in less than 5 minutes. The sessions are preceded by the application of moist heat and analgesic medication for the first several weeks. Most often the physical therapy program can be taught to the spouse, and the physical therapist observes the spouse to ascertain that the fine details of position and technique can be reproduced. The phase II program is generally added at the time of suture removal. The phase III program begins anywhere from 3 to 6 weeks later, depending on the progress of the earlier phases. The last phase incorporates adduction to improve sleep patterns and improves external rotation while the arm is in 90 degrees of abduction.

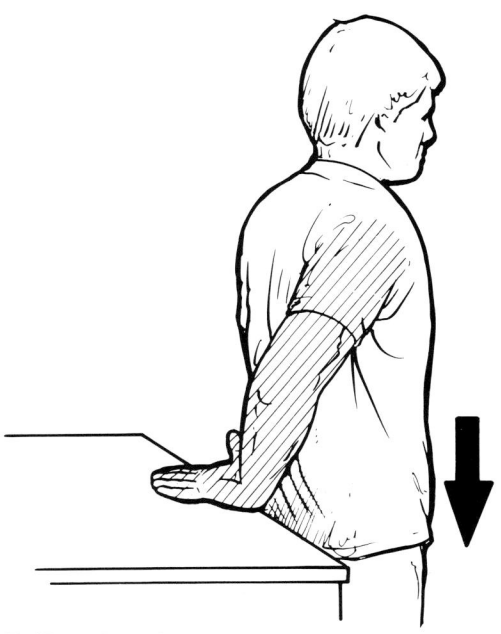

Figure 7–17. The patient stands with the back to a table or ledge approximately at waist level. The arm is held behind the back with the thumb along the spine and rests on the table. As the patient bends the knee, the arm is forced into internal rotation and extension.

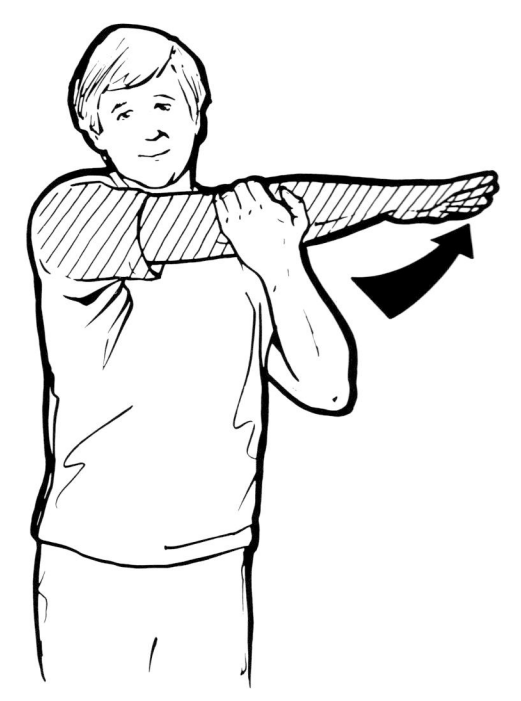

Figure 7–18. The arm is held at shoulder level just under the chin and pulled across the chest to stretch the posterior capsule. This particular exercise seems to improve the patient's positional night pain.

At each follow-up visit the physician should observe patients doing these exercises to be certain that they have not incorporated unacceptable modifications on their own. Rarely are modifications necessary in the stretching program. Occasionally, surgical lengthening of a tight anterior capsule and shortened muscles may dictate a delay in the initiation of external rotation exercises to prevent instability.

Strengthening

As the patient progresses through the stretching program, strengthening exercises may begin. In those patients who have a shoulder arthroplasty for primary osteoarthritis, active motion is not only allowed but also encouraged within 10 to 14 days of the surgical procedure. When there is good strength initially, the phase I and phase II strengthening program may be unnecessary. On the other hand, when shoulder arthroplasty is performed on patients who have rheumatoid arthritis and possible severe rotator cuff deficiencies, then the benefits of the phase I strengthening program to be discussed become very evident.

The phase I strengthening program is designed to gradually and progressively increase the strength of the anterior deltoid and supraspinatus while utilizing the assistance of gravity. The phase II program is designed to strengthen the rotator cuff and deltoid by eccentric contraction, and the phase III program strengthens muscles for use against gravity.

PHASE I STRENGTHENING

These exercises (Figure 7–19) are designed to begin the strengthening process of very weak muscles. Muscle strengthening is a slow process, and the patient must be persistent because it is easy to become discouraged at what may seem like very slow progress. At times, the underlying condition that led to muscle weakness is only aggravated by the protection that must be imposed to allow satisfactory healing if a rotator cuff repair was required at the time of arthroplasty. Like the stretching exercises, the strengthening exercises should be performed at least twice daily every day of the week.

The patient is positioned supine without a pillow under the head. The patient initially attempts to elevate the arm with the elbow flexed, extending the elbow as the arm comes up overhead. The arm is slowly brought down by the side, trying to keep a steady rhythm as the arm descends between 90 degrees of elevation and 0 degrees. In this arc, gravity influences the arm and tries to accelerate it. It is the patient's prevention of this acceleration that results in strengthening of the muscle. The patient then rests a few moments and repeats the exercise. Ideally, the patient works toward repeating the exercise 10 times before proceeding. In those patients who

Figure 7–19. The patient lies supine to minimize the effects of gravity while strengthening the anterior elevators of the shoulder. The patient adds a progressive weight in 1/2-lb increments, being certain that there is no acceleration as the arm descends from the perpendicular to the side.

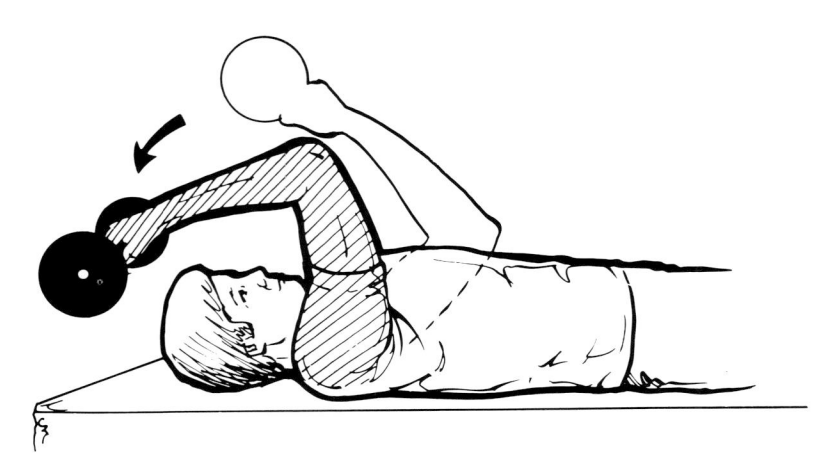

have particularly weak elevators, the uninvolved arm is used to assist in the elevation process, but the patient is to bring the arm back down by the side without any assistance. When this exercise can be performed unassisted from beginning to end at 10 repetitions twice daily, the program is advanced. A 1/2-lb weight is added to the hand and, with the patient supine, the arm is again lifted up overhead and slowly brought back down by the side. When 10 repetitions can be performed without fatigue on a twice daily basis, a 1-lb weight is used. This process is repeated adding 1/2-lb weight increments only when 10 repetitions are possible without fatigue. When the patient is able to perform this exercise with 5 lb, the phase II program is initiated.

PHASE II STRENGTHENING

Whereas the phase I program is performed with the patient positioned supine, minimizing the affect of gravity, the phase II program (Figure 7–20) uses gravity and strengthens muscles in an eccentric fashion. The muscles of the deltoid and rotator cuff are elongating under a contracting force, which tends to improve their strength characteristics.

The patient stands or sits and passively lifts the involved arm with the uninvolved arm to the point of maximum elevation. The affected arm is then released and balanced up overhead with active muscle control. The patient slowly flexes the elbow as the arm descends in the elevation plane, trying to prevent any acceleration as the arm is lowered. Once the arm is lowered down to the side, the patient rests for a few moments and repeats the exercise, making sure that when the arm is released, it actively descends without acceleration. This process is repeated 10 times and the program performed twice daily.

When the patient can do this exercise 10 times without fatigue, a 1/2-lb weight is added to the hand of the involved extremity, which is passively elevated using the uninvolved arm and balanced overhead. The uninvolved arm is once again placed at the side and the involved shoulder is balanced overhead now holding the 1/2-lb weight. Within a few seconds, the elbow is flexed and the arm is brought down by the side, again maintaining a smooth motion without acceleration. When this can be repeated 10 times, a 1-lb weight is held in the hand and the process repeated. This program continues until the patient can actively descend while holding 5 or 6 pounds. In each and every case, the incremental change in weight must be no more than 1/2 pound so the muscles see only a gradual increase in load. When 5 to 6 pounds can be actively brought down to the side 10 times without acceleration, the phase III strengthening program begins.

PHASE III STRENGTHENING

Many patients who have good muscle strength prior to shoulder arthroplasty can initiate the strengthening program with this phase, which utilizes graduated elastic surgical tubing to strengthen the deltoid and individual rotator cuff muscles. In consideration of deltoid strengthening, each of its three heads (anterior, middle, and posterior) is isolated and strengthened separately. Similarly, the subscapularis and infraspinatus are each strengthened individually. To strengthen the anterior deltoid, the patient's back is placed toward the door (Figure 7–21). With the elbow flexed to 90 degrees and starting with the humerus in the sagittal midline of the body, the elastic element is pulled forward approximately 45 degrees. It is then held there for 5 seconds and slowly released. After resting for a few seconds, the exercise is repeated 10 times.

The posterior deltoid is strengthened in a similar manner by having the patient face the door as shown (Figure 7–22). Of primary importance in this exercise is that the arm begins in a 45-degree forward position, allowing the posterior deltoid to pull the arm back against resistance but never beyond the sagittal midline. If the arm is pulled beyond and posterior to the sagittal midline, considerable forces are placed on the anterior capsular repair. This exercise is repeated 10 times twice daily.

Strengthening of the middle deltoid is often best performed in front of a mirror to be certain that symmetry is maintained (Figure 7–23). The patient holds the elastic device in both arms and symmetrically abducts the shoulder in the coronal plane. It is not important that the angular excursion exceed 45 degrees, as shown in the figure.

The internal rotators are strengthened as shown in Figure 7–24. It is important to remind the patient that the elbow must remain tight up against the side, ensuring that only rotational forces are generated. The elbow remains flexed at 90 de-

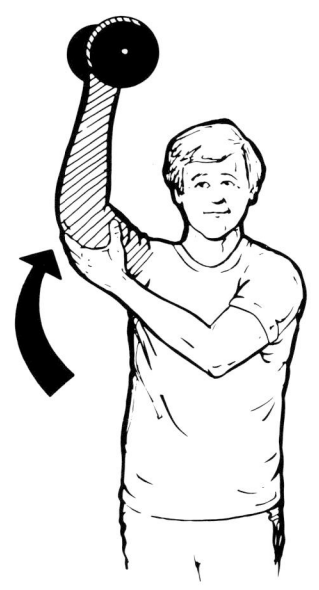

Figure 7–20. The patient now stands or sits and passively elevates the involved arm overhead. The arm is then actively brought down by the side in an eccentric muscle-strengthening fashion.

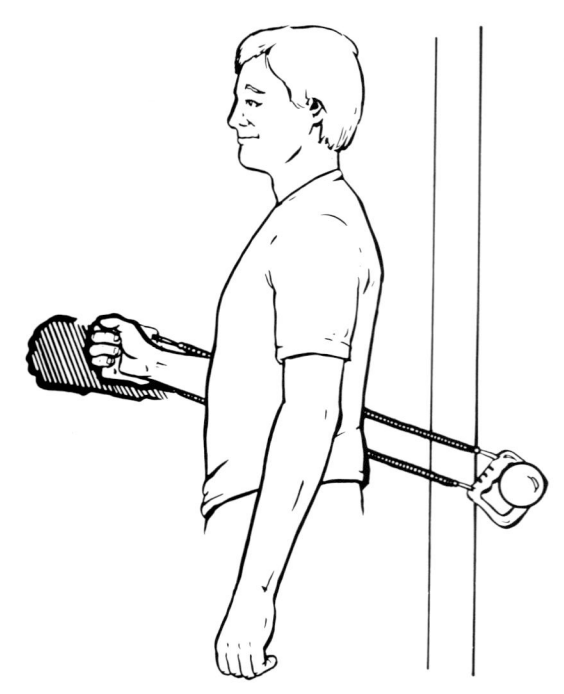

Figure 7–21. The patient stands with the back to the door. The elastic device is pulled forward, held for 5 seconds, and slowly released. The exercise is repeated in sets of 10.

grees, the arm is rotated internally against resistance no more than 45 degrees, and the tension is slowly released.

External rotators are strengthened in a very similar fashion, with the patient facing the opposite direction relative to the door handle, as shown in Figure 7–25. The arm is rotated out 45 degrees, keeping the elbow tight against the side. The infraspinatus is the only effective external rotator, and there is a frequent tendency to abduct the arm away from the side allowing the deltoid to substitute.

Each of these phase III strengthening exercises should be performed twice daily in sets of 10. Once the patient spends 3 months on this program, strengthening of scapular muscles, including the trapezius, rhomboids, latissimus, and pectorals, begins. Depending on the patient's age and activity level, variable intensity is given to this later set of exercises.

CONTINUOUS PASSIVE MOTION

The author has no personal experience in the use of continuous passive motion for shoulder arthroplasty. The patient must be the active agent in the rehabilitation program, and certain personality types will become dependent on the machine and lose sight of the fact that they themselves are responsible for their rehabilitation program.

Certain situations may lend themselves to the use of continuous passive motion. Patients who have bilateral shoulder problems may find continuous passive motion beneficial where self-assisted exercises would be difficult or impossible. However, setting up and removing the apparatus is difficult and usually requires an assistant, particularly in the geriatric population. Craig[11] and Neer et al.[12] reported their experiences with continuous passive motion after reconstructive surgery of the shoulder. For rotator cuff repairs, shoulder arthroplasties, and acromioplasties, they found use of continuous passive motion to result in earlier recovery of motion, diminished pain, and a shorter hospital stay.

Figure 7–22. The patient stands facing the door with the arm flexed out in front, as shown. The arm is pulled back against the elastic resistance, but the elbow never goes beyond the lateral midline. The elastic is held under tension for approximately 5 seconds and slowly released.

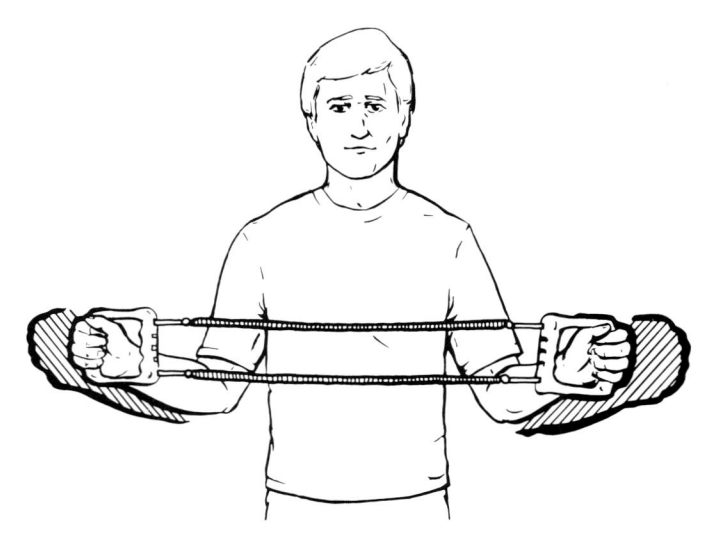

Figure 7–23. The arms are held as shown and abducted in a symmetric fashion. The elastic is held under tension for approximately 5 seconds and slowly released. This exercise is best performed in front of a mirror to maintain symmetry. Adequate instruction is given to be certain the arms are not externally rotating at the shoulder during the exercise.

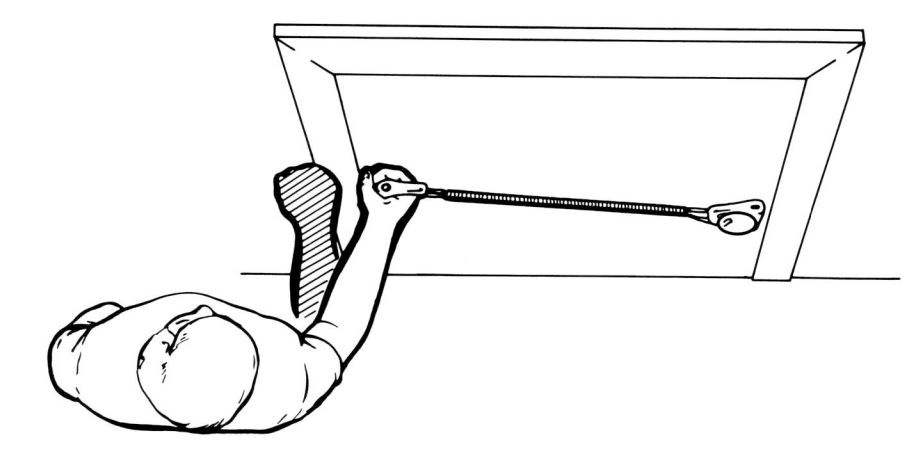

Figure 7–24. The arm is held nearly perpendicular to the frontal plane of the body with the elastic, as shown. The arm is pulled inward no more than 45 degrees, held for 5 seconds, and slowly released.

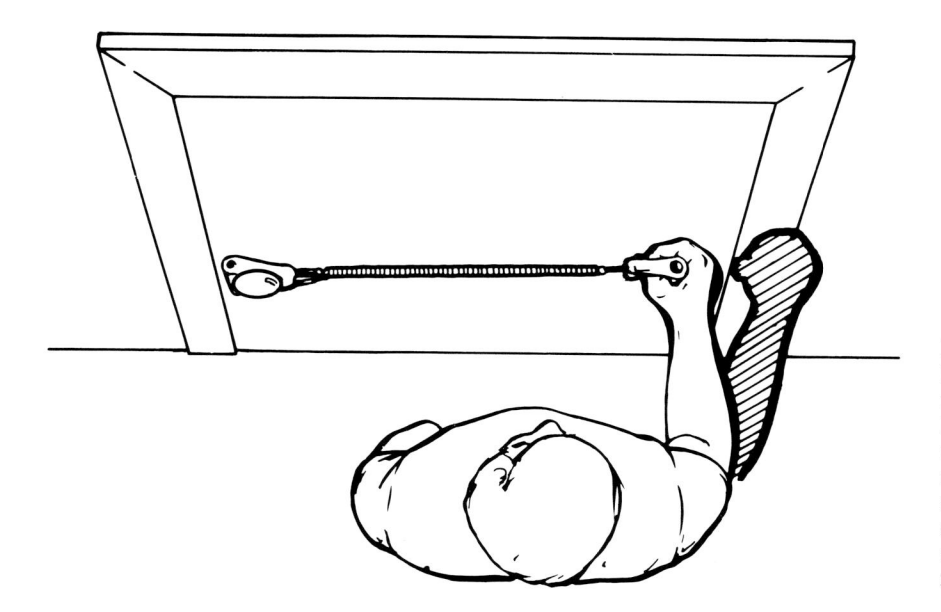

Figure 7–25. The patient stands holding the elastic device with the forearm perpendicular to the body. Keeping the elbow tight against the side, the arm is externally rotated no more than 45 degrees, held for 5 seconds, and slowly released. The elbow must be kept tight against the side at all times to minimize recruitment of the deltoid muscle.

Continuous passive motion machines of many varieties are commercially available. Thorough knowledge of a machine's capabilities and limitations is mandatory if the surgeon is going to use one. The cost/benefit ratio should be evaluated and its use limited to those patients and situations where self-assistance is not possible.

SUMMARY

Proper rehabilitation following total shoulder arthroplasty is not only necessary, but also critical to a successful outcome. The surgeon must direct, modify, and continually evaluate progress with the physical therapy program. Unless specific surgical concerns dictate otherwise, the rehabilitation program should begin no more than 48 hours after the procedure. The rehabilitation program proceeds in a logical and orderly fashion, beginning with joint mobilization to maximize range of motion in the cardinal planes. Strengthening begins when motion allows, and likewise proceeds in a stepwise fashion until maximum strength is achieved. When the principals of surgical technique are combined with the principals of rehabilitation, a successful total shoulder replacement is not just possible, it is predictable.

REFERENCES

1. Donatelli R, ed. *Physical Therapy of the Shoulder*. New York: Churchill-Livingstone, 1987.
2. Travell J, Simons DG. *Myofascial Pain and Dysfunction: The Trigger Point Manual*. Baltimore: Williams & Wilkins, 1983.
3. Gould JA, Simons DG, eds. *Orthopaedics and Sports Physical Therapy*. St Louis: CV Mosby, 1985;2:199–211.
4. Neer CS. In: Shoulder Reconstruction. CS Neer (ed), *Anatomy of Shoulder Reconstruction*. Philadelphia: WB Saunders, 1990:1–10.

5. Rockwood CA. The technique of total shoulder arthroplasty. *Instr Course Lect* 1990;39:437–447.
6. Neer CS. In: Shoulder Reconstruction. CS Neer (ed), *Glenohumeral Arthroplasty*. Philadelphia: WB Saunders, 1990:169–237.
7. Brems JJ, Yoon HJ, Tetzlaff J. Interscalene block anaesthesia and shoulder surgery. *Orthop Trans* 1990;14:250.
8. Kisner C, Colby LA. *Therapeutic Exercise Foundations and Techniques*. 2nd ed. Philadelphia: FA Davis, 1990:241–270.
9. Neer CS. In: Shoulder Reconstruction. CS Neer (ed), *Shoulder Rehabilitation*. Philadelphia: WB Saunders, 1990:487–530.
10. Cofield RH. Degenerative and arthritic problems of the glenohumeral joint. In: Rockwood CA, Matsen FA, eds. *The Shoulder*. Philadelphia: WB Saunders, 1990:735–736.
11. Craig EV. Continuous passive motion in the rehabilitation of the surgically reconstructed shoulder: A preliminary report. *Orthop Trans* 1986;10:219.
12. Neer CS, McCann PD, Macfarlane EA, et al. Earlier passive motion following shoulder arthroplasty and rotator cuff repair: A prospective study. *Orthop Trans* 1987;11:231.

SECTION III

Alternatives to Total Shoulder Arthroplasty

8 Synovectomy of the Shoulder

Jan A. Pahle, M.D., and Lasse Kvarnes, M.D.

Surgical treatment of rheumatoid arthritis is closely related to the development of corrective orthopaedic surgery and synovectomy. Resection arthroplasty was described in the 16th century by Paré, and systematically used from 1750. The first book on joint arthroplasty was published in 1805, and artificial replacement of joint ends was first done by Ollier in 1878. In the last half of the 19th century, the idea of preventive surgical intervention was discussed in several countries.

The most dramatic aspects of rheumatoid arthritis, an autoimmune disease, occur at the innermost layer of the joint capsule, the synovial membrane. It is important to remember that this disease leads to a general attack on all connective tissues in the body. General symptoms such as asthenia and anemia are common and may be present for a long period of time before the joints and other body organs are affected. Among the many visceral organs affected, malfunctioning kidneys represent the most serious problem to the surgeon treating rheumatoid arthritis.

It is still debated whether the target cell in this autoimmune disease is the mesothelial synovial cell or the chondrocyte. However, the pathologic process leads to a thickening of the synovial membrane (Figure 8–1), sometimes more than a hundred times its normal thickness. The production of joint fluid increases and changes in quality, explaining the joint distension seen. At an early stage, this may lead to weakening of the supporting structures about the joint, such as the capsule and ligaments. After a period of time, the diseased synovial membrane starts to expand over its normal boundaries and begins invading and destroying articular cartilage, ligaments, and the capsule. It may also penetrate deep into the bony tissue, causing erosions and cysts. The synovial membrane acts like an invasive tumor, which can invade the tendon sheaths and destroy the tendon fibrils until they rupture, often with a substantial defect, making end-to-end suturing impossible.

Destruction of the joint cartilage leads to increased friction and pain. Ingrowth into the bony tissue, which seems to follow the nutritional vessels, may produce cystic defects that coalesce to form larger cavities and weaken the bone. This leads to collapse of the joint surfaces, resulting in axial distortions. The well-known deformities in rheumatoid arthritis are all explained by this destructive nature of the synovial membrane.

It is unclear whether the ingrowth of granulomatous tissue over the joint cartilage, the so-called pannus formation, is a destructive process, or simply a reparative measure similar to scar formation.[1] The sharply circumscribed extension of the pannus, as depicted in Figure 8–2, suggests that it may be the source of destruction, since it is difficult to explain such a sharp delineation of scar tissue if the destruction of articular cartilage is caused by lysozomal enzymes in the joint fluid.

RATIONALE FOR SYNOVECTOMY

Synovectomy means removal of the pathologically altered synovial membrane, and this may be performed in most joints and tendon sheaths without deleterious adverse effects to the important surrounding structures.[2] The synovial membrane is a primitive organ that can regenerate very rapidly. The regenerated membrane in some cases is entirely without inflammatory features, but usually some signs of inflammation are present, although practically never to the same degree as in the original granulomatous membrane.[3] It is seemingly more resistant to repeat attacks of the disease, which may explain the obvious retardation of the destructive process in the operated joint. In quite a few cases of early synovectomy, what appears to be a total arrest of the destruction is observed.

The first synovectomies were performed in 1877, but the term was not used until 1889 by Mignon. Müller in Achen described synovectomies for rheumatoid arthritis as early as 1888. Successful results were reported in the United States in 1916. In later years, several observers noted that when the diseased membrane is radically removed, less inflammation recurs in the regenerated membrane.[4] Radical synovectomy has become a standard in Scandinavian and continental European clinics dealing with the surgical treatment of rheumatoid arthritis.[5]

Even though it has been more than 100 years since the first synovectomies were performed, the years 1949 to 1951 are recognized as the start of modern rheumatoid arthritis surgery, when the concept of the *combined unit* was created at the Rheumatism Foundation Hospital in Finland under the guidance of the rheumatologist Veikko Laine and the orthopaedic surgeon Kauko Vainio.[6] Vainio became the teacher to a whole generation of surgeons from all over the world. Combined units have since been set up in several countries where rheumatologists and other specialists work together in a team with the orthopaedic surgeon. In such centers, surgeons have developed new techniques that differ in several ways from the standard procedures previously described. This is a result of the fact that one is dealing with a disease that attacks multiple joints simultaneously, as well as other organ systems, with serious consequences.

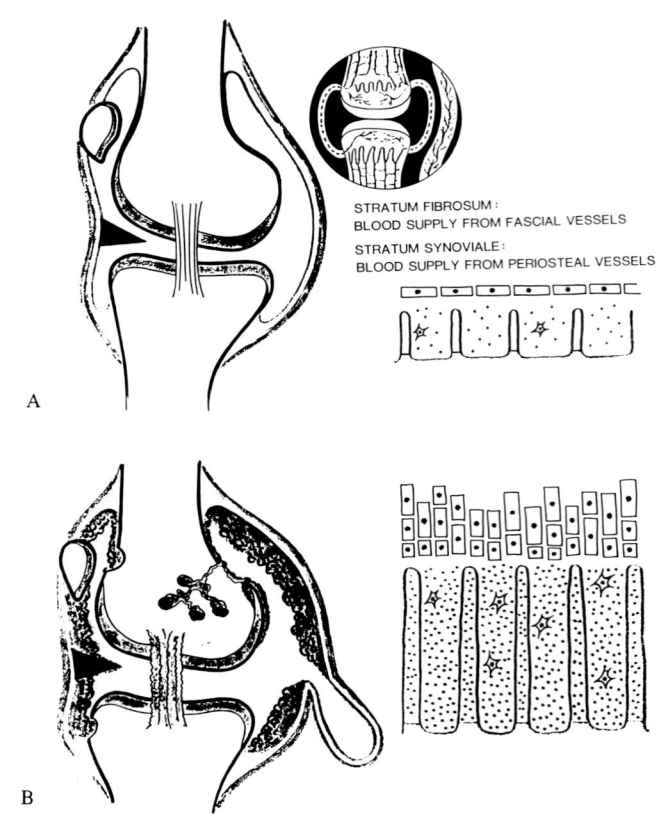

Figure 8–1. **A.** In a normal joint, the synovial membrane is only film-thick, covering the inside of the fibrous capsule, and by a reflection continuing on the periosteum to the edge of the articular cartilage, thereby constituting a closed sac. Although intimately connected to the fibrous capsule, it has its own blood, lymph, and nerve supply. Histologically, there is usually one layer of mesothelial cells upon a thin stroma where short-circuited vascular slings are seen. **B.** The inflammatory changes are conspicuous: The thickening synovial membrane, which grows expansively underneath and over the articular cartilage (pannus), invades the osseous and ligamentous tissue and sometimes penetrates the fibrous capsule (Baker cyst). Histologically, there is an increased number of vascular slings, massive infiltration of mononuclear cells, and a proliferation of mesothelial cells, cylindrical in several layers.

The efficacy of synovectomy is still disputed in many countries. This dispute may be explained by two circumstances. First, there can be a lack of adequate technique guaranteeing radical removal of the diseased synovial membrane. What is called a synovectomy can often vary greatly in technique. Second, in advanced cases of joint destruction, radical removal of the synovium is impossible due to the already present intraosseous and intraligamentous invasion. Therefore, the destroyed cartilage and other joint structures may need additional reconstructive surgery in order to function satisfactorily. Only in clinics that have adopted the combined-unit principle where the rheumatologist and orthopaedic surgeon work closely together will it be possible to get *early* cases referred for synovectomy. In many countries the rheumatologist may continue with conservative therapy beyond the point where a synovectomy can be of maximum benefit, and this may explain the poor reputation synovectomy has achieved in some countries.[7] The rheumatoid arthritis patient should be presented to the experienced rheumatoid arthritis surgeon from the very beginning, even if operative treatment is not planned at that stage.

It is the authors' experience that synovectomy for rheumatoid arthritis in radiologic grades I to III is worthwhile and may at times be curative. There is also, in the authors' opinion, some evidence that removal of the diseased synovial membrane in a sufficient number of large joints may directly influence the total course of the disease and contribute to a general remission. This is in accordance with the fact that local immune processes that have a general influence on the systemic immune apparatus are going on in the synovial membrane. The frequency of complications following synovectomy is less than that seen for many of the cytotoxic medications used. Patients often request to have other affected joints operated upon following a synovectomy, since they have experienced not only a reduction in pain but also improvement in function, leading to an overall improvement in the total capacity of the patient.

There are few reports detailing the results of synovectomy of the shoulder in the world literature. Some reports dealt only with removal of an inflamed subdeltoid or subacromial

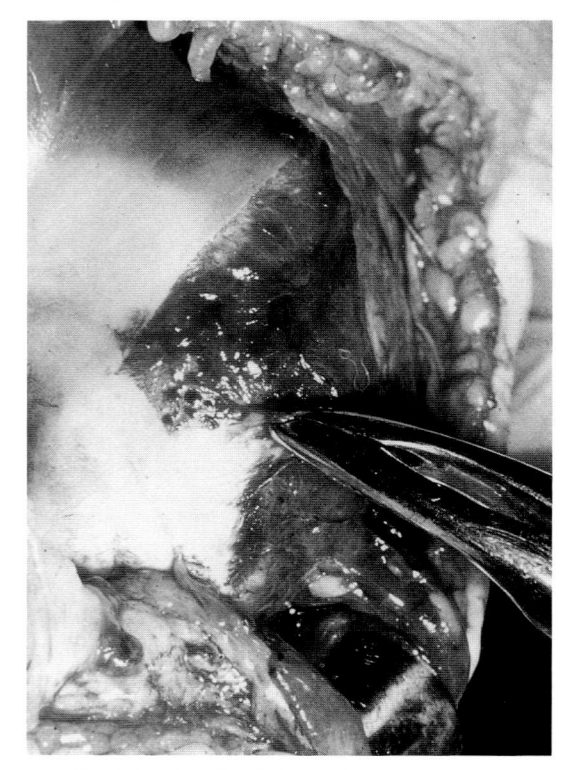

Figure 8–2. The sharply delineated pannus ingrowth is lifted from the cartilage of a femoral condyle and reveals a steplike defect in the cartilage underneath. According to Fassbender,[1] this early stage of pannus is an aggressive granulation tissue, which later will be transformed into a scarlike connective tissue.

bursa.[8] This chapter discusses 24 years of experience with synovectomy of the shoulder for rheumatoid arthritis in the Oslo Sanitetsforening Rheumatism Hospital.

INCIDENCE AND TECHNIQUE

Rheumatoid arthritis of the glenohumeral joint is a common manifestation of the disease, and is often bilateral. Gschwend[9] found frequencies of about 60%, whereas Petersson[10] found that as many as 91% of the patients had shoulder problems. Sbarbaro[11] stated in 1975 that the majority of patients do not develop disabling symptoms, and for this reason synovectomy should not be performed routinely. This is in sharp contrast to many authors' experience, who have observed that rheumatoid arthritis of the shoulder joint will rapidly lead to restricted motion and pain, resulting in severe disability.[12]

In the years 1968 through 1991, 117 synovectomies of the glenohumeral joint (often including the acromioclavicular joint) were performed in the authors' hospital. In the period 1973 through 1991, 179 prosthetic shoulder arthroplasties of the glenohumeral joint were performed. The synovectomy group of patients usually had a history of disease in the shoulder joint about half as long as that for the arthroplasty group (10.5 years versus 18.7 years).[13,14] This waiting time before surgery is definitely too long in either case. The synovectomy group had mostly radiologic grade II or III disease, whereas the arthroplasty group had mainly grade IV or V disease.[15]

Until 1981 the technique always included resection of the lateral part of the acromion after releasing the origin of the deltoid muscle, and then splitting the rotator cuff between the supraspinatus and infraspinatus tendons or using an already existing defect to enter the joint craniodorsally. With internal rotation of the humerus, the head is then subluxed dorsally out of the glenoid fossa.[16] A total of 37 patients were operated on in this way.

Since 1981 the standard approach has been modified in order to facilitate insertion of a prosthesis if necessary, something that is not always possible to decide preoperatively.[17] Since 1987 these operations have been performed with an interscalene brachial plexus block (Figure 8–3), using a catheter that is left in place for postoperative analgesia and physical therapy.[18] With this type of anesthesia, the mean blood loss is reduced approximately 50% compared to patients operated on under general anesthesia.[19] The patient is operated on in a semisitting position, with an arm board for support.

The modified approach is based upon the guidelines of Neer et al.[20] and does not require detachment of the deltoid muscle. The cranial half of the pectoralis major tendon is divided and the rotator cuff inspected (Figure 8–4). Tenosynovectomy (Figure 8–5) of the long head of the biceps is performed in both types of operations by splitting the transverse ligament over the bicipital groove. This frequently ruptured tendon is usually found adherent to the bony walls of the groove, and fixation of the distal stump with sutures to the transverse ligament is necessary only in a few cases. This explains the normal contour of the biceps muscle belly even in cases of tendon disruption. In most cases, tenosynovitis is found to be pronounced, with expansion of the tenosynovium after release of the transverse ligament, indicating that pressure on the tendon must have been severe. This pressure may account for part of the patient's pain. Care must be taken to avoid damaging the ascending lateral branch of the anterior circumflex artery,[21] since osteonecrosis of the humeral head may result.

Subdeltoid and subacromial bursectomies are performed, followed by division of the subscapularis tendon and capsule to permit subluxation of the humeral head with external rotation, adduction, and extension. In this way, good access

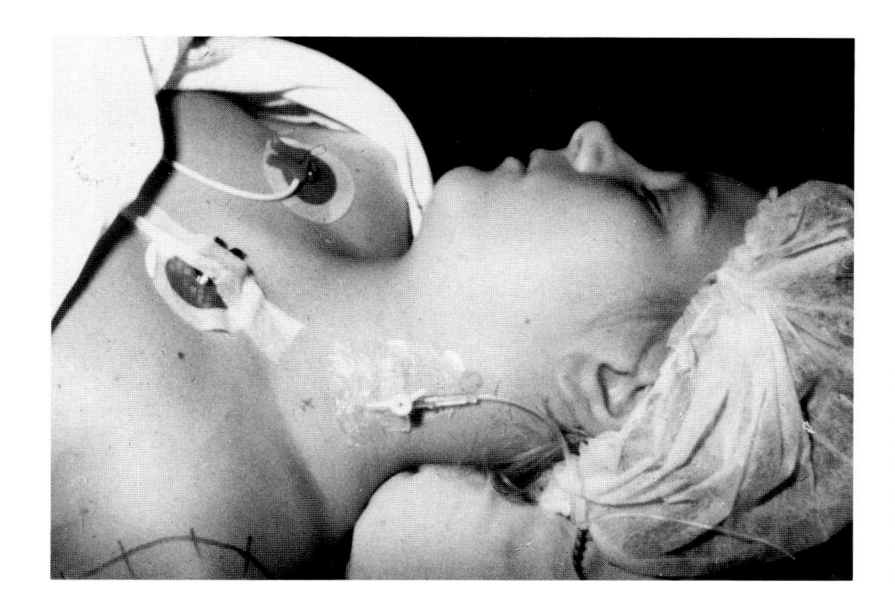

Figure 8–3. Interscalene brachial plexus block via catheter, usually left in situ 2 to 3 days postoperatively for analgesia, facilitating the postoperative training. The average blood loss during the operation is greatly reduced when this type of regional anesthesia is applied. Autotransfusion is used regularly.

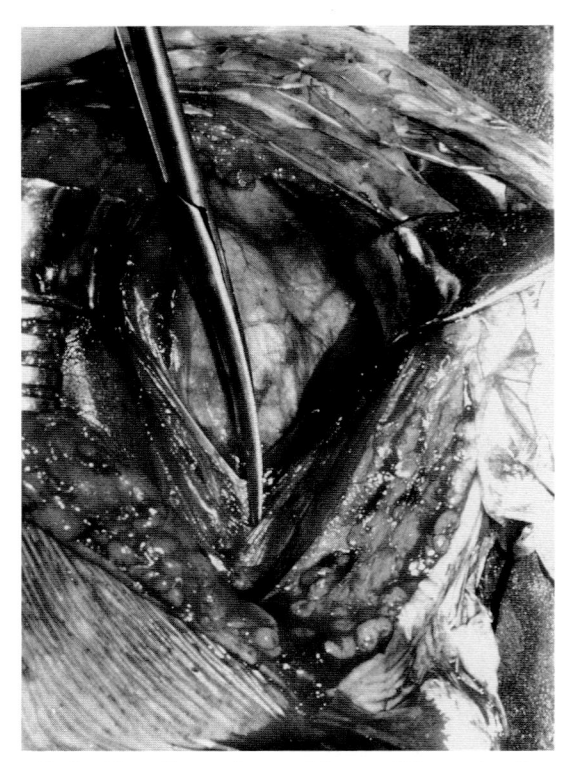

Figure 8–4. By splitting the cranial part of the pectoralis major insertion, good access to the upper end of the humerus is obtained.

the rotators because of the depressor effect they exert on the humeral head. Specific occupational therapy is instituted after 1 week, including "switchboard training." Combined physical and occupational therapy is continued for at least 6 weeks postoperatively.

Whereas the old approach facilitated simultaneous resection of the acromion, releasing the deltoid made the postoperative physical therapy difficult. The postoperative management with preservation of the deltoid origin has resulted in an easier postoperative rehabilitation course.

MATERIALS AND METHODS

The purpose of this review is twofold. First, to examine the long-term results after synovectomy, and second, to compare the outcome of the two different techniques, with or without resection of the acromion and release of the deltoid origin. The material presented here pertains to all patients who underwent synovectomy of the shoulder joint in the authors' hospital from 1978 to 1984, totaling 31 shoulders in 26 patients (Table 8–1). All 26 patients were examined clinically and radiographically between 1990 and 1992, with an average follow-up period of 11 years after the synovectomy. The aim was to compare two groups who were matched with regards to age, sex, duration of disease in the affected

to the entire glenoid and anatomic neck of the humerus is obtained, facilitating radical synovectomy. The stepwise application of medium-size and small retractors is shown in Figure 8–6. Synovectomy around the anatomic neck is performed. Osteophytes and other irregularities are removed and smoothed out with a file and ball drill (Figure 8–7). Ruptures of the rotator cuff are repaired, and sometimes the proximal stump of the long head of the biceps can be used for such repair work. Diverticula of the synovial membrane may reach deep into the axilla through defects between the capsular ligaments, demanding great care when excising the membrane to avoid damaging nearby nerves and vessels. After a thorough synovectomy, the acromioclavicular joint is inspected, and a synovectomy performed if necessary. Adhesions between the subscapularis tendon and the anterior edge of the glenoid are carefully released to ensure a functioning subscapularis muscle (Figure 8–8).

In order to visualize the glenoid, a Hohman retractor is used around the upper and lower borders of the glenoid neck, and a Bankart retractor over the proximal end of the humerus may be pressed laterally and dorsally for exposure. During this procedure adhesions and scarring may be loosened by sharp or blunt dissection.

With this approach the patient is usually up and around after 2 to 3 days, with a light abduction splint set between 30 and 60 degrees for 2 to 3 weeks (Figure 8–9). Isometric exercises of the deltoid and the internal and external rotators are started on the first postoperative day, with emphasis on

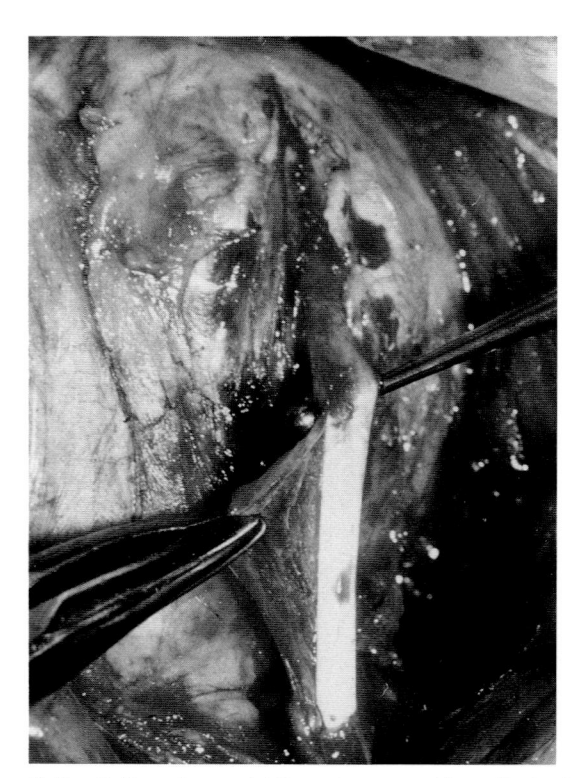

Figure 8–5. Inflamed synovial tissue is removed from the tendon of the long head of the biceps after the transverse ligament is split. In this case, the distal part of the ruptured tendon is adherent to the groove and does not need special fixation.

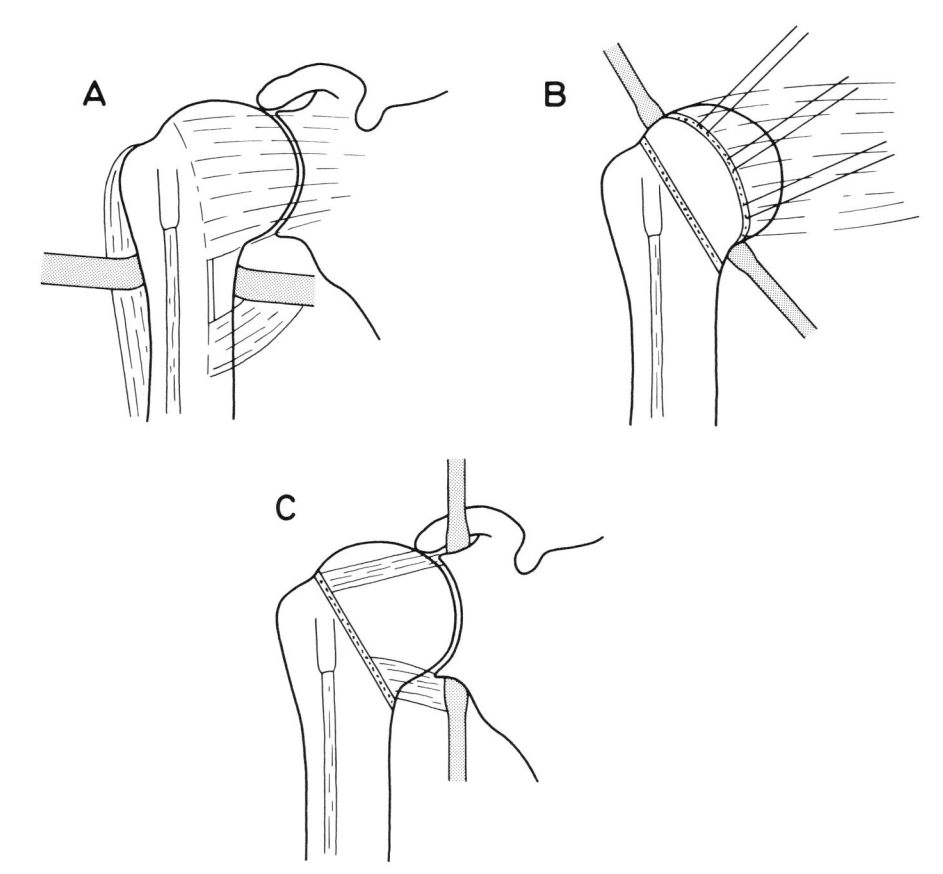

Figure 8–6. **A.** After division of the cranial half of the pectoralis major insertion, a wide Hohman retractor may be introduced around the medial part of the surgical neck. By abducting the humerus, the deltoid muscle may be pulled laterally and backwards by means of another wide Hohman retractor. Good access is obtained to the long head of the biceps, subdeltoid bursa, and rotator cuff. **B.** After the insertion of the subscapularis tendon is split 5 to 10 mm from the lesser tuberosity, the proximal part of the tendon is pulled medially by stay sutures, and two small Hohman retractors are introduced around the anatomic neck. **C.** In the last step, the glenoid is visualized by means of two small Hohman retractors around the upper and lower border of the glenoid neck.

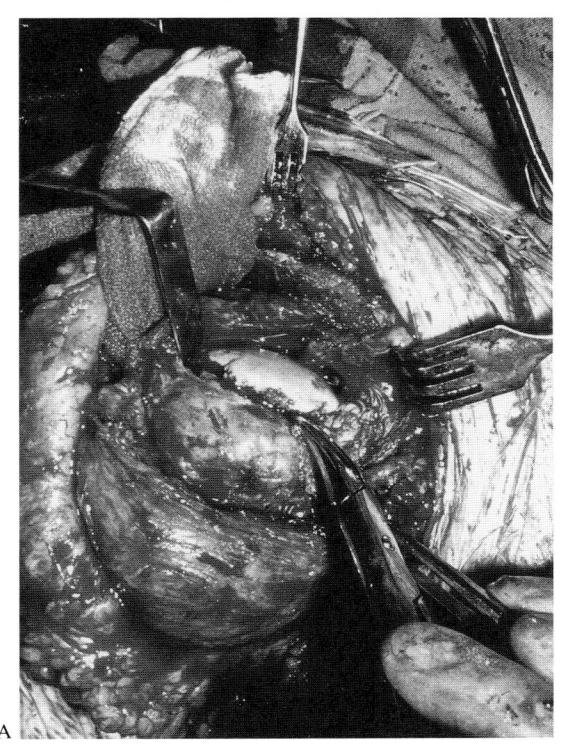

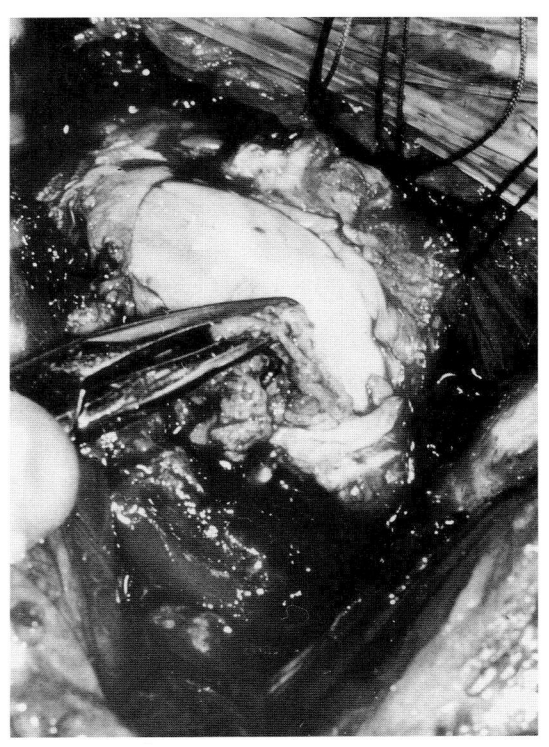

Figure 8–7. **A** and **B.** By externally rotating the humerus, the head is now visible in the opening of the rotator cuff, and Hohman retractors may be introduced around the anatomic neck intra-articularly, whereafter synovectomy is performed. If the defects of the head are large, a prosthetic replacement may be considered at this stage.

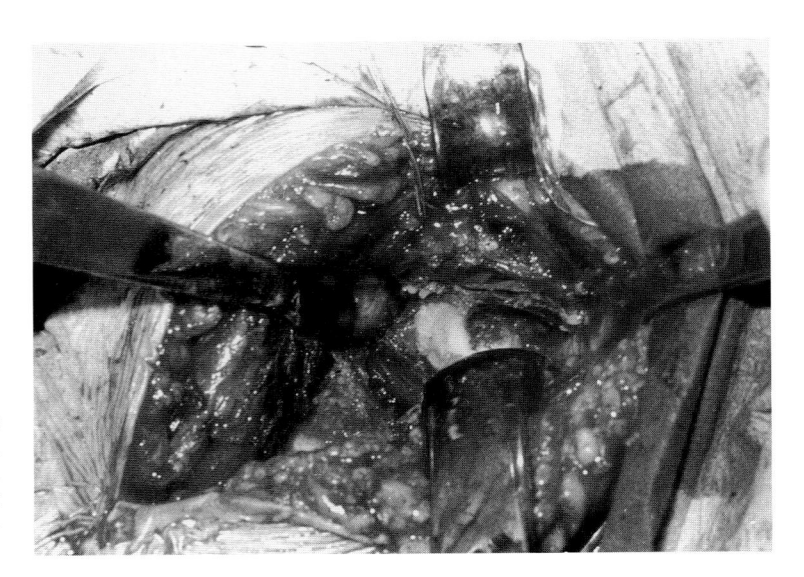

Figure 8–8. A Bankart retractor is positioned over the humeral head, against the posterior edge of glenoid. Good access for cleaning the joint surface of the glenoid is thereby established.

shoulder, and radiologic grade but who underwent different surgical techniques.

In 14 shoulders, the lateral part of the acromion was resected simultaneously. This group is hereafter designated as group A, and the 17 shoulders without resection of the acromion are in group B. The diagnosis (Table 8–2) was definite or classic rheumatoid arthritis according to the American Rheumatism Association criteria in 21 patients; 2 patients had ankylosing spondylitis and 3 had juvenile rheumatoid arthritis.

It must be remembered that juvenile rheumatoid arthritis results in growth disturbances as well as joint destruction, and these growth disturbances, such as blown-up condyles in contrast to slender shafts and changes in version, may cause a greater functional disturbance than the joint destructions[22] (Figure 8–10). The radiologic staging is therefore somewhat inadequate for the juvenile rheumatoid arthritis patient.

Most of the patients were diagnosed preoperatively as being grade II or III, with only 2 shoulders considered grade I (Table 8–3). Shoulders with late disease (grade IV) were also included. In the 7 with late disease where almost all of the articular cartilage was gone, synovectomy was combined with débridement, including removal of osteophytes, release of adhesions, and smoothing of the joint surface. If the joint surfaces could be made spherical and smooth following débridement, then a shoulder prosthesis was not implanted.

RESULTS

As seen in Table 8–4, the long-term results were good, with only 1 shoulder with late disease (grade IV) being a candidate for total shoulder arthroplasty after 10 years. In group A, 1 of 14 shoulders had no signs of osteoarthrosis at the time of follow-up, and had radiographically improved from grade III

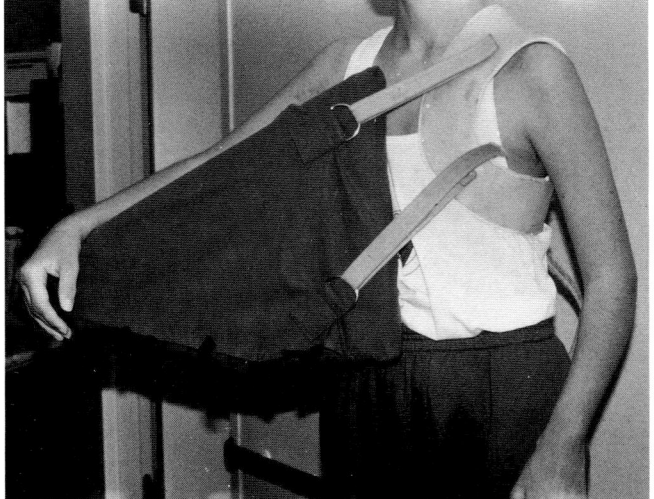

Figure 8–9. After a few days the patient is usually up and around with an abduction splint. The top angle varies between 30 and 60 degrees. Note the fixation of the straps to the plastic ring around the contralateral shoulder. The vertical part of the splint is concave in order to adapt to the thoracic wall.

Table 8–1. Synovectomy of the Shoulder (n = 31; 26 patients)

Females	20
Males	6
Disease duration in the shoulder	11.5 y
Group A (with acromion resection)	14 shoulders
Group B (without acromion resection)	17 shoulders
Average age (range) at operation	
Group A	38.7 y (14–57 y)
Group B	39.8 y (13–57 y)
Average (range) observation time	
Group A	12.3 y (10–16 y)
Group B	9.2 y (7–14 y)

Table 8–2. Diagnosis (n = 31 shoulders, 26 patients)

DIAGNOSIS	NO. OF PATIENTS	AVERAGE AGE (RANGE)	NO. OF GROUP A PATIENTS	NO. OF GROUP B PATIENTS
Juvenile rheumatoid arthritis	3	15 y (13–17 y)	2	1
Rheumatoid arthritis	21	44 y (18–57 y)	12	9
Ankylosing spondylitis	2	25 y	0	2

to II during this time (see Table 8–3). In group B, 2 of 17 shoulders developed no sign of osteoarthrosis during the follow-up period (Figure 8–11).

The osteoarthrosis was diagnosed as severe in only 2 of the 31 shoulders (Figures 8–12 and 8–13). In the remainder, the general findings were reduction of the joint space with slight medialization and cranial subluxation of the humeral head (Figure 8–14). Only 3 of the 31 shoulders did not develop radiologic osteoarthrosis (Figure 8–15). A reduction in the range of motion was found in most cases (Table 8–5), but this reduction was seldom accompanied by pain. This is reflected in the fact that only 3 of the shoulders needed to have a total shoulder arthroplasty (Table 8–6). The mean follow-up time was 12.3 years for group A (range, 10 to 16 years) and 9.3 years (range, 7 to 14 years) for group B.

Aside from recording the range of motion in degrees, a better understanding of function is possible by examining the functional range of motion as demonstrated by activities of daily living, such as reaching behind the back of the neck, combing hair, perineal care, and washing the opposite axilla.[5] (Table 8–7, Figure 8–16). In normal individuals, almost 90% of the daily activities are performed below 90 degrees of abduction. Patients are also concerned about the ability to sleep on the operated shoulder, and only in 7 shoulders were the patients not able to do so.

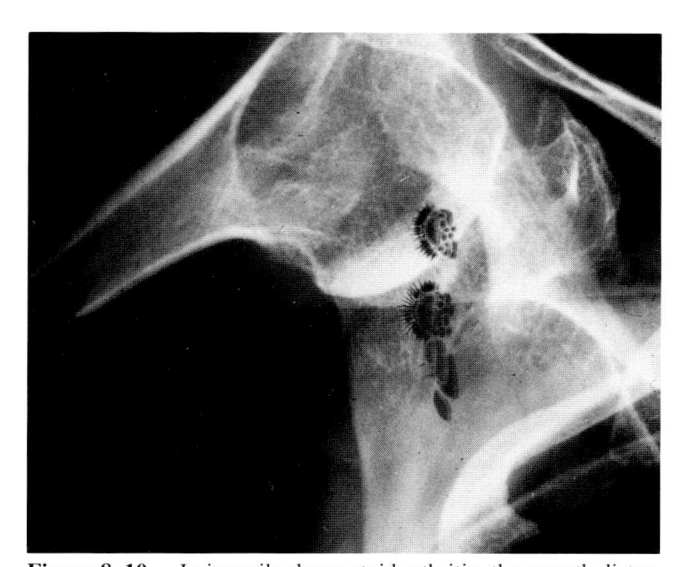

Figure 8–10. In juvenile rheumatoid arthritis, the growth disturbances may account for more functional disturbance than the destructive processes.

Table 8–3. Radiologic Findings According to Larsen et al.[15] (n = 31 shoulders, 26 patients)*

	PREOPERATIVE	POSTOPERATIVE†
Group A		
Grade I	1	0
Grade II	7	5
Grade III	4	3
Grade IV	2	5
Grade V	0	1
Group B		
Grade I	1	1
Grade II	5	1
Grade III	6	9‡
Grade IV	5	4
Grade V	0	2

*Data are number of shoulders.

†For group A, the mean postoperative time was 12.3 years; for group B, 9.3 years.

‡In group A, 1 shoulder in grade II and in group B, 2 shoulders in grade III were without visible osteoarthrosis at the time of follow-up.

Table 8–4. Results for 7 Shoulders with Radiologic Grade IV Preoperatively

Group A: 2 shoulders	X-ray unchanged, *no pain*, can reach head and back to thoracic spine
Group B: 3 shoulders	X-ray unchanged, *no pain*, can reach head and back to thoracic spine
Group B: 1 shoulder	Severe osteoarthrosis and pain, can reach mouth and back
Group B: 1 shoulder	Candidate for total shoulder arthroplasty, 10 y after synovectomy

All patients went through a long postoperative period of physical therapy, starting with 3 weeks in the hospital and continuing for up to 4 months as an outpatient, with emphasis on muscle strengthening and internal and external rotation. These patients were suffering from a polyarticular disease where elbow and hand functions were also affected simultaneously.

PERIOPERATIVE FINDINGS

In 26 shoulders, a bursa was found, often communicating with the joint itself and in some cases containing rice bodies

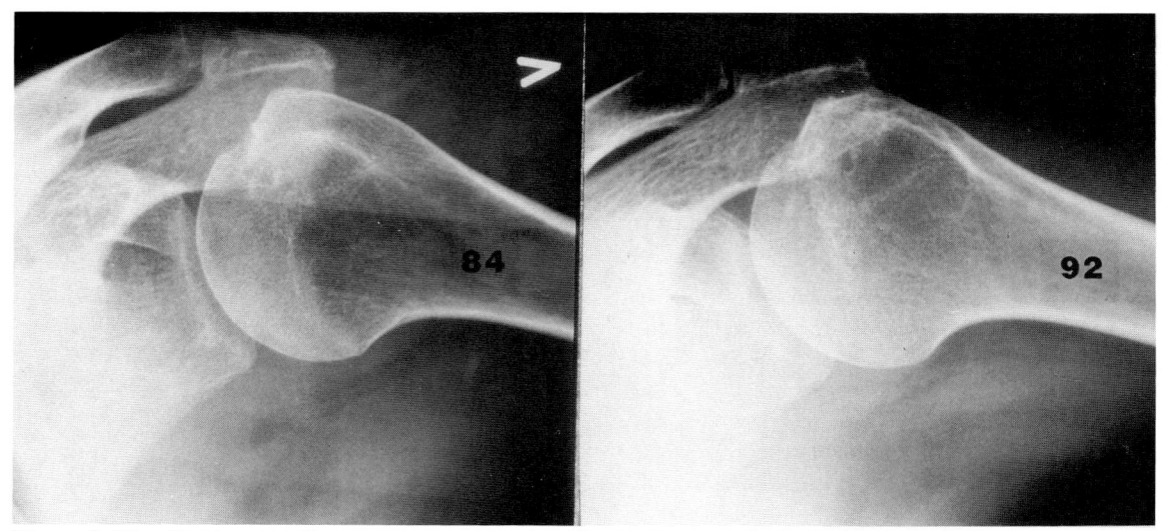

Figure 8–11. Eight years after synovectomy the shoulder is almost unchanged without medialization or upward migration, is pain-free, and is functioning well.

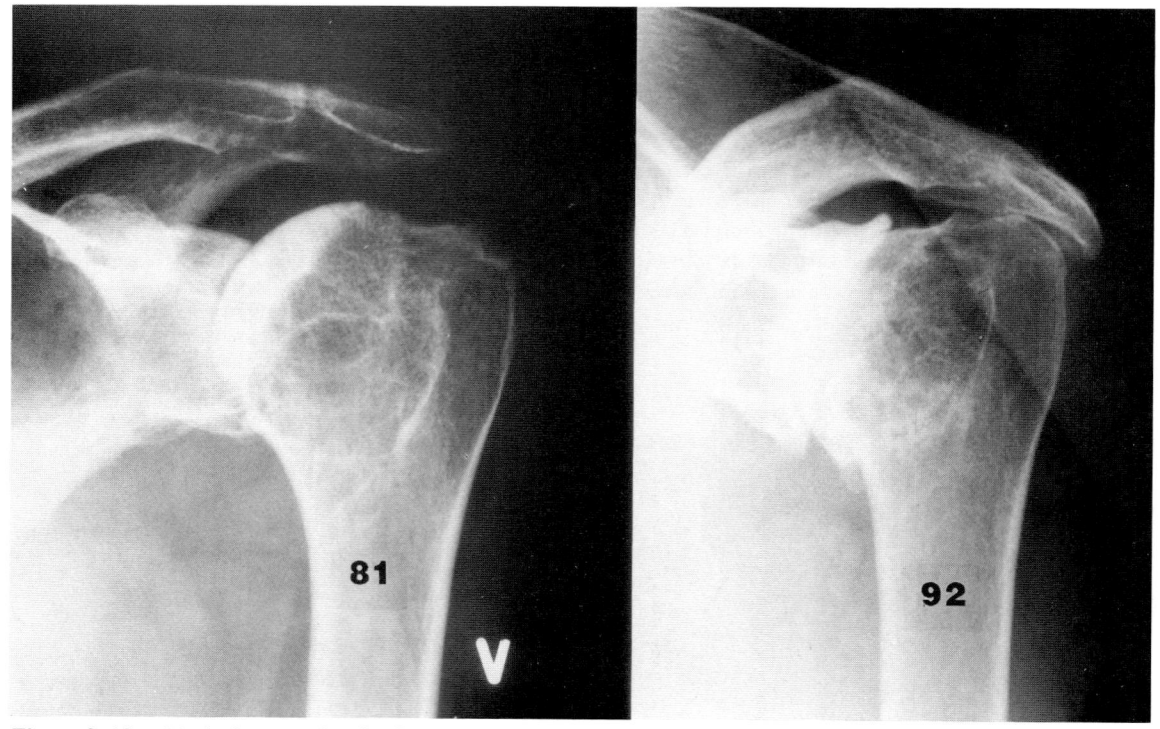

Figure 8–12. Marked osteoarthrosis after 11 years, but the shoulder is pain-free and functioning well.

Synovectomy of the Shoulder 121

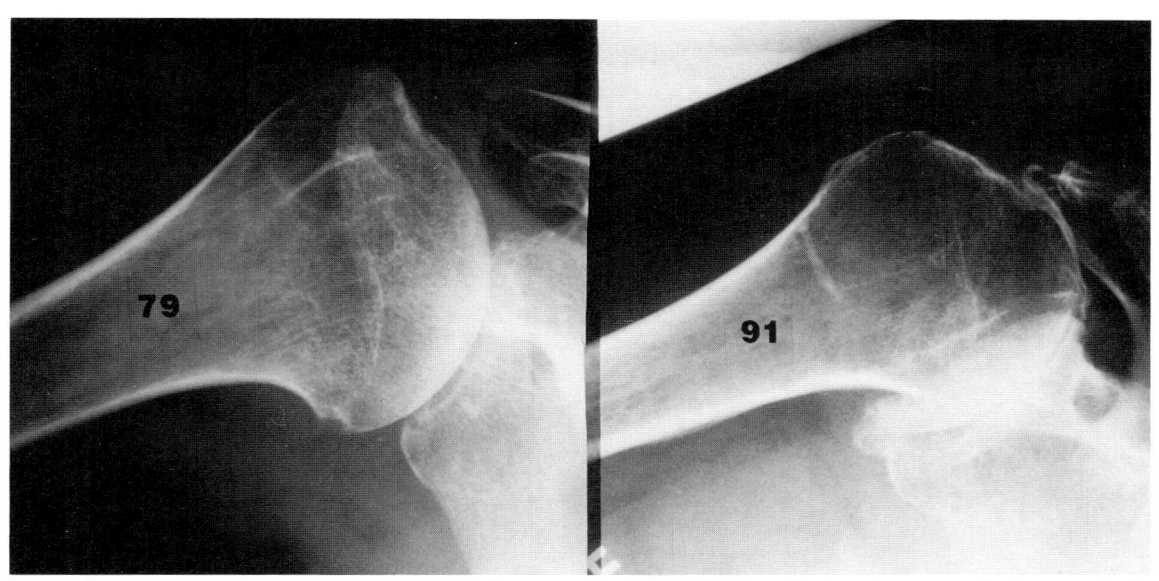

Figure 8–13. Severe osteoarthrosis 12 years after synovectomy, with upward migration, necessitating prosthetic arthroplasty.

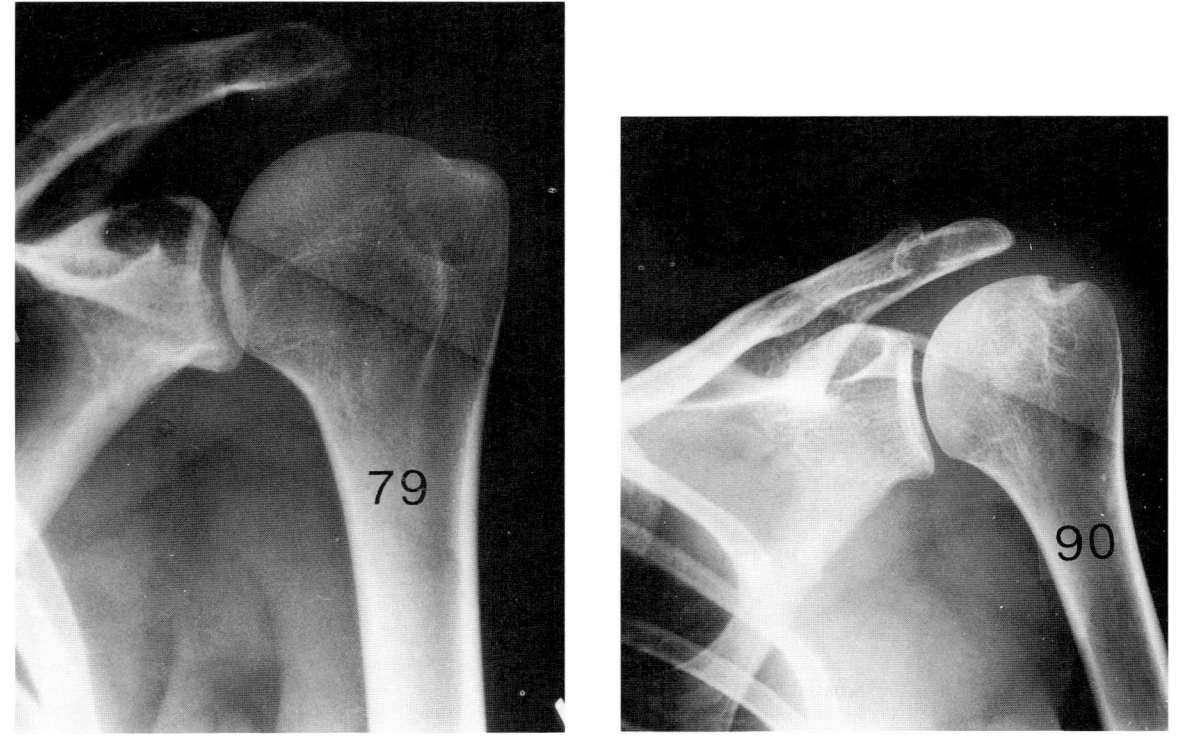

Figure 8–14. After 11 years there is a slight reduction of the joint space and cranial migration. The marginal erosion has deepened, most likely due to the curettage, as there is no clinical sign of recurrence, no pain, and a good range of motion.

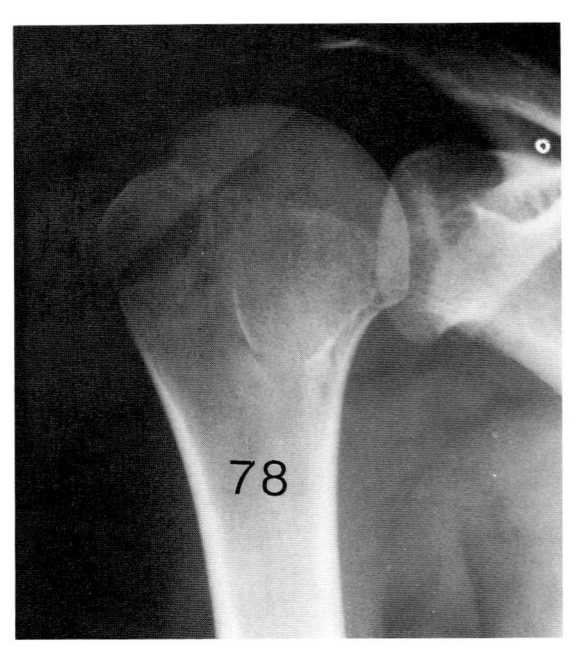

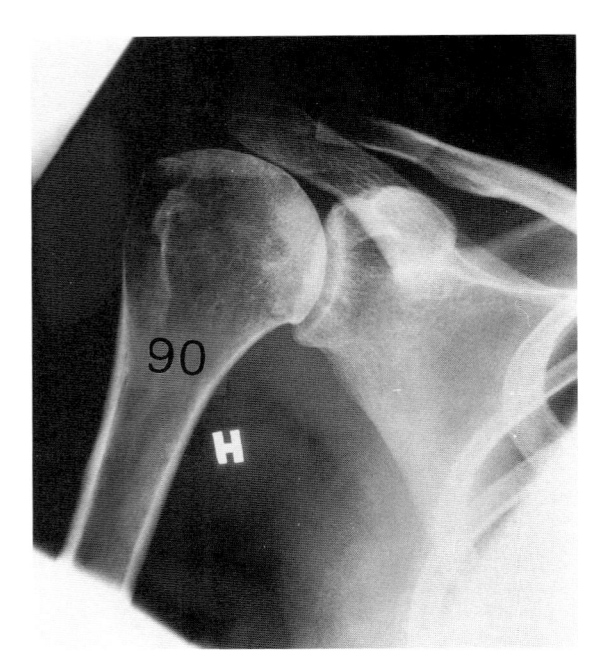

Figure 8–15. Practically unchanged 12 years after synovectomy.

Table 8–5. Active Range of Motion (degrees) (n = 31 shoulders, 26 patients)

	PREOPERATIVE		AT FOLLOW-UP*	
	Mean	Range	Mean	Range
Group A				
Abduction	57.0	30–90	52.8	20–90
Flexion	78.5	60–120	75.3	30–130
Extension	39.6	25–60	31.7	10–40
External rotation	41.0	10–60	19.6	5–50
Internal rotation	62.8	20–90	58.2	30–80
Group B				
Abduction	75.3	45–100	67.3	30–90
Flexion	99.0	55–120	93.2	55–120
Extension	42.6	30–50	51.5	25–60
External rotatiaon	35.0	15–70	23.5	0–60
Internal rotation	70.0	50–90	63.5	30–90

*Mean follow-up time for group A was 12.3 years; for group B, 9.3 years.

Table 8–6. Postoperative Pain and Function after a Mean of 11 Years: Patients' Assessment

Good function, without pain	20 shoulders
Acceptable function with reduced pain	2 shoulders
Fair function with some pain	5 shoulders
Poor function with moderate pain	1 shoulder
No pain, good function 6–9 y postoperatively when a total shoulder arthroplasty was done	3 shoulders
Total	31 shoulders

(First four rows: No further operations necessary)

Table 8–7. Postoperative Functional Assessment (n = 28 shoulders,* 23 patients)

Reach head and neck	17
Reach mouth only	11
Reach opposite axilla	27
Reach back to thoracic spine	20
Reach back to lumbar spine	8

*Three shoulders later had a prosthetic replacement and are therefore not included.

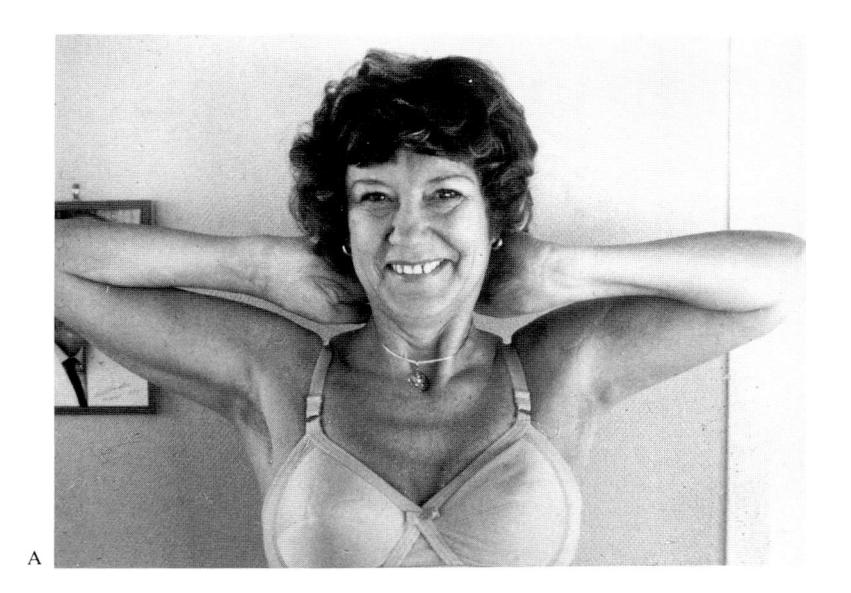

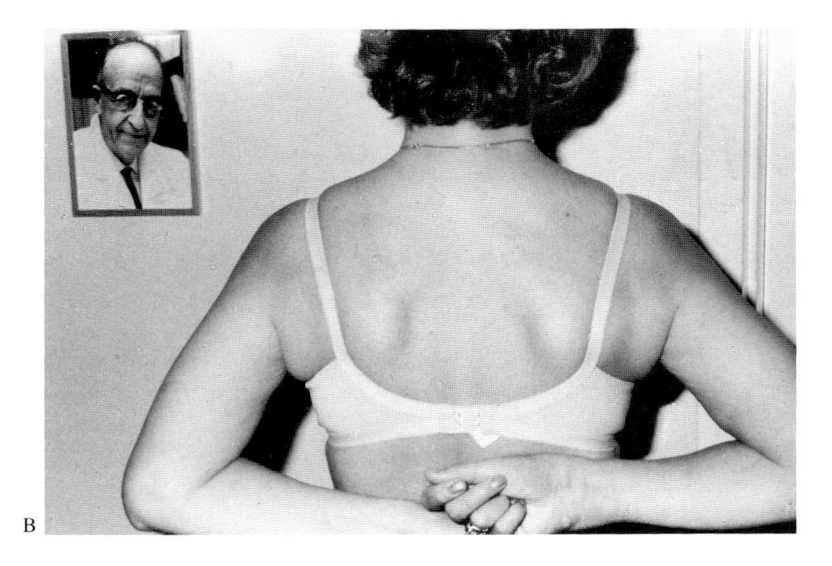

Figure 8–16. A and B. Range of motion 11 years after bilateral shoulder synovectomy.

(Figure 8–17). The subdeltoid bursa was found to be more posterior than expected. Tenosynovitis with a ruptured long head of the biceps was found in 18 shoulders, tenosynovitis without rupture in 12 shoulders, and a normal tendon in 1. Marginal erosions present on the humeral head were often not visualized on standard radiographs. It is necessary to obtain exposure in maximum internal rotation (Figure 8–18) to observe the wide and deep erosions on the dorsal part of the anatomic neck. Undermining of the epiphysis is sometimes severe, often communicating with intraosseous cysts. If this severe erosion is present, one should consider a primary prosthesis.

Marginal erosions were found on the humeral head in 27 shoulders and on the glenoid in 17. In 4 of these 17 glenoids, erosions were also found centrally, varying in degree from crabmeat degeneration to a definite cavitation of the subchondral bone (see Figure 8–8). The glenoid labrum was often degenerated or completely absent. If a degenerated or loose labrum was found, it was better to excise it.

Twenty-seven shoulders had visible swelling preoperatively due to fluid in the bursa, but usually much less than that seen at the onset of the disease. The synovitis and fluid in the joint itself did not account for the palpable swelling in the shoulder region, and therefore a lack of swelling is not a prediction of intra-articular pathology. The presence of swelling and localized tenderness in the intertubercular groove is a better indicator. In only 1 shoulder was postoperative swelling found, necessitating reoperation 1 year after the primary operation.

Eleven of the 31 shoulders had pain postoperatively, but it started as late as 6 years or more after the operation, most likely concurrent with the development of osteoarthrosis (see

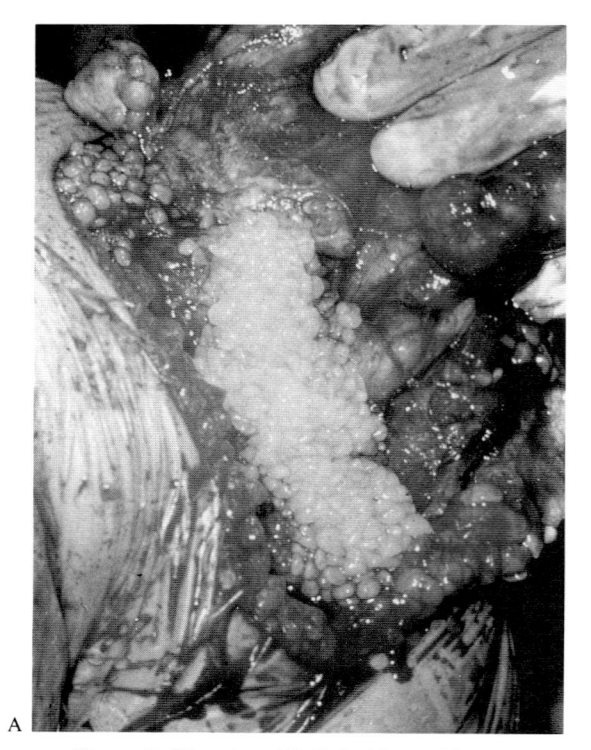

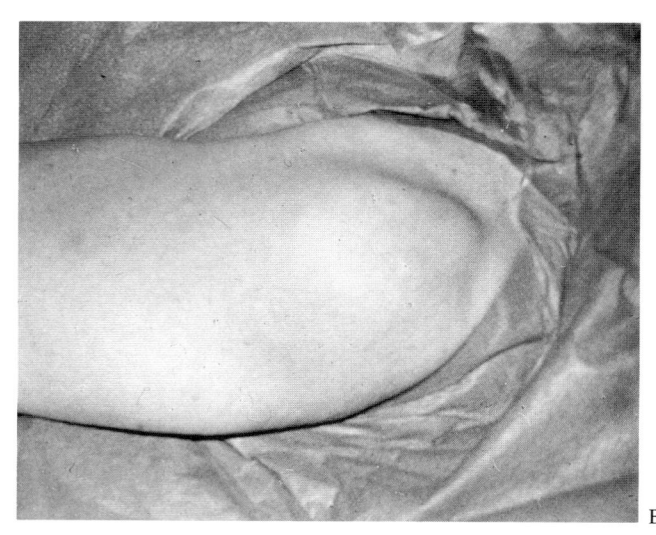

Figure 8–17. **A** and **B.** Palpable swelling of the shoulder region is mostly due to a swollen subdeltoid bursa which may contain rice bodies. The swelling along the tendon of the long head of the biceps in the intertubercular groove may be very pronounced, and is usually tender. The swelling seen in Figure 8–17B is due to the tenosynovitis. The amount of fluid in the glenohumeral joint itself is usually small and not palpable. In the later stages, when there is a palpable medialization and an upward migration of the head of the humerus, the swelling is often absent, and the rotator cuff shrunk.

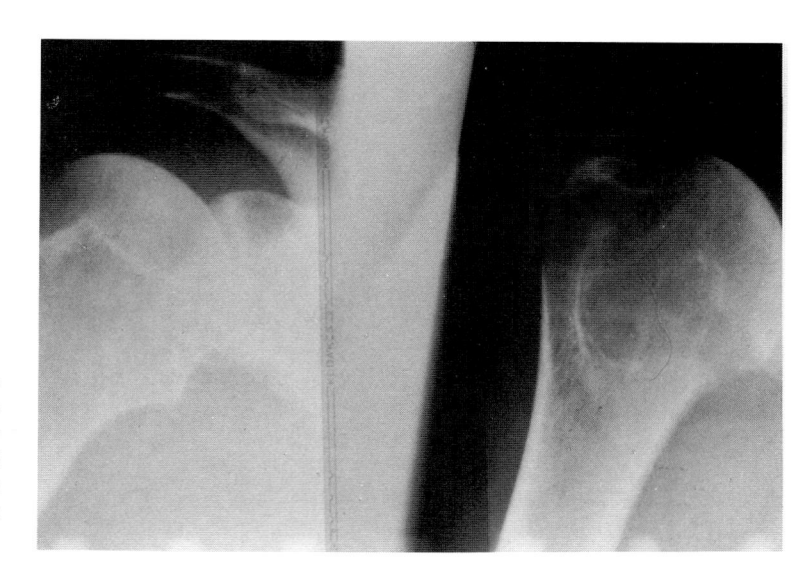

Figure 8–18. On plain radiographs, the erosion along the anatomic neck may be hidden or only minimally visualized. Photographed with maximal inward rotation as seen on the left, the wide and deep erosion posteriorly may be visualized.

Table 8–6). The 3 patients who did not develop osteoarthrosis did not complain of any pain postoperatively. These results may be considered acceptable when only 11 of 31 shoulders developed pain after an average follow-up period of 11 years.

DISCUSSION

Even in shoulders with fairly advanced disease, defined as radiographic grade III or higher, radical synovectomy appears to provide good results, with significant relief of pain and initially an increase in the range of motion, which gradually decreases with the development of osteoarthrosis. Seven shoulders were grade IV preoperatively, and 6 of these shoulders were still functioning well, with 1 patient having pain after 10 years and not being able to lie on the operated shoulder (see Table 8–4). The best results were obtained in the shoulders with early disease, as would be expected. Resection of acromion did not seem to influence the results. Good results, however, depend heavily upon vigorous postoperative physical and occupational therapy. Tenosynovitis of the long head of the biceps tendon is a frequent cause of pain and calls for early intervention.

Radiographic changes are late, and synovectomy should be performed more on the basis of clinical findings. In most cases there was a discrepancy between the preoperative radiographic grade and the perioperative findings. It seems that this operation has in several cases delayed or prevented a total shoulder arthroplasty. Even young patients with juvenile rheumatoid arthritis may have involvement of the shoulder joint, (Pahle JA: Unpublished data, 1992.) and synovectomy in an early stage should be considered the treatment of choice in these individuals.

REFERENCES

1. Fassbender HG. Entzündliche und destruierende Prozesse bei rheumatoider Arthritis. *Verh Dtsch Ges Inn Med* 1983;89:227–238.
2. Vainio K. Surgery in rheumatoid arthritis. *Manitoba Med Rev* 1964;44:548.
3. Goldie IF. Synovectomy in rheumatoid arthritis: A general review and an eight-year follow-up of synovectomy in 50 rheumatoid knee joints. *Semin Arthritis Rheum* 1974;3:219.
4. Moberg E. Cartilage lesions. In: Hijmans W, Paul WD, Herschel H, eds. *Early Synovectomy in Rheumatoid Arthritis.* Amsterdam: Excerpta Medica, 1969:42, 173–177.
5. Allieu Y, Aubriot J-H. Chirurgie de la polyarthrite rhumatoide. Encyclopedie Medico-Chirurgicale, Paris 1991; 14220 B:1–16.
6. Laine V, Vainio K. Orthopedic surgery in rheumatoid arthritis. *Bull Rheum Dis* 1964;15:360–361.
7. McEwen C, et al. Multicenter evaluation of synovectomy in the treatment of rheumatoid arthritis. *Arthritis Rheum* 1977;20:765–771.
8. Ansell BM, Arden GP. Synovectomy of the shoulder. In: Hijmans W, Paul WD, Herschel H, eds. *Early Synovectomy in Rheumatoid Arthritis.* Amsterdam: Excerpta Medica, 1969:12S–128.
9. Gschwend N; Stiasny G, trans. *Surgical Treatment of Rheumatoid Arthritis, Operations in the Region of the Shoulder Joint.* 2nd ed. New York: Thieme, 1980:35–44.
10. Petersson CJ. Painful shoulders in patients with rheumatoid arthritis. *Scand J Rheumatol* 1986;15:275–279.
11. Sbarbaro JL Jr. The rheumatoid shoulder. *Orthop Clin North Am* 1975;6:593–596.
12. Pahle JA. The shoulder in rheumatoid arthritis. In: Lettin AWF, Peterson C, eds. *Rheumatoid Arthritis. Surgery of the Shoulder.* Basel: Karger, 1989;12:15–23.
13. Pahle JA, Kvarnes L. Shoulder synovectomy. *Ann Chir Gynaecol Suppl* 1985;198:37–39.
14. Pahle JA, Kvarnes L. Shoulder replacement arthroplasty. *Ann Chir Gynaecol Suppl* 1985;198:85–89.
15. Larsen A, Dale K, Eek M. Radiographic evaluation of rheumatoid arthritis and related conditions by standard reference films. *Acta Radiol Diagn* 18, 1977;18:481.
16. Pahle JA. Synovektomie des Schultergelenks. *Orthopade* 1973;2:70–72.
17. Pahle JA. Experiences with synovectomy of the shoulder. In: Lettin AWF, Peterson C, eds. *Rheumatoid Arthritis. Surgery of the Shoulder.* Basel: Karger, 1989;12:31–39.
18. Spiechowicz J, Pahle JA, Stubhaug A. Clinical aspects of postoperative continuous regional analgesia in children with juvenile chronic arthritis (JCA). *IMRA* 1991;41–42.
19. Endresen GKM, Spiechowicz J, Pahle JA, Espeland B. Intraoperative autotransfusion in reconstructive hip joint surgery of patients with rheumatoid arthritis and ankylosing spondylitis. *Scand J Rheumatol* 1991;20:28–35.
20. Neer CS, Watson KE, Stanton FJ. Recent experience in total shoulder replacement. *J Bone Joint Surg [Am]* 1982;64:319–337.
21. Gerber C, Schneeberger AG, Tho-Son V. The arterial vascularization of the humeral head. An anatomical study. *J Bone Joint Surg [Am]* 1990;72:1486–1494.
22. Rydholm U. *Surgery for Juvenile Chronic Arthritis. Growth Affection.* Lund, Sweden: Ortolani, 1990:18–27.

9 Osteotomy and Resection Arthroplasty of the Shoulder

Karl Tillmann, M.D., Dieter Braatz, M.D., Wolfgang Rüther, M.D., and Jan Backer, M.D.

OSTEOTOMY OF THE SHOULDER

Juxta-articular osteotomy is a well-established method for the treatment of biomechanically induced joint disorders. In the region of the shoulder, rotational arthroplasty has become popular in Europe for the treatment of recurrent dislocations of the shoulder.[1] External derotation osteotomy has been performed in order to correct internal rotation contractures in rheumatoid patients.[2] More widely used is Benjamin's double osteotomy for the treatment of osteoarthrosis and rheumatoid arthritis of the shoulder.[3]

The place for osteotomy in the correction of deformities, and for double osteotomy in the treatment of osteoarthritis, has been established clinically and experimentally. The alterations of blood circulation in osteoarthrosis are well known.[4,5] Osteotomy has an immediate effect in normalizing the blood flow by lowering the raised intraosseous blood pressure.[4,6–8] However, similar experimental evidence regarding the effects of osteotomy in rheumatoid arthritis is still lacking, so the therapeutic effects are based solely on clinical experience.[9–12]

Indications

Benjamin et al.[10] performed this procedure in both rheumatoid and osteoarthritic patients. Jaffe and Learmont[11] reported their results primarily for rheumatoid arthritis patients. The patients in our series all had rheumatoid arthritis.[12] The mean age of Jaffe and Learmont's patients was about 12 years less than that for both of the other groups mentioned above.

Since the postoperative rehabilitation regimen for this procedure is much less demanding than that after other reconstructive shoulder operations, we reserved double osteotomy mainly for patients with a very low expectation regarding their ability to cooperate. Under certain conditions (sufficient bone stock, intact rotator cuff, good compliance of the patient) we prefer resection and interposition arthroplasty.

Surgical Technique

According to the original description of Benjamin,[3] an anteromedial approach is used, splitting the deltoid muscle about 2.5 cm lateral of the medial border of the deltoid. The cephalic vein is preserved. Usually the coracoid process is osteotomized and the conjoined tendon is retracted medially. The subscapularis muscle is cut by a vertical incision just medial to its insertion. Swollen synovium is removed as necessary in order to provide adequate exposure.

Two small elevators, one cranial and one caudal, are used for exposure of the glenoid. It is osteotomized with a slightly curved osteotome 5 to 10 mm lateral and exactly parallel to the joint surface, running from anteromedial to dorsolateral. The posterior cortex is only cracked by moving the osteotome a little laterally. After this the humerus is osteotomized at the level of the surgical neck, cracking the dorsal cortex in a similar way mentioned above for the glenoid neck (Figure 9–1). Testing the mobility of the joint demonstrates good stability.

After this, the subscapularis tendon and coracoid process are reattached with strong nonabsorbable sutures. Suction drainage is used, running it over the rotator cuff. The fascia and the superficial fibers of the deltoid muscle are gently apposed with thin absorbable sutures. The procedure ends with a meticulous closure of the wound.

No fixation is used after this operation, except for a simple sling and pad in the axilla. The patient is permitted to get up the day after surgery. Suction drainage is removed 48 hours after surgery. No physical therapy is permitted. The patient starts to use the arm according to his or her own feeling and ability. The sling is usually discontinued 8 to 11 days postoperatively.

Results

The clinical experience in our present series[12] is compared with that in two other studies,[10,11] and the data are presented in Tables 9–1 and 9–2. With regards to pain relief and active total abduction of the shoulder, Jaffe and Learmont[11] attained the best results, whereas the results of double osteotomy in our series were not as good. The results of Benjamin's study[11] fell in between those for both of these series. In our series, only one of the osteotomies resulted in nonunion, but no other major complications have occurred. Benjamin et al.[10] reported two delayed unions and two cases with a loss of mobility.

The differences in these three studies are mainly related to differences in patient selection and indications. The excellent result with this procedure attained by Jaffe and Learmont[11] may have been influenced by the lower mean age. Benjamin's superior results in comparison to ours reflects his greater experience and expertise, in addition to having more

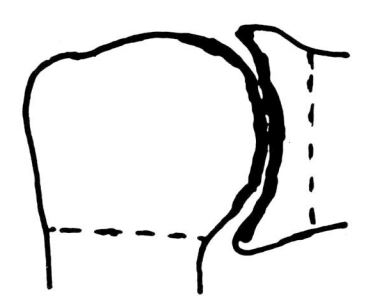

Figure 9–1. Location of the glenoid and humeral osteotomies in the double osteotomy of the shoulder for rheumatoid arthritis.

osteoarthritic patients. Comparing the results of double osteotomy to resection-interposition arthroplasty in nonrandomized, but comparable groups with regards to number and age of the patients, pain relief, active mobility in any direction, and the patient's subjective assessment have been superior after resection-interposition arthroplasty, likely due to our biased selection and indications.[12]

Discussion

With regard to the results of other studies[9–11] and to our selection of problematic patients for double osteotomy, we feel that our results are not a reason to abandon double osteotomy for rheumatoid arthritis patients, as many advantages do exist for the properly selected patient. In terms of the postoperative rehabilitation, there is no less demanding surgery for the severely affected rheumatoid shoulder. The complication rate for this procedure is low. We feel that double osteotomy is a worthwhile surgical procedure for selected rheumatoid arthritis patients.

In order to avoid disappointments, it is necessary to have realistic expectations about this procedure and inform the patients correctly before surgery. This operation generally yields considerable relief of pain and secondarily some improvement in function, especially through improvements in scapulothoracic motion. Benjamin et al.[10] demonstrated radiographically that there is no improvement in glenohumeral mobility. With a few individual patients, improvements were seen both clinically and radiographically (Figure 9–2). In summary, we favor this operation for late cases of rheumatoid arthritis affecting the shoulder with radiologic signs of secondary osteoarthrosis, in patients with limited functional demands and a decreased ability to cooperate fully with a rigorous postoperative rehabilitation protocol.

RESECTION ARTHROPLASTY

The first reports of resection-interposition arthroplasty of the glenohumeral joint were for salvage procedures to treat traumatic, septic, and neoplastic disorders, and generally ended up with either an unstable, flail, or stiff shoulder.[13] However, good results of resection-interposition arthroplasty for the wrist and elbow had been reported. These results coupled with a high rate of failure for constrained total shoulder arthroplasties in the late 1970s, especially with loosening of the glenoid component, led us to adopt the resection-interposition arthroplasty technique for the treatment of the rheumatoid shoulder in 1980.[14] In contrast to Wainwright[15] and Gariepy,[16] instead of resecting the glenoid we remodeled the humeral head and only smoothed out the glenoid, favoring a more lateral center of rotation for the humeral head and therefore a better lever arm for the rotator

Table 9–1. Patients

	NO. OF SHOULDERS				AGE (y) (Range)	FOLLOW-UP (mo)
	OA	RA/JRA	Others*	Total		
Benjamin et al.[10] (1981)	10	19		29	54 (14–74)	13 (12–156)
Jaffe and Learmont[11] (1989)	4	25	3	32	42 (19–72)	35 (8–72)
Tillmann and Braatz[12] (1987)		24		24	54 (39–72)	29 (14–44)

*Ankylosing spondylitis in 2, avascular necrosis in 1.
OA = osteoarthritis; RA = rheumatoid arthritis; JRA = juvenile rheumatoid arthritis.

Table 9–2. Results

	PAIN RELIEF*		GAIN OF ACTIVE ABDUCTION (Degrees)	COMPLICATIONS	
	Preoperative	Postoperative		Nonunion	Delayed Union
Benjamin et al.[10] (1981)	3.0	0.83	+29	1	2
Jaffe and Learmont[11] (1989)	3.0	0.34	+31	2	
Tillmann and Braatz[12] (1987)	2.34	1.51	+8	1	

*Pain: 0 = none; 1 = mild; 2 = moderate; 3 = severe.

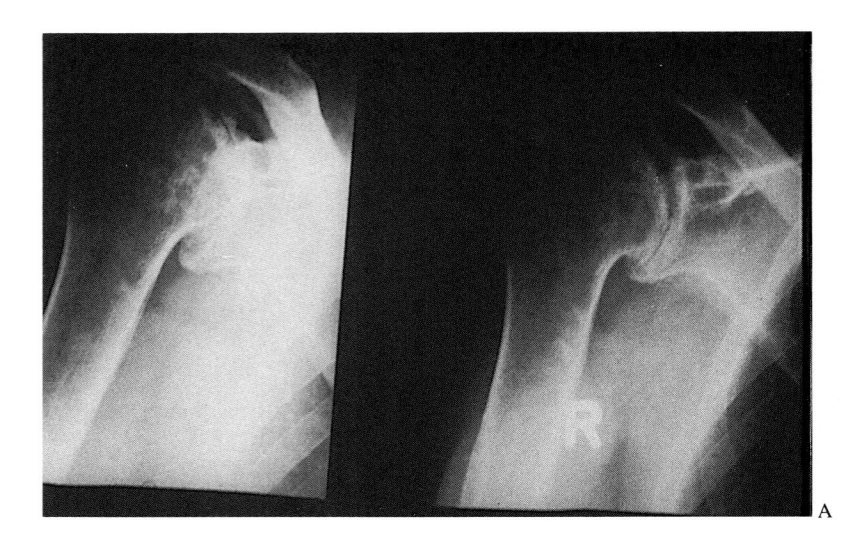

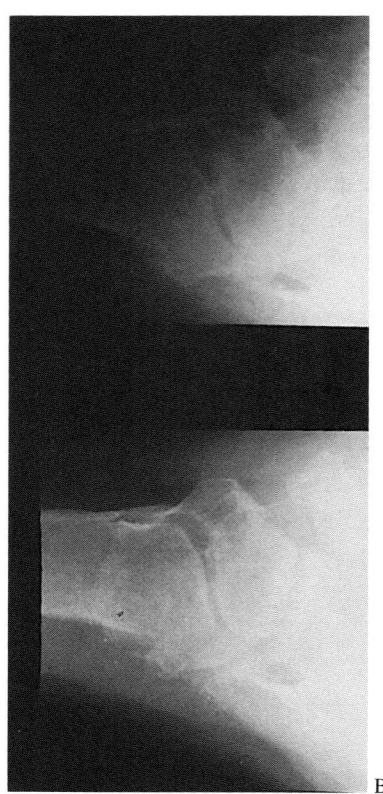

Figure 9–2. A and B. Anteroposterior and axillary radiographs, respectively, of a 54-year-old man with rheumatoid arthritis preoperatively and 13 months postoperatively after a double osteotomy who had a good clinical result.

cuff and deltoid muscles, and at the same time achieving a more cosmetically acceptable result.

The main indication for this procedure, almost exclusively, was the severely destroyed rheumatoid shoulder with a well-preserved rotator cuff. Giant cysts in the humeral head, major defects in the rotator cuff, and limited ability to cooperate with the postoperative rehabilitation protocol were contraindications.

Operative Technique

We prefer a transacromial approach in order to get complete access to the joint. Inflamed bursae are excised. The subscapularis, supraspinatus, and cranial half of the infraspinatus tendons are dissected close to their insertions on the humerus. A radical synovectomy is performed. The humeral head is reshaped, smoothing out the articular surface, diminishing its size and radius (Figure 9–3A), and increasing the

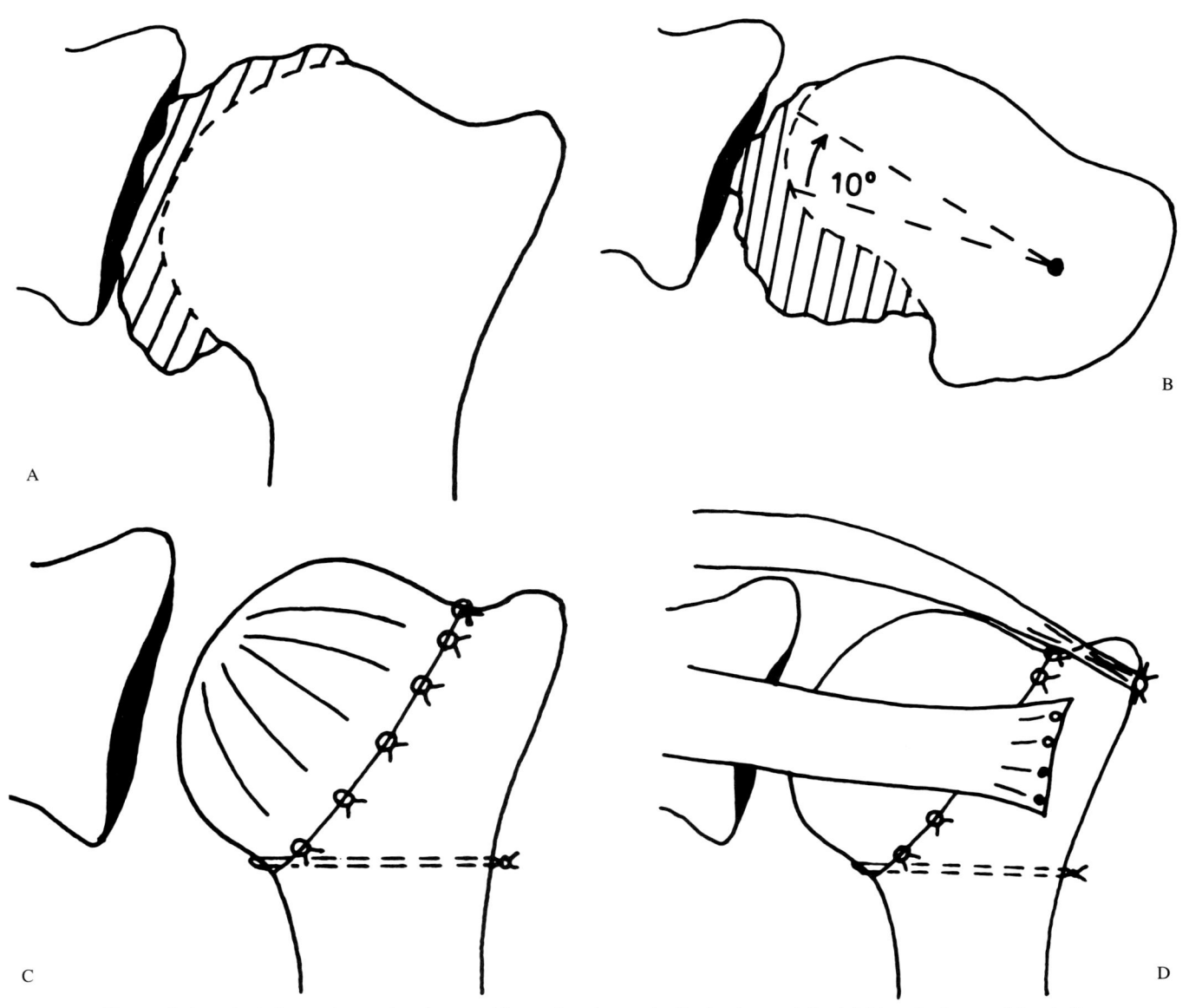

Figure 9–3. Technique of resection-interposition arthroplasty. **A.** Reshaping and diminishing the humeral head. **B.** Increasing the amount of humeral retroversion. **C.** Covering the humeral head with lyophylized dura. **D.** Reattachment of the rotator cuff tendons.

angle of retroversion by about 10 degrees compared to its preexisting position (Figure 9–3B) in order to prevent the newly formed joint from anterior subluxation. The surface of the glenoid is smoothed as necessary. The reshaped humeral head is then covered snugly with lyophylized dura, by drilling two holes through the surgical neck of the humerus and pulling the lower edge of the dura tightly with sutures passed through the drill holes (Figure 9–3C). The surgical procedure has been modified by others to include covering both articular surfaces with lyophylized dura and adding an anterior acromioplasty in cases of cranial subluxation of the humeral head.[17,18]

After this, the rotator cuff is reattached under appropriate tension throughout. Frequently, transosseous fixation of the rotator cuff is necessary (Figure 9–3D). Before the lateral margin of the dissected acromion is reattached and the wound closed, a suction drainage is placed around the rotator cuff. After the wound is dressed, the arm is placed in an abduction splint with the elbow flexed 90 degrees and the wrist in a functional position. It is necessary to keep the elbow anterior to the coronal plane of the body to avoid the humeral head from pressing on the subscapularis tendon repair.

The postoperative physical therapy is very demanding and long-lasting, especially compared to that after a double osteotomy. The abduction splint is exchanged for an individually formed elevation splint two times a day for 6 weeks. This regimen can, of course, be replaced by a continuous passive motion machine. For the first 3 weeks after surgery,

Table 9-3. Resection-Interposition Arthroplasty of the Shoulder

	NO. OF SHOULDERS		AGE	FOLLOW-UP	PAIN RELIEF*		GAIN ACTIVE ROM (Degrees)			
	RA	Others	(y)	(mo)	Preoperative	Postoperative	Abduction	Flexion	IR	ER
Tillmann and Braatz[19] (1989)	22		54 (31–74)	30 (6–57)	2.5	0.8	+24	+32	+13	+15
Miehlke and Thabe[17] (1989)	29	3	48 (24–76)	20 (6–54)	2.8	0.6	+47	+65	+28	+7
Milbrink and Wigren[18] (1990)	10		53 (33–79)	21 (10–30)			+60	+67	+21	+25
Tillmann, Ruther, and Backer[20] (1990)	29		53 (28–77)	74 (48–120)	3.0	0.6	+55	+43	+35	+25

*Pain: 0 = none; 1 = mild; 2 = moderate; 3 = severe.
RA = rheumatoid arthritis; ROM = range of motion; IR = internal rotation; ER = external rotation.

passive range of motion only is performed, followed by 3 weeks of active-assistive range of motion. The abduction splint is discontinued at this point, and daily exercises are carried on by the patient, with a physical therapist supervising at least three times a week, for at least 6 more weeks and often up to 6 months postoperatively.

Results

In order to understand the effects of resection-interposition arthroplasty in rheumatoid arthritis patients, we compared the results of three different follow-up studies[17–19] to our most recent series[20] in terms of pain relief and increase in total active elevation (Table 9–3). All patients suffered from rheumatoid arthritis except three, two having osteonecrosis of the humeral head and the other having ankylosing spondylitis. In one study[17] the mean age of the patients was a little bit lower compared to the others. Our most recent study[20] included 29 shoulders in 26 patients. Of the 37 original patients in the series, 7 had died and 4 had been lost to follow-up. One study[18] used the Swanson shoulder score, which includes relief of pain, to grade their results. In the other series[17,19] a separate pain score has been used.

Comparing the short- and medium-term results, it is evident that there is no deterioration over the years. This was also our experience when grouping the patients in our latest study according to the follow-up time (Table 9–4).[20] The same is true for the gains in active range of motion. In this regard, the results in our first study were somewhat inferior to the others, but when comparing the overall results of medium- and long-term follow-up, there were no marked differences. This was also established by grouping the results of our recent study[20] according to the time of follow-up (Table 9–5).

To assess function and activities of daily living, we tested the patients' ability to reach their neck and back of the head for combing hair (flexion/abduction/internal rotation) and to reach the back of their waist for tying an apron and performing personal hygiene independent of external support. A simple scoring system was used (0 = easily, 1 = with difficulty, 2 = incomplete, 3 = impossible). In the short term, patients' scores improved from a mean of 2.5 to 1.3 for doing hair, and from 2.0 to 0.9 for apron tying."[19] With longer follow-up, the activities of daily living continued to improve rather than deteriorate over time.

In the study of Milbrink and Wigren,[18] only three patients were able to reach their mouth, comb their hair, reach the opposite axilla, place the hand on the neck, and reach their back preoperatively. After surgery, all patients were able to perform these activities of daily living. The authors also determined isometric muscle strength (horizontal and vertical pull as well as horizontal and vertical push) after operation, and compared the results to strength of the contralateral side. They found that all patients had regained muscle power postoperatively to at least the level of the contralateral arm.

A concern regarding this procedure was instability secondary to rotator cuff insufficiency, which was torn in more than

Table 9-4. Resection-Interposition Arthroplasty of the Shoulder

PAIN (total)		FOLLOW-UP (years)		
		4 + 5	6 + 7	8–10
Number		8	9	12
Severe	2	2	—	—
Moderate	2	—	—	2
Mild	7	3	3	1
None	18	3	6	9

Table 9-5. Resection-Interposition Arthroplasty of the Shoulder

RANGE OF MOTION (average)	FOLLOW-UP (years)		
	4 + 5	6 + 7	8–10
Number	8	9	12
Flexion total	80°	100°	90°
Abduction total	80°	90°	70°

two-thirds of the patients at the time of surgery. However, instability occurred only once in the short term[17–19] and was not seen with longer follow-up. Two failures due to insufficiency of the rotator cuff occurred among the 37 patients with 43 joints treated. However, this complication was much less frequent than originally suspected. Other complications included 2 cases of ankylosis, and 6 cases of nonunion of the lateral margin of the acromion secondary to the transacromial approach.[17,18,20] Successful refixation was accomplished in 3 cases, whereas 2 were not significant and did not require revision. The other patient had a severe tear of the rotator cuff and instability required an arthrodesis.

Discussion

With the long-term success of total shoulder arthroplasty, alternative surgical procedures are always subject to controversy. The justification and indications depend on the individual situation of the surgeon who is faced with various problems. Many surgeons are rather reluctant with regard to prosthetic replacement of the shoulder joint in young rheumatoid arthritis patients. At the present we try to avoid prosthetic arthroplasty for as long as possible in favor of alternative procedures. Synovectomy performed early, radically, and meticulously yields much better results compared to any reconstructive surgery. However, a synovectomy is indicated only as long as there is little or no joint destruction and it seems worthwhile to protect the remaining articular cartilage, such as that seen with grade II or III.[21]

With the present state of reconstructive shoulder surgery, we prefer resection-interposition arthroplasty in suitable cases of rheumatoid shoulder destruction for cooperative patients with high functional demands, especially in the younger age group. Prerequisites include sufficient bone stock in order to remodel and create a well-shaped humeral head, and a good rotator cuff, which, if partially torn, can be reconstructed in order to achieve good active and passive mobility and stability.

In the presence of giant cysts, autogenous bone grafting may be possible,[17] but in this situation we usually favor a total shoulder arthroplasty. For patients with a low capacity for postoperative cooperation and minimal functional demands, double osteotomy seems to be more preferable.[10–12] This procedure would also be recommended if significant secondary osteoarthrosis is already present. While the authors have no personal experience, external derotation osteotomy has a similar indication.[2] The above-mentioned procedures offer less complicated alternatives to prosthetic replacement as well as arthrodesis. Resection-interposition arthroplasty has the inherent disadvantage of a demanding postoperative regimen, in contrast to osteotomy.

The indications for resection-interposition arthroplasty and arthrodesis for severely destroyed rheumatoid shoulders can overlap. Presently, arthrodesis is indicated mainly as a salvage procedure for failed resection-interposition arthroplasty and double osteotomy. According to the literature, the functional results are inferior when compared to those after an arthroplasty, but the scapulothoracic motion permits good functional results and excellent pain relief. The main functional disability is a loss of rotation. Another drawback to arthrodesis in the rheumatoid arthritis patient is the lack of any future alternatives in case of increasing disability to the elbow and cervical spine that requires surgical correction. However, it may be more frequently indicated in cases of severe rotator cuff deficiency with arthritis rather than a problematic and risky reconstruction.

The main argument against resection-interposition arthroplasty over the years was the unproved assertion that patients would generally end up with a fibrous ankylosis and that they would have only scapulothoracic motion. If this were true, there should be no difference regarding motion between the results of arthrodesis[22] and also to some extent double osteotomy.[10,12] This becomes especially significant regarding rotation, which is extremely important for upper extremity function.

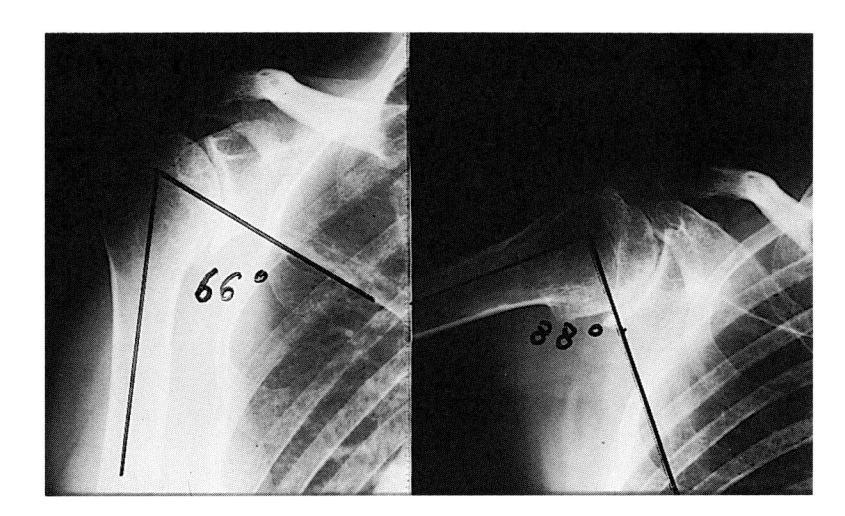

Figure 9–4. Radiographs of a 49-year-old woman 6 years following a resection-interposition arthroplasty for rheumatoid arthritis. Between the resting position (left) and an abducted position (right), there is 70 degrees of active elevation, which includes 20 degrees of glenohumeral motion.

Clinically, even in shoulders with poor motion after resection-interposition arthroplasty, a considerable amount of active and even more passive abduction and rotation are present in the glenohumeral joint, and this was confirmed radiographically (Figure 9–4). In shoulders with good motion, the radiographic findings have been impressive (Figure 9–5). It appears, therefore, that resection-interposition arthroplasty is not a useless procedure that should be abandoned in favor of arthrodesis. The benefit of providing rotation offers a major advantage. As long as prosthetic arthroplasty of the shoulder joint in rheumatoid arthritis patients still has some unsolved problems, resection-interposition arthroplasty has to be regarded as a useful alternative for pain relief and functional restoration of severely damaged rheumatoid shoulder joints.

REFERENCES

1. Weber BG. Operative treatment of recurrent dislocation of the shoulder. *Injury* 1969;1:107–109.
2. Allieu Y, Lussiez B, Desbonnet P, Benichou M. External derotation osteotomy of the humerus in rheumatoid arthritis. In: Lettin AWF, Petersson C, eds. *Rheumatoid Arthritis. Surgery of the Shoulder*. Basel: Karger, 1989;12:60–67.
3. Benjamin A. Double osteotomy of the shoulder. *Scand J Rheumatol* 1974;3:65.
4. Brookes M, Helal B. Primary osteoarthrosis, venous engorgement and osteogensis. *J Bone Joint Surg [Br]* 1968;50:493–504.
5. Helal B. The pain in primary ostoarthritis of the knee. *Postgrad Med J* 1965;41:172–181.
6. Arnoldi CC, Lempberg R, Liderholm H. Immediate effects of osteotomy on the intramedullary pressure in the femoral head and neck in patients with degenerative osteoarthritis. *Acta Orthop Scand* 1971;42:454–455.
7. Lynch A. Venous abnormalities and intraosseous hypertension associated with osteoarthritis of the knee. In: *The Knee Joint. Proceedings of the International Congress Rotterdam Sept. 1973*. Amsterdam: Excerpta Medica, 1973:87.
8. Tillman K. Uberlegungen zur Pathogenese der Arthrosen und ihre Bedeutung fur die operative Therapie. *Acta Rheumatol* 1977;2:53–68.
9. Benjamin A, Hirschowitz D, Arden GP. The treatment of arthritis of the shoulder joint by osteotomy. *Int Orthop* 1979;3:211–216.
10. Benjamin H, Hirschowitz D, Arden GP, Blackburn N. Doppelosteotomie am Schultergelenk. *Orthopade* 1981;10:245–249.
11. Jaffe R, Learmont ID. Double osteotomy for arthritis of the gleno-humeral joint. In: Lettin AFW, Petersson C, eds. *Rheumatoid Arthritis. Surgery of the Shoulder*. Basel: Karger, 1989;12:52–59.
12. Tillmann K, Braatz D. Results of resection arthroplasty and the Benjamin double osteotomy. In: Kölbel R, Helbig B, Blauth W, eds. *Shoulder Replacement*. Berlin: Springer-Verlag, 1987:47–50.

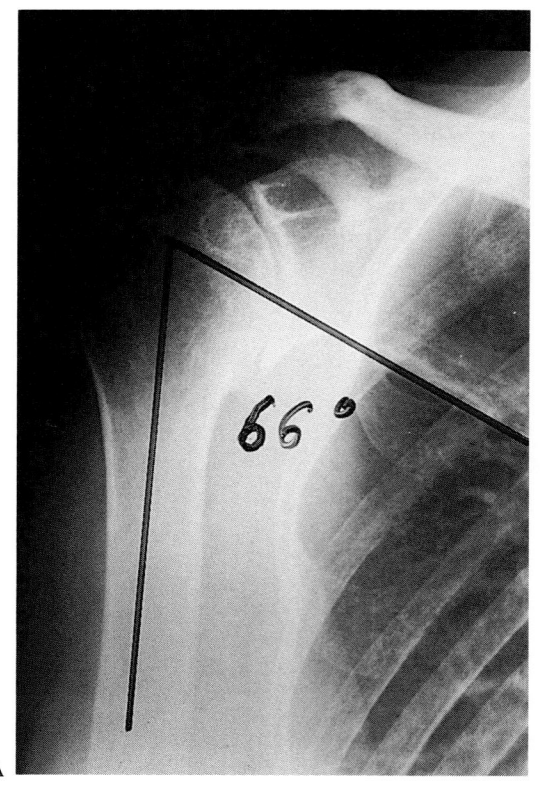

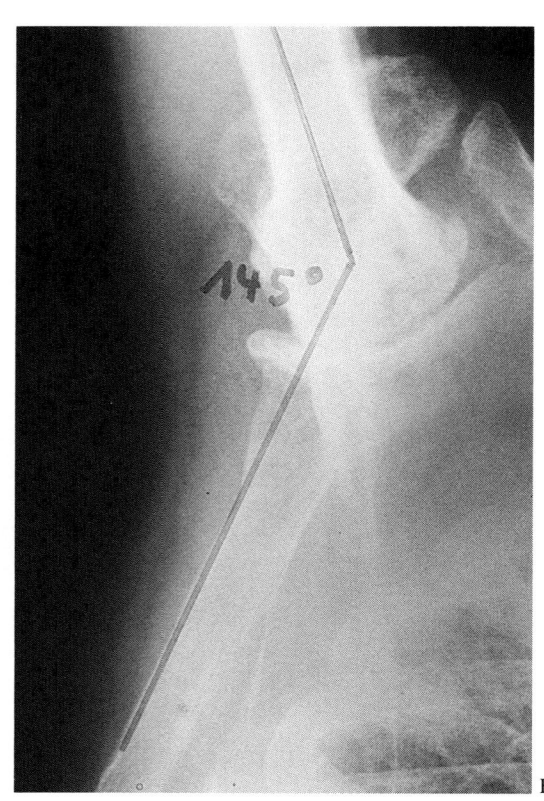

Figure 9–5. Radiographs of a 62-year-old man 8 years following a resection-interposition arthroplasty for rheumatoid arthritis. The patient has excellent motion, with 150 degrees of elevation, including 79 degrees of glenohumeral motion, between the (**A**) resting and (**B**) abducted position.

13. Jäger M, Wirth CJ. Resektions-Interpositionsplastik des Schultergelenkes als Alternative zur Alloarthroplastik und Arthrodese. *Aktuel Probl Chir Orthop* 1977;1:67–76.
14. Tillman K. Die operative Behandlung des rheumatichen Schultergelenkes. *Chir Prax* 1982;30:485–489.
15. Wainwright D. Glenoidectomy: A method of treating a painful shoulder in severe rheumatoid arthritis. *Ann Rheum Dis* 1974;33:110.
16. Gariepy R. Glenoidectomy in the repair of the rheumatoid shoulder. *J Bone Joint Surg [Br]* 1977;58:122.
17. Miehlke RK, Thabe H. Resection interposition arthrolasty of the rheumatoid shoulder. In: Lettin AWF, Petersson C, eds. *Rheumatoid Arthritis. Surgery of the Shoulder*. Basel: Karger, 1989;12:73–76.
18. Milbrink J, Wigren A. Resection interposition arthroplasty of the shoulder in rheumatoid arthritis. A follow-up study. Comprehensive summaries of the Upsala dissertations from the Faculty of Medicine vol. 273, IV. In: Milbrink J, ed. *Surgical Treatment of Rheumatoid Arthritis in the Cervical Spine and Upper Limb*. Upsala: Acta Universitatis Upsaliensis, 1990.
19. Tillmann K, Braatz D. Resection interposition arthroplasty of the shoulder in rheumatoid arthritis. In Lettin AWF, Petersson C, eds. *Rheumatoid Arthritis. Surgery of the Shoulder*. Basel: Karger, 1989;12:68–72.
20. Tillmann K, Rüther W, Backer J. Mid-term results of resection interposition arthroplasty of the shoulder in rheumatic diseases. Presented at the XVIII SICOT Congress; September 14, 1990; Montreal.
21. Larsen A, Dahle K, Eek M. Radiographic evaluation of rheumatoid arthritis and related conditions by standard reference films. *Acta Radiol Diagn* 1977;18:481–491.
22. Hämäläinen M. Arthrodesis of the shoulder joint in rheumatoid arthritis. In: Lettin AWF, Petersson C, eds. *Rheumatic Arthritis. Surgery of the Shoulder*. Basel: Karger, 1989;12:127–135.

10 Shoulder Arthrodesis

Robin R. Richards, M.D., F.R.C.S.(C)

The advent of total shoulder arthroplasty and the refinement of other reconstructive procedures have narrowed the indications for shoulder arthrodesis.[1] Nevertheless, arthrodesis of the glenohumeral joint continues to provide a valuable method of shoulder reconstruction for specific indications.[2-4] Albert first attempted a shoulder arthrodesis in 1881. Since then, a voluminous literature has evolved outlining different indications for the procedure and a variety of surgical techniques to perform shoulder arthrodesis. Controversies regarding the indications for the procedure and the optimum position of shoulder arthrodesis have developed in the literature.[5,6] More recently, discussion has arisen with regard to the functional results that can be achieved with the procedure[7] (Figure 10–1).

This chapter discusses the techniques of shoulder arthrodesis, the optimum position for shoulder arthrodesis, indications and contraindications for the procedure, and the author's preferred technique. Finally, complications and the results of shoulder arthrodesis are discussed. Arthrodesis remains an important method of shoulder reconstruction. The procedure has stood the test of time and continues to deserve a place in the shoulder surgeon's armamentarium. For certain specific indications it provides a reliable method of restoring function to the shoulder.

TECHNIQUE

Many techniques for shoulder arthrodesis have been reported. Some authors have utilized extra-articular arthrodesis, others have reported on methods of intra-articular arthrodesis, and still others have utilized a combination of the two methods. In reviewing the literature it is apparent that internal fixation has been utilized more and more frequently in recent years. Historically, most authors have recommended external immobilization although recent reports of shoulder arthrodesis without external immobilization have appeared.[8,9] Extra-articular arthrodesis, intra-articular arthrodesis, the use of internal fixation, and the use of external fixators are discussed.

Extra-articular Arthrodesis

Extra-articular arthrodesis is primarily a historical procedure used prior to the antibiotic era to treat tuberculous arthritis. This treatment method was used to avoid entering the tuberculous joint and obliterate joint motion without activating and spreading the infection. Watson-Jones[10] described a technique utilizing a Cubbin's approach to the shoulder and decorticating the superior and inferior surfaces of the acromion. A bone flap was then cut into the greater tuberosity and both the clavicle and the acromion were osteotomized. The arm was abducted and the acromion positioned to lie between the two edges of the bone flap in the proximal part of the humerus. A spica cast was applied for 4 months.

Putti[11] described a technique whereby the spine of the scapula and the acromion were exposed subperiosteally. The spine of the scapula was detached, the acromion split, and the medial and lateral portions and the upper end of the humerus exposed. The lateral surface of the humerus was split similar to the method described by Watson-Jones and the spine of the scapula driven down into the humerus with the arm abducted. Spica cast immobilization was necessary following this procedure. Neither Watson-Jones' nor Putti's technique is truly extra-articular since the shoulder joint was usually entered in creating the split in the proximal part of the humerus.

Brittain[12] described a true extra-articular arthrodesis, which used a large tibial graft placed between the medial aspect of the humerus and the axillary border of the scapula. The graft was maintained in position by its "arrow" shape (the pointed end was inserted into the humerus and the opposite, notched end into the axillary border of the scapula). The graft was stabilized by its shape and adduction of the arm, which produced a compressive force along the long axis of the graft. DePalma[13] reported that the failure rate of the arthrodesis was high due to fracture of the long tibial graft.

Intra-articular Arthrodesis

Gill[14] combined intra-articular and extra-articular arthrodeses, utilizing a U-shaped incision centered 2 cm below the acromion combined with a downward limb to the incision. Gill denuded the superior and inferior surfaces of the acromion and excised the rotator cuff. The glenoid fossa was decorticated as was the cartilaginous surface of the humeral head. An osseous flap was elevated from the anterolateral surface of the humerus and a wedge-shaped slice of bone with its base superiorly was removed from the humerus. The arm was then abducted and impacted onto the acromion. The position was maintained by suture of the capsule and rotator cuff to the periosteum on the superior surface of the acromion. This technique is predicated on the assumption that it is desirable to fuse the glenohumeral joint in a large amount of abduction. This can be desirable in children when internal fixation is not used, but is less desirable in adults due to the

SHOULDER FUNCTION
ARTHRODESIS vs. ARTHROPLASTY

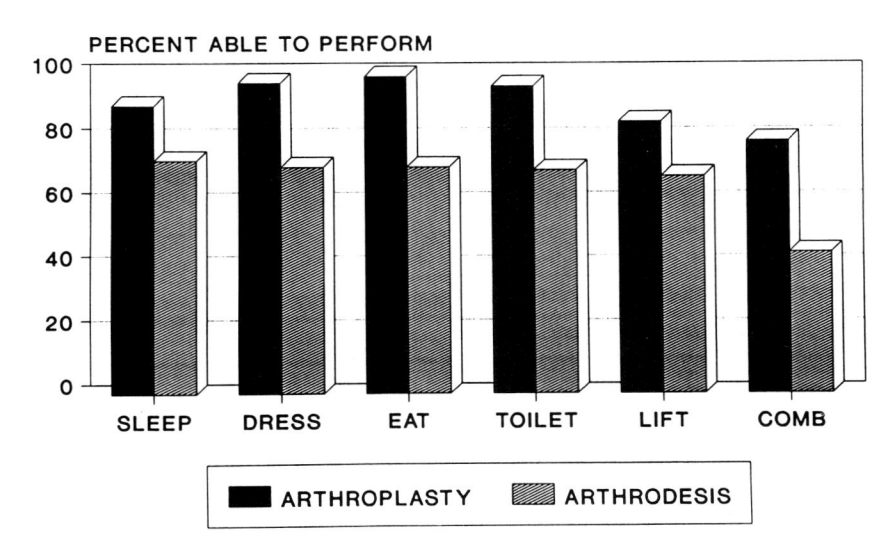

Figure 10-1. Histogram showing that arthrodesis of the shoulder does not give as good a functional result as shoulder arthroplasty. Accordingly, shoulder arthrodesis is reserved for situations where shoulder arthroplasty is not possible or not indicated. Wherever possible, the author prefers to perform shoulder arthroplasty due to the superior functional result and higher level of patient satisfaction than can be obtained with arthrodesis. (Reproduced with permission from Cofield RH, Briggs BT. T Bone Joint Surg 1984; 64A: 889.)

likelihood of excessive abduction being retained following arthrodesis.

Makin[15] reported on a method of shoulder arthrodesis in children which preserves the growth potential of the proximal humeral epiphysis. He fused the shoulder in 80 to 90 degrees of abduction, fixing the humerus to the glenoid with Steinmann pins inserted first into the humerus in a proximal-distal direction and then driven in the reverse direction into the glenoid. Makin followed these children to adult life and noted that there was only a small loss in humeral length and no change in position of the fused shoulder. He recommended this technique, stating that this amount of abduction was necessary to maintain the growth potential of the proximal humeral epiphysis.

Moseley[16] reported dividing the rotator cuff insertion, excising the intra-articular portion of the biceps tendon, and suturing the biceps tendon into the bicipital groove after division of the origin. This is an important step to remember in those patients who have a functioning biceps in order to avoid the unsightly cosmetic deformity identical to that seen in rupture of the long head of the biceps tendon, and to avoid the small loss of elbow flexor and supinator strength that is associated with this pathologic condition. The author performs a biceps tenodesis during shoulder arthrodesis in all patients who have a functional biceps.

Moseley denuded the inferior surface of the acromion as well as the articular cartilage of the humeral head and glenoid fossa. This is an important step in performing shoulder arthrodesis, since the humeral head presents such a small surface area compared to the glenoid, across which fusion can occur. Moseley elevated the humeral head to oppose the undersurface of the acromion and maintained the position with internal fixation. Proximal migration of the humeral head can decrease the contact surface between the humeral head and the glenoid if the zenith of the humeral head is not removed. Attention to this detail must be made when the joint surfaces are prepared.

Beltran et al.[17] performed shoulder arthrodesis through an anterior approach. They osteotomized the coracoid and created a tunnel that crossed the humerus and entered the glenoid cavity. They utilized a screw for internal fixation and in addition used a Cloward reamer to position a fibular graft from the proximal portion of the humerus into the infraglenoid region. Other techniques for shoulder arthrodesis have been described by May[18] and Davis and Cottrell.[19]

Internal Fixation

A variety of methods of internal fixation have been advocated for shoulder arthrodesis. It is generally agreed that internal fixation is desirable, since it maintains the position of the arthrodesis and can decrease the length of time that plaster immobilization is necessary in order to obtain an arthrodesis. As mentioned above, Makin advocates the use of Steinmann pins in children who are undergoing shoulder arthrodesis at an early age.

Carroll[20] reported on the use of a wire loop in order to maintain the position of shoulder arthrodesis, with no. 22 gauge wire passed through the head of the humerus and the anterior-superior lip of the glenoid. He utilized this method of arthrodesis in 15 patients, and all achieved solid bony union between the third and fourth month following surgery. Carroll noted that it was possible to manipulate the shoulder following surgery and change the position of the arthrodesis.

Over time, however, most authors have advocated more rigid forms of internal fixation.

Other authors have reported the use of screws in order to obtain fixation during glenohumeral arthrodesis. May[18] utilized a single stabilizing wood screw crossing the humerus and entering the glenoid fossa. Davis and Cottrell[19] utilized a similar technique and added a muscle pedicle bone graft that was fixed in place with wood screws. Cofield and Briggs[7] and Leffert[21] also reported on the use of compression screw fixation without the use of a plate. Beltran et al.[17] developed a special fixation device utilizing a screw bolt and washer in order to obtain shoulder arthrodesis. In addition, Beltran et al.[17] used an acromial-humeral screw and a fibular graft as methods of internal fixation.

The Arbeitsgemeinschaft für Osteosynthesefragen/Association for the Study of Internal Fixation (AO/ASIF) group first advocated the use of plate fixation in 1970. They described this method of arthrodesis as not requiring supplementary plaster immobilization, and advocated the use of two plates for internal fixation.[22] The first plate was applied along the spine of the scapula and then bent down over the humerus, maintaining a position of 70 degrees of abduction between the vertebral border of the scapula and the humerus. The object of this position was to obtain a clinical position of 50 degrees of abduction, 40 degrees of internal rotation, and 25 degrees of flexion. They anchored this plate to the scapula with a long screw placed down through the plate, the acromion, and into the neck of the glenoid. They also noted that fixation could be improved by the insertion of two long screws through the plate, the humeral head, and into the glenoid, if necessary, to improve the internal fixation.

Kostuik and Schatzker[9] reported on the use of the AO/ASIF technique. They did not utilize external immobilization postoperatively and reported good results in their patients. Riggins[8] reported on shoulder arthrodesis without external immobilization in 1976. Both the AO/ASIF group and Riggins supplemented their arthrodeses with bone grafts. Riggins treated four patients with the use of a plate for internal fixation. Two of the patients had above-elbow amputations. The arthrodesis was successful in each case.

A modified method of shoulder arthrodesis utilizing internal fixation in 14 adult patients with a brachial plexus palsy has been reported by the author.[23] A single 4.5-mm AO/ASIF dynamic compression plate applied over the spine of the scapula onto the shaft of the humerus was used. Two cancellous compression screws are passed through the plate and the proximal part of the humerus into the glenoid first, in order to achieve compression at the glenohumeral arthrodesis site. The plate is anchored to the scapula with a long screw passing through the spine of the scapula into the area of the coracoid base. Anchorage of the plate by this method, as opposed to the AO/ASIF method which involves inserting the screw into the glenoid neck, provides good fixation yet leaves room for the large compression screws in the glenoid, which are felt to be more important in obtaining an arthrodesis.

Initially a postoperative spica cast was used, since adult patients with brachial plexus injuries generally have significant osteoporosis, poor muscle control, and decreased proprioception resulting from their neurologic injury. Bone grafts were not used in this series and no nonunions occurred. More recently, thermoplastic thoracobrachial orthoses have been used after shoulder arthrodeses and spica casts are no longer used.

Recently a modification of the technique described in 1985 was reported, using a single 10-hole, 4.5-mm, AO/ASIF malleable reconstruction plate for internal fixation.[24] This plate, although weaker than the 4.5-mm dynamic compression plate, is much easier to contour in the operating room and much less prominent as it passes over the acromion onto the shaft of the humerus. None of the 11 patients whose shoulders were arthrodesed with this method complained of plate prominence. Arthrodesis was obtained in each instance without failure of the internal fixation device. External cast immobilization was used for 6 weeks postoperatively.

External Fixation

Charnley and Houston[25] reported a method for compression arthrodesis of the shoulder utilizing two Steinmann pins. The first Steinmann pin was inserted posterosuperiorly into the base of the acromion and then into the main mass of the scapula just proximal to the glenoid. The second pin was inserted posterolaterally in relation to the shaft of the humerus and perpendicular in relation to the axis of the humerus, in order to transfix the region of the surgical neck. A compression apparatus was then applied to the two pins, and a plaster spica cast applied and worn for an average of 4.8 weeks. After removal of the pins and compression clamp, a second plaster cast was applied for an average of 5.3 weeks. Other methods of external fixation have been reported.[26–29]

At the present time, the indications for shoulder arthrodesis using external fixation are limited. The author has used this method occasionally in patients with active septic arthritis of the shoulder. Pins are placed through the clavicle and acromion and a second set of pins inserted in a separate plane into the spine of the scapula and neck of the glenoid. Two half-frames are then constructed in order to stabilize the shoulder, and can be cross-connected for increased stability. This technique is desirable if there is an open infected wound draining from the shoulder joint, since it allows for dressing changes and care of the soft tissues without the increased dissection and soft-tissue disruption necessary to place an internal fixation device.

OPTIMUM POSITION

A number of different positions for glenohumeral arthrodesis have been advocated in the literature. Perusal of the literature reveals that no two authors agree on exactly the same optimum position for shoulder arthrodesis. There was sufficient controversy in the literature that the American Orthopaedic Association established a committee to determine, among other things, the optimum position for shoulder arthrodesis. In 1942, this committee concluded that the optimum position for shoulder arthrodesis was 45 to 50 degrees of abduction (measured from the vertebral border of the scapula), 15 to 25 degrees of forward flexion from the plane of the scapula, and 25 to 30 degrees of internal rotation.[5] This report caused a great deal of controversy in the literature following its publication, partly revolving around the method used to measure abduction. Some authors recommended using the angle formed by the vertebral border of scapula and the axis of the humerus in order to determine abduction while others argued that the angle between the arm and the side of the body was more appropriate to measure (clinical abduction).

Rowe[6] noted in 1974 that the amount of abduction that had been recommended was excessive for adults. This position had been recommended primarily for patients who were having their shoulders arthrodesed as children in whom internal fixation was not used. In this situation, the amount of abduction present at the time of surgery was commonly lost during the period required for the arthrodesis to become secure, and later as growth occurred. If the same position was utilized in adults, excessive scapular winging would occur and the scapula would not comfortably rest at the side. Furthermore, Rowe[6] noted that the measurement of clinical abduction was more practical and recommended this method rather than measuring abduction from the vertebral border of the scapula. Rowe[6] further recommended that the arm be placed closer to the center of gravity of the body with enough abduction to clear the axilla and sufficient flexion and internal rotation to bring the hand to the midline of the body.

Other authors have recommended a variety of positions for shoulder arthrodesis. All agree that abduction and forward flexion are desirable, and most have recommended internal rotation (Figure 10–2). The author believes that the optimum position for shoulder arthrodesis is one that brings the hand to the midline anteriorly so that, with elbow flexion, the mouth can be reached. The amount of abduction should not be excessive so that the arm can rest comfortably at the side. This can be accomplished with 30 degrees of abduction (measured clinically), 30 degrees of forward flexion, and 30 degrees of internal rotation. The so-called 30-30-30 position is easily obtained in the operating room and provides patients with the ability to reach their mouth, their front pocket, and their back pocket in the majority of instances (Figure 10–3). It must be recognized that the position cannot be measured exactly at the time of surgery, but it is usually possible to arthrodese the shoulder within 10 degrees of the above position.

INDICATIONS

Shoulder arthrodesis can effectively restore shoulder function to patients with certain specific disorders. Patient selec-

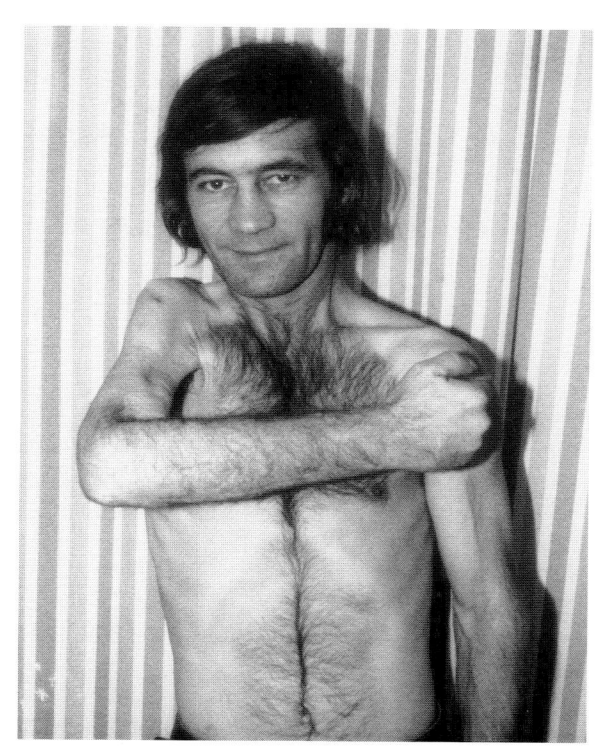

Figure 10–2. This patient's shoulder has been fused in excessive internal fixation. The functional position for shoulder arthrodesis is one that allows the arm to drop comfortably to the side, brings the arm forward to place it in an effective position for work at bench level, and is of sufficient internal rotation so that when the patient bends his or her elbow the hand will reach the mouth. The author recommends a position of 30 degrees of abduction, 30 degrees of flexion, and 30 degrees of internal rotation. This patient required an external rotation osteotomy to place the hand in a more functional position.

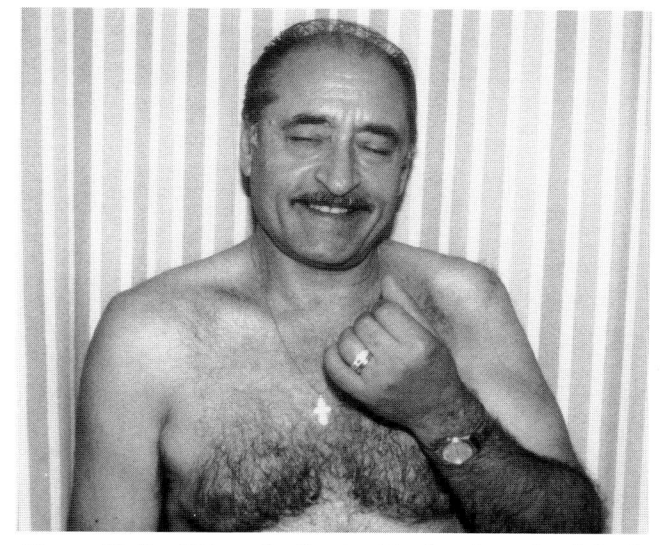

Figure 10–3. This patient's shoulder has been fused in the "30-30-30" position. This position brings the hand to the midline anteriorly so that, with elbow flexion, the patient can reach the mouth.

tion is important in determining whether or not the procedure will be beneficial. The procedure results in the effective sacrifice of all rotation through the glenohumeral joint. Wherever possible, shoulder arthroplasty is preferable to shoulder arthrodesis if there is a choice for the patient between the two procedures. Shoulders can be arthrodesed if an arthroplasty fails, although in this situation it is a technical challenge. The indications for surgery in the author's personal series are illustrated in Figure 10–4.

Paralysis

All authors agree that the presence of a flail shoulder is an indication for shoulder arthrodesis. Patients with anterior poliomyelitis, patients with severe proximal root and upper trunk brachial plexus lesions, and some patients with isolated axillary nerve paralysis are candidates for shoulder arthrodesis. These patients have good function in their elbows and hands but are unable to optimize their upper extremity function due to their inability to place their hand in space. If such a patient has good function in the periscapular musculature, particularly the trapezius, levator scapulae, and serratus anterior, glenohumeral arthrodesis stabilizes the extremity and allows effective hand function.[30] Such patients can then fully utilize their upper extremity potential and work effectively at bench level. In addition, many patients with flail shoulders develop inferior subluxation of the glenohumeral joint due to periarticular paralysis. This condition is uncomfortable and, in some patients, frankly painful. Such patients often find that they must keep their arm in a sling to avoid injuring it. Painful inferior subluxation at the shoulder

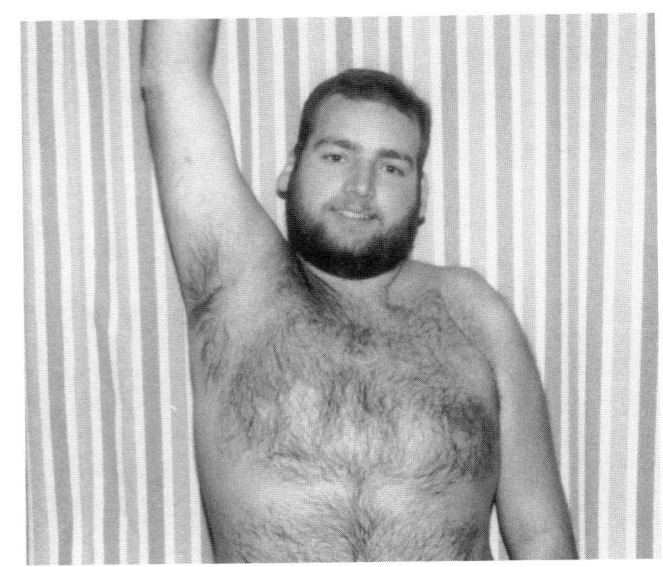

Figure 10–5. A male patient, 24 years old, with an irreparable lesion of the brachial plexus. Brachial plexus exploration and sural nerve grafting were not successful in restoring shoulder function 18 months after the procedure. The shoulder is flail and the glenohumeral joint remains subluxated inferiorly if the arm is not supported in a sling. Although the patient has effective hand and wrist function, the upper extremity is ineffectual due to his inability to move or otherwise control his shoulder. This type of patient would benefit greatly from arthrodesis of the shoulder. Shoulder arthroplasty is contraindicated in patients with a flail shoulder.

provides another indication for stabilization of the glenohumeral joint (Figure 10–5).

Patients who have the combination of a flail shoulder and elbow need reconstruction of both. In this situation, glenohumeral arthrodesis combined with elbow flexorplasty improves the result of the elbow flexorplasty. Without shoulder stabilization, elbow flexion tends to drive the humerus posteriorly, resulting in shoulder extension rather than elbow flexion. Arthrodesis of the shoulder in some flexion and abduction helps to eliminate the effect of gravity and optimizes the result that can be achieved with the elbow flexorplasty. Patients with flail shoulders often have a tendency to internally rotate their upper extremity to their chest when some internal rotation function remains (pectoralis major, latissimus dorsi) and no function remains in the external rotators. Shoulder stabilization in the form of either arthrodesis or a L'Episcipo tendon transfer reduces this undesirable tendency (Figures 10–6 and 10–7).

There is a wide degree of variability in the disability caused by axillary nerve paralysis, and there are patients who have virtually full motion following paralysis of the axillary nerve providing the rotator cuff musculature is undisturbed (endurance is never normal). Patients with isolated paralysis of the axillary nerve can be treated by either muscle or tendon transfer or glenohumeral arthrodesis. Numerous reports exist in the literature on the value of muscle and muscle-tendon transfers to restore shoulder function following paralysis of

SHOULDER ARTHRODESIS PREOPERATIVE DIAGNOSIS

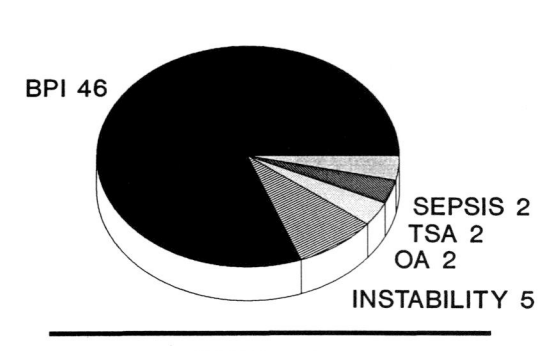

BPI 46
SEPSIS 2
TSA 2
OA 2
INSTABILITY 5

TOTAL = 57

Figure 10–4. Pie chart showing the indication for shoulder arthrodesis in the author's personal series of 57 procedures. The vast majority of procedures were performed for brachial plexus injuries. A lesser number of procedures were performed for recalcitrant shoulder instability, osteoarthritis in young people, failed total shoulder arthroplasty, and sepsis.

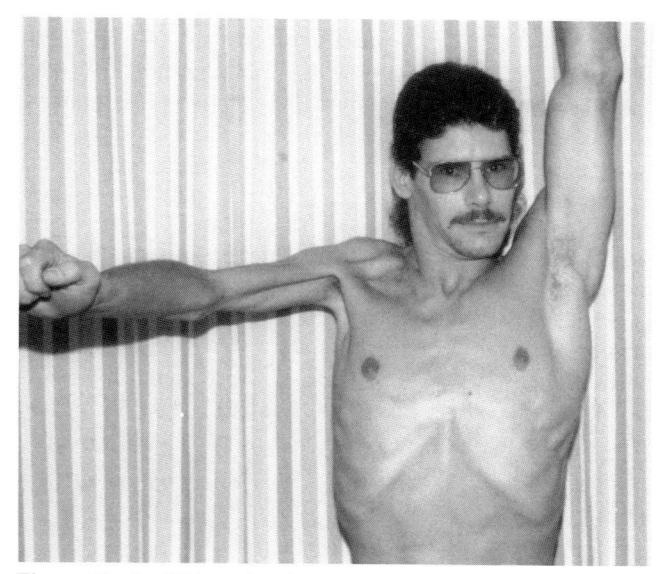

Figure 10–6. This patient had a flail elbow and shoulder prior to surgery, due to an irreparable lesion of the brachial plexus. At the same sitting he underwent shoulder arthrodesis combined with pectoralis to biceps tendon transfer utilizing a fascia lata graft. Shoulder arthrodesis optimizes the function of the pectoral transfer in this situation, since all movement resulting from contraction of the transferred muscle acts on the elbow rather than on the elbow and shoulder combined. Furthermore, shoulder arthrodesis allows the patient to flex his arm against gravity and thus further augments the weak flexor power that is present in the transfer. In this patient's situation the transfer would be much less effective if the shoulder had not been stabilized.

the axillary nerve.[31] Multiple transfers are necessary to restore deltoid function, and significant problems can occur with gliding of transfers over the acromion. It is often necessary to harvest autogenous tissue such as fascia lata to lengthen the transfers, and the process of rehabilitation is challenging following such procedures. Such transfers are indicated primarily for pediatric patients and adults who have only partial paralysis of the axillary nerve.[31] However, it must be noted that pediatric patients do well with shoulder arthrodesis, and some authors feel they are better able to adapt to the procedure.[32] If total paralysis of the axillary nerve is present and significant limitation of shoulder function ensues, glenohumeral arthrodesis is recommended, recognizing that the alternative of muscle transfers may be available in carefully selected patients. Glenohumeral arthrodesis is useful in such patients provided their symptoms justify the procedure.

Reconstruction Following Tumor Resection

En bloc resection of periarticular malignant tumors often requires sacrifice of the rotator cuff and/or the deltoid. If the resection requires sacrifice of these tissues, reconstruction of the shoulder with an arthroplasty is inadvisable, due to the high risk of instability if a nonconstrained prosthesis is used, and the certainty of loosening if a constrained prosthesis is used. Shoulder arthrodesis is the procedure of choice to reconstruct the shoulder following wide resection of periarticular malignancies. Specific techniques have been recommended for shoulder arthrodesis following tumor resection.[33] These include the use of specialized fixation devices and bone-grafting techniques. Vascularized bone grafts and massive allografts are sometimes necessary due to the large defects created by tumor resection.

Shoulder Joint Destruction due to Infection

Destruction of the shoulder joint due to septic arthritis remains an indication for shoulder arthrodesis. In the past, tuberculous arthritis was a common indication for shoulder arthrodesis. Worldwide, this condition remains prevalent, although in the Western world it has become extremely uncommon. Septic arthritis continues to occur, and when it does, the shoulder joint can be destroyed, with resultant pain and limitation of function. Most surgeons would agree that in a young patient with shoulder dysfunction due to sepsis, arthrodesis of the shoulder, as opposed to total shoulder

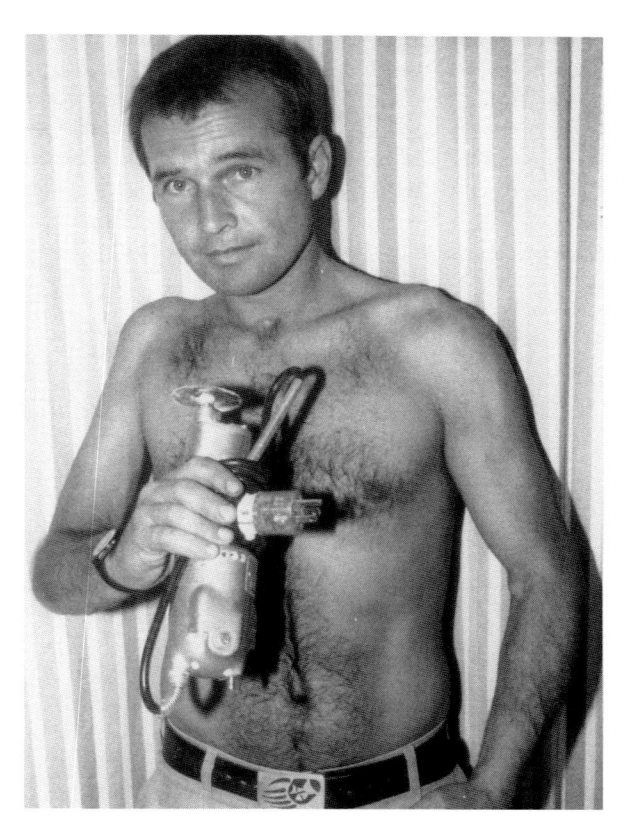

Figure 10–7. This patient has had a shoulder arthrodesis and Steindler flexorplasty. The two procedures were performed a few days apart. The Steindler procedure was done first, since it is difficult to perform technically once the shoulder has been fused. Shoulder arthrodesis improves elbow function after the Steindler procedure since there is not a tendency for the humerus to be driven posteriorly (shoulder extended) when the patients flexes his elbow. In the presence of a flail shoulder, elbow flexion is not as effective in placing the hand in a functional position.

arthroplasty, would be indicated. Although total shoulder arthroplasty can be performed in patients with a remote history of sepsis, if there is a recent history of sepsis or if the patient is young, arthrodesis provides a more satisfactory alternative.

Failed Total Shoulder Arthroplasty

The author has seen several patients who have had multiple unsuccessful shoulder arthroplasties. Although the results of shoulder arthroplasty are generally good, there are some patients in whom loosening, sepsis, and implant breakage occurs. These patients often have severe loss of humeral and glenoid bone stock. In this situation, the surgeon must choose between attempting a repeat revision of the shoulder arthroplasty and obliteration of the shoulder joint by arthrodesis. The results of revision total shoulder arthroplasty are suboptimal when compared to the results of primary arthroplasty performed for other reasons (Figure 10–8). The decision between these two alternatives must be made on the basis of the patient's age, the presence or absence of sepsis, the bone stock that remains in the proximal portion of the humerus and the glenoid, the symptoms the patient is experiencing, and the technical experience and expertise of the surgeon. In several patients who were significantly disabled, the author carried out glenohumeral arthrodesis following failed total shoulder arthroplasty and found it to be a gratifying procedure. The author believes shoulder arthrodesis must be considered when the reconstructive surgeon is confronted with a patient who has a history of multiple failed total shoulder arthroplasties.

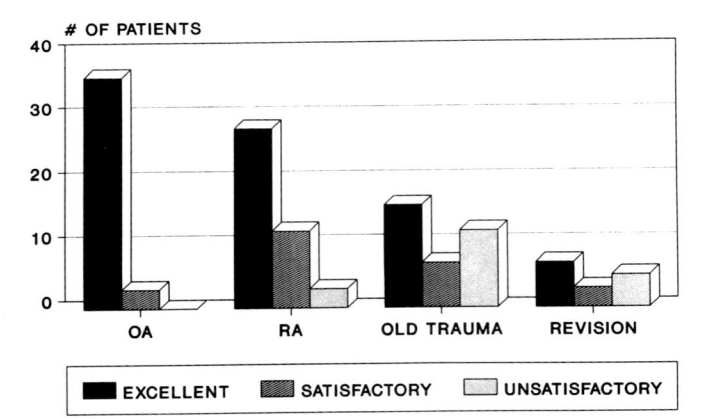

Figure 10–8. Histogram showing the results of total shoulder arthroplasty for different indications. Neer[1] found the results to be most satisfactory for patients with osteoarthritis and least satisfactory for patients undergoing revision arthroplasty. The author's experience has been similar. Accordingly, if patients require revision of their arthoplasty, arthrodesis can be considered in certain instances. It can be difficult to obtain arthrodesis in this situation due to deficiency in either glenoid and/or humeral bone stock. (Reproduced with permission from Neer.[1])

Shoulder Instability

The vast majority of patients with shoulder instability can be treated by soft-tissue or bony reconstructive procedures in order to stabilize the glenohumeral joint. Rarely a patient will present with chronic shoulder instability after multiple attempts at surgical stabilization. If every surgical therapeutic alternative has been exhausted, the patient's shoulder remains symptomatically unstable, and the patient does not wish to wear a thoracobrachial support, arthrodesis can be indicated to restore shoulder stability. In this situation, careful assessment of the patient's psychological makeup must be carried out to be certain the patient has a full understanding of the procedure's implications. Much has been written about the difficulties in managing such patients[34] (Figure 10–9).

Rotator Cuff Tear

Severe shoulder dysfunction can result from massive rotator cuff tears. The great majority of rotator cuff tears can be managed by coracoacromial decompression and repair of the rotator cuff. In patients who have massive rotator cuff tears that cannot be repaired, some authors reported good results with debridement of the cuff tear and coracoacromial decompression.[35] Long-standing rotator cuff tears can lead to rotator cuff tear arthropathy as reported by Neer et al.,[36] who treated this entity with total shoulder arthroplasty and rotator cuff reconstruction. This is predicated on the surgeon's ability to repair the rotator cuff by cuff transfer and/or the use of exogenous materials. Neer et al.[36] reported that such patients must have "limited goals," since this is a difficult form of reconstruction. Shoulder arthrodesis should be kept in mind as a possible alternative form of reconstruction in such patients where the technical skill of the surgeon does not permit rotator cuff reconstruction and the patient is sufficiently symptomatic to exchange the loss of glenohumeral motion for the relief of pain. In the author's experience, this situation rarely, if ever, develops.

Malunion

Glenohumeral arthrodesis is rarely indicated for posttraumatic deformity. Most patients with posttraumatic deformities such as osteonecrosis of the humeral head, chronic fracture-dislocations, tuberosity impingement, or a malunion of the proximal part of the humerus are best treated by shoulder reconstruction using either osteotomy, arthroplasty, or a combination of both. If these procedures are not possible, then glenohumeral arthrodesis can be considered.

Osteoarthritis

The presence of glenohumeral osteoarthritis in an otherwise normal shoulder is an indication for total shoulder arthroplasty, and the vast majority of patients are of sufficient age that they are excellent candidates. If the patient was to develop osteoarthritis at a relatively young age, then glenohumeral arthrodesis might be considered.[37] However, the

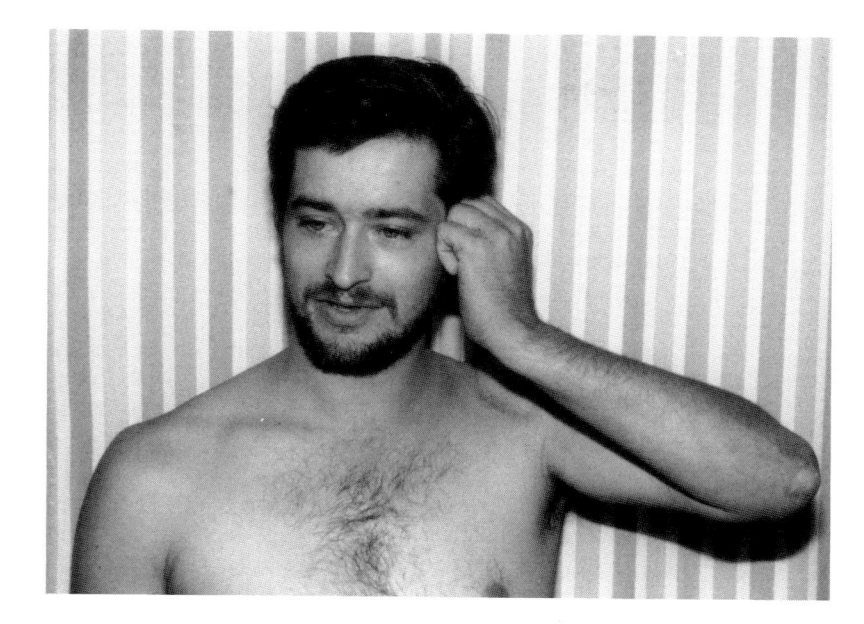

Figure 10–9. This 28-year-old patient had undergone five stabilization procedures to treat multidirectional shoulder instability. He underwent shoulder arthrodesis, recognizing that it would compromise his glenohumeral motion but prevent episodes of instability from occurring in the future. Patients who have their shoulder fused for this indication are less satisfied than those who undergo arthrodesis for other indications. However, the procedure does have a role to play for certain specific individuals. Shoulder arthroplasty would be considered contraindicated by most surgeons in the presence of instability.

results of total shoulder arthroplasty are so much superior that in the author's experience, the operation is rarely indicated for patients with this diagnosis.

Rheumatoid Arthritis

Patients with rheumatoid arthritis affecting the glenohumeral joint commonly have multiple problems in their upper extremity. Shoulder arthrodesis is recognized as a procedure that can decrease pain arising from the glenohumeral joint.[38–40] Obliteration of glenohumeral motion has a negative influence on their upper extremity function. Frequently both upper extremities are involved. Patients with rheumatoid arthritis are much more effectively treated by total shoulder arthroplasty.[41] Favorable reports of combined shoulder and elbow arthroplasties have appeared in the literature and the author would advocate this method of reconstruction for such patients.

CONTRAINDICATIONS

Shoulder arthrodesis should not be performed if an alternative method of shoulder reconstruction is available. Many patients are amenable to arthroplasty reconstruction, which preserves glenohumeral motion and has greater potential to restore function. Shoulder arthrodesis should be reserved for those situations that are not amenable to reconstruction by any other means, as it places a significant functional demand on the patient and requires a major effort to rehabilitate the shoulder following surgery and strengthen the scapulothoracic musculature.

The procedure is contraindicated in a patient who cannot cooperate with such a program of rehabilitation. The author has not performed shoulder arthrodesis on elderly patients for this reason. Similarly, the procedure is contraindicated in any patient with a progressive neurologic disorder who may experience paralysis of the trapezius, levator scapulae, and/or serratus anterior muscles following the procedure. Glenohumeral arthrodesis relies on these muscles to motor the extremity and significant weakness will grossly impair shoulder function following the procedure.

AUTHOR'S PREFERRED SURGICAL TECHNIQUE

The operative technique and postoperative protocol are similar to those previously described. The patient is placed in the semi-sitting position, and the arm is draped free.[42] An incision extends from the spine of the scapula to the anterior part of the acromion and down the anterior aspect of the shaft of the humerus. Uematsu[43] recommended a posterior approach when performing shoulder arthrodesis. The deltoid muscle is detached from the anterior part of the acromion and its fibers are split distally. The rotator cuff is resected. The glenoid fossa, the undersurface of the acromion, and the humeral head are decorticated. An attempt is made to obtain arthrodesis of both the glenohumeral and acromiohumeral articulations, since the glenoid fossa offers such a small area for arthrodesis with the humeral head. Decortication of the undersurface of the acromion increases the potential area. A 10-hole, 4.5-mm AO/ASIF pelvic reconstruction plate is used for internal fixation during the procedure (Figure 10–10).

After resection of the rotator cuff and decortication of the joint surfaces, the shoulder is supported in 30 degrees of flexion, 30 degrees of abduction, and 30 degrees of internal rotation. Abduction is measured from the side of the body. Although this method of measurement does not accommodate for individual variations in muscle mass or body fat,

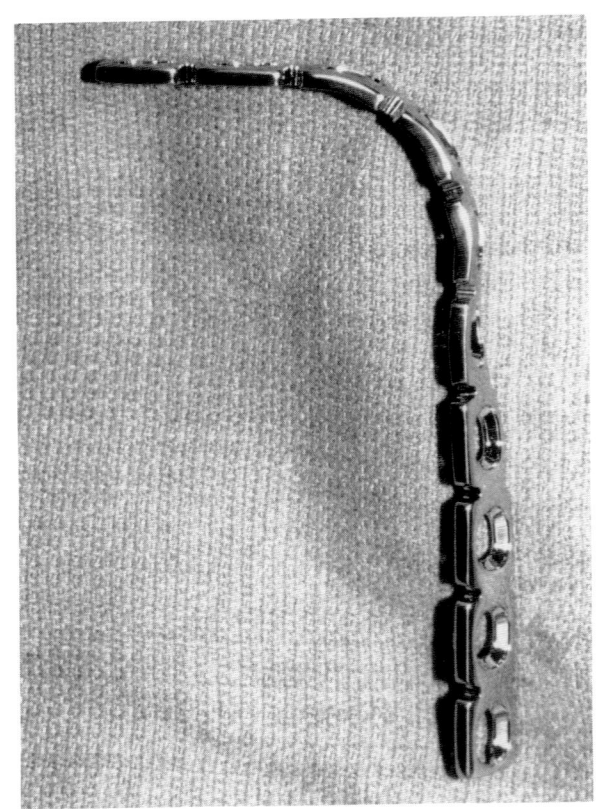

Figure 10–10. A 10-hole pelvic reconstruction plate for 4.5-mm screws is used for internal fixation. This plate can be contoured easily in the operating room and when combined with 6 weeks of postoperative immobilization in a thermoplastic orthosis, provides adequate stability to obtain arthrodesis. The union rate in the author's personal series of 57 procedures is over 96% with single-plate fixation. Bone grafting is not performed routinely.

clinical experience has shown it to be accurate to within 10 degrees in any plane. The humeral head is brought proximally to appose the decorticated undersurface of the acromion. When the humerus is abducted and flexed 30 degrees, the humeral head apposes both the undersurface of the acromion and the glenoid fossa. The position is maintained by supporting the arm with sterile folded sheets, and an assistant is assigned to maintain the position while the plate is contoured (Figure 10–11). Thirty degrees of internal rotation brings the hand to the midline. The author has not found it necessary to measure abduction radiographically.

Hand-held bending irons are used to contour the plate along the spine of the scapula, over the acromion, and down onto the shaft of the humerus. The malleable nature of the plate allows precise intraoperative contouring of the implant to the specific local anatomy in any given patient (Figure 10–11). The plate must be gently bent 60 degrees over the acromion and twisted 20 to 25 degrees just distal to the bend to appose the shaft of the humerus. The reconstruction plate has holes that allow angulation of the screws as they are passed through the plate.

The screws passing through the plate and the humeral head into the glenoid fossa are inserted first. Two or three screws can be inserted in this fashion, compressing the arthrodesis site. A screw should be directed next from the spine of the scapula into the base of the coracoid process. Due to the nature of the cortical bone in this region, care must be taken not to break the drill bit when drilling into the scapula. Another cancellous screw is placed across the acromiohumeral fusion site and the remaining holes of the plate are secured with cortical screws.

The acromion is not osteotomized since it is used to augment fixation of the scapula to the humerus. Autogenous bone graft is not used routinely. If there is a deficiency of the glenoid and/or humerus, bone graft should be used, which is often the situation when the procedure is performed for failed total shoulder arthroplasty.

The arm of the patient is supported postoperatively with a pillow and swathe. A thermoplastic thoracobrachial orthosis is applied 24 to 48 hours postoperatively. If possible, the orthosis can be fabricated preoperatively and then adjusted in the postoperative period as necessary. The orthosis is worn for 6 weeks postoperatively, but can be removed for short periods of time while the patient showers, providing the arm is supported. Six weeks postoperatively, the patient is examined radiographically and the stability of the arthrodesis is tested manually in a gentle fashion.

If there are no radiographic signs of the internal fixation loosening 6 weeks postoperatively, the arm is placed in a sling. Gentle range-of-motion exercises are allowed until radiographic union is achieved. It is difficult to be certain

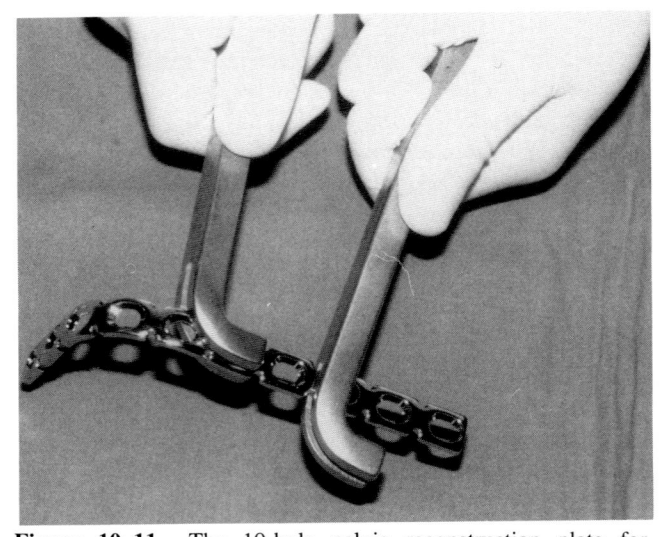

Figure 10–11. The 10-hole pelvic reconstruction plate for 4.5-mm screws is contoured with hand-held bending irons. The plate must be bent as it crosses the acromion and twisted just past the bend so that it lies flush with the surface of the humerus. It is much easier to contour the malleable pelvic reconstruction plate in the operating room than the standard dynamic compression plates for 4.5-mm screws. Use of this plate decreases operative time and reduces the prominence of the plate as it crosses the acromion.

when fusion occurs radiographically since the fixation is sufficiently rigid that very little callus forms around the arthrodesis site (Figure 10–12). Muscle strengthening is encouraged after removal of the orthosis, but return to strenuous activity is delayed for at least 16 weeks postoperatively. Scapulothoracic strengthening and mobilization exercises can be started 3 months following surgery.

COMPLICATIONS OF GLENOHUMERAL ARTHRODESIS

Nonunion

Nonunion following shoulder arthrodesis is surprisingly infrequent in view of the magnitude of the procedure, the high stresses across the arthrodesis site, and the problems with postoperative immobilization. In Cofield and Briggs' series (1979)[7] of 71 shoulder arthrodeses, only 3 patients went on to nonunion, but all showed successful fusions following a second operative procedure. If nonunion occurs following shoulder arthrodesis, a repeat operation with revision of the internal fixation device is indicated, and bone grafting should be used to augment the arthrodesis site. On occasion, a small number of patients will obtain an acromiohumeral fusion but not a solid fusion at the glenohumeral joint. In one such patient the internal fixation device failed and bone grafting was necessary.

Infection

Infection is relatively uncommon following shoulder arthrodesis due to the excellent vascularity of the periarticular tissues. Infection following shoulder arthrodesis should be treated with surgical drainage and the appropriate parenteral antibiotics. The internal fixation device should not be removed if it is providing stability and rigid fixation at the arthrodesis site. An attempt should be made to obtain a solid arthrodesis prior to removal of any fixation device.

Malposition

Excessive abduction of the extremity during shoulder arthrodesis can place a significant strain on the scapulothoracic musculature. Adult patients have great difficulty adapting to

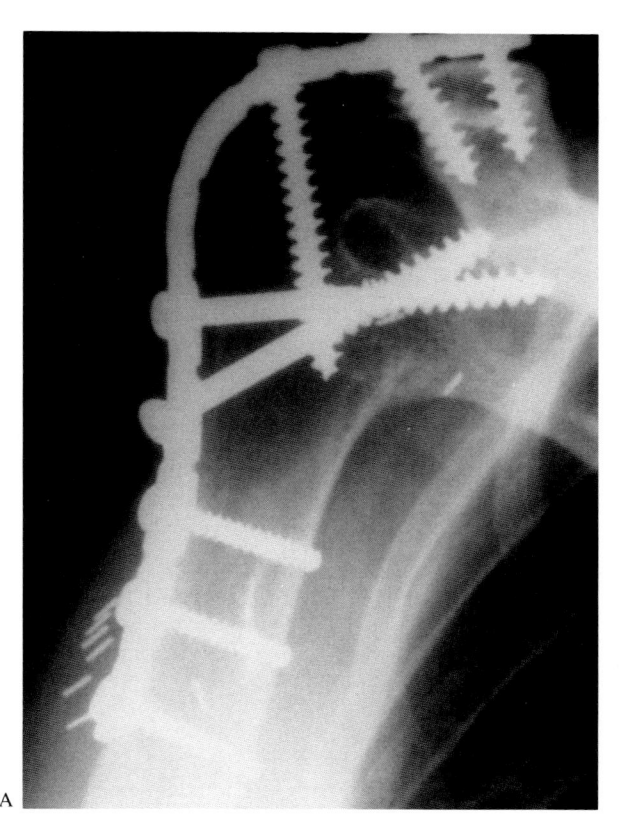

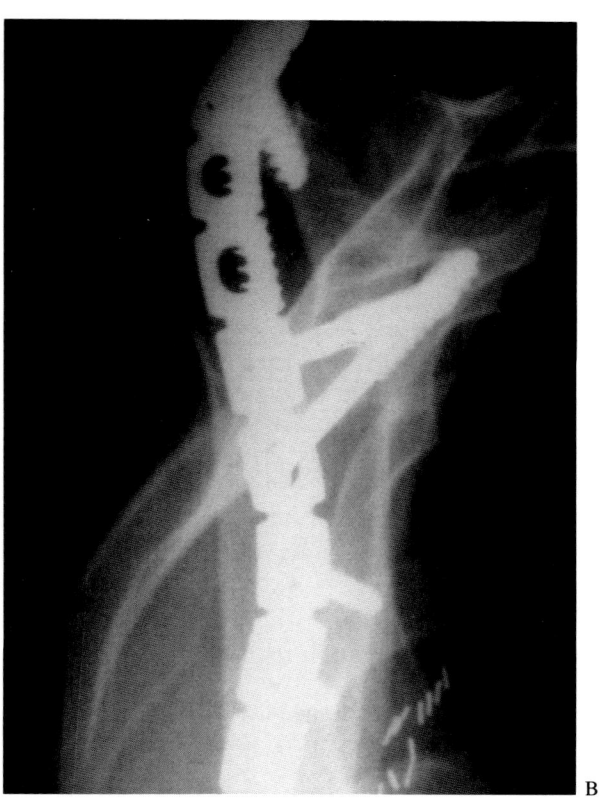

Figure 10–12. **A.** Anteroposterior radiograph showing solid arthrodesis 4 months postoperatively in a patient with an irreparable lesion of the brachial plexus. The two screws running from the plate into the glenoid should be inserted first. These screws compress the arthrodesis site. It is usually possible to insert two or three screws in this fashion. The remaining screws are inserted after the compression screws have been applied. **B.** Lateral radiographic view of the same patient, showing that the plate is contoured in more than one plane. The humerus is flexed in relation to the scapula. When inserting the compression screws into the glenoid, it is wise to place one's finger anterior to the glenoid as a directional guide. Since the glenoid is thin, it is relatively easy to inadvertently exit the glenoid and/or break a drill bit when drilling these holes.

positions of greater than 45 degrees of abduction. Hyperabduction at the arthrodesis site causes significant winging of the scapula, making it difficult for the arm to drop to the patient's side. Indeed, in some patients the arm will not approximate the trunk if the shoulder has been arthrodesed in too much abduction. Women are unhappy with the cosmetic appearance of a shoulder that has been arthrodesed in too much abduction, due to the significant prominence of the scapula that is created when the arm is adducted.

Arthrodesis of the shoulder in too much internal rotation can occur, and the patient cannot easily bring his or her hand to the mouth or reach either front or back pockets. Rotational osteotomy of the humerus may be necessary for patients whose extremities have been positioned in too much internal rotation.

Prominence of the Internal Fixation Device

Many patients who have had internal fixation devices applied over the spine of the scapula have significant skin tenderness over the appliance. This can be particularly troublesome when the patient must wear a prosthetic harness, with skin irritation and ulceration having been reported.[23] Cofield and Briggs[7] reported a significant incidence of tenderness over the internal fixation device that required its removal in 17 of their patients. The author has had a similar experience, although use of a malleable reconstruction plate has decreased skin tenderness and made the need for hardware removal less frequent.[24]

Fracture of the Humerus

Fracture of the humerus at the distal end of the internal fixation device is sufficiently common that the AO/ASIF group has recommended prophylactically bone grafting this area.[22] Cofield and Briggs[7] reported a fracture in the arthrodesed extremity in 10 of 71 patients. This complication occurred in the author's series as well in association with significant trauma to the arthrodesed shoulder. If an unstable fracture occurs at the end of the internal fixation device, it should be removed followed by internal fixation of the fracture if the arthrodesis site had solidly healed. If the fracture is relatively nondisplaced, it can be treated by closed means, but this is uncommon.

RESULTS

The author has carried out 57 shoulder arthrodeses. The ages of the patients ranged from 19 to 64 years. Forty-six patients were operated on for irreparable lesions of the brachial plexus; 5 patients, for recalcitrant shoulder instability; 2 patients, for osteoarthritis; 2 patients, for failed total shoulder arthroplasties; and 2 patients, for sepsis. The technique utilized was that of combined glenohumeral and acromiohumeral arthrodesis as described above. Only 2 patients had bone grafts at the time of the initial surgery and both of these patients had failed total shoulder arthroplasties.

Solid arthrodesis was obtained in 55 (96%) of 57 shoulders. Two patients developed an acromiohumeral arthrodesis only. One of these had a broken screw and underwent a secondary bone-grafting procedure. Infection occurred in only 1 patient. Clinical examination showed all shoulders arthrodesed within 10 degrees of the desired position. The author has not used special techniques to assess the position of the arthrodesis.[44] Twelve patients required surgery for plate removal and 2 patients sustained fractures of the humerus distal to the plate.

Five patients who had neurogenic pain preoperatively continued to complain of significant neurogenic pain postoperatively. Several other patients who had compensable injuries continued to complain of postoperative pain in spite of a solid arthrodesis. Most patients can reach both their front and back pockets following surgery and many have returned to fairly heavy occupations. These occupations have included tool and dye manufacture, gardening, heavy equipment operation, and brick laying. Patients who had shoulder arthrodesis for compensable injuries did not return to their previous occupations.

No acromioclavicular joint problems were encountered following shoulder arthrodesis. Some authors recommend excision arthroplasty of the acromioclavicular joint following arthrodesis, in an effort to maximize shoulder motion.[45] It has not been necessary to perform this adjunctive procedure in this series of patients. In the following paragraphs, arthrodesis, function, and pain following shoulder arthrodesis are discussed in more detail.

Arthrodesis

The success rates for shoulder arthrodesis are high. Most older series do not report any nonunions. Recent series utilizing internal fixation devices also report high union rates. It is often difficult to judge radiographic union in patients who have had internal fixation, since the fixation device commonly obscures the arthrodesis site and rigid internal fixation prevents the formation of periarticular new bone. External immobilization is empirically discontinued at 6 to 8 weeks, and the shoulder is examined clinically. Assuming the patient is comfortable, the patient is placed in a sling at this time. No attempt is made to mobilize the scapulothoracic musculature until at least 3 months after the arthrodesis. Using this method of postoperative rehabilitation, delayed union and nonunion are distinctly uncommon.

Function

The amount of improvement in shoulder function following arthrodesis is dependent on the function that was present preoperatively. Patients who have flail shoulders experience a significant improvement in glenohumeral function following arthrodesis, since they can actively position their extremities in space. Shoulder subluxation is relieved and function is significantly improved. Most, but not all, patients can use their extremity to lift, dress, tend to personal hygiene, eat, and comb their hair. In Cofield and Brigg's series,[7] hair combing was the most difficult task to perform following arthrodesis of the glenohumeral joint.

Pain

Pain relief is not universal following shoulder arthrodesis. In fact, some pain is commonly present in patients whose shoulders have been successfully arthrodesed. The presence of moderate to severe pain following a successful shoulder arthrodesis is difficult to explain. It is thought that such pain is related to the contiguous soft tissues. Shoulder arthrodesis places a significant strain on the periscapular musculature and requires the patient to make a profound functional adjustment. Pain surrounding successful fusions has also been reported following hip and knee arthrodeses. Most patients experience less pain with longer follow-up periods, and this suggests that with time the periscapular musculature adjusts to the changes imposed on it by glenohumeral arthrodesis.

Patients with neurogenic pain due to brachial plexus injuries will not experience pain relief following glenohumeral arthrodesis. Shoulder function is improved in these patients, but they should understand fully that the procedure is being performed to improve function and not to relieve pain. It has been the author's impression that if function is improved, such neurogenic pain is generally better tolerated by the patient. Therefore, one should concentrate on restoration of limb function rather than on relief of pain by neurosurgical means.

Acromioclavicular Joint Pain

Acromioclavicular joint pain has been reported following shoulder arthrodesis. Some methods of shoulder arthrodesis require osteotomy of the acromion. Such osteotomies disturb the normal acromioclavicular relationships. If pain arises from the acromioclavicular joint postoperatively, excision arthroplasty is indicated if local injections confirm that the pain is arising from the acromioclavicular joint. Some authors have reported anecdotally that excision arthroplasty of the acromioclavicular joint improves motion following shoulder arthrodesis. In the author's experience, acromioclavicular joint pain is rare following glenohumeral arthrodesis when the acromion is left in the anatomic position. For this reason, acromial osteotomy is not recommend in order to approximate the acromion to the superior surface of the humeral head.

Bone Grafting

Bone grafting during shoulder arthrodesis is advocated by some authors, while others routinely do not. The AO/ASIF group recommends prophylactic bone grafting at the termination of a plate if a plate is used for internal fixation. Eleven of Cofield and Brigg's 71 patients had autogenous bone grafts placed at the time of their initial procedure.[7] Richards et al.[24] obtained successful arthrodeses without primary bone grafts in patients with significant osteoporosis. Bone grafting is indicated to fill large defects in patients who are undergoing glenohumeral arthrodesis following failed total shoulder arthroplasty. Nonunion of shoulder arthrodeses should be treated by revision of the arthrodesis combined with bone grafting. An attempt must be made to obtain rigid internal fixation during the arthrodesis. This method of treatment has, in the author's experience, been successful when used.

SUMMARY

Shoulder arthrodesis remains an important procedure that should be part of every shoulder surgeon's armamentarium. The procedure is indicated for patients with paralytic disorders; those who require en bloc resection of their glenohumeral joint together with the rotator cuff and/or deltoid; and less commonly those with old septic arthritis, failed total shoulder arthroplasties, shoulder instability, failed rotator cuff repairs, periarticular malunions, osteoarthritis, or rheumatoid arthritis.

Although a variety of different positions for glenohumeral arthrodesis have been advocated in the literature, a position of 30 degrees of abduction (measured clinically), 30 degrees of flexion, and 30 degrees of internal rotation is recommended. This position brings the hand to the midline anteriorly so with elbow flexion, the patient can reach his or her mouth. With the shoulder arthrodesed in this position, the arm drops comfortably to the side. Arthrodesis of both the acromiohumeral and glenohumeral articulations and the use of internal fixation are recommended. Complications following shoulder arthrodesis are relatively infrequent, and most can be dealt with successfully if they do occur.

The improvement in shoulder function following shoulder arthrodesis is dependent on the patient's preoperative shoulder function. Patients with flail shoulders experience a significant improvement in function. Patients with significant mechanical pain in the glenohumeral joint experience pain relief following the procedure. Shoulder arthrodesis is primarily indicated to restore function. In general, bone grafting is not routinely necessary. The procedure is contraindicated in any patient with a progressive neurologic disorder affecting the periscapular musculature.

REFERENCES

1. Neer CS II, Watson KC, Stanton FJ. Recent experience in total shoulder replacement. *J Bone and Joint Surg [Am]* 1982; 64:319–337.
2. De Velasco PG, Cardoso MA. Arthrodesis of the shoulder. *Clin Orthop* 1973;90:178–182.
3. Hawkins RJ, Neer CS. A functional analysis of shoulder fusions. *Clin Orthop* 1987;223:65–76.
4. Wilde AH, Brems JJ, Boumphrey FR. Arthrodesis of the shoulder: Current indications and operative technique. *Orthop Clin North Am* 1987;18:463–472.
5. Barr JS, Freiberg JA, Colonna PC, Pemberton PA. A survey of end results on stabilization of the paralyzed shoulder. Report of

the Research Committee of the American Orthopaedic Association. *J Bone Joint Surg* 1942;24:699–707.
6. Rowe CR. Re-evaluation of the position of the arm in arthrodesis of the shoulder in the adult. *J Bone Joint Surg [Am]* 1974;56:5:913–922.
7. Cofield RH, Briggs BT. Glenohumeral arthrodesis. *J Bone Joint Surg [Am]* 1979;61:668–677.
8. Riggins RS. Shoulder fusion without external fixation. *J Bone Joint Surg [Am]* 1976;58:1007–1008.
9. Kostuik JP, Schatzker J. Shoulder arthrodesis—AO technique. In: Bateman JE, Welsh RP, eds. *Surgery of the Shoulder*. St. Louis: CV Mosby, 1984:207–210.
10. Watson-Jones R. Extra-articular arthrodesis of the shoulder. *J Bone Joint Surg* 1933;15:862–871.
11. Putti V. Arthrodesis for tuberculosis of the knee and shoulder. *Chir Organi Mov* 1933;18:217.
12. Brittain HA. *Architectural Principles in Arthrodesis*. 3rd ed. Edinburgh: E and L Livingstone, 1952.
13. DePalma AF. *Surgery of the Shoulder*. 3rd ed. Philadelphia, JB Lippincott, 1983:132–143.
14. Gill AB. A new operation for arthrodesis of the shoulder. *J Bone Joint Surg* 1931;13:287.
15. Makin M. Early arthrodesis for a flail shoulder in young children. *J Bone Joint Surg [Am]* 1977;59:317–321.
16. Moseley HF. Arthrodesis of the shoulder in the adult. *Clin Orthop* 1961;20:156–162.
17. Beltran JE, Trilla JC, Barjan R. A simplified compression arthrodesis of the shoulder. *J Bone Joint Surg [Am]* 1975;57:538–541.
18. May VR. Shoulder fusion: A review of fourteen cases. *J Bone Joint Surg [Am]* 1962;44:65–76.
19. Davis JB, Cottrell GW. A technique for shoulder arthrodesis. *J Bone Joint Surg [Am]* 1962;44:657–661.
20. Carroll RE. Wire loop in arthrodesis in the shoulder. *Clin Orthop* 1957;9:185–189.
21. Leffert RD. *Brachial Plexus Injuries*. New York: Churchill-Livingstone, 1985:193–210.
22. Muller ME, Allgower AM, Willenegger H. *Manual of Internal Fixation*. 2nd ed. Berlin: Springer-Verlag, 1979.
23. Richards RR, Waddell JP, Hudson AR. Shoulder arthrodesis for the treatment of brachial plexus palsy. *Clin Orthop* 1985;198:250–258.
24. Richards RR, Sherman RMP, Hudson AR, Waddell JP. Shoulder arthrodesis using a modified pelvic reconstruction plate: A review of eleven cases. *J Bone Joint Surg [Am]* 1988;70:416–421.
25. Charnley J, Houston JK. Compression arthrodesis of the shoulder. *J Bone Joint Surg [Br]* 1964;46:614–620.
26. Johnson CA, Healy WL, Brooker AF Jr, Krackow KA. External fixation shoulder arthrodesis. *Clin Orthop* 1986;211:219–223.
27. Kocialkowski A, Wallace WA. Shoulder arthrodesis using an external fixator. *J Bone Joint Surg [Br]* 1991;73:180–181.
28. Nagano A, Okinaga S, Ochiai N, Kurokawa T. Shoulder arthrodesis by external fixation. *Clin Orthop* 1989;247:97–100.
29. Schrader HA, Frandsen PA. External compression arthrodesis of the shoulder joint. *Acta Orthop Scand* 1983;54:592–595.
30. Richards RR. Operative treatment for irreparable lesions of the brachial plexus. In: Gelberman RH, ed. *Operative Nerve Repair and Reconstruction*. Philadelphia: JB Lippincott, 1991:1303–1328.
31. Goldner JL. Muscle-tendon transfers for partial paralysis of the shoulder girdle. In: Evarts CM, ed. *Surgery of the Musculoskeletal System*. New York: Churchill-Livingstone, 1983;3:167–184.
32. Mah JY, Hall JE. Arthrodesis of the shoulder in children. *J Bone Joint Surg [Am]* 1990;72:582–586.
33. MacDonald W, Thrum CB, Hamilton SGL. Designing an implant by CT scanning and solid modelling: Arthrodesis of the shoulder after excision of the upper humerus. *J Bone Joint Surg [Br]* 1986;68:208–212.
34. Rowe CR, Pierce DS, Clark JG. Voluntary dislocation of the shoulder: A preliminary report on a clinical, electromyographic and psychiatric study of twenty-six patients. *J Bone Joint Surg [Am]* 1973;55:445–460.
35. Rockwood CA, Burkhead WZ. The management of patients with massive rotator cuff defects by acromioplasty and radical cuff debridement. Presentation to the Orthopaedic Associations of the English Speaking World; May 1987; Washington, DC.
36. Neer CS II, Craig EV, Fukuda H. Cuff tear arthropathy. *J Bone Joint Surg [Am]* 1983;65:1232–1244.
37. Barton NJ. Arthrodesis of the shoulder for degenerative conditions. *J Bone Joint Surg [Am]* 1972;54:1759–1764.
38. Rybka V, Raunio P, Vainio K. Arthrodesis of the shoulder in rheumatoid arthritis: A review of forty-one cases. *J Bone Joint Surg [Br]* 1979;61:155–158.
39. Raunio P. Arthrodesis of the shoulder joint in rheumatoid arthritis. *Reconstr Surg Traumatol* 1981;18:48–54.
40. Jonsson E, Brattstrom M, Lidgren L. Evaluation of the rheumatoid shoulder function after hemiarthroplasty and arthrodesis. *Scand J Rheumatol* 1988;17:17–26.
41. Friedman RJ, Ewald FC. Arthroplasty of the ipsilateral shoulder and elbow in patients who have rheumatoid arthritis. *J Bone Joint Surg [Am]* 1987;69:661–666.
42. Bateman JE. *The Shoulder and Neck*. 2nd ed. Philadelphia, WB Saunders, 1978:273–274.
43. Uematsu A. Arthrodesis of the shoulder: Posterior approach. *Clin Orthop* 1979;139:169–173.
44. Jonsson E, Lidgren L, Rydholm U. Position of shoulder arthrodesis measured with Moire photography. *Clin Orthop* 1989;238:117–121.
45. Pipkin G. Claviculectomy as an adjunct to shoulder arthrodesis. *Clin Orthop* 1967;54:145–160.

SECTION IV

Indications for Total Shoulder Arthroplasty

11 Glenohumeral Osteoarthritis

Keith Watson, M.D.

Primary osteoarthritis of the shoulder, although not as common as that of the hip or knee, occurs with sufficient regularity that its unique characteristics and presentation should be familiar to those who treat shoulder problems. While advances have been made in the area of pathogenesis, underlying biomechanical and biochemical alterations, and treatment, it continues to be a challenging condition. Historically, shoulder problems have been given a low priority, but with improved diagnostic and treatment options, interest and enthusiasm in this area of orthopaedics have mushroomed.

PATHOPHYSIOLOGY

The contribution of trauma as a component in the development of glenohumeral osteoarthritis is unclear.[1] There is often a history of macrotrauma. Previous microtrauma and surgery are contributing factors in some cases.[2] At the cellular level, there is an increase in water content and softening of the articular cartilage, leading to a decrease in density and weakening of its biomechanical function to withstand compressive forces.[3] Despite the fact that the shoulder is considered a non–weight-bearing joint, it has been shown that the reactive force across the glenohumeral joint with the arm abducted to 90 degrees approaches one times the body weight.[2] In light of this, it is surprising that articular cartilage degeneration in the shoulder does not occur more frequently.

The pathology of this condition is very consistent. There is thinning of the articular cartilage, most severe where contact occurs between the humeral head and the glenoid in the position of greatest joint reaction force, 60 to 100 degrees of abduction in the scapular plane. In this area there is eburnation of bone. There may be subchondral cysts and a peripheral ring osteophyte around the articular margin, with the largest being inferior and obliterating the calcar of the humerus. Changes on the glenoid side include smooth eburnation of the glenoid face, flattening and posterior erosion, and marginal osteophyte formation within the remnants of the labrum and capsule.[4]

Frequently there will be osteochondral loose bodies and distension of the subscapularis bursa and biceps sheath distal to the transverse humeral ligament by excessive joint fluid. Rarely is there a rotator cuff tear, as it is recognized that the forces responsible for the production of these structural changes requires a functioning rotator cuff (Figure 11–1). In long-standing cases, there may be loss of subscapularis excursion resulting in an internal rotation contracture, even after resection of a bony osteophyte.

CLINICAL PRESENTATION

The clinical course of this condition is one of gradual loss of mobility associated with increasing discomfort. While it occurs in some individuals during middle age without preexisting evidence of joint disease, there is an increasing incidence with age.[5] In addition, there are known metabolic causes such as ochronosis, gout, and pseudogout. Traumatic causes include previous dislocation, an injury of some magnitude in the past, or previous surgery for such a condition (Figure 11–2). Irradiation for breast cancer may damage the articular cartilage or lead to radiation necrosis (Figure 11–3). Congenital causes such as dysplasia or subluxation/dislocation are known to be precipitating factors[6] (Figure 11–4). Osteoarthritis has characteristics that set it apart from rheumatoid arthritis, traumatic arthritis, and massive rotator cuff defects with glenohumeral arthritis (Table 11–1).

History

Typically, the patient notices a gradual loss of mobility in the shoulder associated with occasional episodes of discomfort and pain. This increases in frequency, along with dull aching and soreness accompanying vigorous use, until the symptoms cause the patient to seek medical attention. Often, there is a history of old macrotrauma, such as a dislocation or severe injury to the shoulder that may or may not have been treated, or microtrauma such as repetitive heavy use at a specific occupation. There may have been previous surgery involving the shoulder, and in many cases, multiple injections into the glenohumeral joint. It is important to assess the cervical spine and adjacent articulations such as the acromioclavicular joint, as arthritic degeneration of these areas may be a concomitant condition (Figure 11–5). Although the glenohumeral joint shows evidence of arthritic degeneration, it may not be the primary source of the patient's symptoms.[7] The patient may give a history of the arm catching or grating, having difficulty sleeping on that side, or the activities of daily living being severely restricted, particularly if the dominant extremity is involved.

Physical Examination

There will frequently be some degree of atrophy of the deltoid and/or the rotator cuff muscles, tenderness at the

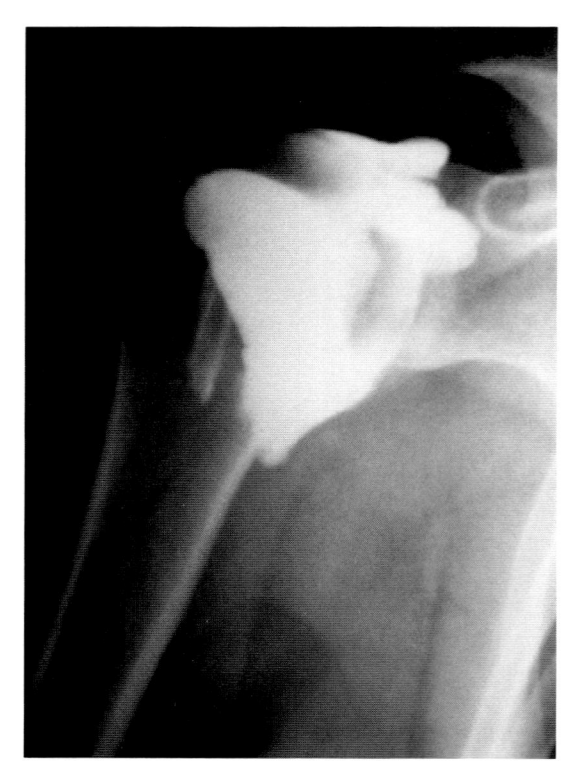

Figure 11–1. Arthrography in osteoarthritis rarely reveals rotator cuff defects.

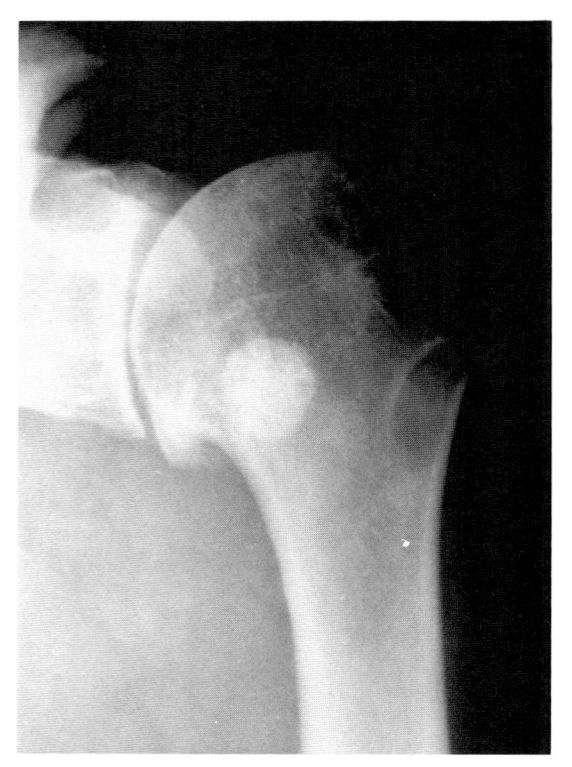

Figure 11–2. Arthritis of instability. Note the large osseous loose body as well as the inferior osteophyte and joint space narrowing.

posterior joint line, and decreased active and passive range of motion, especially to rotation in abduction. There may be a hard crepitus or ratcheting with forward flexion as the humeral head slides backward on the flattened and eburnated glenoid surface, resulting in a posterior fullness secondary to the pseudosubluxation that develops in osteoarthritis.[8] Despite significant restriction of mobility, patients retain good power because the rotator cuff is intact. False weakness may be encountered if there is guarding due to pain. Intra-articular injection with a local anesthetic may improve the validity of the examination by localizing the symptoms to the glenohumeral joint.

Radiography

Initial evaluation must include a true anteroposterior view of the glenohumeral joint in internal and external rotation, and an axillary lateral view. The inferior osteophytes are best

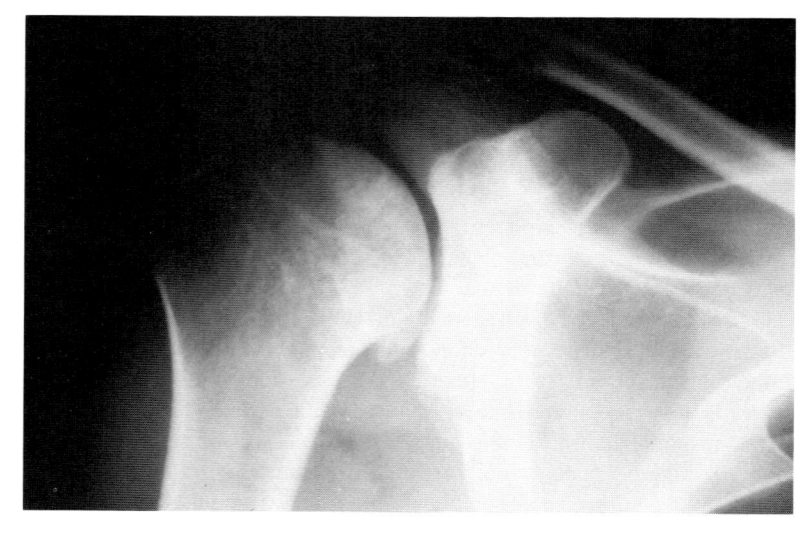

Figure 11–3. Postirradiation arthritis, which is frequently seen following irradiation for breast carcinoma. Patients may exhibit lymphedema or dermal atrophy. This case, which was rapid in development and markedly symptomatic, would suggest an effect on the articular cartilage similar to chondrolysis.

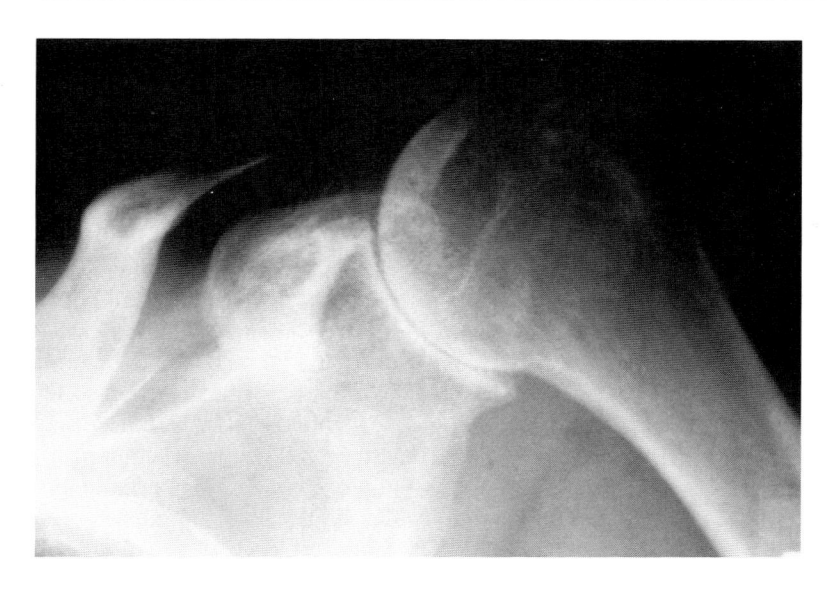

Figure 11-4. Congenital dysplasia of the glenoid, with secondary radiographic changes involving mainly the humeral head.

Table 11-1. Comparison Between the Common Forms of Arthritis That Affect the Glenohumeral Joint

FEATURE	OSTEOARTHRITIS	RHEUMATOID ARTHRITIS	TRAUMATIC ARTHRITIS
Bone density	Good	Poor	Variable
Osteophytes	Large	Small	Variable
Rotator cuff	Intact	50% deficit	Scarred
Loose bodies	Osseous	Cartilaginous	Osseous
Synovitis	Degenerative	Inflammatory	Degenerative
Glenoid wear	Posterior	Central	Variable
Contiguous joints affected	Occasional	Frequent	Rarely
Age	Older	Variable	Younger

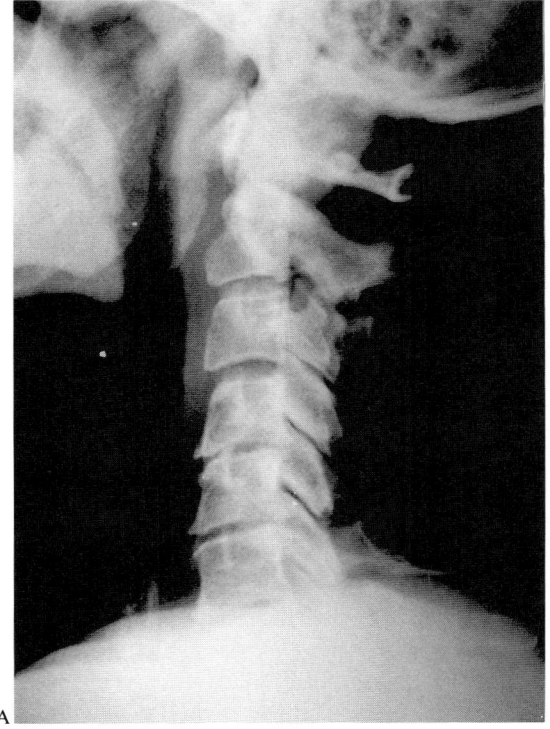

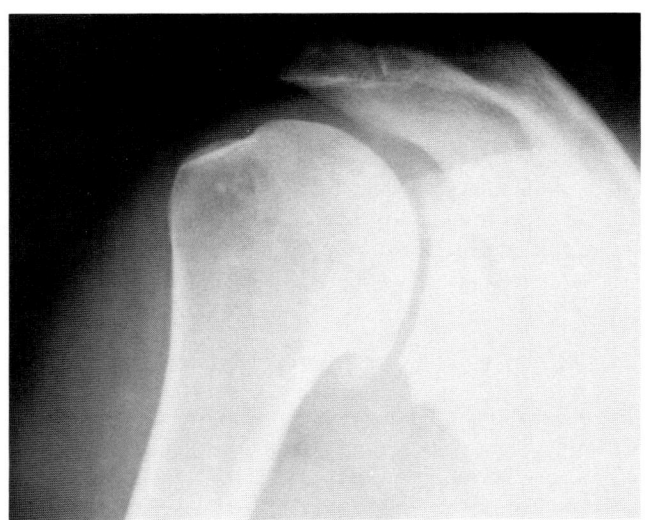

Figure 11-5. Osteoarthritis may affect contiguous areas such as the cervical spine (**A**) and acromioclavicular joint (**B**), which may be sources of pain. There are degenerative lesions in the cervical spine and distal aspect of the clavicle.

seen on the external rotation view in full profile (Figure 11–6). The axillary lateral view shows narrowing of the joint space and asymmetric wear of the glenoid. An arthrogram is not likely to be helpful, since in the majority of cases the rotator cuff will be intact. A computerized tomography scan may be helpful to better evaluate the extent of articular cartilage narrowing and glenoid wear.[9] Classic radiographic findings include narrowing or obliteration of the joint space, subchondral sclerosis in the superior and middle portion of the humeral head, subchondral cysts on both the humeral and the glenoid side, significant peripheral osteophyte formation best seen at the inferior margin and the region of the calcar, osteocartilaginous loose bodies, and, occasionally, posterior migration of the humeral head with asymmetric wear on the glenoid.[4,10] Radiographic changes are frequently advanced before symptoms are incapacitating.

CONSERVATIVE TREATMENT

Conservative treatment is indicated in almost all patients initially, as the degenerative changes are frequently advanced before the patient experiences truly disabling symptoms. In addition, while the radiographic findings may be intriguing, it must be determined that they are indeed responsible for the patient's symptoms. Many patients with primary osteoarthritis will be well managed with conservative measures, and while there are no medications that will reverse the disease process, nonsteroidal anti-inflammatory drugs will often have a reasonable effect in decreasing pain early on. Physical therapy cannot be expected to overcome the advanced bony alterations of the anatomy, but isometric exercises may improve muscle tone and blood flow, and range-of-motion exercises may minimize further losses.

Intra-articular corticosteroid injections are not recommended on a regular basis; however, if meticulous care and aseptic technique are used, the argument can be made that an occasional intra-articular injection is worthwhile, especially if it will reduce the attendant synovitis and decrease the patient's dependence on medication for a period of time. In these advanced cases, there is little concern for the detrimental effects of cortisone on the articular cartilage since it is already destroyed. The usefulness of this treatment modality must be balanced with concern for the possible introduction of an iatrogenic septic arthritis, while placement of local anesthetic into the joint itself may afford the patient and the clinician the opportunity to determine more precisely whether the arthritic degeneration of the shoulder is the major cause producing the patient's symptoms.

OPERATIVE TREATMENT

A number of operative options are possible in the treatment of osteoarthritis. Debridement of the glenohumeral joint with resection of the peripheral osteophytes, removal of the osteocartilaginous loose bodies, and concomitant synovectomy have been performed in the past. While there is little information in the literature, it would suggest that results with this approach are poor.[4,6] If indeed, these are adaptive changes, the removal of any stabilizing influence the osteophytes provide would allow for increased wear, greater migration, and progressively more pain. In addition, the attendant scar formation from such surgery might interfere with subsequent operative options such as arthroplasty.

There has been nothing published about arthroscopic debridement for osteoarthritis. This might be indicated in the early stages of the condition, before the osteophytes became massive. However, at this stage most patients are not sufficiently painful or disabled to warrant such intervention, and once the condition becomes severe enough to require surgery, the magnitude of the procedure, if done arthoscopically, would be formidable. While arthroscopic synovectomy for rheumatoid disease may be a reasonable rational approach, the synovitis of osteoarthritis is largely secondary and degenerative in nature rather than inflammatory, and it is doubtful that this would have sufficient impact on the progression of the disease process as to be meaningful. Resection arthroplasty has been attempted in the past and results have been very poor. With the options available to the surgeon today, resection arthroplasty should be reserved only for infection or extensive bone loss.[11]

Arthrodesis is a consideration in the treatment of osteoarthritis, but should be reserved for certain select conditions such as extensive nerve palsy, failed prior arthroplasty, and septic complications following repair of a fracture.[11] Humeral head replacement or hemiarthroplasty is a reasonable choice in young patients, particularly if glenoid wear is minimal. Prior to the introduction of ultra-high-molecular-weight polyethylene glenoid components, the early results of treatment for osteoarthritis with humeral head replacement alone were remarkably good, consistent, and durable (Figure 11–7). Therefore, this must be a consideration in the patient with limited glenoid involvement.[4,7]

Total shoulder arthroplasty has proved to be an effective treatment for primary osteoarthritis of the glenohumeral joint.[6–8,12–15] This treatment option is ideal for this condition because there is, in general, both adequate and good-quality bone stock with an intact well-functioning rotator cuff. A congruent glenohumeral joint and functioning rotator cuff are essential for normal shoulder function, and can often be achieved in osteoarthritis with total shoulder arthroplasty.[8]

Indications are primarily for pain relief, with improved function being a secondary consideration. Contraindications are infection, paralysis, and preexisting neuropathy. The decision to use a glenoid component must be made on the basis of damage to the glenoid itself. If there is excessive wear with flattening or erosion, so that the humeral component would not be well contained or the version of the glenoid component would not match that of the humeral component, then consideration must be given to resurfacing both sides. In this day and age, a constrained device is not acceptable. It has been well documented that the durability of constrained

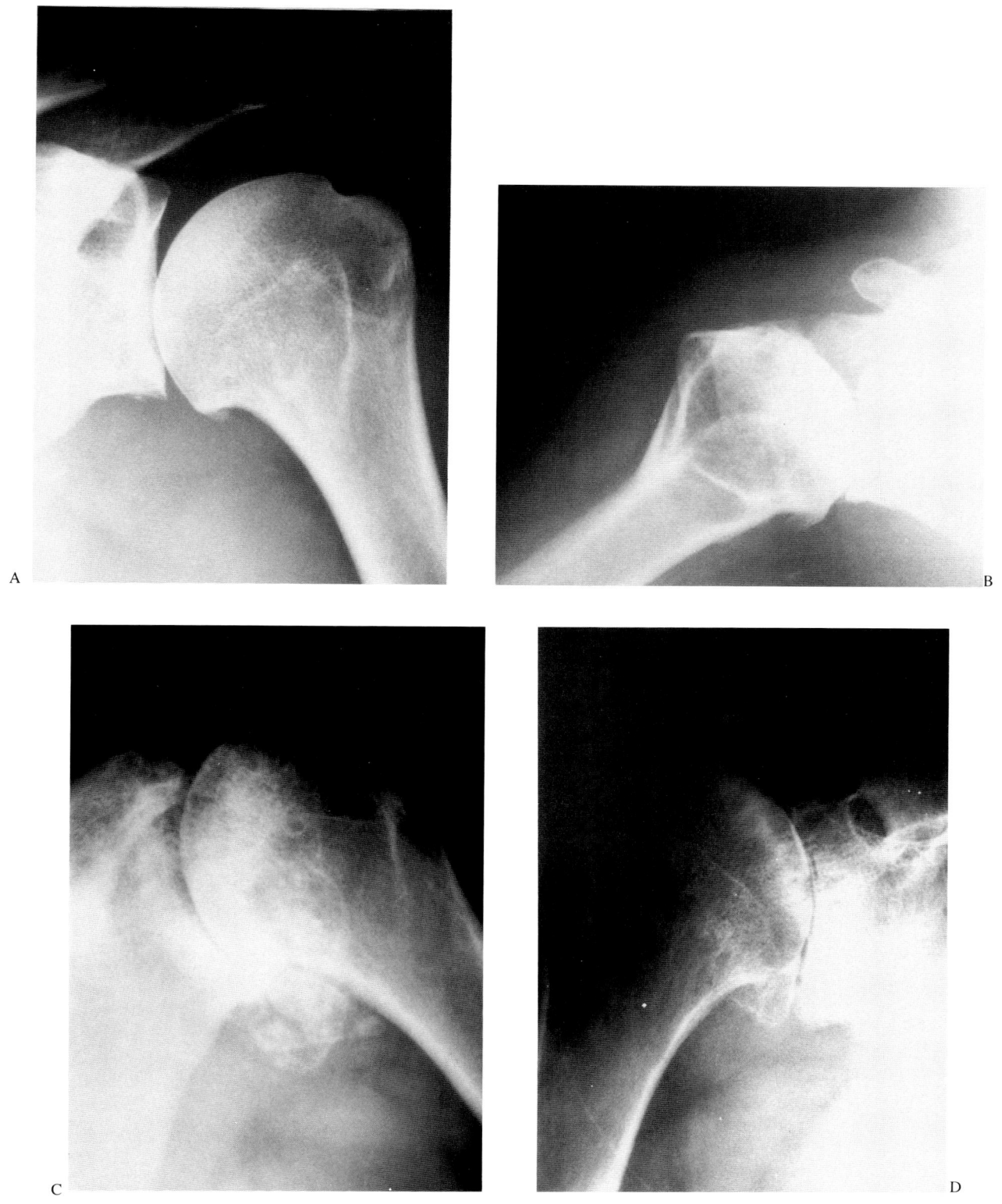

Figure 11–6. Radiographic changes seen in osteoarthritis of the glenohumeral joint. **A.** Small osteophytes of early osteoarthritis, best appreciated on the anteroposterior view in external rotation. **B.** Narrowing of the joint space best appreciated on the axillary view **C.** Subchondral sclerosis on both the glenoid and the humeral side. **D.** Subchondral cysts on both sides of the joint.

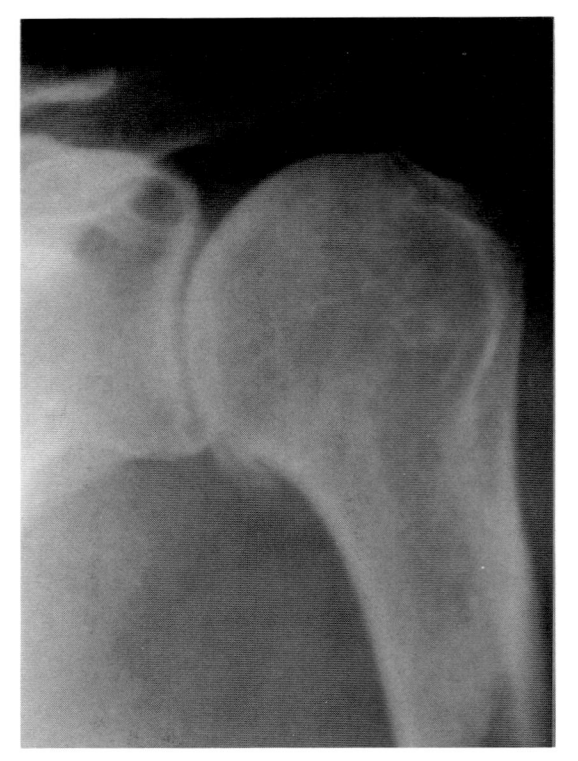

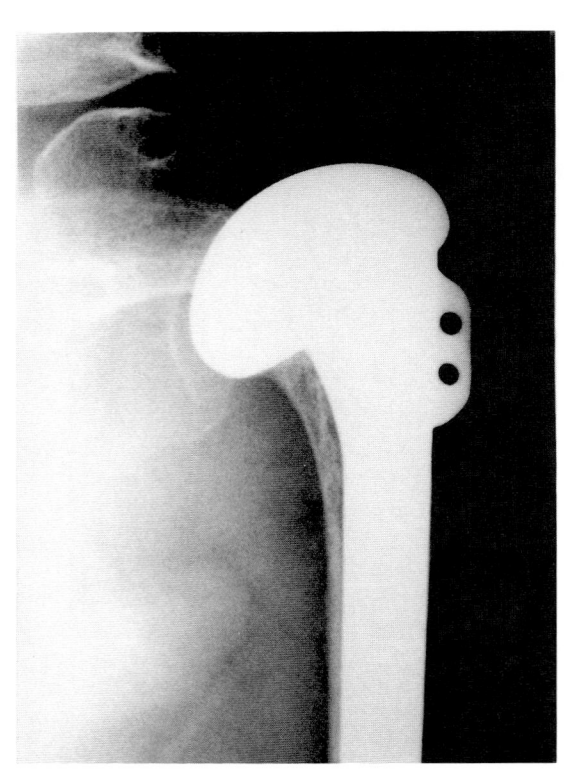

Figure 11-7. Humeral hemiarthroplasty for limited involvement.

devices is inadequate given the limitations imposed by the unique anatomy of the shoulder (Figure 11-8).[16-21]

The goal of a nonconstrained total shoulder arthroplasty is approximate restoration of normal anatomy, and while there are several different designs available, the concepts and general principles are the same. This will necessarily place greater demands on the surgeon's skill at repairing, reconstructing, and rehabilitating the soft tissues. Fortunately, in osteoarthritis, the soft tissues are generally in reasonably good condition. Problems in glenohumeral arthroplasty for osteoarthritis will usually fall into two areas: humeral difficulties and glenoid difficulties.

On the humeral side, there are two problems produced by the marginal or peripheral ring osteophytes. They can obscure the true humeral head and its normal version, thus making precise resection of the articular portion difficult. It is helpful to remove the ring osteophytes and expose the calcar of the humeral head before making the first cut. In addition, failure to remove the posterior osteophytes will result in a tight posterior capsule, leading to the selection of a smaller-than-appropriate humeral head, and thus limiting rotation and elevation. The magnitude of these osteophytes is often not appreciated until the articular surface cut has been made.

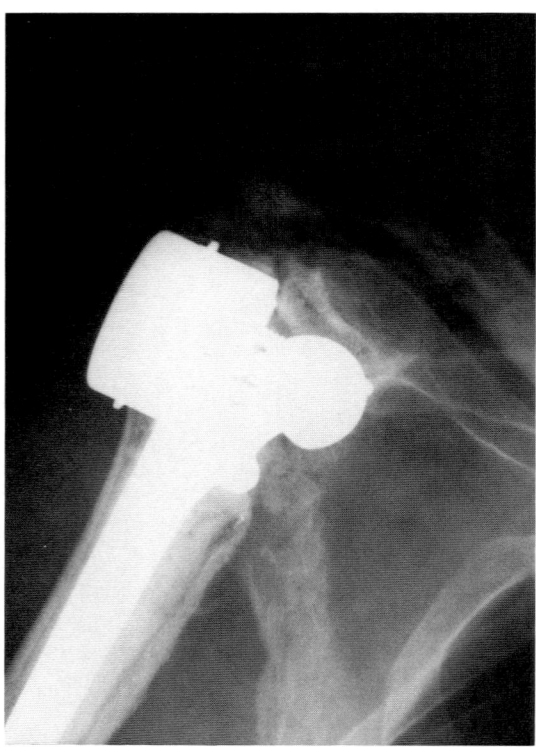

Figure 11-8. Constrained devices have demonstrated an unacceptable failure rate, such as the dislocation shown here.

On the glenoid side, erosion may occur without an appreciation of the change in version that this signifies, making placement of a keeled glenoid hazardous. Perforation of the cortex will undoubtedly occur, and at the same time, incorrect version will result. Often the anterior glenoid cartilage will be minimally affected, and probing with a needle will reveal substantial remaining articular cartilage. However, probing the posterior aspect of the glenoid will reveal only bare bone.

Failure to recognize such asymmetric posterior wear may result in the placement of a humeral component alone, with resulting inadequate pain relief. Uneven wear of the glenoid may be dealt with by burring down the anterior rim if the amount of resection necessary is not too great, allowing placement of the glenoid component in proper version. If it is not possible to correct the retroversion adequately by this method, then consideration must be given to bone grafting using a portion of the resected humeral head anchored with screws to adequately support the glenoid component, or using an augmented prosthesis.[22] Filling in the space between the glenoid component and the subchondral bone with cement is considered a violation of technique, as this does not provide adequate support for the prosthesis against the subjacent bone (Figure 11–9).[23]

With good-quality bone in osteoarthritis, the humeral component may be press-fit in most cases. Within 6 months in the active patient, there will often be a silhouette of cancellous bone condensation outlining the shaft of the prosthesis (Figure 11–10). This signifies adaptive changes in the surrounding bone, indicating that the mechanical stresses at the bone-implant interface are acceptable. Recent design modifications have incorporated bone-ingrowth potential.[24-26]

CONTRAINDICATIONS

Active or recent infection is an obvious contraindication to prosthetic arthroplasty for osteoarthritis. While previous surgical complications such as poor wound healing, splitting of sutures, or a history of a suture granuloma are all warning signs, suspicion should also be raised for patients with unusual reactions to or a history of multiple cortisone injections. Any concern should initiate an infection workup, with a complete blood cell count, sedimentation rate, aspiration arthrogram with culture and sensitivity, indium scanning, and perhaps even an open biopsy prior to implantation in difficult cases.

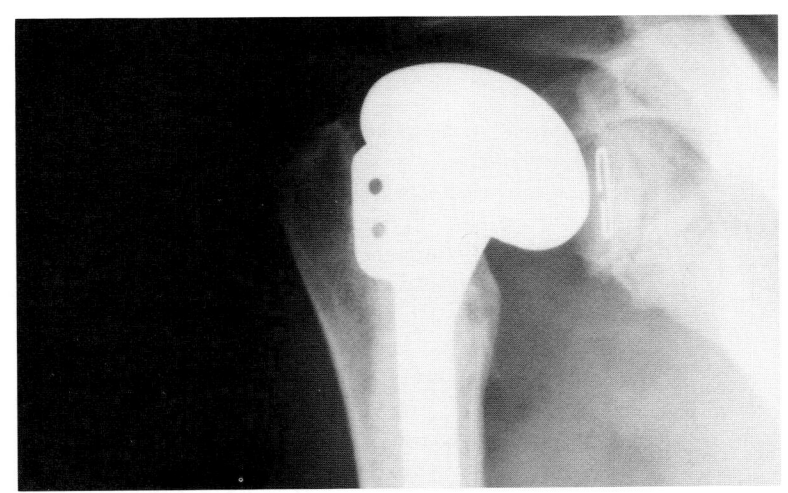

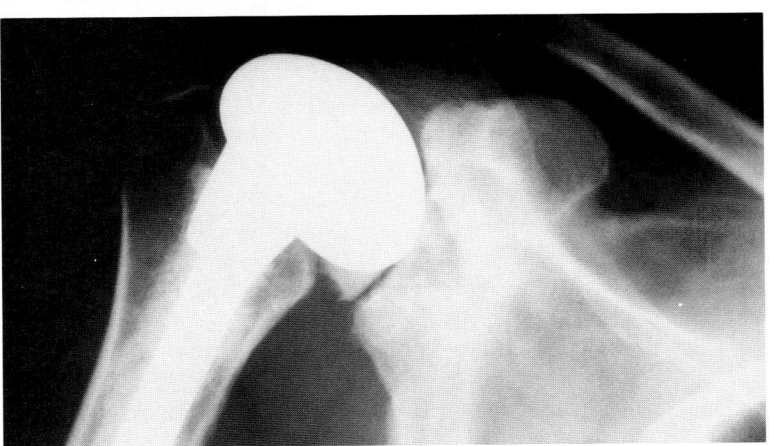

Figure 11–9. Anteroposterior radiographs reveal a violation of technique. Unrecognized posterior glenoid erosion resulted in the glenoid component being supported by a shelf of cement, which subsequently cracks and displaces. The unsupported polyethylene glenoid component fatigues and fails.

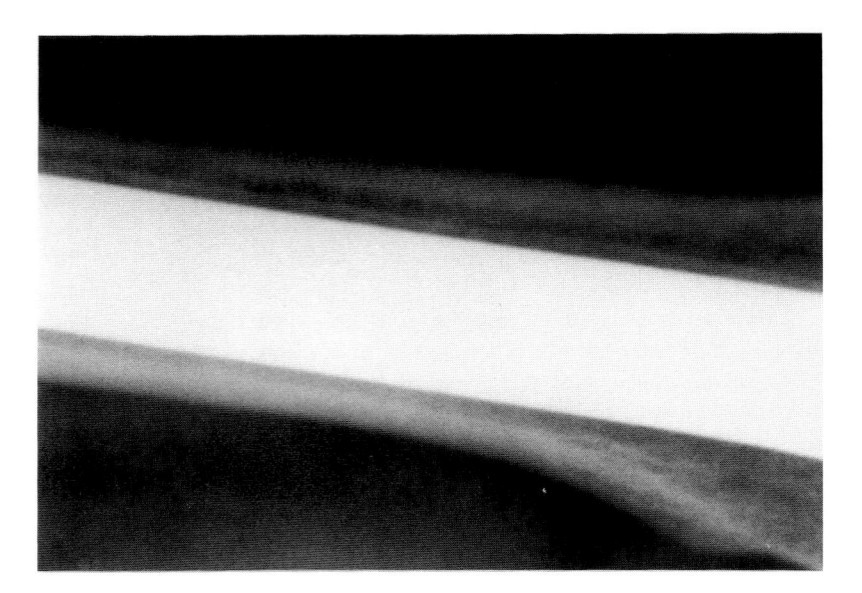

Figure 11-10. Radiograph shows a line of condensation around the prosthetic stem, indicating acceptable mechanical stresses.

Extensive brachial plexus injury or other neurologic deficits should be approached cautiously. These are not likely to be encountered in the treatment of true osteoarthritis. Neuropathic degeneration of the shoulder, on the other hand, may be difficult to distinguish from osteoarthritis.[27] With a neuropathy, there is often a discrepancy between the degree of joint destruction and the magnitude of symptoms. Patients are usually younger, and the rate of joint deterioration is more rapid compared to the relatively slowly evolving osteoarthritis (Figure 11-11). Complete neurologic workup should be undertaken if there are any suspicions. Although a cervical syrinx is probably the most likely cause of a neuropathic shoulder joint in this day and age, unrecognized seizure activity can produce a similar picture.

COMPLICATIONS

Major complications of surgery for osteoarthritis fall into three areas: infection, instability, and component failure. Reported series do not break down complications by diagnosis, but the overall complication rate reported by 13 different authors from 1982 through 1989 is 11.3%.[19]

The shoulder enjoys a better environment than the hip and knee with regard to late infection. Whereas late hematogenous infection in hip and knee replacements occurs with regularity, this has been reported infrequently in the shoulder. Still, it is prudent to require prophylactic antibiotic coverage for patients undergoing dental or urologic procedures. The most commonly reported pathogen by far is *Staphylococcus aureus*, unless there is preexisting immune system compromise. Postoperative infections following total shoulder arthroplasty are also more likely when there has been previous surgery such as open reduction and internal fixation and are therefore more common in cases of posttraumatic arthritis.

Instability of a shoulder arthroplasty is most likely to occur when the condition existed preoperatively or as a result of rotator cuff insufficiency. Chronic distortion of the soft tissues will require special treatment and alterations of the usual rehabilitation protocol.

There is a subset of individuals with distortion of the soft tissues who present with osteoarthritis and must be addressed with care. These are patients with Parkinson's disease or Parkinson-like symptoms who exhibit a persistent involun-

Figure 11-11. Degree of destruction produced within 6 weeks after prosthetic replacement of a neuropathic joint.

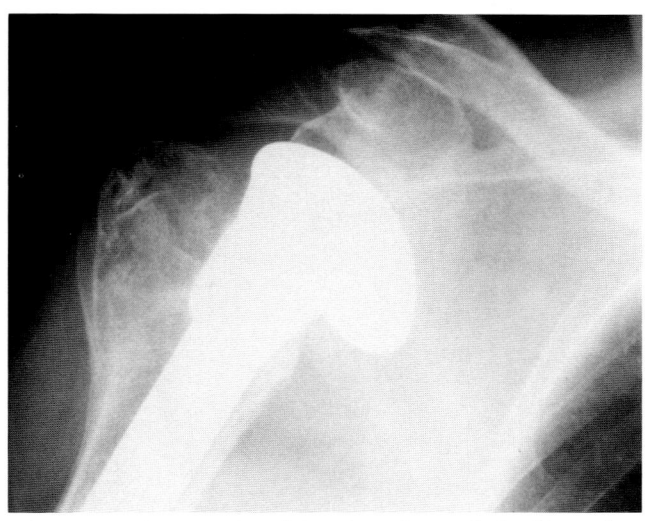

Figure 11–12. Anterior dislocation of a total shoulder arthroplasty in a patient with Parkinson's disease.

tary tremor-like activity of their shoulder (which may play a role in the development of the osteoarthritis). Their shoulders act in some respects like neuropathic joints, with a gradual stretching of their anterior structures. After several months, they will present with an anterior dislocation of the components (Figure 11–12). Revision procedures with altered version of components and reconstruction of the anterior structures provide only temporary stability. In actuality, these patients may represent a relative contraindication to total shoulder arthroplasty and should be recognized, if possible, beforehand.

Component failure falls into two categories: technical failure and design failure. Technical failures on the humeral side are most often seen with inadequate or excessive resection of the humeral head. Both situations (prosthesis too proud or tuberosities too proud) result in improper tensioning of the rotator cuff and poor function. Humeral version in osteoarthritis is usually the normal 35 to 40 degrees of retroversion. Unless there are unusual problems with wear or rotator cuff deficiency, usually seen with rheumatoid or traumatic arthritis, the normal anatomic retroversion of the humeral head will be most appropriate. Inappropriate version may be suspected if at the time of trial reduction, the humeral component hinges open on the glenoid rather than rotates around a fixed center. Frequently, in these cases, unappreciated posterior osteophytes will cause the surgeon to resect the head with too little retroversion.

Design failures are specific to individual prosthetic designs but are characterized by the increasing complexity built into such prostheses. The more complicated the design, the higher the likelihood of component failure. Specific bonding problems, such as the polyethylene glenoid insert separating from the metal backing, have affected some designs.[19] In some modular designs, separation of the modular humeral head from the humeral component has occurred. Recognition of these types of mechanical failure could influence the choice of prosthetic design.

Complications on the glenoid side also fall into two areas. As mentioned above, failure to recognize asymmetric glenoid wear can cause incorrect alignment of the glenoid. With a keel design or central peg, this is likely to cause perforation of the scapular neck cortex and lead to less-than-optimal fixation. The glenoid may be inserted without congruent subchondral bony support, which will allow toggle or fatigue, resulting in component failure.

The incidence of glenoid component loosening as a cause for revision has ranged from 3.6 to 10.9%.[26] Some differences are due to design variations and others to patient variables (e.g., predominance of osteoporotic rheumatoid arthritic patients), but a better understanding of the constraints on glenoid fixation has come about because of these experiences. It is recommended that minimal bone resection be carried out, and as much subchondral bone as possible should be preserved to support the glenoid component.[6] If an excessive amount of glenoid resection is required to achieve proper version, then bone grafting the glenoid should be considered.[22] Careful cementing technique has been recommended with as dry a field as possible. Cement pressurization has been used by some investigators, but its efficacy in the glenoid is not yet clearly established. In every case, the quality of the glenoid fixation should be rigorously assessed at the time of implantation and if any question remains, then reimplantation should be performed immediately. In addition, an unusually high incidence of glenoid loosening has been identified in that group of patients with large rotator cuff tears who continue to exhibit proximal humeral migration even after repair of the cuff defect.[23] While this condition is quite unusual in primary osteoarthritis, consideration of hemiarthroplasty alone may prove prudent in such cases.

The occurrence of radiolucent lines at the bone-cement interface of the glenoid component has been noticed and discussed by most authors with experience in total shoulder arthroplasty.[14] In the majority of cases, these radiolucencies exist without progression and appear to have no detrimental impact on the clinical course of the patient.[6] In many instances, the radiolucencies can be identified on the immediate postoperative radiographs and are thought to be related to the surgical technique.[8] Radiolucencies that are seen to progress undoubtedly do represent true loosening, and these patients must be observed closely although not all will require revision surgery.

DIFFICULTIES

The following conditions are referred to as difficulties rather than complications since they are often encountered and appreciated preoperatively, but require continued postoperative treatment to successfully overcome them.

Stiffness following total shoulder arthroplasty for osteoarthritis is usually due to inadequate resection of osteophytes, inadequate capsular release, and inadequate rehabilitation.

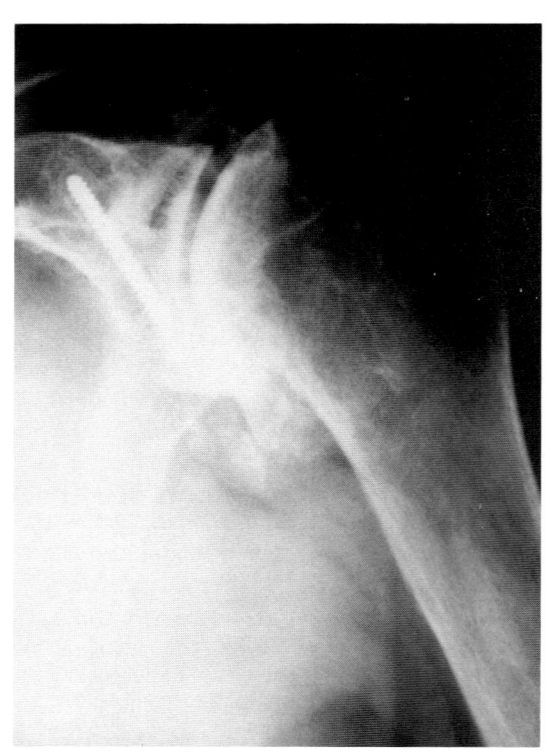

Figure 11–13. Anteroposterior radiograph shows advanced osteoarthritis. The screw was placed to repair a coracoid osteotomy done for exposure at the time of debridement 10 years previously.

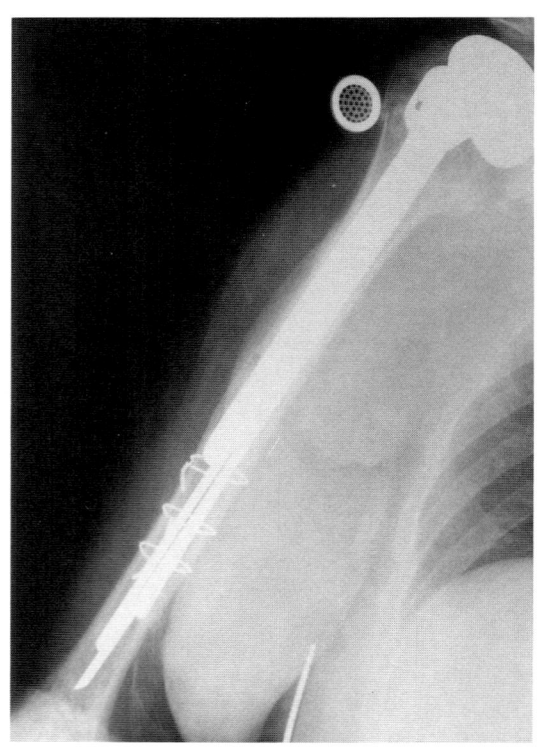

Figure 11–14. Anteroposterior radiograph reveals a fracture of the humeral shaft and successful repair with intramedullary reinforcement.

Heterotopic bone formation rarely occurs following total shoulder arthroplasty for osteoarthritis. Ectopic bone is much more likely to affect the results of shoulder hemiarthroplasty following a fracture. There is one type of patient with osteoarthritis who may prove to be somewhat difficult with respect to mobility (Figure 11–13). This is the patient who has undergone prior glenohumeral débridement with subsequent scarring of the rotator cuff, especially the subscapularis and anterior capsule, presenting a formidable challenge to both the surgeon and the physical therapist.

Fracture of the humeral shaft during surgery is more likely to occur in conditions of rheumatoid and traumatic arthritis, since such patients are more likely to exhibit disuse osteoporosis (Figure 11–14). Even with good-quality bone, rotating the arm for exposure before adequate soft-tissue release and osteophyte resection have been performed can result in a fracture.[28] This problem will challenge the surgeon's abilities in fracture repair. A spiral fracture pattern means the radial nerve must be protected and, if methylmethacrylate is incorporated, shielded from thermal damage should there be leakage (Figure 11–15).

REHABILITATION

Of all the conditions for which shoulder athroplasty is performed, osteoarthritis is one of the most pleasing. The elimination of painful bony incongruence and deformity

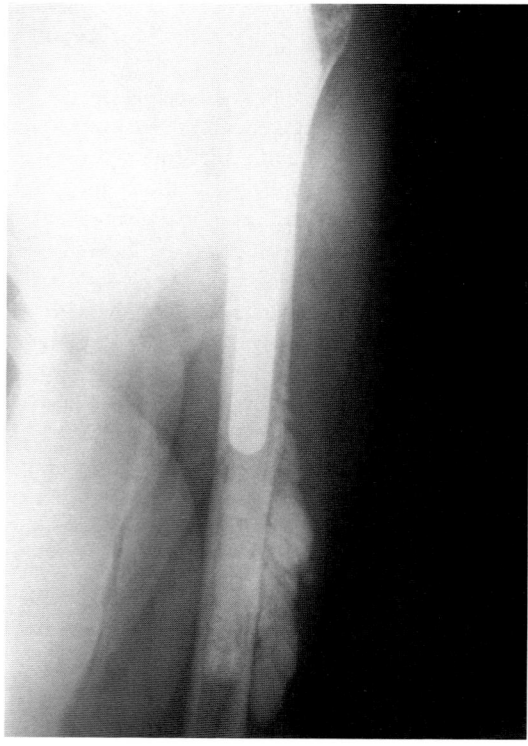

Figure 11–15. Anteroposterior radiograph shows leakage of methylmethacrylate following attempted repair of an intraoperative fracture. Permanent radial nerve palsy resulted.

allows recovery of function by the attendant soft tissues, and therefore rehabilitation is paramount to the success of the surgery. While there is no precise program for rehabilitation following shoulder arthroplasty, osteoarthritis probably comes close. In general, a secure repair of the subscapularis is achievable, thus allowing institution of immediate passive exercises. At times, continuous passive motion machines are used in the recovery room or soon thereafter.[13] While it has not been shown that the use of continuous passive motion has any ability to affect the subsequent functional result, it does allow early mobilization of the soft tissues, can be applied frequently without a physical therapist, and the patient perceives rapid progress. Patients are quickly advanced from pendulum pulley exercises to passive range-of-motion exercises at home, under the supervision of a physical therapist. Active-assisted range-of-motion exercises can often be instituted within 2 weeks, but passive range of motion is still emphasized in the early stages. Maturation of the suture line at 3 to 4 weeks allows initiation of gradual isometric strengthening exercises. At 6 to 12 weeks, fine-tuning is accomplished with stretching into diagonals and adduction. Increased demands according to the patients' life-style are accommodated gradually after 3 months.

RESULTS

Pain relief following nonconstrained total shoulder arthroplasty, regardless of diagnosis, has been excellent in 84 to 98% of patients. It is the functional recovery following total shoulder arthroplasty that sets osteoarthritis apart from all other groups.[6,8,13,14,19] The better functional results with regard to active and passive range of motion and strength improvements in osteoarthritis reflect the good quality of the rotator cuff muscles in these patients. With careful attention to the technical details of surgery, appropriate patient selection, and a well-directed rehabilitation program, the osteoarthritic patient can achieve a nearly normal functional recovery.

REFERENCES

1. Handley CJ. Experimental osteoarthritis in relation to human pathology. In: *Articular Cartilage and Osteoarthritis.* New York: Raven Press, 1991:411–413.
2. Neer CS II. Degenerative lesions of the proximal humeral articular surface. *Clin Orthop* 1961;20:116–125.
3. Kimura JH. Some thoughts on the physical properties of cartilage. In: *Articular Cartilage and Osteoarthritis.* New York: Raven Press, 1991:351–354.
4. Neer CS II. Replacement arthroplasty for glenohumeral osteoarthritis. *J Bone Joint Surg [Am]* 1974;56:1–13.
5. Peterson CJ. Degeneration of the glenohumeral joint. *Acta Orthop Scand* 1983;54:277–283.
6. Neer CS II. Glenohumeral arthroplasty. In: *Shoulder Reconstruction.* Philadelphia: WB Saunders, 1990:143–271.
7. Cofield RH. Symposium: Shoulder joint replacement. *Contemp Orthop* 1982;5:99–127.
8. Neer CS II, et al. Recent experience in total shoulder replacement. *J Bone Joint Surg [Am]* 1982;64:319–336.
9. Friedman RJ, Hawthorne KB, Genez BM. Evaluation of glenoid bone loss with computerized tomography. *J Bone Joint Surg [Am]* 1992;74:1032–1037.
10. Kerr R, et al. Osteoarthritis of glenohumeral joint: A radiologic-pathologic study. *AJR* 1985;144:967–972.
11. Cofield RH. Shoulder arthrodesis and resection arthroplasty. *Instr Course Lect* 1985;34:268–277.
12. Cofield RH. Total shoulder arthroplasty with the Neer prosthesis. *J Bone Joint Surg [Am]* 1984;66:849–906.
13. Craig CV. Total shoulder replacement. *Orthopedics* 1988;11:125–136.
14. Weiss AC, et al. Unconstrained shoulder arthroplasty—A five year average follow-up study. *Clin Orthop* 1990;257:86–90.
15. Brenner BC, et al. Survivorship of unconstrained total shoulder arthroplasty. *J Bone Joint Surg [Am]* 1989;71:1289–1296.
16. Caughlin MJ, et al. The semi constrained total shoulder arthroplasty. *J Bone Joint Surg [Am]* 1979;61:574.
17. Lettin AWF, et al. The Stanmore total shoulder replacement. *J Bone Joint Surg [Am]* 1982;64:47.
18. Post M, et al. Total shoulder replacement with a constrained prosthesis. *J Bone Joint Surg [Am]* 1980;62:327.
19. Cofield RH. The shoulder. Results and Complications. In: Morrey BG, ed. *Joint Replacement Arthroplasty.* New York: Churchill-Livingstone, 1991;pg 437–453.
20. Post M. Constrained TSR. *Instr Course Lect* 1985;34:287.
21. Brostrom LA, et al. The Kessel prosthesis in total shoulder arthroplasty: A five year experience. *Clin Orthop* 1992;277:155.
22. Neer CS, Morrison DS. Glenoid bone grafting in total shoulder arthroplasty. *J Bone Joing Surg [Am]* 1988;70:1154–1162.
23. Barrett WP, et al. Total shoulder arthroplasty. *J Bone Joint Surg [Am]* 1987;69:865.
24. Copeland S. Cementless total shoulder replacement. In: Post M, Morrey, Hawkins, eds. *Surgery of the Shoulder.* St. Louis: Mosby-Year Book, 1990:289.
25. Faludi DD, Weiland AJ. Cementless total shoulder arthroplasty: Preliminary experience with thirteen cases. *Orthopedics* 1983;6:431.
26. Cofield RH. Uncemented total shoulder arthroplasty. *Orthop Trans* 1990;14:254.
27. Cofield RH, Edgerton BC. Total shoulder arthroplasty: Complications and revision surgery. *Instr Course Lect* 1990;39:449.
28. Bonutti PM, Hawkins RJ. Fracture of the humeral shaft associated with total replacement arthroplasty of the shoulder. *J Bone Joint Surg [Am]* 1992;74:617–618.

12 Total Shoulder Arthroplasty in Rheumatoid Arthritis

Richard J. Friedman, M.D., F.R.C.S.(C)

Rheumatoid arthritis of the glenohumeral joint is a common clinical problem and may be present in 50 to 60% of persons with polyarticular disease.[1,2] Patients may complain of pain, swelling, and decreased function, which are often much more serious to the patient than the physician may realize. Pain is at times severe and frequently interferes with sleep. The ability to perform simple activities of daily living such as eating, dressing, and personal hygiene can be greatly impaired, making the patient dependent upon others.

Involvement of the shoulder can lead to a rapid restriction of motion and severe deformity. Anatomically, the shoulder joint comprises four separate articulations that work in concert.[3] Three of these, the glenohumeral, acromioclavicular, and sternoclavicular articulations, can be involved in the early stages of rheumatoid arthritis with synovitis, whereas later on, the glenohumeral and acromioclavicular joints are mainly affected by severe rheumatoid destruction. The scapulothoracic articulation allows for compensatory flexion and abduction, but not rotation.

Despite frequent involvement, the shoulder is often overlooked. Historically, there has been a much greater interest in the treatment of the hip, knee, hand, and foot for which the treatment options are better understood. The shoulder is less conspicuous, and patients may complain less and present later because they are able to compensate with scapulothoracic motion and continue functioning to various degrees. Physicians should seek out shoulder involvement in their patients, as early diagnosis and treatment are the key to obtaining the best results possible. End-stage disease involving the glenohumeral joint may render the soft tissues and bone unsuitable for reconstruction, thereby compromising the physician's ability to provide the best possible care for the patient.

FEATURES OF RHEUMATOID DISEASE

Several important differences exist between rheumatoid arthritis patients and others with arthritis of the glenohumeral joint and must be considered when weighing the treatment options. Some of these are a result of the disease process, while others are secondary to treatment with medications such as corticosteroids.

Skin and Bone

The skin in a rheumatoid arthritis patient is often thin and atrophic. It must be handled very meticulously, and incisions should be carefully planned. Skin breakdown and subsequent wound problems can be devastating. The bone quality is often poor, due to secondary osteopenia from disuse or medications, which compromises the ability for the cortical and cancellous bone to support a prosthesis under the expected loads. A nonconstrained prosthesis, which minimizes the transfer of stresses at the bone-cement or bone-prosthesis interface, is best suited for this situation.

Subchondral Cysts

Another factor contributing to weakened bone is the presence of subchondral cysts, which are much more common in rheumatoid arthritis compared to osteoarthritis. They can be quite large and are often filled only with granulation tissue. It is important that they are recognized, either preoperatively with computerized tomography or intraoperatively, and then curetted and filled with bone graft or methylmethacrylate to strengthen the bone supporting a prosthesis.[4]

Soft-Tissue Contractures

Soft-tissue contractures that limit elevation and rotation develop around the shoulder joint. These contractures must be recognized intraoperatively and released, both to obtain adequate exposure for the surgical procedure and to improve motion postoperatively. One aims to restore a functional range of motion to the shoulder, which includes 125 degrees of elevation and 30 degrees of external rotation.[2,5]

Active Rheumatoid Synovitis

The proliferative synovitis seen in rheumatoid arthritis releases degradative enzymes that result in cartilage destruction and erosive changes of the joint surface.[1] Recurrent episodes of synovitis cause pain, with eventual loss of motion and decreased function. If all the remaining articular surfaces in a joint are removed at the time of a procedure such as a total shoulder arthroplasty, then recurrence of active rheumatoid synovitis can be prevented.[6]

Rotator Cuff

The glenohumeral joint is the most mobile in the body. Stability is provided by the surrounding musculotendinous cuff, as there is very little inherent bony stability between the humeral head and the glenoid. The subacromial space is a common site for rheumatoid involvement, often leading to erosions and eventual rupture of the rotator cuff tendons and rarely the long head of the biceps as they pass under the subacromial arch.[7] Previous studies using arthrography have found rotator cuff tears in 46% of patients.[8] Thinning, or attenuation, and weakening of the rotator cuff occur in many more patients, but are not demonstrated arthrographically.[9] Of patients undergoing total shoulder arthroplasty, 30 to 40% have rotator cuff tears, and many more have attenuation of the cuff muscles.[10,11] This is much higher than the 1 to 5% incidence of rotator cuff tears seen in patients with osteoarthritis.[12]

Rotator cuff tears, however, are not a contraindication to total shoulder arthroplasty and do not necessarily lead to postoperative instability. In a study of patients who had severe rheumatoid arthritis and class IV function, only 25% had a normal rotator cuff.[11] Thirty-seven percent had an attenuated rotator cuff and 38% had minor or major tears of the rotator cuff. All tears were repaired at the time of total shoulder arthroplasty. At a mean follow-up of 4.5 years, there was no significant difference in the ability to elevate the arm between those that had a normal or attenuated cuff and those that had the rotator cuff repaired. Pain, motion, and function were all significantly improved in both groups. There were no episodes of instability.

Medical Condition

The mean age of rheumatoid patients undergoing total joint arthroplasty is less than that of patients with osteoarthritis. While rheumatoid patients may have fewer medical problems related to their cardiovascular and pulmonary systems, other medical concerns exist. In general, they should be screened to ensure an adequate nutritional status,[13] have their medical condition optimized, and be placed on the lowest maintenance dose of drugs that their condition will allow.[14]

Patients with rheumatoid arthritis are often taking a first-line treatment drug such as aspirin or a nonsteroidal anti-inflammatory medication, both of which can interfere with platelet function and increase the bleeding time. Aspirin's effect lasts for the life of the platelet, while the effects of the nonsteroidal anti-inflammatory agents are reversible and last only as long as the drug is present. Those patients with more severe disease are likely to be taking other antirheumatic agents, such as corticosteroids, methotrexate, azathioprine, and cyclophosphamide. These agents all have potential serious and life-threatening side effects, and patients must be followed very carefully while on these medications.

Patients with rheumatoid arthritis are two to three times more likely to develop a postoperative infection compared to those with osteoarthritis.[15] They are immunocompromised from both their disease process and immunosuppressive drugs, making them more susceptible to infection. Also, rheumatoid patients often have recurrent sources of infection that must be dealt with prior to total shoulder arthroplasty. Rheumatoid foot deformities frequently result in repeated episodes of skin breakdown with or without underlying osteomyelitis and may require surgical correction prior to total joint arthroplasty. A careful survey is needed preoperatively to rule out any active or potential sources of infection.

CLINICAL EXAMINATION

Clinically, patients with rheumatoid arthritis of the glenohumeral joint will present with pain and decreased range of motion. The onset is usually insidious, and patients complain of acute exacerbations that leave them with further shoulder stiffness. As this progresses, they may complain of significant functional impairment, including personal hygiene and dressing. The pain may also interfere with their sleep at night. The pain is poorly localized and often radiates widely up into the neck, over the scapula, and down the arm to the elbow.

The physical examination should begin with the patient seated comfortably and both shoulders fully exposed. As part of any shoulder examination, the cervical spine, scapula, elbow, wrist, hand, and sternoclavicular, acromioclavicular, and glenohumeral joints should be thoroughly evaluated. Often rheumatoid patients have many joints involved, and the cervical spine and complete upper extremity must be examined in order to confirm the diagnosis and determine the most appropriate choice and sequence of treatments.

The shoulder region is inspected, noting particularly any muscle atrophy, and then palpated for swelling, synovial thickening, tenderness, and warmth. Motion is measured both in the sitting and in the supine position, according to the American Shoulder and Elbow Surgeons evaluation form.[16] Total elevation rather than abduction and forward elevation is recorded, as this is more practical from a functional point of view. If patients wish to reach above the horizontal, they will turn their body in line with the position of the arm that has the greatest amount of elevation, be that at the side or in front of the body.

Loss of motion, particularly elevation, begins early in the course of the disease. However, the available range of motion is much greater than the functional range of motion, and therefore the initial loss is not likely to cause any great functional disability.[2,5] Gradually, elevation will be restricted to less than 90 degrees, and both internal and external rotation may also become significantly limited. If left untreated, the most severe cases will progress to a complete loss of shoulder elevation.

Biomechanical studies have shown that patients lose glenohumeral motion to a much greater extent than scapulothoracic motion, as the disease process progresses about the glenohumeral joint.[17] As a result, the normal ratio of glenohumeral to scapulothoracic motion is reversed from 2:1 to 1:2. This is associated with significant pain, decreased motion, and therefore decreased function, and likely represents the patient's attempt to immobilize the glenohumeral joint for pain relief, and at the same time maximize shoulder motion through the scapulothoracic joint.

Stability and strength are next evaluated, with particular attention to the deltoid and the rotator cuff muscles. To assess the patients' functional level, and how disabled they are by their disease process, one can ask about simple activities of daily living, such as reaching to the back pocket and opposite axilla, combing the hair, using the hand at arm level and overhead, and eating with utensils.

RADIOGRAPHIC EVALUATION

The routine roentgenographic evaluation of a patient with rheumatoid arthritis should include views in the anteroposterior plane of the glenohumeral joint with the arm in internal and external rotation, and a true axillary view. The scapula and, therefore, the plane of the articular surfaces lie on the posterior chest wall inclined approximately 30 to 40 degrees anterior to the coronal plane of the body when viewed in the transverse plane (see Figure 2–1).[18] In order to obtain the anteroposterior view of the glenohumeral joint, the roentgenographic beam must be angled a corresponding amount. Doing so allows one to evaluate the condition of the articular surfaces with no overlap between the humeral head and glenoid fossa (see Figure 4–1).

In early cases of rheumatoid arthritis, nothing more than osteopenia may be seen on roentgenographic examination.[19] As the disease progresses, erosions of the joint margins occur, particularly around the anatomic neck of the proximal part of the humerus and in the greater tuberosity under the supraspinatus insertion (see Figure 4–7). Erosions of the subchondral bone plate, loss of articular cartilage with symmetric joint space narrowing, and occasionally osteophyte formation indicate significant joint involvement (Figures 12–1 and 12–2). In severe end-stage disease, gross destruction of the contours of the humeral head and glenoid fossa can occur, along with large cyst formation and subchondral sclerosis from secondary osteoarthritis (Figures 12–3 and 12–4). The glenoid itself may be eroded down to the base of the coracoid process, making it impossible to use a glenoid prosthesis for a total shoulder arthroplasty (Figure 12–5).

With rotator cuff involvement, there may be a superior subluxation of the humeral head on the glenoid. Initially, this may just represent attenuation of the rotator cuff muscles, but can signify rupture of the cuff tendons in more advanced disease. Eventually the humeral head can come to articulate with the undersurface of the acromion and the upper one-third of the glenoid, creating a secondary or false eburnated socket.

Posterior erosions of the glenoid and posterior subluxation

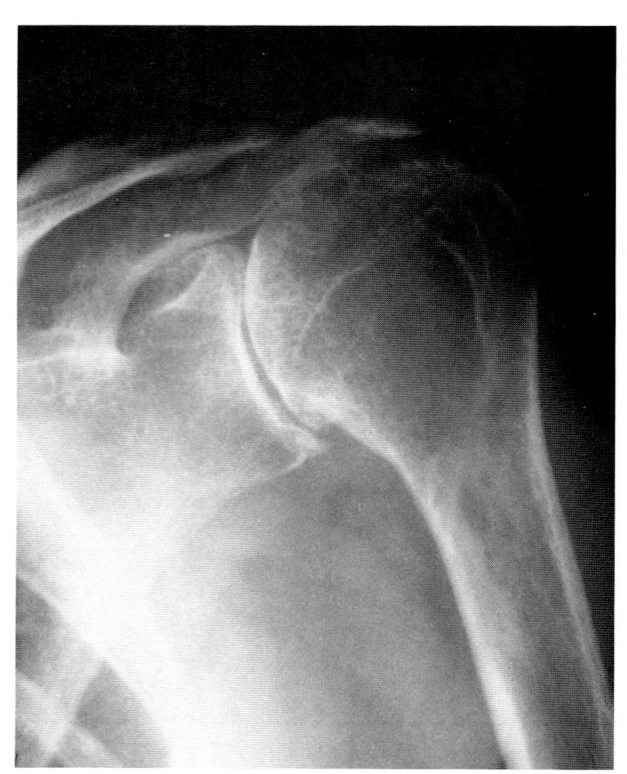

Figure 12–1. Anteroposterior radiograph of the left glenohumeral joint in a 64-year-old woman with rheumatoid arthritis, showing loss of articular cartilage, subchondral sclerosis, and superior subluxation.

of the humeral head can be seen on the axillary view, but are best evaluated with computerized tomography (Figure 12–6). Computerized tomographic scans can demonstrate uneven wear of the glenoid surface, osteophytes, large cysts, and posterior displacement of the humeral head.[4] Glenoid retroversion is increased in rheumatoid arthritis, and computerized tomographic scans can accurately determine the degree and pattern of bone erosion, helping the surgeon decide if glenoid augmentation will be needed during total shoulder arthroplasty.

Preoperative computerized tomographic scanning can play an important role in evaluating rheumatoid arthritis patients for a total shoulder arthroplasty, because it provides an accurate depiction of the bony anatomy and can contribute to operative success by revealing to the surgeon the extent of the patients' disease and the need for modification of the surgical technique. Computerized tomographic scanning provides objective assessment of the proximal part of the humerus and glenoid fossa, something anteroposterior and axial roentgenograms and intraoperative visualization are not able to do accurately. The computerized tomographic scan may be accomplished with great patient comfort, low radiation exposure, and ease in performing because it is relatively free of operator dependence.

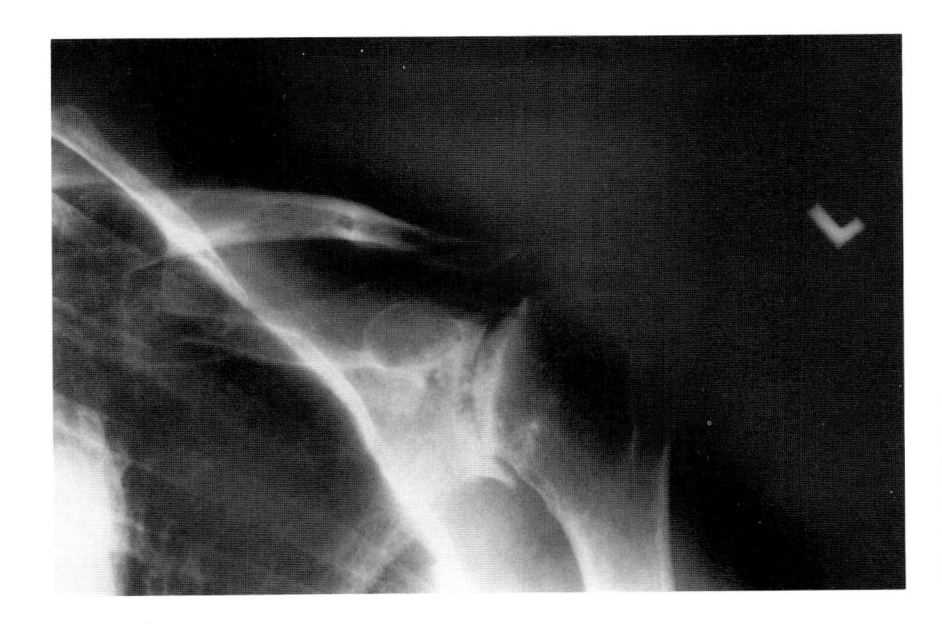

Figure 12–2. Anteroposterior radiograph of the left glenohumeral joint in a 56-year-old woman with rheumatoid arthritis, demonstrating symmetric loss of the joint space, subchondral sclerosis and cyst formation, and an inferior glenoid osteophyte.

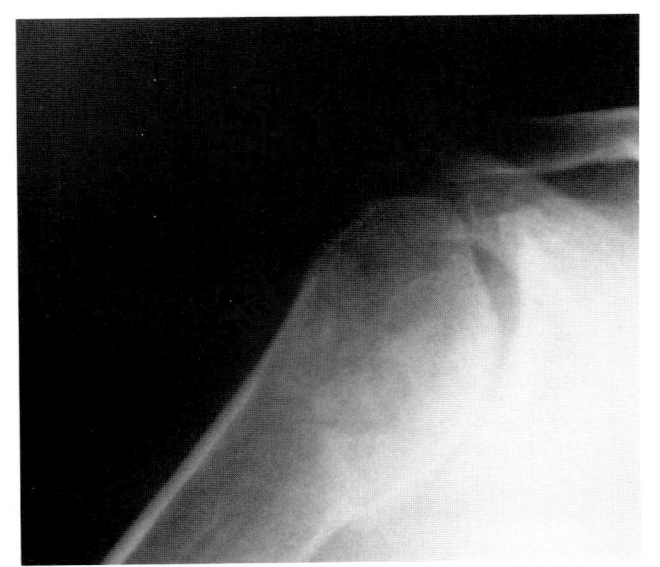

Figure 12–3. Marked deformity of the right humeral head with loss of articular cartilage in a 31-year-old woman with juvenile rheumatoid arthritis.

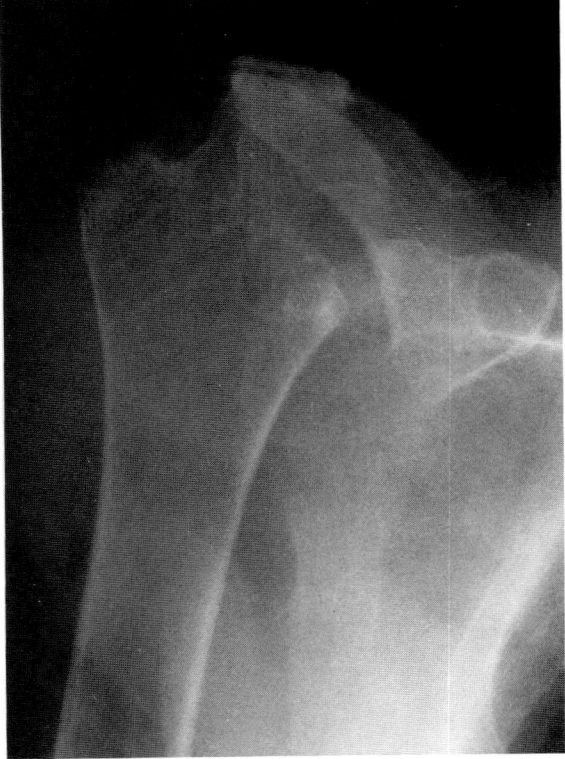

Figure 12–4. Severe erosions of the right humeral head with superior subluxation in a 28-year-old woman with rheumatoid arthritis.

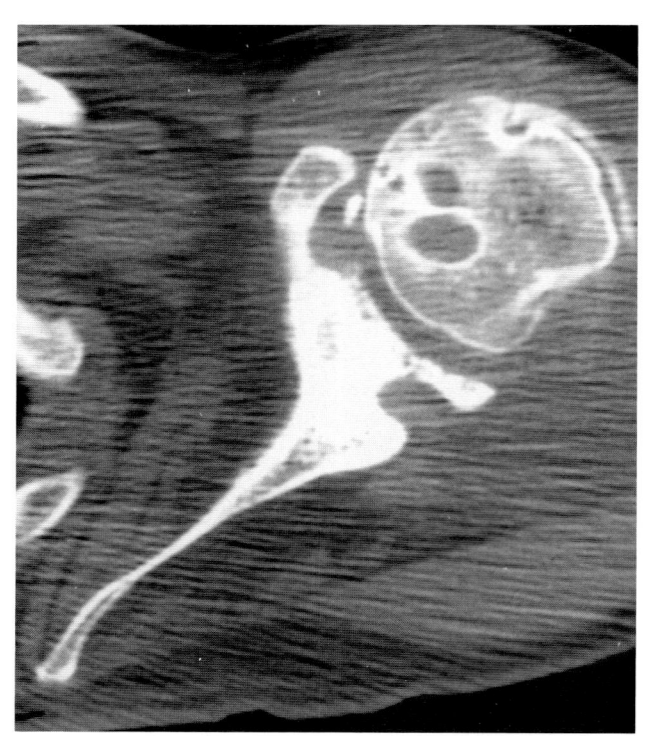

Figure 12–5. Computerized tomographic scan of the left glenohumeral joint in a 72-year-old man with rheumatoid arthritis, showing the glenoid fossa worn down to the base of the coracoid process, with very little scapular neck remaining for the stem of a glenoid prosthesis.

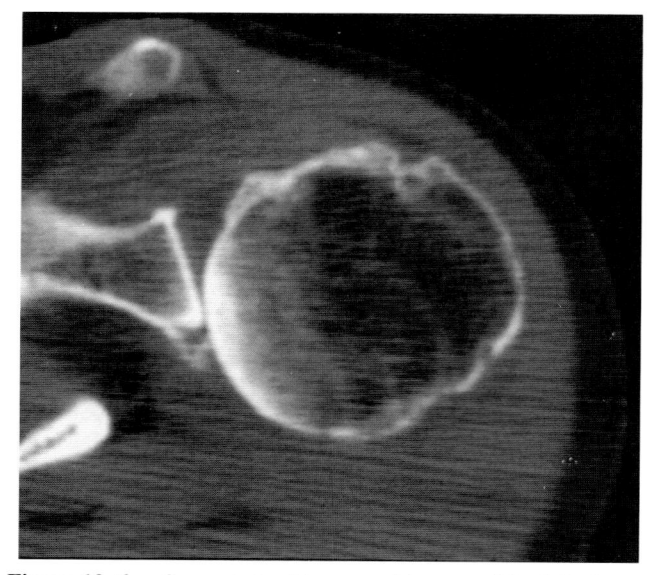

Figure 12–6. Computerized tomographic scan of the left glenohumeral joint in a 69-year-old woman with rheumatoid arthritis, demonstrating posterior subluxation not seen on the axillary radiograph.

CONSERVATIVE TREATMENT

The principles of conservative treatment for rheumatoid involvement of the glenohumeral joint are the same as in other joints afflicted with rheumatoid arthritis. A multidisciplinary team approach is best suited to accomplish the goals of conservative treatment, aiming to control pain and maintain function through the safest methods available. A rheumatologist usually coordinates the patient's care with the physical therapist and the orthopaedic surgeon, as well as other arthritis health care professionals. Medications, including nonsteroidal anti-inflammatory drugs, corticosteroids, and immunosuppressive therapy, are managed by the rheumatologist to control pain and inflammation and to minimize the activity of the rheumatoid process. Subacromial and intra-articular injections of lidocaine (Xylocaine) with or without corticosteroids may be beneficial in the short term, but repetitive use is limited by the potential risks of damage to the articular cartilage and rotator cuff tendons.[7]

Physical therapy is necessary to maintain motion through the glenohumeral and scapulothoracic joints and strengthen the shoulder muscles. Patients with a painful shoulder tend to hold the arm at their side, in a protective position, with the arm clasped to the chest wall in internal rotation. This guards against painful movements, but also leads to stiffening of the joints and loss of motion, especially elevation and external rotation. If they then try to move the arm, they will experience pain at the extremes of motion, secondary to the stiffness that has occurred. As a result, they become less likely to move the extremity, leading to more stiffness and more pain. This cycle is very difficult to interrupt and can lead to a frozen shoulder, as well as contractures at the elbow, wrist, and hand. Also, with decreased joint motion or immobilization, the articular cartilage does not get properly bathed and nourished by the synovial fluid, resulting in another deleterious effect on the joint surfaces.

Ideally, physical therapy should begin early, prior to the onset of shoulder stiffness. Initially, passive, active-assistive, and active range-of-motion exercises are directed at maintaining or regaining elevation and external rotation, aiming for 140 degrees of the former and 40 degrees of the latter.[20] Once this has been reached, then stretching exercises are added. To help restore strength, isometric exercises can be used initially while the shoulder is still irritated and painful. All exercises should be performed three or four times a day. The patient may wish to use heat and analgesics as adjunctive treatment either before or after the exercises. Abduction bracing may prove helpful to maintain the arm away from the body between exercises and prevent loss of motion during an acute flare-up of synovitis. Assistive exercises can also be done with the brace on initially.

Surgical intervention has a small but important role in the management of the rheumatoid shoulder. Early consultation and evaluation by the orthopaedic surgeon can help determine the most appropriate timing for surgical intervention, in an attempt to limit irreversible joint damage and deformities when the above therapeutic measures are no longer effective. In the early stages of the disease process, surgery is aimed at prolonging the life of the joint surfaces and limiting damage to the soft tissues. With advanced disease, the aims are to decrease pain and restore function through reconstruction of the joint, which has been severely damaged by the disease process.

INDICATIONS AND TIMING FOR SURGICAL INTERVENTION

The timing of surgical intervention in the patient with rheumatoid arthritis of the shoulder is of the utmost importance to the success of any procedure, whether being done early or late in the course of the disease. One must determine not only the absolute time to intervene, but also the most appropriate order when multiple procedures are required. Many factors will influence these decisions, such as the activity and progress of the disease, the age of the patient, and the functional and social demands of the patient.[21]

In general, for rheumatoid patients, shoulder arthroplasty is indicated when there is structural damage, sufficient pain, and disability not controlled by conservative measures to warrant the risks of surgery. One tends to intervene earlier in the upper extremity compared to the lower extremity, because of the importance of the surrounding soft-tissue structures and their role in restoring function. Shoulder arthroplasty should not be delayed past the point where the rotator cuff tendons have become severely involved or ruptured, or that the bone has been destroyed by rheumatoid granulations so that insufficient bone stock remains to seat the prosthetic components, making a successful arthroplasty difficult.

An absolute contraindication to total shoulder arthroplasty is active infection, either locally or remotely. Relative contraindications include poor bone stock, neurologic deficit involving the deltoid or rotator cuff muscles, and an inability by the patient to follow the postoperative rehabilitation program.

At any age, the goals of surgery are to relieve pain and restore function so that simple activities of daily living such as personal hygiene, perineal and rectal care, personal grooming, eating, and sleeping can be carried out independently. While pain relief is the main indication for surgical intervention, increasing motion and improving function are secondary indications that depend on the condition of the soft-tissue structures. The amount of pain relief is reliable and consistent. However, the increase in motion and therefore the improvement in function are variable, and depend on the surgeon's ability to restore or reconstruct the surrounding musculotendinous cuff, and on the patient's ability to cooperate with the postoperative rehabilitation protocol.

The surgeon must be very wary to operate on patients with a painless, ankylosed shoulder, since the conditions of the soft tissues may be such that the desired improvements in function may not be possible, and therefore the patients will be disappointed. However, if they are not able to carry out simple activities of daily living, then they may wish to undergo surgical reconstruction, if fully informed of the potential outcomes, to make themselves more independent.

Shoulder arthroplasty in younger rheumatoid patients carries the risk of later loosening and the inevitable need for multiple revision surgeries during their lifetime. It is imperative that patients be fully informed of all the risks, benefits, and alternatives so that they can make a well-informed decision. Most patients will chose a definitive procedure such as an arthroplasty that will allow them to enjoy some of their recreational activities, and permit them to maintain employment and be financially and socially independent. At the other extreme, shoulder arthroplasty can be performed in patients well into their ninth and tenth decades if indicated. A successful arthroplasty can allow them to remain independent at home instead of being placed into a nursing home.

Regarding the relative timing of multiple procedures, there are some basic guidelines that can be followed, but these must be individualized to each patient. It is important that the physician gain the confidence of patients early on, so that they are amenable to further procedures. When both the upper and lower limbs are involved, the one causing the greatest amount of pain and/or functional limitation should be considered first. It must be kept in mind that crutches, walkers, and canes will be required for some period of time following hip and knee arthroplasty, and the upper extremities must be able to withstand the expected loads. Otherwise, surgery on the upper extremity should be considered first, followed 3 months later by the lower extremity reconstructive surgery.

In the early years of rheumatoid surgery, attention was focused on the hand and wrist. With the success of shoulder and elbow arthroplasties over the last 15 years, the surgical options have greatly expanded. It would serve little purpose to reconstruct the rheumatoid hand and wrist only, if the elbow or shoulder were so severely involved that the hand could not be raised to the mouth for feeding.

In general, any program of reconstructive surgery should consider beginning with the larger proximal joints.[21] When both the shoulder and the elbow are involved, the joint that causes the most pain and disability should be operated on first. If both joints appear to be equally involved, it has been recommended that the elbow be operated on first, as this seems to result in greater functional improvement and allows a longer interval between arthroplasties when compared to doing them in the reverse order.[22] Improvements in pain, motion and function are not compromised when the two arthroplasties are performed in the same extremity.

ALTERNATIVE PROCEDURES TO SHOULDER ARTHROPLASTY

The most frequent procedure done today for rheumatoid arthritis of the glenohumeral joint is a total shoulder arthroplasty, followed by a shoulder hemiarthroplasty.[9] Alternative procedures to a shoulder arthroplasty include synovectomy, glenohumeral arthrodesis, osteotomy, and resection arthroplasty. While these are discussed elsewhere in great detail, certain points can be made with an emphasis on patients with rheumatoid arthritis.

Synovectomy

Synovectomy and debridement of the glenohumeral joint, combined with a bursectomy of the subacromial space when needed, has been much more popular in Europe than North America. This requires early intervention before any significant destruction of the articular surfaces has occurred, and both rheumatologists and surgeons have been somewhat reluctant to consider these patients for surgery in the very early stages of their disease process. The early cases that would benefit from synovectomy are followed by the rheumatologists, and unless they are referred for early surgical consultation, the orthopaedic surgeon seldom sees them. As a result, a potentially valuable surgical treatment may be underutilized.

The goals of shoulder synovectomy are relief of pain and prevention of disease progression. Clinically, a diagnosis of early synovitis of the glenohumeral joint should be made, but this can be difficult, as pain is not a reliable indicator specific to the glenohumeral joint. Waiting for the onset of visible swelling with bursitis may allow the disease to progress too far. A functional range of motion should be maintained. Patients should have minimal changes on their roentgenograms with good preservation of the articular surfaces, as described by Larsen stage I or II.[23]

Shoulder synovectomy is performed through an anterior deltopectoral approach, which provides good access to the glenoid and anatomic neck of the proximal part of the humerus.[24] A subacromial bursectomy, debridement and/or resection of the acromioclavicular joint, debridement of osteophytes, and repair of any rotator cuff tears can be accomplished at the same time.

The results in 54 patients followed for a mean of 5.3 years (range, 1 to 16 years) showed that only 10 still had some pain after synovectomy, and 6 of them eventually went on to total shoulder arthroplasty.[25] The remaining patients were doing well, with improved function and minimal radiographic progression, even after 10 years. It was felt that the best results were obtained in patients with early disease.

More recently, arthroscopic synovectomy has been proposed.[26] Despite using power instruments, the procedure is technically difficult. Significant bleeding occurs, and a double irrigation system is needed. The short-term results were good, with 9 of 11 patients having significant improvements in pain and motion. However, longer follow-up is required to determine the value of this less invasive procedure.

Glenohumeral Arthrodesis

Glenohumeral arthrodesis has been advocated for the treatment of severe end-stage rheumatoid arthritis of the glenohumeral joint, but this was prior to the recent successful results of total shoulder arthroplasty.[27,28] Even then, however, there was a reluctance to perform this procedure on rheumatoid patients for many reasons, despite the success in relieving pain and restoring pain-free shoulder girdle function.[2]

Until recently, most techniques of shoulder arthrodesis required some form of external immobilization and support for approximately 3 months. This prolonged period of immobilization can have deleterious effects on the function of the ipsilateral elbow, wrist, and hand. Arthrodesis eliminates internal and external rotation, which is needed for activities of daily living such as perineal hygiene, and was felt not to be warranted in rheumatoid patients who may have contralateral shoulder disease. Concerns have existed about the difficulties with hardware fixation in the osteopenic rheumatoid bone, but arthrodesis appears to be a reliable procedure with a high rate of fusion.[28,29]

The exact role of glenohumeral arthrodesis for the primary treatment of rheumatoid arthritis remains controversial, with most surgeons cautiously recommending its use in the patient for whom conservative therapy has failed and in whom prosthetic replacement is contraindicated.[30] Glenohumeral arthrodesis has a valuable role, though, in the salvage of the failed shoulder arthroplasty.[31] While the procedure is more difficult and fusion harder to achieve, it can provide the patient with a pain-free, stable shoulder.

Osteotomy

Double osteotomy of the shoulder joint, through the neck of the glenoid and the surgical neck of the proximal part of the humerus, is a relatively straightforward procedure performed through a deltopectoral approach.[32,33] Similar concerns exist for this procedure as with arthrodesis. Osteopenic bone may lead to fixation problems. Any period of prolonged immobilization may have a deleterious effect on the ipsilateral joints.

With this procedure, bone stock is preserved and does not preclude another operation such as a shoulder arthroplasty in the future. Motion is not significantly improved, but pain is relieved in about 80% of patients.[33] Overall function is improved due to the pain relief. However, total shoulder arthroplasty offers more consistent and reliable results in terms of pain relief, increased motion, and improved function, and is performed much more frequently than an osteotomy.[10] The double osteotomy may be indicated in a patient who has incapacitating pain from the glenohumeral joint but in whom joint destruction has not progressed far enough to justify an arthroplasty.

Resection Arthroplasty

Historically, a resection arthroplasty of the glenohumeral joint has produced inconsistent relief of pain, relieving pain being the main indication for performing the procedure.[9,34] The patient is left with a flail shoulder, and resection arthroplasty is generally regarded as a salvage procedure following a failed shoulder arthroplasty.

Glenoidectomy has been advocated in the past as a surgical alternative.[35,36] Given the success of total shoulder arthroplasty, there remains little indication for this procedure. Being irreversible, it precludes a future shoulder arthroplasty and the superior functional results that are obtainable with a total shoulder arthroplasty.

Recently, a resection-interposition arthroplasty using dura mater has been reported.[37] As with similar procedures in the elbow, prosthetic joint replacement offers more consistent and reliable long-term results. Resection-interposition arthroplasty may be indicated in certain patients not ready for a prosthetic replacement, and does not preclude one in the future.

SURGICAL TECHNIQUE

Total shoulder arthroplasty, particularly in patients with rheumatoid arthritis, is a demanding procedure and requires a surgeon skilled and experienced in shoulder surgery to obtain optimal results. Meticulous handling and repair of the soft tissues, in addition to precise, accurate techniques for implanting the prosthetic components, is necessary to ensure a satisfactory outcome. The details of the surgical procedure are outlined elsewhere. However, certain points are emphasized here with regards to the rheumatoid arthritis patient.

Preoperatively, patients are instructed in physical therapy so they are aware of what will be expected of them following surgery. One week prior to surgery, patients stop taking their nonsteroidal anti-inflammatory medications to allow the bleeding time to return to normal. Those who are unable to do so because of a flare-up of their symptoms can be given nonacetylated salicylates, which do not prolong the bleeding time. Surgical scrubs with an antiseptic cleanser should be performed the day prior to surgery. Antibiotic prophylaxis with 1 gm of cefazolin is started immediately prior to the procedure and continued for 24 hours postoperatively. Vancomycin, 500 mg, is given in patients with an allergy to cephalosporins.

The patient is placed in a beach-chair position on the operating room table, utilizing a special extension or headrest that is cut out for the shoulder region, yet supports the spine and contralateral shoulder. Regional anesthesia with an interscalene block is the author's preferred technique in these patients, since many of them have significant cervical spine disease that makes endotracheal intubation difficult and risky. The patient's blood is typed and cross-matched, but intraoperative and postoperative transfusions are uncommon, and the intraoperative blood loss is usually not sufficient to justify the use of a cell-saver unit.

A standard deltopectoral incision is used, taking care to preserve the cephalic vein with either the deltoid or pectoralis major muscle.[10] It is unnecessary to detach the origin of the deltoid for exposure. The clavipectoral fascia is divided, and the subscapularis is exposed. The axillary nerve can be palpated running along the inferior border of the subscapularis muscle, and externally rotating the arm will move the nerve more medially away from the arthrotomy site. The subscapularis tendon, tagged with stay sutures, and the capsule are divided as a single layer approximately 1 cm medial to the lesser tuberosity.

The capsule often must be released or excised anteriorly, inferiorly, and posteriorly along with release of scar tissue and lysis of adhesions, to obtain adequate exposure and increase the range of motion in abduction and external rotation. The humeral head is delivered into the wound with adduction, extension, and external rotation of the arm. Synovium and bursa are debrided as necessary to expose the humeral head. The bone is usually osteopenic, and the humeral head is detached with an osteotome in 30 to 40 degrees of retroversion at the level of the anatomic neck. Care must be taken to stay medial to the greater tuberosity, and remove a minimal amount of bone.

With the humeral head removed, the rotator cuff muscles and the subacromial space can be inspected. The coracoacromial ligament is divided if exposure is needed, or excised if there is evidence of rotator cuff pathology. Should an acromioclavicular arthroplasty or anterior acromioplasty be indicated, it may be performed at this point, and no further exposure is required. The rotator cuff is inspected and if found to be torn, it is mobilized and closed so that the rotator cuff tendons can be reattached through drill holes into the greater tuberosity. The tendons often require release not only superficially, but also from around the base of the coracoid and the joint capsule. The soft-tissue repair can be difficult but is of paramount importance to the functional outcome of the arthroplasty.

Exposure of the glenoid cavity requires the proximal end of the humerus to be displaced posteriorly. This is facilitated by releasing any posterior capsular scarring and contractures. Great care must be taken not to fracture or crush the proximal end of the humerus during retraction. The glenoid cavity must be debrided of all soft tissue, including rheumatoid granulations on what remains of the articular surface, and the margins of the glenoid clearly defined.

Large bone cysts detected on computerized tomographic scanning are important to identify, as these often need to be curetted and filled with either bone graft or methylmethacrylate to support the glenoid component and prevent early failure. Large osteophytes clearly delineated on the computerized tomographic scan must be resected intraoperatively to allow accurate placement of the glenoid prosthesis keel or fixation pegs into the scapular neck, and have the component well supported by medullary bone instead of resting on thin unsupported osteophytes.

Meticulous care must be taken to prepare and dry the glenoid surface prior to injection of methylmethacrylate and implantation of the component. Problems with glenoid component fixation may occur when there is anterior, posterior, or superior erosion. Bone graft, augmented components, or the use of excess bone cement may be necessary to stabilize the glenoid component.[4,10,38] Bone erosions can progress down to the base of the coracoid process, leaving insufficient bone in the glenoid neck in which to seat a prosthesis. In rheumatoid patients with severe destruction of the glenoid cavity where grafting or augmenting will not provide a stable fulcrum for the component, a hemiarthroplasty with a large-head humeral component is preferred.

The size of the humeral component's head and neck can be adjusted to obtain appropriate tensioning of the deltoid and rotator cuff muscles. The humeral component may be implanted with a press-fit, if the bone stock is adequate and satisfactory rotational stability is obtained. Often this is not the case; methylmethacrylate, with a distal cement restrictor, cement gun, and pressurizer, is used to anchor the humeral prosthesis.

The subscapularis tendon is repaired following implantation of the components. All scarring and adhesions are released, and the underlying capsule excised to mobilize the tendon and obtain maximum external rotation. If external rotation was limited preoperatively to less than 30 degrees, then lengthening the tendon should be considered. One method is to perform a coronal Z-plasty during exposure of the glenohumeral joint. An alternative method is to remove the subscapularis tendon from its insertion on the lesser tuberosity during the exposure, and reattach it more medially through drill holes in bone, thereby effectively lengthening it.

The postoperative exercise protocol must be individualized to each patient, and will largely be determined by the status of the rotator cuff muscles. Patients with an intact rotator cuff, or those in whom a secure repair was obtained, are treated in a similar manner.[11] In general, to restore motion and prevent postoperative scarring and adhesive capsulitis, passive exercises are begun the day of surgery, and the patient is progressed to active-assisted range-of-motion exercises as tolerated.[9,10] Active range-of-motion and gentle isometric muscle-strengthening exercises are started at approximately 2 weeks, but are delayed for 6 weeks if the rotator cuff had a tenuous repair. Resistive and stretching exercises are the last to be added to the protocol.[20]

Rehabilitation of the soft tissues through an exercise regimen is of paramount importance to the long-term results of a total shoulder arthroplasty, especially in rheumatoid patients. They must be taught that the exercise program should become a way of life, and that it can take 6 months or longer to obtain maximum function.

RESULTS

Total shoulder arthroplasty has become the procedure of choice for the treatment of rheumatoid arthritis when disease has destroyed the articular surfaces and the patient has disabling pain. It is a well-established procedure, accepted as reconstructive rather than salvage surgery with reproducible results. However, when evaluating these results, care must be taken to separate those with rheumatoid arthritis from patients in other diagnostic categories. Very few studies report exclusively on rheumatoid patients, or with the results separated from other diagnoses.[11,16,22,39–51]

The most common type of prosthesis used today for a patient with rheumatoid arthritis is a nonconstrained one. The success of this type of prosthesis, which attempts to recreate normal anatomy and relies on the surrounding musculotendinous cuff for stability, depends on disease severity and condition of the deltoid and rotator cuff muscles, both of which can be severely involved in rheumatoid arthritis. The nonconstrained prosthesis introduced by Neer

Table 12–1. Results of Total Shoulder Arthoplasty in Rheumatoid Arthritis

AUTHOR(S)	FOLLOW-UP (y)	NO. OF SHOULDERS	PAIN RELIEF (% of shoulders)	MEAN ELEVATION (degrees)	MEAN EXTERNAL ROTATION (degrees)	CUFF TEAR (# of shoulders)	CUFF ATTENUATION (# of shoulders)
Bade et al.[52] (1984)	4.5	13		93			
Barrett et al.[45] (1989)	5	140	93	90	40	45	50
Barrett et al.[16] (1987)	3.5	11	100	100			
Brenner et al.[51] (1989)	6	25	88	93	44	2	6
Cofield[48] (1984)	3.8	29	92	103	35	7	17
Frich et al.[50] (1988)	2.3	35	94	78	20		
Friedman and Ewald[22] (1987)	5	35	94	87	37		
Friedman et al.[11] (1989)	4.5	24	92	81	51	9	9
Hawkins et al.[49] (1989)	3.3	34	91	100	35		
Kelly et al.[41] (1987)	3	40	88	75	40	8	26
McCoy et al.[47] (1989)	3.1	29	93	76		7	4
Petersson[44] (1986)	2	7	100	89	21	2	0
Vahvanen et al.[46] (1989)	1.7	41	98	105	43	13	28

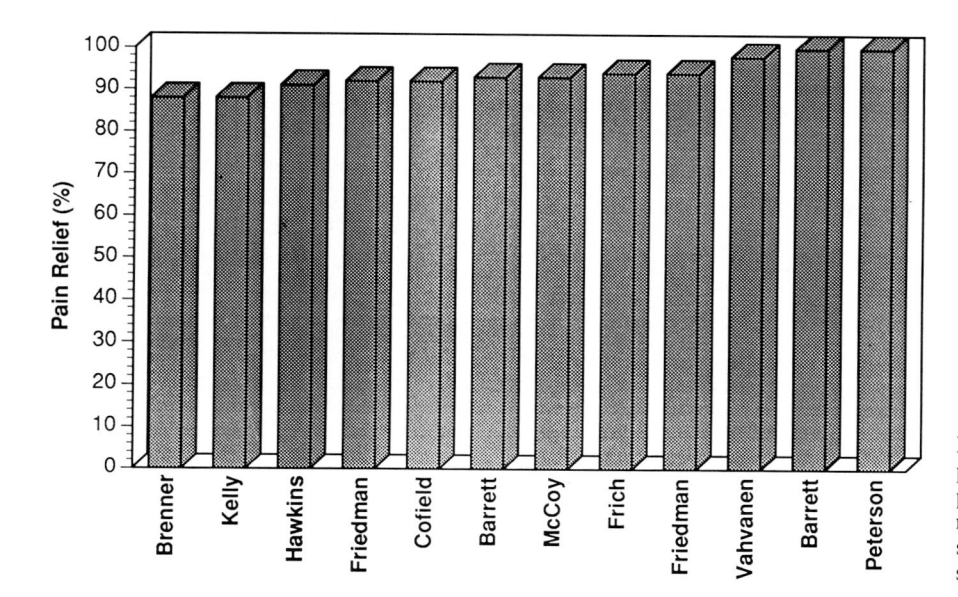

Figure 12–7. Graph showing the percentage of rheumatoid arthritis patients with good or excellent pain relief following nonconstrained total shoulder arthroplasty, based on the series presented in Table 12–1.

in 1973 has been widely used and reported on for patients with rheumatoid arthritis.[10]

Achieving relief of pain, the main indication for total shoulder arthroplasty, has been highly successful in patients with rheumatoid arthritis. In a review of published series using the Neer prosthesis, 94% of patients had satisfactory pain relief, ranging from 88 to 100% (Table 12–1, Figure 12–7).[11,16,22,41,44–52] The mean follow-up time was 4 years, and 463 patients were included. This improvement occurred independent of the changes in motion or function.

The improvements in motion are much less dramatic and not as consistent as those with pain relief. This relates directly to the condition of the surrounding soft-tissue structures and the delay before shoulder arthroplasty.[45] The mean active elevation, either abduction or forward flexion, following total shoulder arthroplasty was only 90 degrees (Table 12–1, Figure 12–8).[11,16,22,41,44–52] External rotation, however, averaged 37 degrees in this group of patients, enough to carry out most activities of daily living.

Eight of the series detailed the status of the rotator cuff muscles.[11,41,44–48,51] The rotator cuff was reported as normal in only 30% (102/335) of the patients. Forty-two percent (140/335) had attenuation, or thinning, of the cuff muscles. Twenty-eight percent (93/335) had a rotator cuff tear, varying in size from less than 1 cm to massive, complete tears that could not be repaired. When the rotator cuff can be repaired, the relief of pain and improvements in motion and function are comparable to those obtained in patients with a normal or attenuated rotator cuff.[11,44]

Rheumatoid arthritis patients with class IV function have severe restrictions of motion and function preoperatively, and this has a direct effect on the outcome of surgery.[11,44]

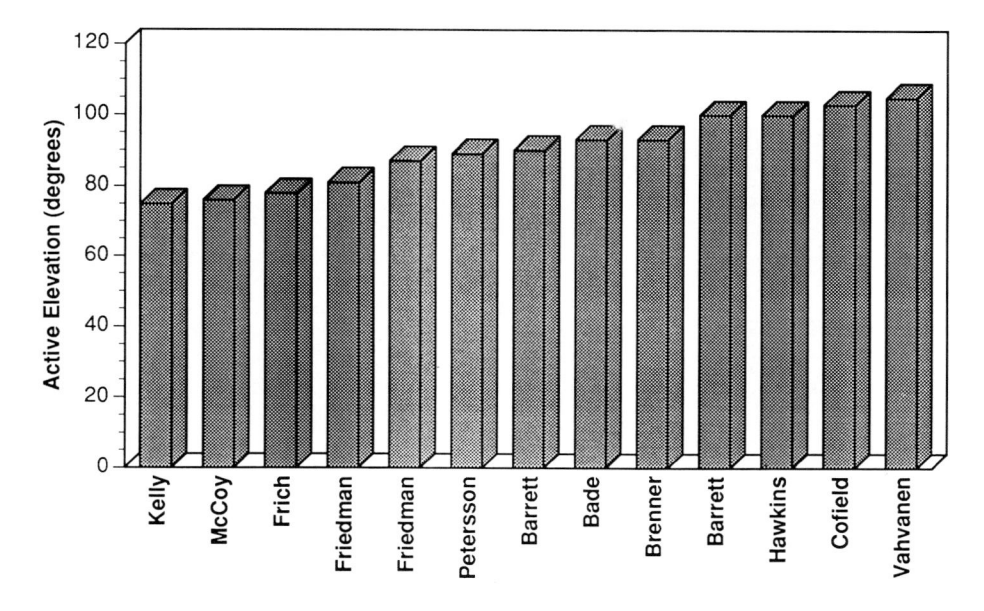

Figure 12–8. Graph demonstrating the mean active elevation in rheumatoid arthritis patients following nonconstrained total shoulder arthroplasty, based on the series presented in Table 12–1.

While pain relief is comparable, the improvements in motion and function are less than those reported for patients who have less severe rheumatoid disease.[10,16,40,45,48] However, these patients do not appear to have a higher incidence of rotator cuff tears, and the pathologic changes in the cuff muscles do not correlate with the severity of the rheumatoid disease.

With relief of pain and improvements in motion, particularly rotation, patients show major functional gains after total shoulder arthroplasty.[53] Even with limited motion compared to normals or osteoarthritics following total shoulder arthroplasty, function is improved to the point where patients can perform a wider variety of the activities of daily living than they did preoperatively.[2,10,39,45,54] The improvements in function, pain relief, and motion with other nonconstrained prosthetic designs parallel the results of the Neer arthroplasty system.[42,55-57]

The roentgenographic results of total shoulder arthroplasty done for rheumatoid arthritis do not differ significantly from those reported for other conditions. The glenoid component is secured almost exclusively with methylmethacrylate in rheumatoid patients. Radiolucent lines around the glenoid component at the bone-cement interface are quite common, with the incidence ranging from 30[10] to 80%.[41] Most of these are present on the initial postoperative roentgenogram, are less than 1 mm in thickness, and are not progressive. Some will develop later and progress in width and extent. Eventually, a shift in the position of the glenoid component may be noted between successive roentgenograms, indicating loosening of the component.

Currently, the incidence of glenoid loosening requiring revision surgery is extremely low.[9] Neer reported on his personal series of 143 rheumatoid shoulders treated with a Neer II total shoulder arthroplasty, with an average 5-year follow-up. The incidence of radiolucent lines remained at 33%, and no shoulders have undergone revision for loosening. A comprehensive review of the literature found only 10 glenoid components revised for loosening in over 1000 arthroplasties performed.[9]

If appropriate, the humeral component can be inserted using a press-fit technique or methylmethacrylate. The reported use of methylmethacrylate varies greatly in the literature, ranging from 25[45] to 90%.[46] The reported 12% incidence of radiolucent lines and 5% subsidence rate about the humeral component is much less than that around the glenoid component.[45] Revision surgery for a loose humeral component is rare.

Based on the results of total hip and knee arthroplasty, the presence of radiolucent lines does not mean that clinical failure of the components is imminent. The same appears to be true for total shoulder arthroplasty. While the roentgenographic findings are of concern, clinically the success rate is high and the revision rate for loosening is low. Longer follow-up is needed to determine the incidence of later component loosening.

SUMMARY

Function is dependent on the preservation or reconstruction of the rotator cuff. It is clear that in neglected rheumatoid shoulders with long-standing disease resulting in severe bone loss and/or rotator cuff tears, the outcome will be compromised. End-stage disease in the rheumatoid shoulder may leave the bone and soft tissues unsuitable for reconstruction. Polyarticular involvement with weak musculature and extensive soft-tissue contractures may compromise the end result.

While patients will have excellent relief from their pain and gain sufficient function to live independently, they will not have near-normal motion or function of the shoulder. Total shoulder arthroplasty in the rheumatoid patient cannot be deferred as safely as arthroplasty of the hip or knee, since these joints do not rely on a musculotendinous cuff for stability, and bone loss does not preclude implantation of components.

A nonconstrained total shoulder arthroplasty provides pain relief and restoration of function necessary for the activities of daily living in patients with rheumatoid arthritis of the shoulder. It can prove to be an extremely difficult challenge for even the most experienced of shoulder surgeons. Strict attention to technical details during the surgery and postoperative rehabilitation is necessary to achieve the optimum result for the patient.

REFERENCES

1. Riordan J, Dieppe P. Arthritis of the glenohumeral joint. *Baillieres Clin Rheumatol* 1989;3:607–625.
2. Souter WA. The surgical treatment of the rheumatoid shoulder. *Ann Acad Med Singapore* 1983;12:243–255.
3. Sarrafian SK. Gross and functional anatomy of the shoulder. *Clin Orthop* 1983;173:11–19.
4. Friedman RJ, Hawthorne KB, Genez BM. Evaluation of glenoid bone loss with computerized tomography. *J Bone Joint Surg [Am]* 1992;74:1032–1037.
5. Reeves B. Total shoulder replacement. In: Dowson D, Wright V, eds. *Introduction to the Biomechanics of Joints and Joint Replacement*. London, Mechanical Engineering Publications, 1981.
6. Boyd AJ, Thomas WH, Scott RD, Sledge CB, Thornhill TS. Total shoulder arthroplasty versus hemiarthroplasty. *J Arthroplasty* 1990;5:329–336.
7. Copeland S. Surgery of the rheumatoid shoulder. *Baillieres Clin Rheumatol* 1989;3:681–691.
8. Ennevaara K. Painful shoulder joint in rheumatoid arthritis. *Acta Rheumatol Scand* 1967;11:1–116.
9. Neer CS. The shoulder. In: Kelly WN, Harris ED, Ruddy S, Sledge CB, eds. *Textbook of Rheumatology*. 3rd ed. Philadelphia: WB Saunders, 1989:2013–2026.
10. Neer CSII, Watson KC, Stanton FJ. Recent experience in total shoulder replacement. *J Bone Joint Surg [Am]* 1982;64:319–337.
11. Friedman RJ, Thornhill TS, Thomas WH, Sledge CB. Nonconstrained total shoulder replacement in patients who have rheumatoid arthritis and class-IV function. *J Bone Joint Surg [Am]* 1989;71:494–498.

12. Neer CS. Replacement arthroplasty for glenohumeral osteoarthritis. *J Bone Joint Surg [Am]* 1974;56:1–13.
13. Jensen J, Jensen T, Smith T, Johnston D, Dudrick S. Nutrition in orthopaedic surgery. *J Bone Joint Surg [Am]* 1982;64:1263–1272.
14. Corman L, Bolt R, eds. *Medical Evaluation of the Preoperative Patient*. Philadelphia: WB Saunders, 1979:1129–1357.
15. Poss R, Thornhill TS, Ewald RC, Thomas WH, Batte NJ, Sledge C. Factors influencing the incidence and outcome of infection following total joint arthroplasty. *Clin Orthop* 1984;182:117–126.
16. Barrett WP, Franklin JL, Jackins SE, Wyss CR, Matsen F III. Total shoulder arthroplasty. *J Bone Joint Surg [Am]* 1987;69:865–872.
17. Friedman R. Total shoulder biomechanics before and after total joint arthroplasty. In: *Proceedings of the 17th SICOT Meeting*. 1990;25:350.
18. Saha A. Dynamic stability of the glenohumeral joint. *Acta Orthop Scand* 1971;42:491–505.
19. Crossan J, Vallance R. Clinical and radiological features of the shoulder joint in rheumatoid arthritis. *J Bone Joint Surg [Br]* 1980;62:116.
20. Hughes M, Neer C II. Glenohumeral joint replacement and postoperative rehabilitation. *Phys Ther* 1975;55:850–858.
21. Souter WA. Present attitudes on timing of surgical interventions in the treatment of rheumatoid disease. *Ann Chir Gynaecol Suppl* 1985;198:19–25.
22. Friedman RJ, Ewald FC. Arthroplasty of the ipsilateral shoulder and elbow in patients who have rheumatoid arthritis. *J Bone Joint Surg [Am]* 1987;69:661–666.
23. Larsen A, Dale K, Eek M. Radiographic evaluation of rheumatoid arthritis and related conditions by standard reference film. *Acta Radiol Diagn* 1977;18:481–491.
24. Pahle JA. The shoulder joint in rheumatoid arthritis: Synovectomy. *Reconstr Surg Traumatol* 1981;18(33):33–47.
25. Pahle JA, Kvarnes L. Shoulder synovectomy. *Ann Chir Gynaecol Suppl* 1985;198(37):37–39.
26. Ogilvie-Harris D, Wiley A. Arthroscopic surgery of the shoulder. *J Bone Joint Surg [Br]* 1986;68:201–207.
27. Vainio K. Orthopaedic surgery in the treatment of rheumatoid arthritis. *Ann Clin Res* 1975;7:216–224.
28. Rybka V, Raunio P, Vainio K. Arthrodesis of the shoulder in rheumatoid arthritis: A review of forty-one cases. *J Bone Joint Surg [Br]* 1979;61:155–158.
29. Cofield R, Briggs B. Glenohumeral arthrodesis. Operative and long term functional results. *J Bone Joint Surg [Am]* 1979;61:668–677.
30. Gschwend N. *Surgical Treatment of Rheumatoid Arthritis*. Philadelphia: WB Saunders, 1980:35–44.
31. Neer C, Kirby R. Revision of humeral head and total shoulder arthroplasties. *Clin Orthop* 1982;170:189–195.
32. Benjamin A. Double osteotomy of the shoulder. *Scand J Rheumatol* 1974;3:65.
33. Benjamin A. The place of osteotomy in rheumatoid arthritis. *Ann Acad Med Singapore* 1983;12:185–190.
34. Neer CSII, Hawkins R. A functional analysis of shoulder fusions. *J Bone Joint Surg [Br]* 1977;59:508.
35. Wainwright D. Glenoidectomy in the treatment of the painful arthritis shoulder. *J Bone Joint Surg [Br]* 1976;58:377.
36. Gariepy R. Glenoidectomy in the repair of the rheumatic shoulder. *J Bone Joint Surg [Br]* 1977;59:122.
37. Milbrink J, Wigren A. Resection arthroplasty of the shoulder. *Scand J Rheumatol* 1990;19:432–436.
38. Neer CSII, Morrison D. Glenoid bone grafting in total shoulder arthroplasty. *J Bone Joint Surg [Am]* 1988;70:1154–1162.
39. Clayton ML, Ferlic DC, Jeffers PD. Prosthetic arthroplasties of the shoulder. *Clin Orthop* 1982;164:184–191.
40. Pahle JA, Kvarnes L. Shoulder replacement arthroplasty. *Ann Chir Gynaecol Suppl* 1985;198(85):85–89.
41. Kelly IG, Foster RS, Fisher WD. Neer total shoulder replacement in rheumatoid arthritis. *J Bone Joint Surg [Br]* 1987;69:723–726.
42. Thomas BJ, Amstutz HC, Cracchiolo A. Shoulder arthroplasty for rheumatoid arthritis. *Clin Orthop* 1991;265:125–128.
43. Paradis DK, Ferlic DC. Shoulder arthroplasty in rheumatoid arthritis. *Phys Ther* 1975;55:157–159.
44. Petersson CJ. Shoulder surgery in rheumatoid arthritis. *Acta Orthop Scand* 1986;57:222–226.
45. Barrett WP, Thornhill TS, Thomas WH, Gebhart EM, Sledge CB. Nonconstrained total shoulder arthroplasty in patients with polyarticular rheumatoid arthritis. *J Arthroplasty* 1989;4:91–96.
46. Vahvanen V, Hamalainen M, Paavolainen P. The Neer II replacement for rheumatoid arthritis of the shoulder. *Int Orthop* 1989;13:57–60.
47. McCoy SR, Warren RF, Bade H III, Ranawat CS, Inglis AE. Total shoulder arthroplasty in rheumatoid arthritis. *J Arthroplasty* 1989;4:105–113.
48. Cofield R. Total shoulder arthroplasty with the Neer prosthesis. *J Bone Joint Surg [Am]* 1984;66:899–906.
49. Hawkins RJ, Bell RH, Jallay B. Total shoulder arthroplasty. *Clin Orthop* 1989;242:188–194.
50. Frich LH, Moller BN, Sneppen O. Shoulder arthroplasty with the Neer Mark-II prosthesis. *Arch Orthop Trauma Surg* 1988;107:110–113.
51. Brenner BC, Ferlic DC, Clayton ML, Dennis DA. Survivorship of unconstrained total shoulder arthroplasty. *J Bone Joint Surg [Am]* 1989;71:1289–1296.
52. Bade H, Warren R, Ranawat C,, Inglis A. Long term results of Neer total shoulder replacement. In: Bateman J, Welsh R, eds. *Surgery of the Shoulder*. St. Louis: CV Mosby, 1984:249–252.
53. Kelly IG. Surgery of the rheumatoid shoulder. *Ann Rheum Dis* 1990;2:824–829.
54. Weiss AP, Adams MA, Moore JR, Weiland AJ. Unconstrained shoulder arthroplasty. A five-year average follow-up. *Clin Orthop* 1990;257:86–90.
55. Amstutz H, Thomas B, Kabo M, Jinnah R, Dorey F. The DANA total shoulder arthroplasty. *J Bone Joint Surg [Am]* 1988;70:1174–1182.
56. Roper BA, Paterson JM, Day WH. The Roper-Day total shoulder replacement. *J Bone Joint Surg [Br]* 1990;72:694–697.
57. Gristina AG, Romano RL, Kammire GC, Webb LX. Total shoulder replacement. *Orthop Clin North Am* 1987;18:445–453.

13 Osteonecrosis

Robert H. Cofield, M.D.

There are three major diagnostic categories accounting for most patients who have shoulder arthroplasty. These are osteoarthritis, rheumatoid arthritis, and arthritis secondary to old trauma, such as fractures, dislocations, and fracture-dislocations. Three other diagnostic categories contribute most of the remaining diagnostic indications for this procedure—osteonecrosis, rotator cuff disease with arthritis, and failed reconstructive surgery. The contribution of osteonecrosis of the humeral head to the overall diagnostic categorization of patients who have prosthetic shoulder arthroplasty can be very much underestimated, for, as will be explained, it may be tabulated within other diagnostic groups such as secondary osteoarthritis, old trauma, and cuff tear arthropathy.[1]

Osteonecrosis has been of major importance in the development of prosthetic shoulder arthroplasty, since the early implant designs were made to address this problem following severe trauma. Of historical interest is the 1951 report by Krueger[2] who used a custom-made chromium cobalt humeral head replacement for the treatment of osteonecrosis of the humeral head, and the 1952 description by Richard, Judet, and Rene[3] of an acrylic implant to replace the humeral head in various traumatic conditions. However, the genesis of the current arthroplasty methodology appeared the following year, 1953, in an article by Neer, Brown, and McLaughlin[4] presenting treatment options for fractures of the neck of the humerus with dislocation of the head fragment. These authors theorized about how prosthetic replacement represented a logical possibility and may prove of value. A newly designed humeral head articular replacement was illustrated.

The first series of patients undergoing surgery with an articular replacement for the humeral head using a metal implant was published in 1955.[5] Of the 12 patients undergoing analysis, 3 were treated for humeral head osteonecrosis. At follow-up periods of 14, 20, and 23 months, none of the 3 had pain, and range of motion was excellent in 1 and good in 2. These cases marked the beginning.

The concept of prosthetic replacement for the shoulder was slow in gaining acceptance. Only a few additional reports appeared in the 1960s and 1970s, most relating to trauma.[6,7] Then in 1974, Neer again published on this subject.[8] Forty-eight shoulders with glenohumeral osteoarthritis treated with humeral head replacement were reviewed. At an average follow-up of 6 years, pain relief and restoration of function occurred in nearly all patients. Osteonecrosis was present in at least 7. The possibility of adding glenoid resurfacing was illustrated in this article, and also reported by other authors during that year.[9] Innumerable early reports on total shoulder arthroplasty subsequently followed.[10]

Osteonecrosis was often one of the diagnoses in these diverse patient series reported, but only a few have appeared isolating this problem as a focus for study. This chapter explores the processes underlying the development of osteonecrosis of the humeral head, illustrates and describes the variations in clinical presentation, presents treatment options with their results and complications, and finally, outlines an approach to patient evaluation and treatment based upon this information and experience.

ETIOLOGY

It is useful to consider the etiology of osteonecrosis of the humeral head as (1) related to trauma or (2) associated with various disease processes. Clinically, cell death is often related to a lack of vascularity or occlusion of the arterial blood supply. There have been several studies of both the extraosseous and intraosseous courses of the major blood vessels supplying the humeral head. Laing[11] studied the arterial supply of the adult humerus. He recognized a rich periosteal blood supply, but most importantly identified a consistent artery on the anterolateral aspect of the humeral head—an ascending branch of the anterior humeral circumflex artery. This ascending branch entered the bone at the upper end of the bicipital groove or by its branches into the adjacent greater and lesser humeral tuberosities. Once inside the bone, a single vessel or multiple vessels pursue a curving posteromedial course just below the obliterated epiphyseal line. This vessel was called the arcuate artery.

Recently, Gerber et al.[12] studied the arterial vascularization of the humeral head in greater detail. This anatomic study confirmed and reemphasized the importance of the ascending branch of the anterior humeral circumflex vessel (Figure 13–1). These investigations clearly defined the extent of the intraosseous distribution of the branches of this vessel, which is responsible for most of the arterial blood supply within the humeral head (Figure 13–2).

Proximal Humeral Fractures

Proximal humeral fractures interrupt the arterial blood supply to the humeral head by tearing this major vessel and disrupting vessels entering from the bone surface or the medullary canal of the humerus. Series evaluating the frequency of osteonecrosis in complex proximal humeral frac-

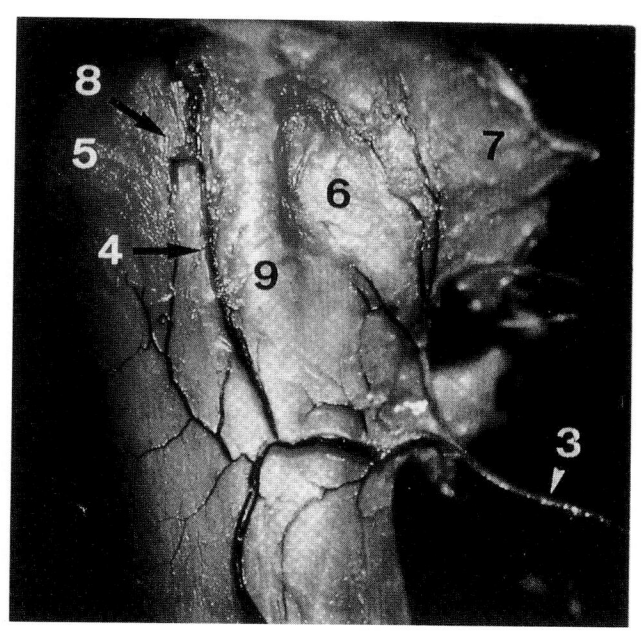

Figure 13–1. Anatomic dissection of the ascending, anterolateral branch of the anterior humeral circumflex artery with its sites of penetration into the humeral head. Anterior aspect of the humeral head. Anterior humeral circumflex artery = 3; anterolateral branch of the anterior circumflex artery = 4; greater tuberosity = 5; lesser tuberosity = 6; constant site of entry of the anterolateral branch into bone = 8; intertubercular groove = 9. (Reproduced with permission from Gerber et al.[12])

tures are shown in Table 13–1.[7,13–25] While there is the potential for osteonecrosis to develop in any type of proximal humeral fracture, it is much more common in those with four-part displacement or anatomic neck fractures (Figure 13–3).[26] If these complex fractures have no surgery or minimal surgical intervention, the frequency of osteonecrosis may be lessened.[13,25] However, the clinical result will be poor unless satisfactory reduction is obtained and maintained.[7] Table 13–2 outlines the potential effects of surgery on the frequency of osteonecrosis in proximal humeral fractures. Osteonecrosis seems to develop more commonly when internal fixation is applied with a plate and screws.

Systemic Diseases

Increased intraosseous pressure is thought to be one mechanism leading to the development of osteonecrosis of the femoral head.[27] This might occur because of elevated bone marrow pressure in association with a variety of conditions or because of venous abnormalities within or extrinsic to the bone. Ficat and Arlet[28] have stressed the importance and diagnostic utility of bone marrow pressure measurements in the diagnosis of osteonecrosis. In fact, intraosseous pressure measurements are thought to be quite useful in diagnosis.[29] These measurements are usually supplemented by venography, characterized in the abnormal state by poor or absent visualization of major efferent veins, delayed drainage of the dye from bone, and reflux of the dye into the diaphysis of the proximal part of the femur. It is reasonable to believe these findings in the femoral head have some relevance to osteonecrosis of the humeral head; however, knowledge is less complete for the shoulder.[30]

Many conditions are associated with necrosis of bone. These include, first and foremost, the use of glucocorticoids.[27,31] Steroid use increases serum lipids; there are fatty changes in the liver followed by fat embolization to multiple tissues, including bone. In this setting, focal osteocyte death occurs.[32] Osteonecrosis may even occur with short-term steroid therapy.[33–35] Recently, two cases of multifocal os-

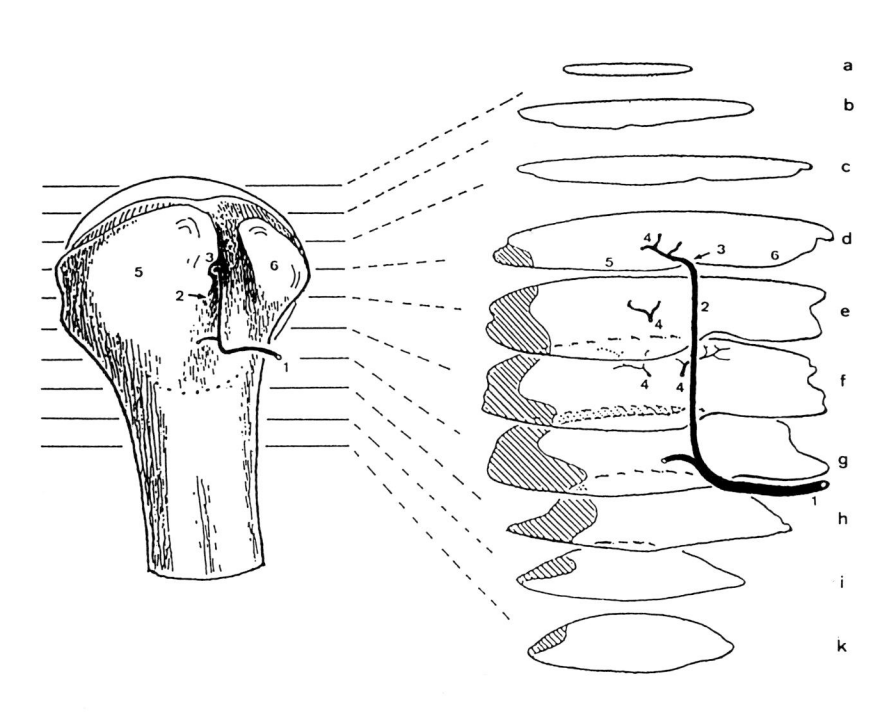

Figure 13–2. Artist's representation of the distribution of the blood supply to the humeral head after injection of the anterior humeral circumflex artery and humeral head sectioning. Anterior humeral circumflex artery = 1; anterolateral ascending branch of the anterior circumflex artery = 2; entry of the branch into the humeral head = 3; main stem of arcuate artery = 4; greater tuberosity = 5; lesser tuberosity = 6. The anterior circumflex artery supplies all of the bone within the humeral head except the areas indicated by hatched marks. (Reproduced with permission from Gerber et al.[12])

Table 13–1. Osteonecrosis in Proximal Humeral Fractures

AUTHOR(S)	FRACTURE TYPE	NO. WITH OSTEONECROSIS/ TOTAL NO. (%)
Neer, 1970[7]	3 part	4/50
	4 part	3/11 Closed treatment
	4 part	6/8 Open treatment
Lee and Hansen, 1981[13]	4 part	0/19
Sturzenegger et al., 1982[14]	3 and 4 part	6/27
Lim et al., 1983[15]	Comminuted	4/12
Leyshon, 1984[16]	4 part	6/8
Hagg and Lundberg, 1984[17]	4 part	7/15
Stableforth, 1984[18]	4 part	4/32
Siebler and Kuner, 1985[19]	4 part	4/21
Hawkins et al., 1986[20]	3 part	2/15
Kristiansen and Christensen, 1986[21]	3 and 4 part	4/26
Mouradian, 1986[22]	4 part	3/7
Seemann et al., 1986[23]	4 part	(19)
Kristiansen and Christensen, 1987[24]	3 part	2/7
	4 part	4/9
Jacob et al., 1991[25]	4 part	5/19

Table 13–2. Proximal Humeral Fractures: The Effect of Surgery on the Development of Osteonecrosis

AUTHOR(S)	FRACTURE TYPE	NO. WITH OSTEONECROSIS/ TOTAL NO.*
Lee and Hansen, 1981[13]	4 part	0/12 (wires or pin)
Sturzenegger et al., 1982[14]	Comminuted	5/17 (plates)
		1/10 (wires or screws)
Siebler and Kuner, 1985[19]	4 part	4/21 (3 plate, 1 minimal IF)
Hawkins et al., 1986[20]	3 part	2/15 (wires)
Kristiansen and Christensen, 1987[24]	3 part	2/7 (plates)
	4 part	4/9 (IF in 5)
Jacob et al., 1991[25]	4 part	5/19 (minimal IF)

*Type of internal fixation (IF) is in parentheses.

teonecrosis developed in association with intra-articular corticosteroid injections![36] Cruess[37] analyzed the etiologic considerations regarding osteonecrosis and related those to his experience with steroid-induced necrosis of the humeral head.

The list of associated diseases and conditions is long, and most importantly includes alcoholism, dysbaric phenomena, Cushing's syndrome, Gaucher's disease, hemoglobinopathies, irradiation, and thermal injuries.[27,31] In addition, there are other probable associations: chemotherapy, gout-hyperuricemia, hyperlipidemia, myxedema, pancreatitis, peripheral vascular disease, pregnancy, and systemic lupus erythematosus.[27-31]

In spite of these many possible causes or associations, for many patients there is no evidence of a risk factor; the condition is idiopathic. Kenzora and Glimcher[38] postulated a multifactorial etiology for so-called idiopathic osteonecrosis. They argued that cell death occurs because of an accumulation of stresses to cell viability. For example, an individual has an underlying systemic disease, such as chronic renal failure, the cells are not functioning normally, and then systemic steroids are added. The cells are overwhelmed by a combination of toxic effects, and necrosis occurs.

CLASSIFICATION

Experience with osteonecrosis of the hip has clearly shown the value of a staging system related to the degree of bony

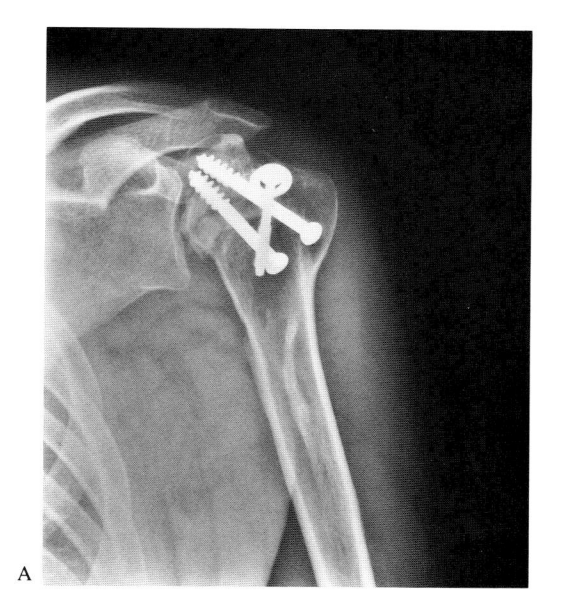

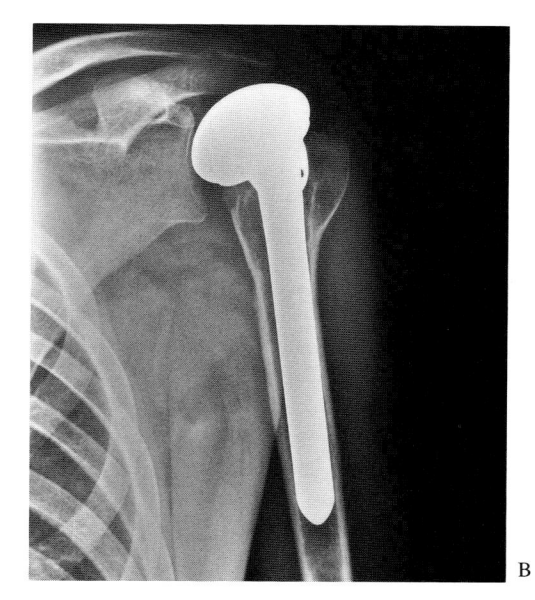

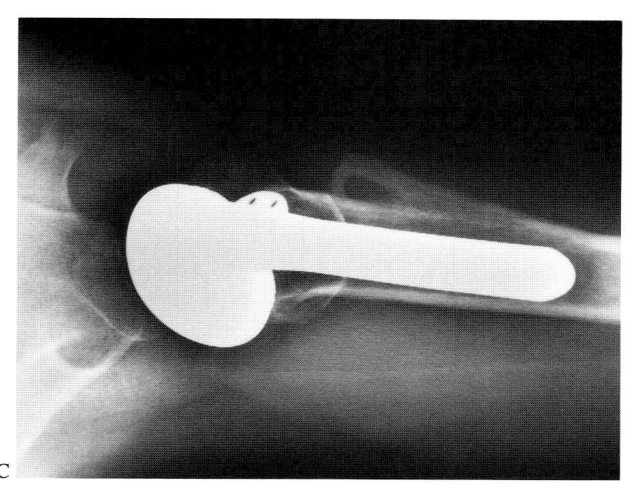

Figure 13–3. **A.** Osteonecrosis of the humeral head in a 17-year-old man following a comminuted, proximal humeral fracture with posterior dislocation. The fracture was openly reduced and internally fixed, but unfortunately osteonecrosis developed and posterior subluxation recurred. **B** and **C.** Anteroposterior and axillary radiographs, respectively, following humeral head replacement arthroplasty.

changes identified on standard radiographs. These changes in turn direct treatment and often dictate the prognosis. A method of classification was introduced by Ficat and Arlet,[39] and modified by Cruess[37] to reflect contemporary treatment considerations.

In stage 1, the radiographs appear essentially normal (Figure 13–4); however, changes may be identified on bone scanning or magnetic resonance imaging. Stage 2 radiographic changes most typically include a segment of sclerosis in the juxta-articular portion of the humeral head, often superior-central. There is, however, no fracture of the subchondral bone. The presence or absence of this fracture is best defined by anteroposterior tomography of the humeral head with the arm in external rotation.

Stage 3 shows the humeral head segment with sclerosis but in addition, there is a subchondral bone fracture extending to the joint surface. On a plain radiograph, the fracture is gently curved, creating the so-called crescent sign. It is best seen on the anteroposterior view with the arm in external rotation, or on the axillary view. There may be no displacement of the joint surface or the segment can be depressed one to several millimeters. Occasionally, this flap of cartilage and sclerotic subchondral bone will become elevated from its bony bed and create an internal derangement within the joint.

In stage 4, the fragment has become displaced into the joint or more commonly has collapsed into the softened adjacent necrotic bone. Thus, the humeral head aspect of the joint surface has a distorted contour, setting the stage for secondary traumatic arthritis or osteoarthritis. Stage 5 reflects these changes plus wear with cartilage loss on the glenoid side of the joint.

The evaluation of osteonecrosis would thus include, in addition to the history and physical examination, the standard shoulder radiographs plus appropriate laboratory testing to identify the presence or absence of any of the conditions or associated diseases outlined above. Importantly, accurate

Staging of Humeral Head Osteonecrosis

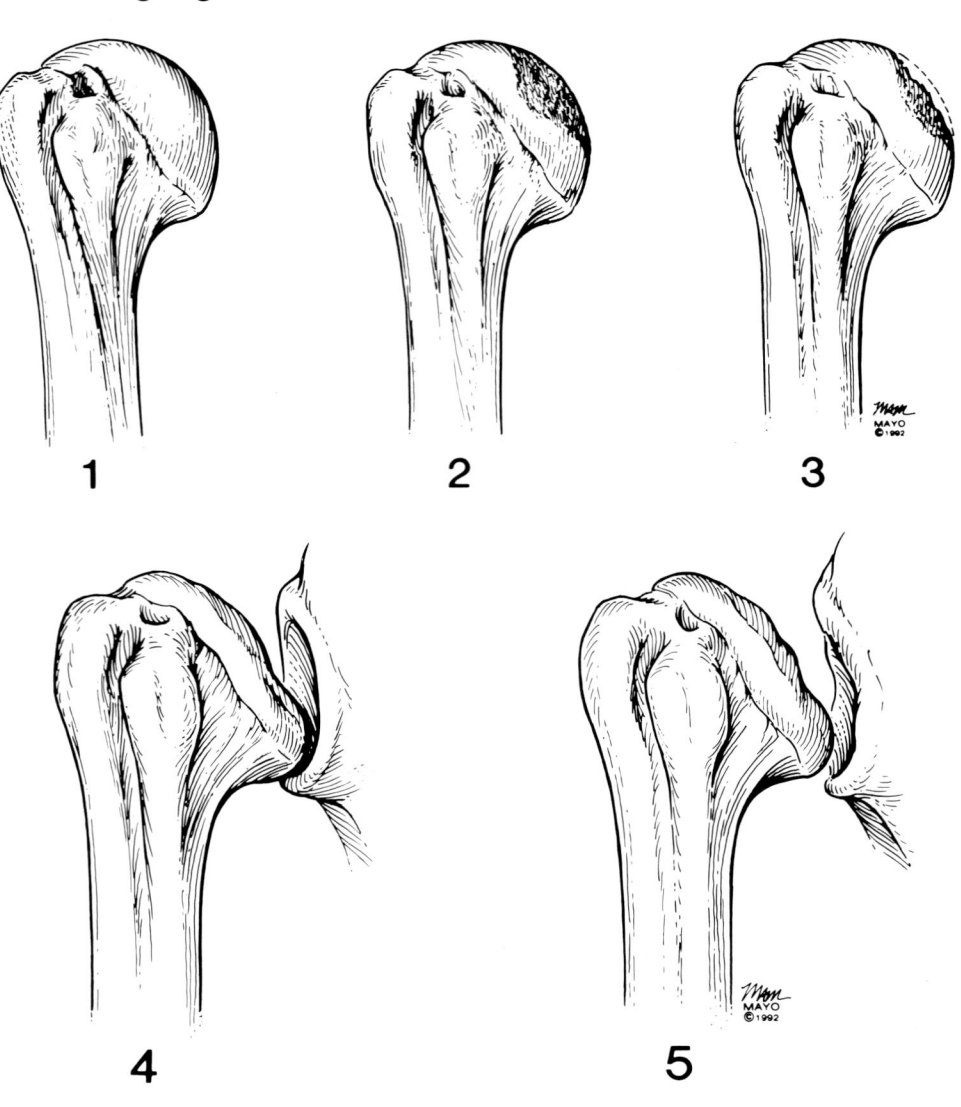

Figure 13-4. Staging of humeral head osteonecrosis. Stage 1: The bone appears normal by plain x-ray film and would appear normal on gross inspection. Marrow changes can be identified on magnetic resonance imaging. Stage 2: On plain films, a segment of sclerosis would be seen. A fracture line is not visible, nor is there any bony collapse. Stage 3: On plain films, a gently curving, subchondral fracture is identified. Radiographically, this crescent sign is represented by a gently curved sliver of bone—often sclerotic. Its outer surface is the subchondral bone plate, while its inner surface is the fracture through necrotic and partially revascularized bone. On visual inspection, the articular surface may be slightly distorted (as illustrated); the fracture often extends through a portion of the articular cartilage. Displacement is limited to a few millimeters. Stage 4: There has been collapse of the humeral head articular surface. The area of collapse is typically superior-central. Stage 5: The humeral head collapse has occurred as in stage 4 but with the addition of glenoid cartilage damage.

staging may be enhanced by tomography or magnetic resonance imaging, which shows the marrow changes quite dramatically. Unfortunately, to date there have been no studies indicating the value of magnetic resonance imaging over and above standard radiographs with tomography as needed once the diagnosis has been made. Thus, magnetic resonance imaging or bone scanning may be instrumental in the early diagnosis but plain radiographs, with or without tomography, are most effective for staging osteonecrosis. In turn, staging directs the treatment.

TREATMENT

Nonoperative treatment considerations are not addressed in any detail here. However, several observations are important when considering the indications for prosthetic arthroplasty.

Until recently, it was generally agreed that nonoperative treatment was appropriate for stages 1 and 2 osteonecrosis. Several centers have investigated the use of electrical stimulation for these prefracture stages. However, no clear direction for its use has emerged, and its place in the treatment regimen is uncertain.

More importantly, core decompression has been considered for humeral head osteonecrosis, as it has been for the femoral head. In a recent report of 30 shoulders, 14 had stage 1 or 2 disease and all had good or excellent results.[30] Follow-up averaged 5 to 6 years for the entire study group (range, 2 to 14 years). In this study, core decompression was associated with excellent results in 7 of 10 shoulders with stage 3 disease, but for 5 of 6 shoulders with stage 4 disease it failed. Based on their experience, these authors concluded that core decompression was a successful procedure for stage

1, 2, or 3 osteonecrosis of the humeral head. Whether or not to consider core decompression is still somewhat of a dilemma. Another study reviewing 16 shoulders at an average of 4.5 years following presentation found that 9 of 11 with stage 2 or 3 disease at presentation had no clinical progression.[40] All 5 shoulders with stage 4 or 5 disease worsened. These authors concluded, based upon their experience, that nonoperative treatment is adequate for stage 1 or 2 disease and can be adequate for stage 3 disease (Figure 13–5).

Physicians will always need to advise and treat patients with less complete information than they might wish to have. In this setting, like most others involving elective reconstructive surgery, physicians will consider prosthetic shoulder arthroplasty surgery for patients with significant symptoms (pain plus functional limitations) and sufficient pathology, which includes stage 5, stage 4, and perhaps stage 3 disease.

Literature Review

Almost one-half of the approximately 50 reported series on prosthetic shoulder arthroplasty included some patients who underwent surgery for osteonecrosis (Table 13–3).[1,41–57] Many of these more general series reporting outcome of an arthroplasty (either humeral head hemiarthroplasty or total shoulder arthroplasty) did not separate the results of those treated for osteonecrosis from the remaining large patient groups such as rheumatoid arthritis or osteoarthritis patients but several did (Table 13–4).[42,43,45,46,50,56]

Analyzing the information in Table 13–3, approximately 5% of patients who require prosthetic shoulder arthroplasty will have the surgery performed for the treatment of osteonecrosis. It is unfortunate that osteonecrosis is so small a subgroup of this entire population, for the details of these patients' results or complications are not always reported separately from the entire study group. When they are, however, the results are quite good (Table 13–4).

Pain relief occurs in more than 90% of patients, and return of active motion is more than three-fourths normal. However, it must be recalled that the number of patients studied and reported is small, and, in a parallel sense, complications are seldom reported selectively for this patient group. Of those complications reported, Kay and Amstutz[50] related two shoulders with postoperative subluxation. Aliabadi et al.[41] detailed the radiographic findings, suggesting that no particular radiographic differences exist between the patients with osteonecrosis and others who have had total shoulder arthroplasty.

Only a few reports specifically addressed the treatment of osteonecrosis of the shoulder. The first and most important was by Cruess.[58] Of 95 patients with steroid-induced osteonecrosis of bone, 18 had humeral head involvement. The steroids were prescribed for renal transplantation in 8; lupus erythematosus in 5; asthma in 2; and glomerulonephritis, hypopituitarism, and Guillain-Barré syndrome in 1 each. All had had steroid therapy for at least 6 months before the onset of shoulder symptoms. At the time of evaluation, the patients fell into one of three groups. The first group of 8 patients had

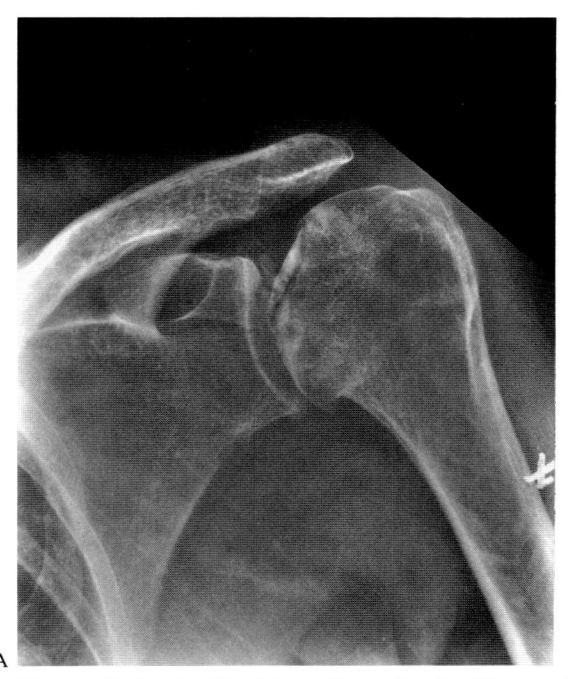

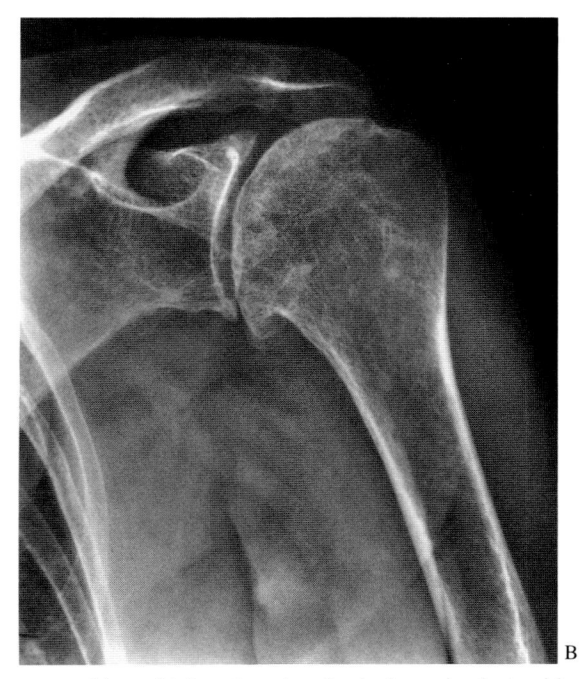

Figure 13–5. **A.** Shoulder radiograph of a 56-year-old woman with multiple sclerosis who had received steroid treatment. The radiographs shows the subchondral fracture with slight collapse of the articular surface. Symptoms were mild, and treatment was conservative. **B.** Radiograph of the same shoulder 9 years later. Her symptoms continue to be minor, and no further treatment was required.

Table 13-3. Prosthetic Arthroplasty for Osteonecrosis of the Shoulder

AUTHOR(S)	NO. OF SHOULDERS IN SERIES	NO. OF SHOULDERS WITH OSTEONECROSIS
Aliabadi et al., 1988[41]	98	5
Amstutz et al., 1988[42]	46	3
Bade et al., 1984[43]	34	5
Bell and Geschwend, 1986[44]	28	3
Boyd et al., 1990[45]	(193)*	(11)*
Boyd et al., 1991[46]	131	6
Cofield, 1983[47]	184	1
Gristina et al., 1987[48]	132	6
Hawkins et al., 1989[49]	70	2
Kay and Amstutz, 1988[50]	15	3
Kjaersgaard-Andersen et al., 1989[51]	63	2
Neer et al., 1982[1]	261	5
Ranawat et al., 1980[52]	40	6
Roper et al., 1990[53]	25	2
Steffee and Moore, 1984[54]	69	4
Tanner and Cofield, 1983[55]	28	8
Warren et al., 1982[56]	21	5
Weiss et al., 1990[57]	46	5

*Number of patients.

a mild anatomic deformity and could return to essentially full activity without surgical intervention. The second group of 6 had more severe deformity, but a sedentary life-style. All in this group continued with steroid therapy and did not require specific treatment for their shoulders. In the third group of 4 patients, 5 shoulders required humeral head replacement using the Neer prosthesis. All experienced relief of pain at the time of follow-up, ranging from 1 to 6 years postoperatively. Range of motion approached normal, and no complications were encountered. In all cases, the glenoid articular cartilage appeared normal or near normal at the time of surgery.

In the second report by Rutherford and Cofield,[40] 13 patients with 17 affected shoulders were available for evaluation between 2.0 and 6.5 years after surgery. Seven patients with 10 shoulders had normal glenoid surfaces or only minor changes, and underwent a humeral head hemiarthroplasty. In addition, 1 patient with loss of glenoid cartilage and bony erosion did not have enough scapular bone remaining to support a glenoid component and had humeral head replacement alone. Five patients with 6 affected shoulders who had stage 5 disease underwent total shoulder arthroplasty. Postoperatively, 16 (94%) of 17 shoulders had mild or no pain. Active abduction averaged 161 degrees in those with humeral head replacement and 150 degrees in those with total shoulder arthroplasty. Overall, all patients with humeral head replacement had excellent or satisfactory results. Four of 6 with total shoulder arthroplasty had excellent or satisfactory results. Two developed postoperative rotator cuff tears, one of whom had further surgery.

In assessing the above literature, it would appear that those patients with no humeral head deformity or only a mild deformity will do well with nonoperative treatment. For those who require surgical treatment, humeral head replace-

Table 13-4. Results of Prosthetic Arthroplasty for Osteonecrosis

AUTHORS	NO. OF SHOULDERS WITH OSTEONECROSIS	NO. WITH PAIN RELIEVED (%)	ACTIVE ABDUCTION (degrees)	EXTERNAL ROTATION (degrees)
Amstutz et al., 1988[42]	3	3 (100)	160	60
Bade et al., 1984[43]	5		170	
Boyd et al., 1990[45]	11	11 (100)		
Boyd et al., 1991[46]	6	5 (83)		
Kay and Amstutz, 1988[50]	3	3 (100)	143	
Warren et al., 1982[56]	5	5 (100)		

ment alone is appropriate when the glenoid cartilage is normal or near normal, as in stage 4 disease (Figure 13–6). Total shoulder arthroplasty is indicated when the glenoid is involved. The results should be quite good, as the capsule and rotator cuff are not destroyed by the disease process. Pain will be relieved in more than 90% of patients, and range of motion will be above average for those patients undergoing prosthetic arthroplasty of the shoulder joint. However, these are major procedures, and significant complications, as with surgery for the other diagnostic categories, will occasionally occur.

Author's Preferred Approach

Treatment is, of course, predicated on an accurate diagnosis. To obtain this, one obtains a history and physical examination, plain radiographs, adjunctive laboratory studies as suggested by the potential presence of associated diseases as

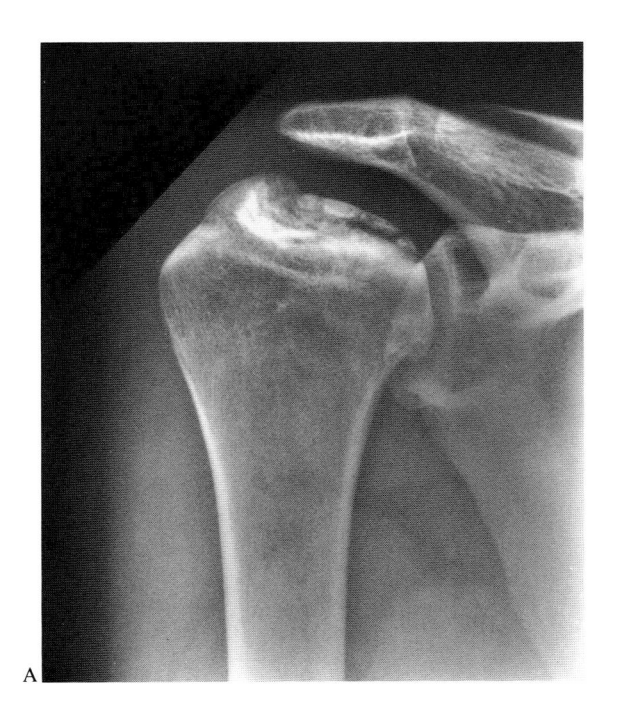

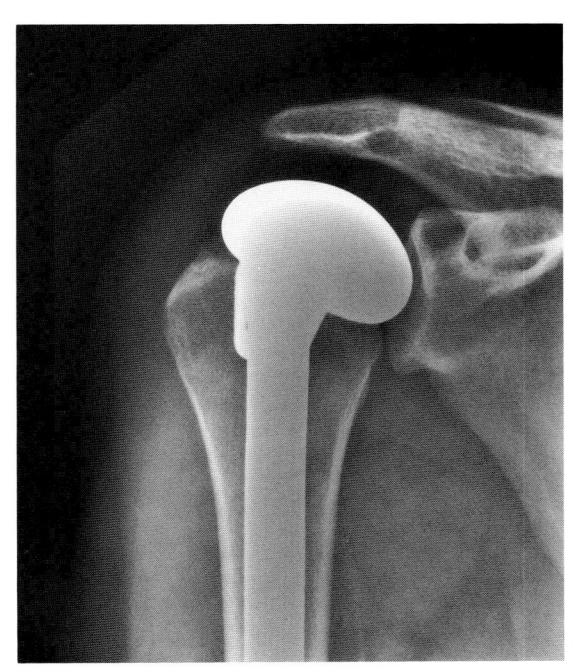

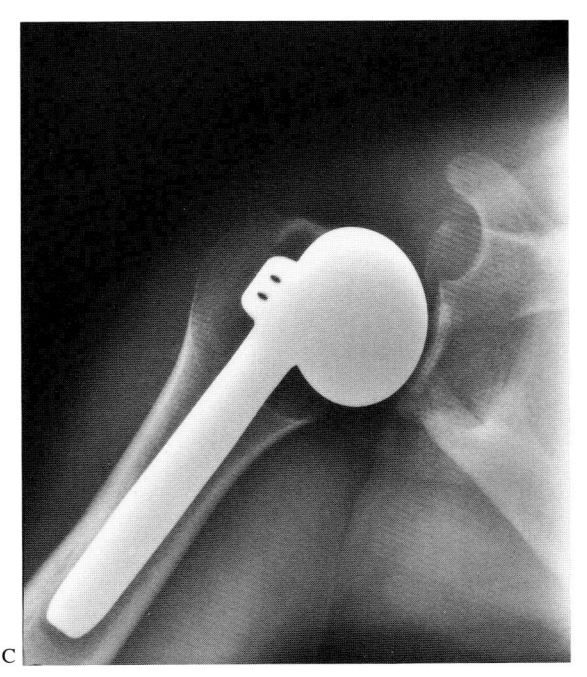

Figure 13–6. A. Osteonecrosis of the right humeral head, stage 4, in a 29-year-old man treated with systemic steroids for gastrointestinal problems. B and C. Anteroposterior view and axillary view, respectively, following humeral head replacement. Five years after surgery, there was mild discomfort and more than 90% of normal motion.

outlined above, and imaging studies. The imaging studies are performed to help accurately stage the disease process. This may be possible with plain radiographs, or it may be necessary to supplement these with tomography. Occasionally, magnetic resonance imaging may also be helpful.

Physical examination will disclose the presence of an associated periarthritic-like response involving the shoulder capsule and rotator cuff. This is particularly important to recognize in stage 2 and stage 3 disease without significant joint surface involvement. These patients may continue to be treated nonoperatively with a reasonable expectation that unless further collapse occurs, operative intervention may not be necessary. However, for patients with persistent, significant symptoms and stage 3 disease, or those who have stage 4 or 5 disease, prosthetic arthroplasty seems to be indicated as the best treatment option.

The surgical approach is through the deltopectoral interval, as outlined elsewhere in this book. As an alternative, the deltoid can be retracted from the cephalic vein, which is allowed to fall medially. Branches from the deltoid to the cephalic vein are cauterized or ligated. In addition, the two major arteriovenous groups from the thoracoacromial axis crossing the deltopectoral interval are cauterized. The subdeltoid and subacromial spaces are freed of scar. The rotator cuff is inspected. Typically, the rotator cuff will be intact. At this point, examination of the shoulder for range of motion is again repeated, and any residual tightness is noted. The shoulder in this situation may have an excellent range of motion, or indeed, there may be some limitations of motion, typically in elevation and external rotation.

The arthrotomy is performed by an incision in the subscapularis and shoulder capsule over the capsular insertion on the humeral head. The incision is continued superiorly in the rotator interval area and inferiorly along the humeral neck. If there are limitations of elevation, the inferior shoulder capsule is released from the humeral neck. Of course, the axillary nerve is identified and protected during this very careful process of capsular release.

The humeral head is then subluxated forward, the lesion is identified, and utilizing a humeral resection guide, the humeral head osteotomy is performed with 35 degrees of retroversion. The remaining metaphyseal bone surface is inspected, and any loosened, soft, necrotic or partially revascularized bone is removed. The metaphysis is trimmed of osteophytes as needed, and the humeral canal is prepared.

If there is an internal rotation contracture, the anterior-superior shoulder capsule is released from the glenoid rim, and this release continues laterally along the edge of the superior band of the inferior glenohumeral ligament. This will allow the anterior-superior shoulder capsule and the subscapularis to have greater flexibility, while protecting the inferior glenohumeral ligament from damage.

The glenoid is then inspected. One can be fooled by the presence of very smooth bone appearing to represent the shape of a normal glenoid. If the cartilage is normal or near normal, the glenoid should probably not be resurfaced. If the glenoid cartilage is absent or as more typically happens in this condition, a segment of the glenoid is eroded and deformed by rubbing against the irregular humeral head, glenoid resurfacing will be needed (Figure 13–7).

Following placement of the glenoid component and after trial reduction and assessment of motion, the proximal part of the humerus is further prepared. It may be possible to press-fit the component if the remaining metaphyseal bone is of good quality. If the bone is of poor quality with cavities created by the necrotic and reparative process, the humeral component will need to be fixed into position with methylmethacrylate.

The subscapularis is then repaired, and motion is carefully assessed and recorded in the operative report so that physical therapy can be appropriately planned. The wound is then closed in a typical fashion, and the arm is positioned in a shoulder immobilizer.

On the day following surgery, active range of motion is started for the hand, wrist, forearm, and elbow. On the subsequent day, a passive motion program is outlined based upon the movements recorded at surgery. Typically, a patient might have 70 degrees of external rotation with the arm at the side, 100 degrees of internal rotation, and flexion or abduction to 165 degrees. The physical therapist is then directed to undertake a passive motion program with external rotation, for instance, to 40 degrees and flexion to 140 degrees. This passive motion program is continued for the first 3 to 6 weeks. At 3 to 4 weeks, assisted pulley exercises in flexion might be added, and at 4 to 6 weeks isometrics can be commenced. At 8 weeks, elastic resistance tubing strengthening is added, and stretching is performed as needed. At 12 to 16 weeks, light weight-lifting may be included as a part of the program.

As outlined in the section reviewing the literature, very little is recognized regarding complications for treatment of this condition. Certainly, there are a few patients who have had humeral head replacement alone who will require subsequent total shoulder arthroplasty (Figure 13–8). This is recognized as being uncommon, but in fact does occur. More importantly, a common problem following any type of prosthetic shoulder arthroplasty is an aberration in healing of the rotator cuff, and the potential for humeral head subluxation. These potential problems, of course, are best addressed by careful patient selection, patient education, proper positioning of the components at surgery, capsule and rotator cuff repair, and then integration of the rehabilitation program into the overall care of the patient. Usually, this will be successful in avoiding these latter complications, but unfortunately success does not always occur.

SUMMARY

In this chapter, the etiologic considerations in osteonecrosis of the humeral head have been presented. Most importantly, these include multipart fractures of the proximal part of the

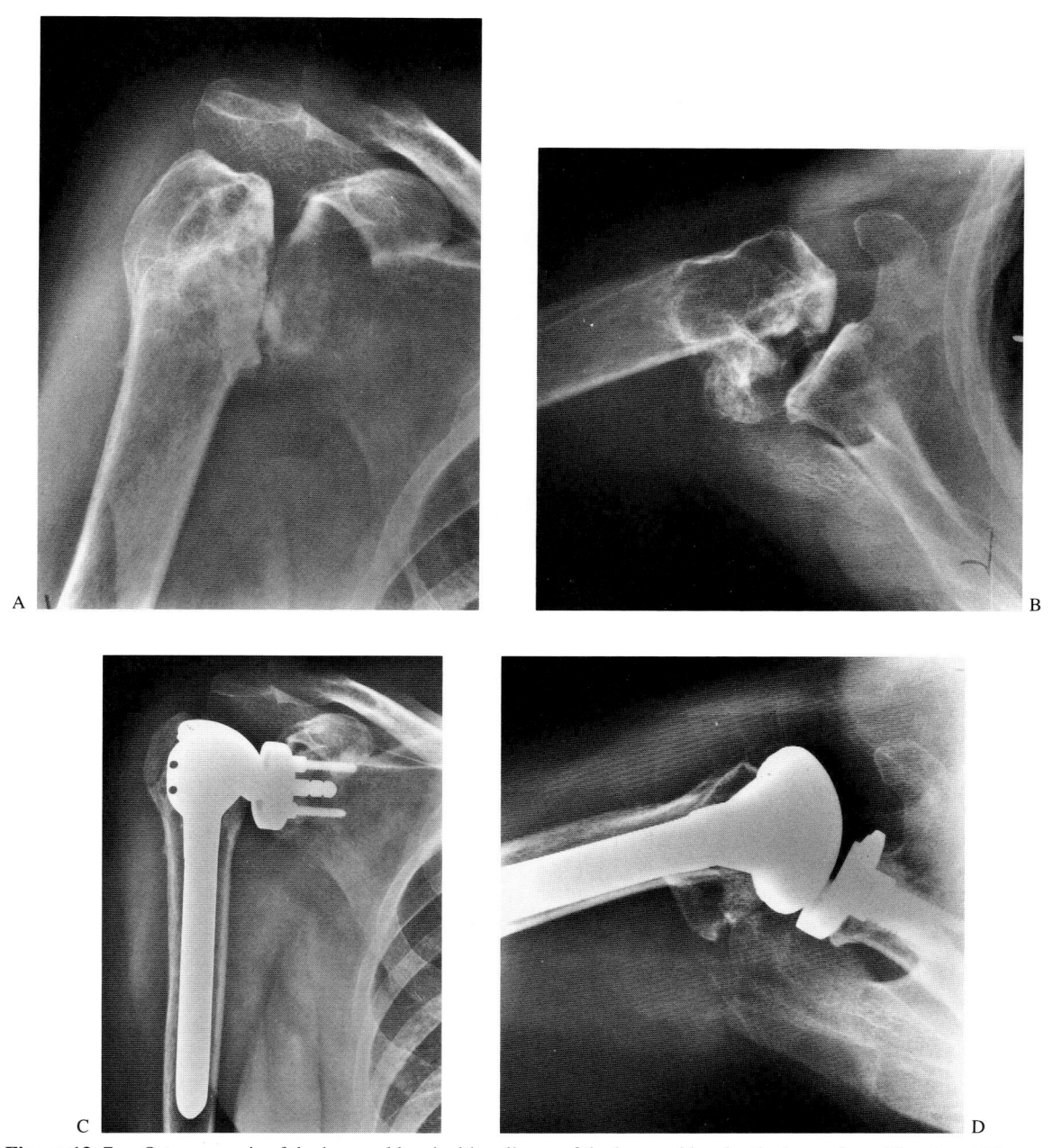

Figure 13-7. Osteonecrosis of the humeral head with collapse of the humeral head articular surface. The glenoid does not appear normal, and at surgery the glenoid cartilage was severely damaged—stage 5 disease. **A** and **B.** Anteroposterior and axillary views, respectively. **C** and **D.** Radiographic appearance following total shoulder arthroplasty.

humerus or anatomic neck fractures of the humeral head. Many disease processes are also associated with osteonecrosis of the humeral head, the most common being treatment with systemic corticosteroids. It has become apparent that staging of the disease process is quite important, as this then directs treatment and prognosis. For stage 1, stage 2, and perhaps stage 3 disease without bone collapse, core decompression of the humeral head might be a consideration. However, it is not clear that this is distinctly more effective than conservative treatment alone, considering the natural course of the disease process for these stages of the disease. In patients with continually symptomatic stage 3 or stage 4 disease, humeral head hemiarthroplasty alone seems to be quite effective. When stage 5 disease is present, with destruction of the glenoid articular surface, total shoulder arthroplasty is the treatment of choice.

The results of humeral head replacement or total shoulder arthroplasty are quite good in this condition, as the capsule and rotator cuff are often normal or near normal. It is important to recognize that osteonecrosis represents about

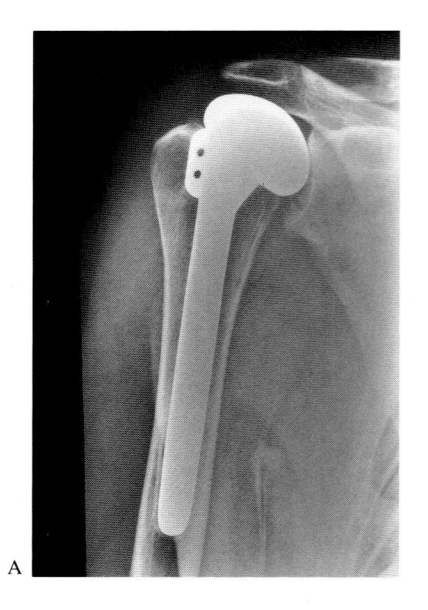

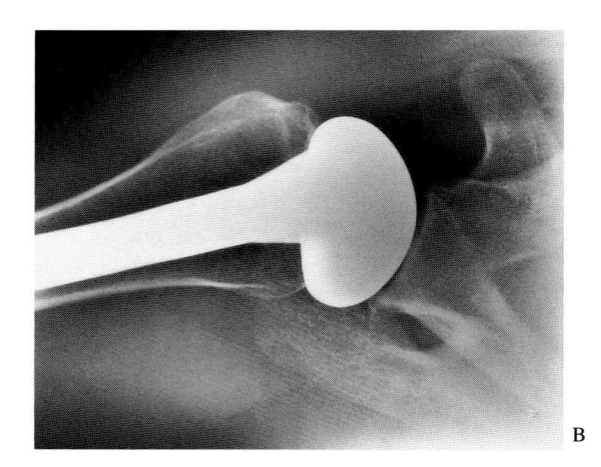

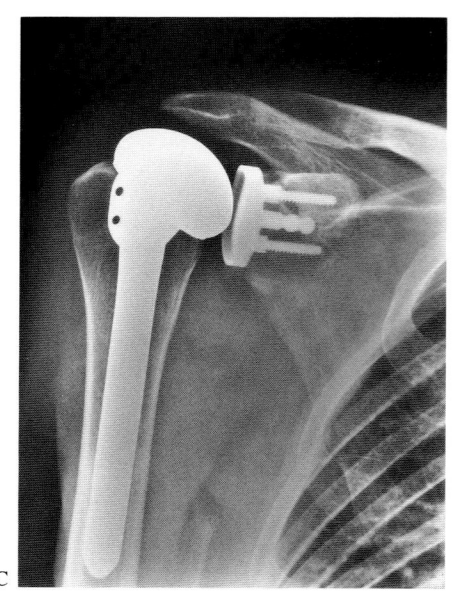

Figure 13–8. **A** and **B.** Radiographs of the shoulder of the patient illustrated in Figure 13–6, now 9 years after surgery. The anteroposterior view (**A**) and the axillary view (**B**) show glenoid cartilage loss with slight superior and posterior humeral subluxation. Shoulder pain was severe. **C.** The humeral head replacement was revised to a total shoulder arthroplasty with excellent pain relief. Approximately 80% of normal movement was regained.

5% of all patients who have prosthetic arthroplasty of the glenohumeral joint. Thus, the disease process, although uncommon, is not rare, and the characteristics of the process will need to be appreciated to effect adequate surgical care. On the other hand, the number of patients who have had prosthetic arthroplasty for this condition is relatively small, and the exact frequency of success and the incidence of complications are difficult to appreciate at this point in time.

REFERENCES

1. Neer CS II, Watson KC, Stanton FJ. Recent experience in total shoulder replacement. *J Bone Joint Surg [Am]* 1982;64:319–337.
2. Krueger FJ. A vitallium replica arthroplasty on the shoulder. A case report of aseptic necrosis of the proximal end of the humerus. *Surgery* 1951;30:1005–1011.
3. Richard A, Judet R, Rene L. Reconstruction prothetique acrylique de l'extremite superieure de l'humerus specialement d cours des fractures-luxations. *J Chir* 1952;68:537–547.
4. Neer CS, Brown TH Jr, McLaughlin HL. Fracture of the neck of the humerus with dislocation of the head fragment. *Am J Surg* 1953;85:252–258.
5. Neer CS. Articular replacement for the humeral head. *J Bone Joint Surg [Am]* 1955;37:215–228.
6. Neer CS II. Follow-up notes on articles previously published in the journal. Articular replacement for the humeral head. *J Bone Joint Surg [Am]* 1964;46:1607–1610.
7. Neer CS II. Displaced proximal humeral fractures. Part II. Treatment of three-part and four-part displacement. *J Bone Joint Surg [Am]* 1970;52:1090–1103.

8. Neer CS II. Replacement arthroplasty for glenohumeral osteoarthritis. *J Bone Joint Surg [Am]* 1974;56:1–13.
9. Kenmore PI, MacCartee C, Vitek B. A simple shoulder replacement. *J Biomed Mater Res* 1974;8:329–330.
10. Cofield RH. Degenerative and arthritic problems of the glenohumeral joint. In: Rockwood CA Jr, Matsen FA III, eds. *The Shoulder*. Philadelphia: WB Saunders, 1990:678–749.
11. Laing PG. The arterial supply of the adult humerus. *J Bone Joint Surg [Am]* 1956;38:1105–1116.
12. Gerber C, Schneeberger AG, Vinh TS. The arterial vascularization of the humeral head. *J Bone Joint Surg [Am]* 1990;72:1486–1494.
13. Lee CK, Hansen HR. Post-traumatic avascular necrosis of the humeral head in displaced proximal humeral fractures. *J Trauma* 1981;21:788–791.
14. Sturzenegger M, Fornaro E, Jakob RP. Results of surgical treatment of multifragmented fractures of the humeral head. *Arch Orthop Trauma Surg* 1982;100:249–259.
15. Lim TE, Ochsner PE, Marti RK, Holscher AA. The results of treatment of comminuted fractures and fracture dislocations of the proximal humerus. *Neth J Surg* 1983;35:139–143.
16. Leyson RC. Closed treatment of fractures of the proximal humerus. *Acta Orthop Scand* 1984;55:48–51.
17. Hagg O, Lundberg B. Aspects of prognostic factors in comminuted and dislocated proximal humeral fractures. In: Bateman JE, Welsh RP, eds. *Surgery of the Shoulder*. Philadelphia: BC Decker, 1984:51–59.
18. Stableforth PG. Four-part fractures of the neck of the humerus. *J Bone Joint Surg [Br]* 1984;66:104–108.
19. Siebler G, Kuner EH. Sp tergebnisse Nach Operativer Behandlung Proximaler Humerusfrakturen bei Erwachsensen. *Unfallchirurgie* 1985;11:119–127.
20. Hawkins RJ, Bell RH, Gurr K. The three-part fracture of the proximal part of the humerus. *J Bone Joint Surg [Am]* 1986;68:1410–1414.
21. Kristiansen B, Christensen SW. Plate fixation of proximal humeral fractures. *Acta Orthop Scand* 1986;57:320–323.
22. Mouradian WH. Displaced proximal humeral fractures. Seven years' experience with a modified Zickel supracondylar device. *Clin Orthop* 1986;212:209–218.
23. Seemann WR, Siebler G, Rupp HG. A new classification of proximal humeral fractures. *Eur J Radiol* 1986;6:163–167.
24. Kristiansen B, Christensen SW. Proximal humeral fractures. Late results in relation to classification and treatment. *Acta Orthop Scand* 1987;58:124–127.
25. Jakob RP, Miniaci A, Anson PS, Jaberg H, Osterwalder A, Ganz R. Four-part valgus impacted fractures of the proximal humerus. *J Bone Joint Surg [Br]* 1991;73:295–298.
26. Neer CS II. Displaced proximal humeral fractures. Part I. Classification and evaluation. *J Bone Joint Surg [Am]* 1970;52:1077–1089.
27. Hungerford DS, Lennox DW. The importance of increased intraosseous pressure in the development of osteonecrosis of the femoral head: Implications for treatment. *Orthop Clin North Am* 1985;16:635–654.
28. Ficat RP, Arlet J. The physiology of bone, and functional investigation of bone under normal conditions. In: *Ischemia and Necrosis of Bone*. Baltimore: Williams & Wilkins, 1980:11–52.
29. Hungerford DS, Zizic TM. Alcoholism associated ischemic necrosis of the femoral head. *Clin Orthop* 1978;130:144–153.
30. Urquhart MW, Mont MA, Maar DC, Lennox DW, Krackow KA, Hungerford DS. Results of core decompression for avascular necrosis of the humeral head. *Orthop Trans* 1992;16:780.
31. Jones JP Jr. Osteonecrosis. In: McCarty DJ, ed. *Arthritis and Allied Conditions*. Philadelphia: Lea & Febiger, 1985:1356–1373.
32. Fisher DE, Bickel WH, Holley KE, Ellefson RD. Corticosteroid-induced aseptic necrosis. II. Experimental study. *Clin Orthop* 1972;84:200–206.
33. Anderton JM, Helm R. Multiple joint osteonecrosis following short-term steroid therapy. *J Bone Joint Surg [Am]* 1982;64:139–141.
34. Fast A, Alon M, Weiss S, Zer-Aviv FR. Avascular necrosis of bone following short-term dexamethasone therapy for brain edema. *J Neurosurg* 1984;61:983–985.
35. Taylor LJ. Multifocal avascular necrosis after short-term high-dose steroid therapy. A report of three cases. *J Bone Joint Surg [Br]* 1984;66:431–433.
36. Laroche M, Arlet J, Mazieres B. Osteonecrosis of the femoral and humeral heads after intraarticular corticosteroid injections. *J Rheumatol* 1990;17:549–551.
37. Cruess RL. Experience with steroid-induced avascular necrosis of the shoulder and etiologic considerations regarding osteonecrosis of the hip. *Clin Orthop* 1978;130:86–93.
38. Kenzora JE, Glimcher MJ. Accumulative cell stress: The multifactorial etiology of idiopathic osteonecrosis. *Orthop Clin North Am* 1985;16:669–679.
39. Ficat P, Arlet J. Necrosis of the femoral head. In: *Ischemia and Bone Necrosis*. Baltimore: Williams & Wilkins, 1980:53–75.
40. Rutherford CS, Cofield RH. Osteonecrosis of the shoulder. *Orthop Trans* 1987;11:239.
41. Aliabadi P, Weissman BN, Thornhill T, Nikpoor N, Sosman JL. Evaluation of a nonconstrained total shoulder prosthesis. *AJR* 1988;151:1169–1172.
42. Amstutz HC, Thomas BJ, Kabo M, Jinnah RH, Dorey FJ. The DANA total shoulder arthroplasty. *J Bone Joint Surg [Am]* 1988;70:1174–1182.
43. Bade HA III, Warren RF, Ranawat CS, Inglis AE. Long term results of Neer total shoulder replacement. In: Bateman JE, Welsh RP, eds. *Surgery of the Shoulder*. Philadelphia: BC Decker, 1984:294–302.
44. Bell SN, Gschwend N. Clinical experience with total arthroplasty and hemiarthroplasty of the shoulder using the Neer prosthesis. *Int Orthop* 1986;10:217–222.
45. Boyd AD, Thomas WH, Scott RD, Sledge CB, Thornhill TS. Total shoulder arthroplasty versus hemiarthroplasty. *J Arthroplasty* 1990;5:329–336.
46. Boyd AD, Aliabadi P, Thornhill TS. Postoperative proximal migration in total shoulder arthroplasty. Incidence and significance. *J Arthroplasty* 1991;6:31–37.
47. Cofield RH. Unconstrained total shoulder prostheses. *Clin Orthop* 1983;173:97–108.
48. Gristina AG, Romano RL, Kammire GC, Webb LX. Total shoulder replacement. *Orthop Clin North Am* 1987;18:445–453.
49. Hawkins RJ, Bell RH, Jalay B. Total shoulder arthroplasty. *Clin Orthop* 1989;242:188–194.
50. Kay SP, Amstutz HC. Shoulder hemiarthroplasty at UCLA. *Clin Orthop* 1988;228:42–48.
51. Kjaersgaard-Andersen P, Frich LH, Sojbjerg JO, Sneppen O. Heterotopic bone formation following total shoulder arthroplasty. *J Arthroplasty* 1989;4:99–104.
52. Ranawat CS, Warren R, Inglis AE. Total shoulder replacement. *Orthop Clin North Am* 1980;11:367–373.
53. Roper BA, Paterson JMH, Day WH. The Roper-Day total shoulder replacement. *J Bone Joint Surg [Br]* 1990;72:694–697.
54. Steffee AD, Moore RW. Hemi-resurfacing arthroplasty of the shoulder. *Contemp Orthop* 1984;9:51–59.
55. Tanner MW, Cofield RH. Prosthetic arthroplasty for fractures and fracture-dislocations of the proximal humerus. *Clin Orthop* 1983;179:116–128.
56. Warren RF, Ranawat CS, Inglis AE. Total shoulder replace-

ment, indications and results of the Neer nonconstrained prosthesis. In: Inglis AE, ed. *American Academy of Orthopaedic Surgeons Symposium, Total Joint Replacement of the Upper Extremity*. St. Louis: CV Mosby, 1982:56–67.
57. Weiss APC, Adams MA, Moore JR, Weiland AJ. Unconstrained shoulder arthroplasty. *Clin Orthop* 1990;257:86–90.
58. Cruess RL. Steroid-induced avascular necrosis of the head of the humerus. Natural history and management. *J Bone Joint Surg [Br]* 1976;58:313–317.

14 Shoulder Arthroplasty for Proximal Humeral Fractures

Gregory P. Nicholson, M.D., Evan L. Flatow, M.D., and Louis U. Bigliani, M.D.

The vast majority of proximal humerus fractures are nondisplaced or minimally displaced, and can be effectively treated with nonoperative methods.[1–7] The four-segment classification of proximal humerus fractures developed by Neer in 1970,[8] which he later simplified,[5,9] made the descriptive account of proximal humerus fractures by Codman[10] clinically relevant, and has become the most widely accepted classification scheme. The classification has prognostic significance, and can guide the treatment of these fractures.[5,8]

Severely displaced fractures of the proximal part of the humerus have not achieved consistently acceptable results when treated with conservative methods[3,6,8,11,12] or open reduction and internal fixation.[8,11–14] Based on the poor results with these forms of treatment, Neer[15] introduced prosthetic arthroplasty for severe fractures of the proximal part of the humerus, and numerous reports in the literature have documented the results of this procedure.[3,8,11,12,16–24] In this chapter, shoulder arthroplasty for fractures of the proximal part of the humerus is discussed, including the evaluation, indications for surgery, operative techniques, complications, and rehabilitation of these difficult injuries.

EVALUATION

The clinical evaluation of the injured limb may be difficult due to pain and swelling. The neurovascular status of the limb must be assessed with a high index of suspicion, as associated injuries are not infrequent.[19] Injuries to the axillary artery are limb-threatening, and should be evaluated with emergency arteriography and vascular surgery consultation. Closed injuries to the brachial plexus or peripheral nerves are initially treated conservatively. Electromyography is obtained at 3 to 4 weeks after injury to help clarify the extent of the injury. A neurologic deficit should not delay definitive management of the fracture. Most injuries are neurapraxias and will resolve sufficiently over time to allow adequate function.[19,25]

To determine if a humeral head replacement is the best treatment option for a proximal humerus fracture, the fracture pattern must be clearly delineated. This is best accomplished with the radiographic trauma series of the shoulder, consisting of three views at right angles to one another.[8] This includes a true anteroposterior view of the scapula (taken 30 to 40 degrees oblique to the coronal plane of the body) and a transscapular lateral or Y-view of the shoulder. The axillary view is extremely important to correctly identify the fracture fragments. This view is taken by abducting the arm 20 to 30 degrees and placing the tube in the axilla with the x-ray plate above the shoulder, without the need to fully abduct the arm. Alternatively, a Velpeau axillary view[26] can be obtained with the patient remaining in a sling and leaning back over the plate and the tube directed downwards.

In the majority of cases, with these three views, the surgeon can identify the fragments and their positions. The guideline for a fracture fragment being classified as a "part" is displacement greater than 1 cm or angulation greater than 45 degrees.[8,9] The critical determination is the status of the head fragment. The loss of blood supply to the head due to fracture displacement can lead to osteonecrosis.[2,5,8,11,13,16,27–29] The head may also be split or have a significant impression defect (greater than 40% involvement) in it (Figure 14–1). Often, this is appreciated only on the axillary radiograph or computerized tomographic scan (Figure 14–2).

In a valgus impacted four-part fracture, the articular segment is rotated down and impacted onto the shaft[30,31] (Figure 14–3). The tuberosities overlie the joint surface, and the articular surface of the head is out of contact with the glenoid. In true fracture-dislocations, the head fragment is completely displaced from the glenoid, anteriorly, posteriorly, or inferiorly. The other fragments or parts are classified based on their position relative to the head fragment. If the head fragment is displaced from both the shaft and the tuberosities, it is a four-part fracture (Figure 14–4). Occasionally, the head is displaced from the shaft and the tuberosities, which remain attached to each other. Since the head has been totally displaced from all bone and soft-tissue attachments, this is classified as a four-part fracture because of the high risk for osteonecrosis. Careful examination of the radiographs and understanding of the guidelines of the classification will help the surgeon correctly classify the injury, assess the risk of osteonecrosis, and thus guide proper treatment.

INDICATIONS FOR SHOULDER ARTHROPLASTY

The acute proximal humerus fractures for which shoulder arthroplasty is indicated are (1) four-part fractures and

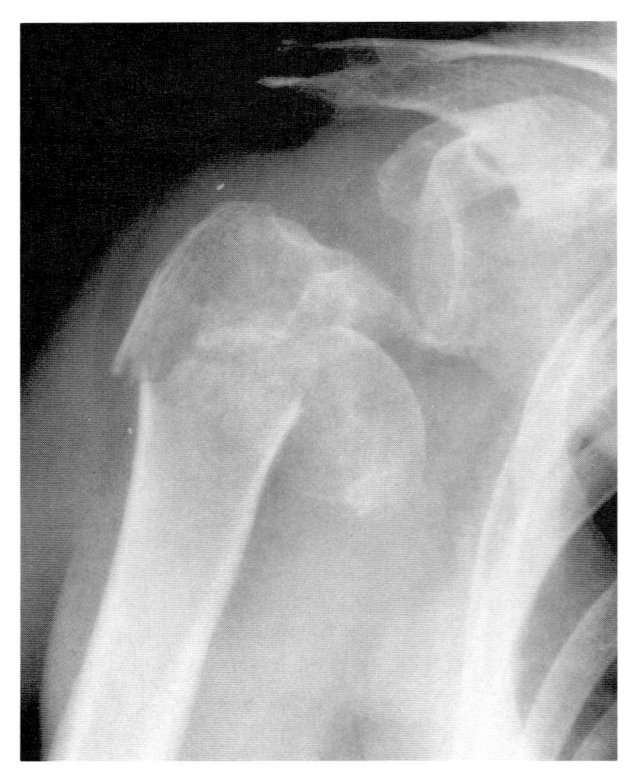

Figure 14–1. In a head-splitting fracture, the articular segment is split with displacement.

fracture-dislocations, (2) head-splitting fractures, (3) impression fractures involving more than 40% of the articular surface, and (4) selected three-part fractures in older patients with osteopenic bone stock. The great majority of severely displaced proximal humerus fractures occur in the older population, with a female predominance.[6,15,17–19,21,23,25] In this population, the bone stock is usually osteopenic and may not hold even minimal internal fixation such as sutures or wires. Medical evaluation of these patients should be expeditious but thorough, so that surgery can be performed ideally within 14 days. This avoids the problems of excessive scarring, contracture, and bony deformity. The surgery is technically easier in the acute setting and pain relief is more predictable.[6,18]

Four-Part Fractures

The literature can be somewhat misleading in regard to the outcome of different treatment methods for four-part fractures, due to the fact that less severe fractures have been included along with the more severe fractures in many series. When only true four-part fractures from the literature are evaluated using a consistent grading scale,[32] a clearer picture evolves. Conservative management of 97 four-part fractures from five series resulted in five (5%) satisfactory outcomes.[3,6,11,12,15] Fifty-six four-part fractures treated with open reduction and internal fixation from five other series were evaluated, and only 17 (30%) satisfactory outcomes were noted.[11–15] Nine series of humeral head replacements for four-part fractures (171 shoulders) were evaluated in the same way, and 136 (80%) satisfactory results were obtained.[4,6,11,12,18,20,22–24,33]

Critical reading of the literature supports shoulder arthroplasty as the best treatment option for four-part fractures and fracture-dislocations regardless of age. Some authors have advocated disimpaction and elevation of the articular segment in valgus impacted four-part fractures, with fixation of the tuberosities below the head.[30,31] In selected young patients, an attempt at open reduction and internal fixation may be reasonable, but the risk of osteonecrosis is high, and the results have not been comparable to those of humeral head replacement.[4,11,12,24,27,33] Those patients who physically or mentally cannot participate with the postoperative care or rehabilitation can be treated conservatively, because the results of surgery with poor aftercare are often worse than those with no surgery at all.[19,25]

Head-Splitting Fractures

Head-splitting fractures, in which the articular surface is split and the fragments displaced, are more common than previously thought.[19] Reducing and holding these fracture fragments with internal fixation is difficult. Head-splitting fractures may or may not have additional displaced parts as components to the injury, but part analysis is difficult. For example, if half the head is with the greater tuberosity, half with the lesser tuberosity, and both are displaced from the shaft, there are three fragments. However, this would not be classified as a three-part fracture, but rather as a head-splitting fracture. The authors' preference is for prosthetic replacement in most of these severe injuries.

Head Impression Fractures

Fractures that result in large impression defects of the articular surface are usually due to posterior fracture-dislocations. The size of the defect will determine treatment. If the lesion involves more than 40% of the surface, a prosthesis should be utilized.[2,4,16]

Three-Part Fractures

Three-part fractures and fracture-dislocations may be the most uncommon type of displaced proximal humerus fractures. In younger patients, open reduction and internal fixation with wire or heavy sutures can achieve satisfactory outcomes.[34,35] However, in older patients with poor bone stock, the ability to achieve stable fixation that allows for early motion is often compromised. Prosthetic replacement with tuberosity reconstruction can achieve a solid construct and allow early motion, thus avoiding prolonged immobilization in this elderly population.

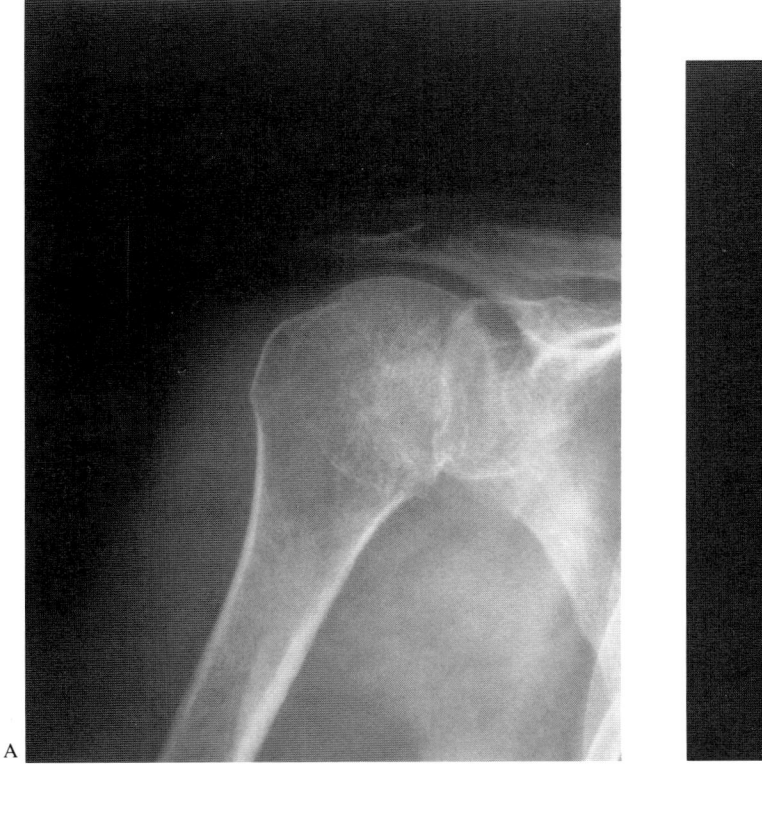

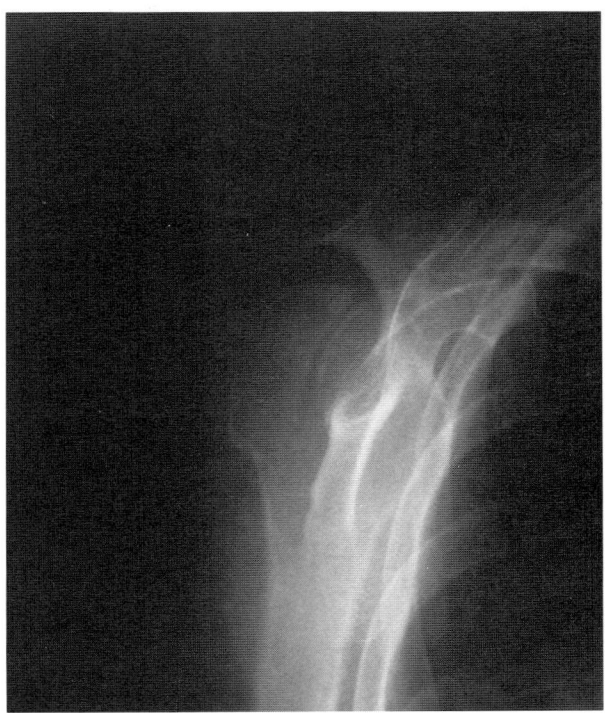

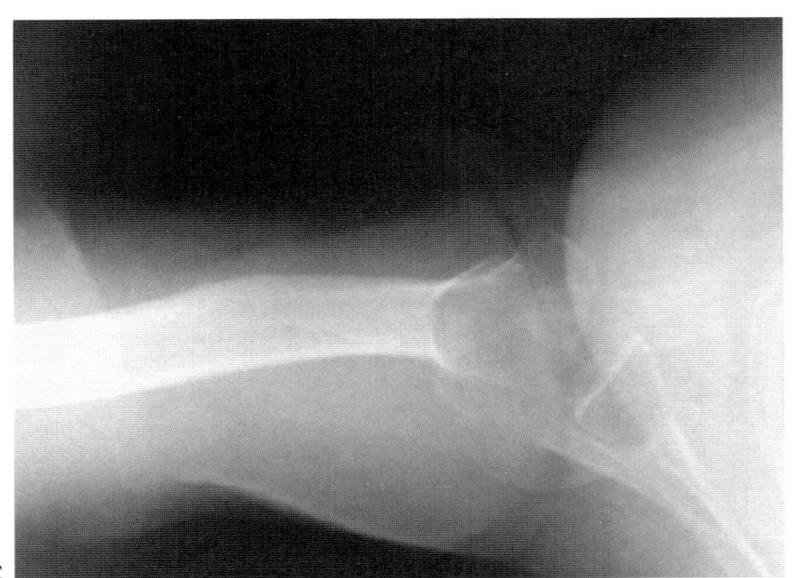

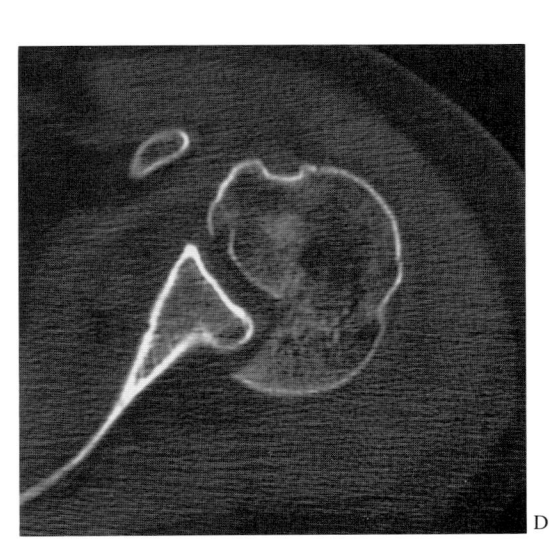

Figure 14–2. A head impression or impaction fracture may not be easily identified on routine anteroposterior (**A**) and lateral (**B**) radiographs. The axillary view (**C**) and computerized tomographic scan (**D**) delineate this injury clearly. This is a posterior fracture-dislocation with significant impaction of the joint surface. This injury requires open reduction of the dislocation, and hemiarthroplasty. There may or may not be significantly displaced parts associated with a head impression fracture.

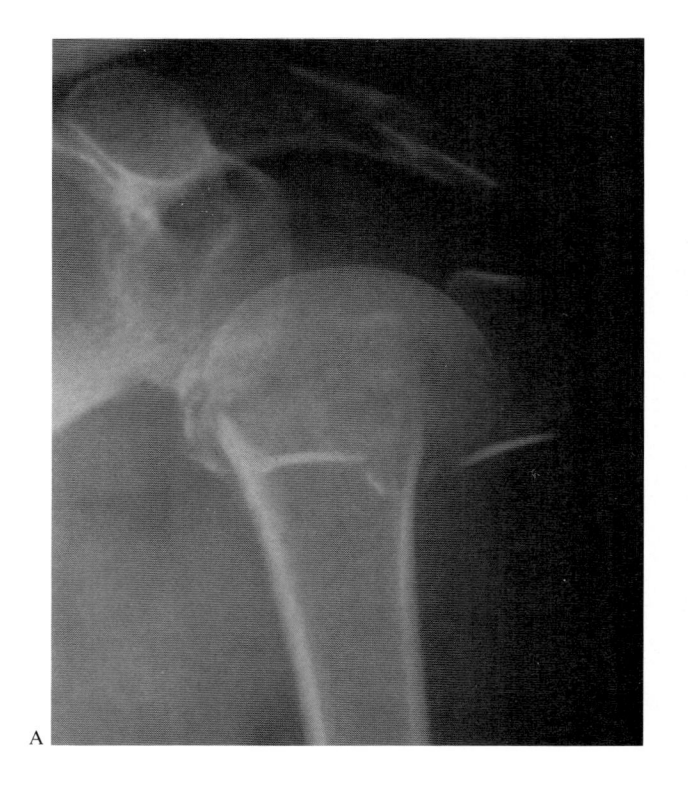

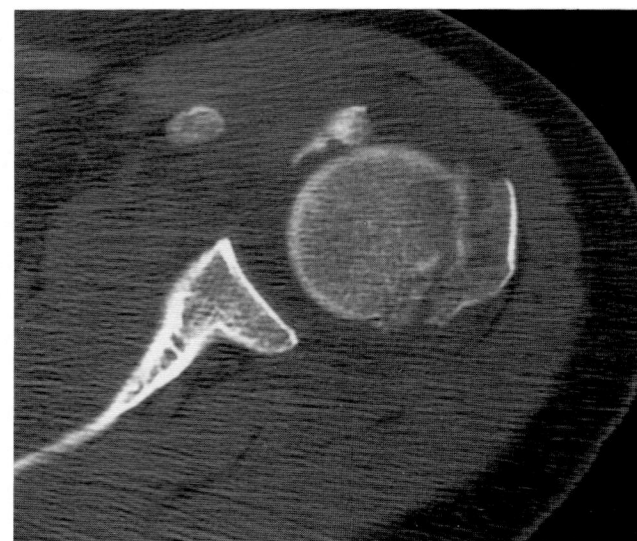

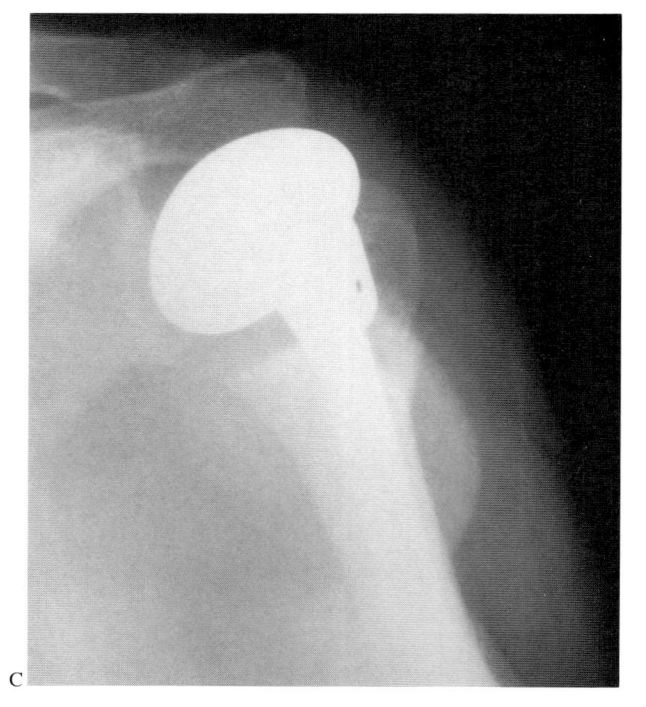

Figure 14–3. **A.** This type of fracture has been termed a "valgus impacted" four-part fracture. The head segment is "impacted" and laterally rotated at least 45 degrees. The tuberosities are displaced and overlie the head. Although this injury initially can appear less displaced than classic four-part fracture-dislocations, it may behave biologically as a four-part fracture as the head is significantly displaced from its blood supply. **B.** The computerized tomographic scan in this type of fracture may be misleading, as the displacement of the head in relation to the glenoid and the tuberosities is underestimated. This is because transverse cuts do not properly demonstrate that the tuberosities are above and overlying the articular surface. **C.** Humeral head replacement was performed, with tuberosity reconstruction below the prosthetic head.

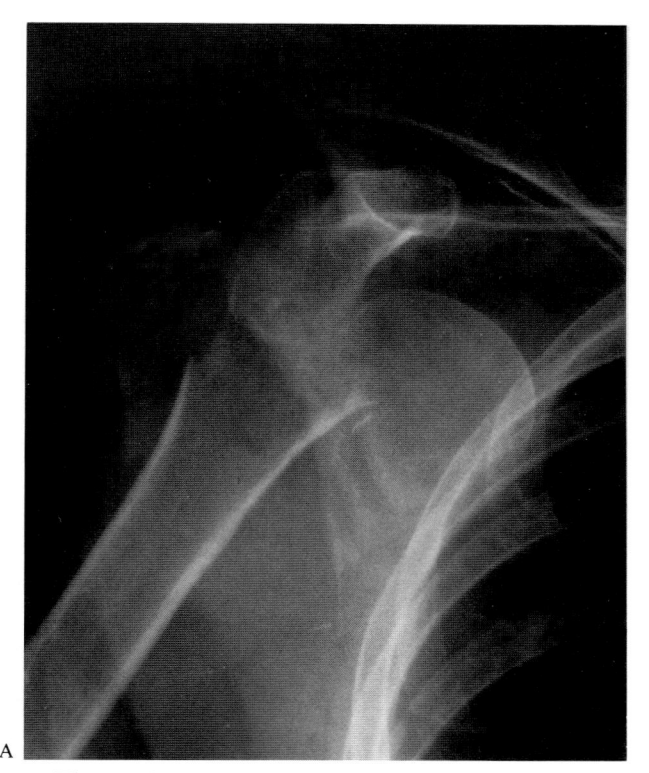

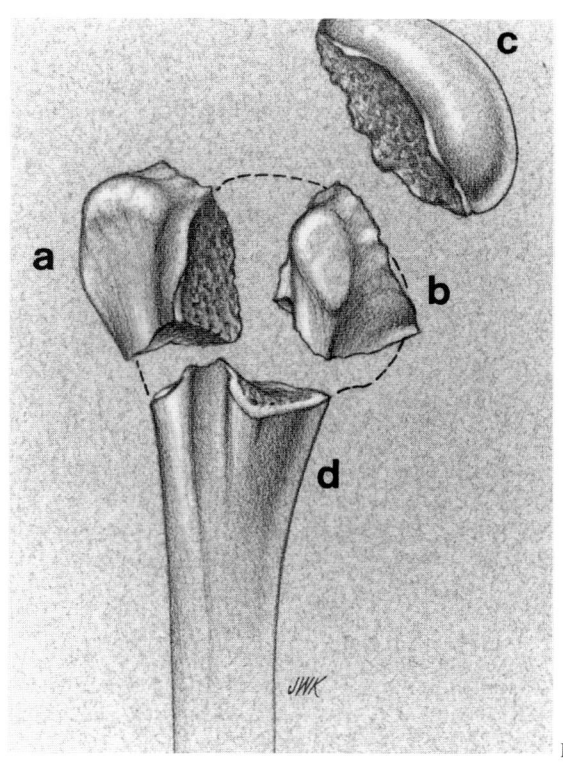

Figure 14-4. **A.** In a classic four-part fracture-dislocation, the head segment is dislocated from the glenoid and separated from all soft-tissue attachments. **B.** The four major anatomic segments are the greater tuberosity (a), lesser tuberosity (b), articular head (c), and humeral shaft (d).

SURGICAL TECHNIQUE

Once the surgeon has determined that surgical intervention is necessary and a shoulder arthroplasty is the best treatment option, certain critical technical factors can influence the outcome.[5,21] The patient is placed in a beach-chair position with the arm draped free so that it can be repositioned during surgery. Interscalene regional block anesthesia is used; it gives excellent muscle relaxation and facilitates exposure. A small roll is placed under the medial border of the scapula to hold it forward. A headrest is used and the operated limb is supported by a short armboard that can be moved to provide maximum mobility to the limb. Prophylactic broad-spectrum antibiotics are administered preoperatively and continued for 48 hours postoperatively.

A long deltopectoral approach is made with an incision from the clavicle over the edge of the coracoid to the area of the deltoid insertion. The deltopectoral interval is utilized with preservation of the cephalic vein. The deltoid origin is preserved. If proximal shaft comminution exists or more exposure is needed, the pectoralis major insertion can be partially released. Instead of elevating the deltoid insertion up to 1 cm as needed, the arm can be abducted to relax the deltoid and provide exposure, thus maintaining the deltoid insertion intact.

The clavipectoral fascia lateral to the conjoint tendon is then incised, exposing the hemorrhagic bursa and fracture hematoma. The coracoid muscles are gently retracted medially and the bursa and hematoma removed to expose the rotator cuff and fracture site. The anterior fascicle of the coracoacromial ligament can be excised to facilitate exposure superiorly. The identification of the fracture fragments may not be easy due to humeral head dislocation. The long head of the biceps will guide the surgeon to the rotator cuff interval, since the greater tuberosity lies lateral and the lesser tuberosity medial to the biceps tendon and groove. The biceps tendon is preserved and the tuberosities with their accompanying rotator cuff tendons are identified. Stay sutures are placed through the tendon-bone junctions, and around the tuberosities. The tendon may be stronger and hold suture fixation better than small comminuted or osteopenic fracture fragments will.

The fracture site is entered by retracting the subscapularis and lesser tuberosity medially. If the head segment has been posteriorly dislocated, the shaft and greater tuberosity are gently retracted laterally so that it can be removed. If the head has been dislocated anteriorly, care must be taken to identify the position of the neurovascular structures prior to pulling the head fragment free. The head fragment may be under or against the neurovascular bundle, and adhesions may be present, especially in the subacute setting. Careful blunt dissection around the head fragment is used to free it up and allow safe removal. The head fragment is saved and used for cancellous bone graft if needed. No other bone cuts or bone débridement are performed.

The armboard is moved up the table to allow the limb to be extended and externally rotated. This maneuver brings the shaft into the wound, and the medullary canal is prepared with sequential rasps and reamers. The prosthetic trials are used to determine the proper stem size, head size, retroversion, and height of the implant. The proper height and retroversion will restore the length and tension to the myofascial sleeve, and allow placement of the tuberosities under the prosthetic head. If the prosthesis is placed down on the remaining shaft, this will almost always be too low. The tuberosities will not fit below the prosthesis, and the myofascial sleeve will be lax. Conversely, the joint should not be stuffed or overtightened, as stiffness may result. The shoulder should have about 50% push-pull, in both anterior-posterior and superior-inferior directions with the trial prosthesis in place. The head should be positioned in 30 to 40 degrees of retroversion to maximize stability (Figure 14–5). This position can be identified by comparing the head position with the distal epicondylar axis of the humerus.

The proper head diameter should allow stability and closure of the rotator cuff around the prosthesis without undue tension. The previously placed sutures in the tendon-tuberosity parts aid in mobilization and reduction of the tuberosity–rotator cuff units, helping to determine proper head size and height. If there is proximal shaft comminution, this must be reduced and held with sutures or wires to reconstruct the proximal bony envelope.

In most fracture cases, a secure press-fit with rotational stability cannot be obtained, and methylmethacrylate is recommended. Prior to cementing, drill holes are made in the proximal shaft and nonabsorbable no. 2 or 5 sutures are placed. These will be used to secure the tuberosities to the humeral shaft, and need to be placed prior to cementing the prosthesis into place. Three to four sutures are used for the greater tuberosity, and two to three for the lesser tuberosity. The prosthesis is then cemented into place, with proper retroversion and height maintained. Excess cement is removed from the bone edges, so as not to impede healing of the tuberosities to the shaft.

The next critical step is to secure the tuberosity reconstruction. This is accomplished utilizing the previously placed large nonabsorbable sutures. The tuberosities are reduced below the level of the prosthetic head and secured to the fin of the prosthesis, to each other, and most importantly, to the shaft of the humerus (Figure 14–6). The tuberosities must be

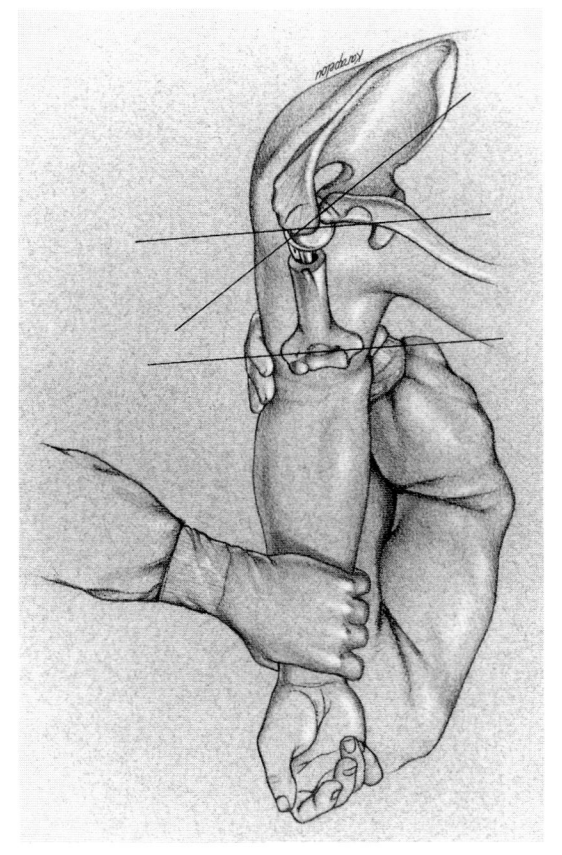

Figure 14–5. The prosthesis should be placed in 30 to 40 degrees of retroversion for acute fractures. This position can be determined by palpating the distal epicondylar axis of the humerus and positioning the prosthesis accordingly.

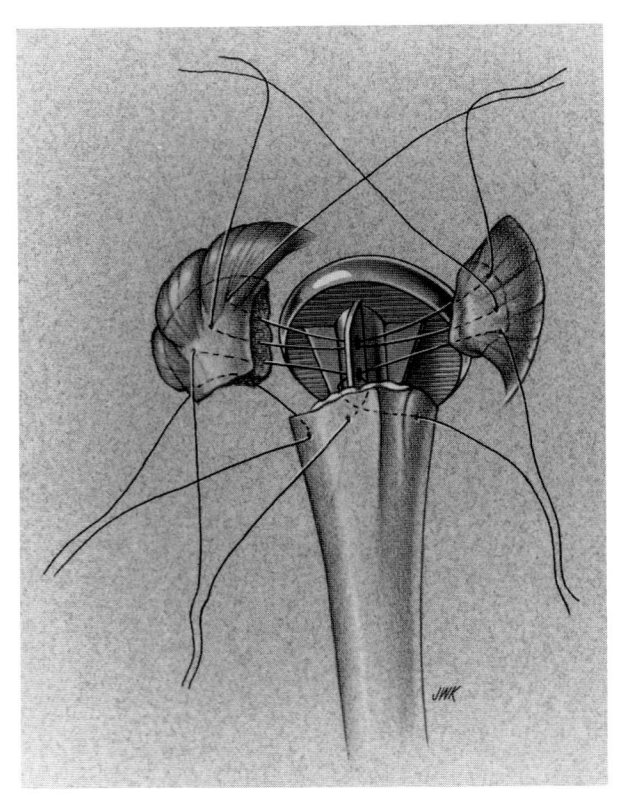

Figure 14–6. With the prosthesis placed with the proper height and retroversion, the tuberosities must fit below the head. The previously placed "pull-down" sutures are now used to secure the tuberosity segments to the shaft. The tuberosities are also secured to the prosthetic fin and to each other.

secured below the prosthetic head or impingement in the subacromial space will occur with attempted elevation of the limb. The tuberosity sutures prevent the muscle forces of the rotator cuff from elevating the tuberosity fragments off the shaft and above the head. The tuberosities should also be fixed through the holes in the prosthetic fin and to each other with heavy sutures.

The rotator cuff interval between the supraspinatus and subscapularis is closed with no. 0 nonabsorbable sutures and the biceps tendon is placed back in the groove, completing the reconstruction (Figure 14–7). If any bone graft is needed, it can be placed under the tuberosity segments prior to definitive fixation. The arm is placed through a careful range of motion and the reconstruction observed. The surgeon can assess the stability of the tuberosity reconstruction and limit postoperative motion accordingly. Suction drains are placed in the subdeltoid space and the deltopectoral interval is reapproximated. Following skin closure, the limb is immobilized in a sling and swathe.

The critical technical points were discussed by Neer and McIlveen.[21,22] The origin of the deltoid is preserved and not elevated. Minimal bone is resected, and any bone graft needed is taken from the head segment that has been removed. The proper height and retroversion of the implant restore the mechanical advantage of the shoulder joint, allowing proper tension in the myofascial sleeve and stability of the construct. The tuberosity repair must be secure, with nonabsorbable suture fixation of the tuberosities to the prosthesis, to each other, and most importantly, to the humeral shaft. Lastly, but most importantly, early passive motion is begun under physician supervision.

REHABILITATION

Proper postoperative rehabilitation is essential because adequate motion of the shoulder is required for optimum function of the limb. The most widely used protocol is the three-phase system devised by Hughes and Neer.[36] The physician directs the therapy throughout the postoperative period, and each patient has the program individualized to his or her specific needs. Compliance with therapy may indeed have a greater affect on the ultimate outcome than any other single factor.[19]

Passive shoulder motion is begun early on the first postoperative day, as are passive and active range-of-motion exercises for the ipsilateral elbow and hand. The surgeon determines the limits to early motion based on the intraoperative assessment of stability following shoulder reconstruction. Consideration is given to the quality of the bone, the status of the rotator cuff muscles and deltoid, and the strength of the tuberosity fixation to the shaft and prosthesis.

The patients' ability to participate in physical therapy and understand the restrictions on activity is crucial. The first goal of therapy is to restore and then maintain motion of the glenohumeral complex. The patient must understand that this is accomplished with only passive motion in the early postoperative period. The desire of the patient (and physical therapist) to begin active or light strengthening exercises must be overcome. Regaining strength of the shoulder girdle must be delayed until healing of the tuberosities has occurred. This becomes evident on radiographs at around 6 to 8 weeks. A greater tuberosity pulloff will lead to a poor result.[19,23]

After surgery, a sling is worn, except while exercising, for 6 weeks. Gravity-assisted pendulum exercises are done to warm up and obtain confidence. Passive elevation in the scapular plane and supine passive external rotation limited to 20 to 30 degrees are begun. The therapist then begins working with the patient on the second day. The exercises are continued in the passive mode only for 6 weeks, with no internal rotation or pulley exercises employed. This is to allow the tuberosities to adequately heal. Prior to discharge from the hospital, the patient should achieve 140 degrees of scapular plane elevation and 30 degrees of external rotation.

When there is evidence of tuberosity healing at approximately 6 weeks, active-assisted elevation with a pulley and isometric strengthening exercises for the rotator cuff are initiated. At approximately 8 weeks active elevation of the

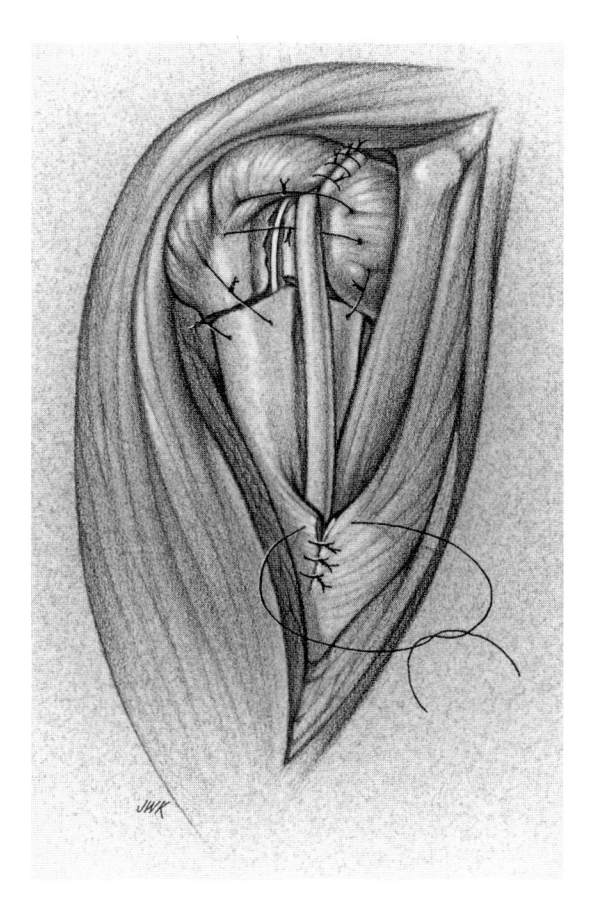

Figure 14–7. The rotator cuff interval is closed and the biceps tendon, which has been preserved, is placed back in the groove. If the pectoralis major tendon was released, it can also be repaired.

arm is begun. Activities of daily living such as personal hygiene, eating, and washing are allowed, and these help build early muscle strength and endurance. Gentle stretching is allowed in this phase to make sure that motion is being maintained. These stretches are gentle and emphasize full glenohumeral and scapulothoracic elevation. Placing the hand on the wall or on a door jam and leaning in to stretch the arm up into elevation are excellent exercises.

Resistive strengthening exercises are begun at about 12 weeks. Graduated rubber bands and light hand weights of 1 to 3 lb will be used and are instituted if the patient has near-full range of motion and is experiencing no pain with therapy. Functional activity is encouraged to a greater extent during phase III. The patient must be encouraged at every phase, and understand that therapy should continue for at least 6 months, and preferably 1 year, to achieve optimum functional results.

PROSTHETIC REPLACEMENT FOR CHRONIC FRACTURES

Prosthetic replacement can also be utilized for the reconstruction of fractures that have gone on to pain and impaired function. Fracture malunions may result in poor motion due to impingement of a prominent or malunited greater tuberosity, poor rotator cuff function, or pericapsular stiffness. The surgery in chronic malunion cases is technically demanding due to distorted bony anatomy and soft-tissue scarring, with greater blood loss, higher complication rates, and less predictable function postoperatively.[6,18] Pain relief is good but not as reliable as in the acute fracture setting.

If surgery is needed in a chronic malunion case, it is important the patient understands that pain relief is the primary goal, and functional improvement is secondary. A malunited greater tuberosity fragment may be prominent and impinge superiorly against the acromion. Tuberosity osteotomy could be performed if necessary to place the prosthesis above the level of the tuberosity, but it is usually better to avoid osteotomy if possible (Figure 14–8). Often, an acromioplasty can also be utilized to enlarge the subacromial space, and the prosthesis set above the tuberosity. Soft-tissue adhesions in the subdeltoid space should be lysed and the rotator cuff inspected and repaired if necessary. Early motion is again under direct physician supervision.

Nonunions of the surgical neck can occur with two-part fractures or as a component in a more severe fracture pattern. The few cases in the literature have been primarily treated with open reduction, internal fixation, and iliac crest bone grafting.[25,37,38] In a recent review of 20 surgical neck nonunions treated surgically at the New York Orthopaedic Hospital, humeral head replacement was found to be comparable in treatment outcome to open reduction, internal fixation, and bone grafting, but without the subsequent hardware problems that followed the internal fixation cases (Bigliani, LU and Flatow, EL, unpublished data 1992). In those cases that had a failed early attempt at fracture fixation, humeral head replacement was clearly superior to another attempt at open reduction and internal fixation with bone grafting. The surgical neck nonunion is a challenging reconstructive problem, and in this review, humeral head replacement was comparable if not superior to open reduction and internal fixation, providing 60 to 80% satisfactory results.

The osteopenic bone stock of the head, often eroded by the pseudoarthrosis, the pericapsular stiffness of the glenohumeral joint, and the difficulty in obtaining stable fixation with hardware between the head fragment and the shaft are all problems that can compromise the outcome of surgery for a malunited fracture. These problems can be overcome with the use of a hemiarthroplasty. The osteopenic, usually malpositioned humeral head itself is removed. Ample cancellous bone is left on the tuberosity segments that are created by osteotomy from the head segment. The rotator cuff insertions are preserved on their respective tuberosity segments and the rotator cuff is mobilized. A prosthesis is cemented in place and the tuberosities are fixed to the shaft of the humerus. The pericapsular scar and stiffness must be aggressively released to restore motion (Figure 14–9). Hardware removal is not required, and the need for fracture fixation in an osteopenic head fragment is eliminated. Most importantly, prolonged immobilization of the shoulder girdle is not required, and early passive motion may be instituted.

COMPLICATIONS

The causes of failure after prosthetic replacement for proximal humerus fractures were recently examined by Bigliani et al.[39] Almost all failed cases had multiple causes, but the most common single identifiable reason was greater tuberosity displacement.[39] Tanner and Cofield[23] identified greater tuberosity displacement as the most common complication in their series. When greater tuberosity displacement occurs, the results are poor.[19,23,39] Proper surgical technique with meticulous tuberosity fixation and the use of only passive motion until evidence of tuberosity healing is seen radiographically can reduce the risk of this complication.

Loosening of the prosthesis itself has been identified as a cause of failure.[39] In the series by Bigliani et al.,[39] all cases of aseptic loosening occurred after uncemented implantation. These fractures generally occur in older shoulders with wide, osteoporotic medullary canals, and all proximal bone support important for rotation stability is lost due to comminution. Therefore, methylmethacrylate should be routinely used, and the immediate stability obtained will allow early motion and muscle rehabilitation, which are the keys to success.

Neurovascular injuries usually occur at the time of injury. Injury to the axillary artery can occur, especially in anterior fracture-dislocations. A high index of suspicion should be maintained and an arteriogram obtained if there is any question of a vascular injury. A careful preoperative assess-

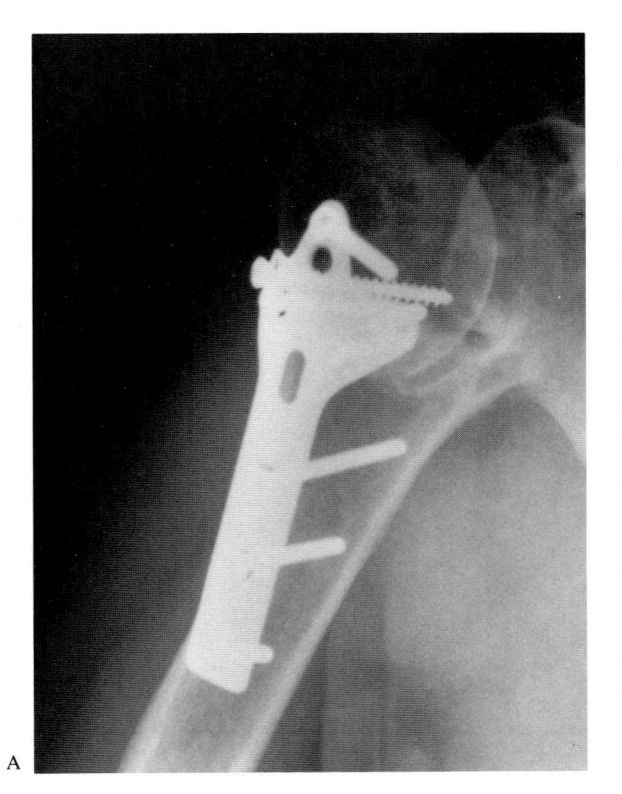

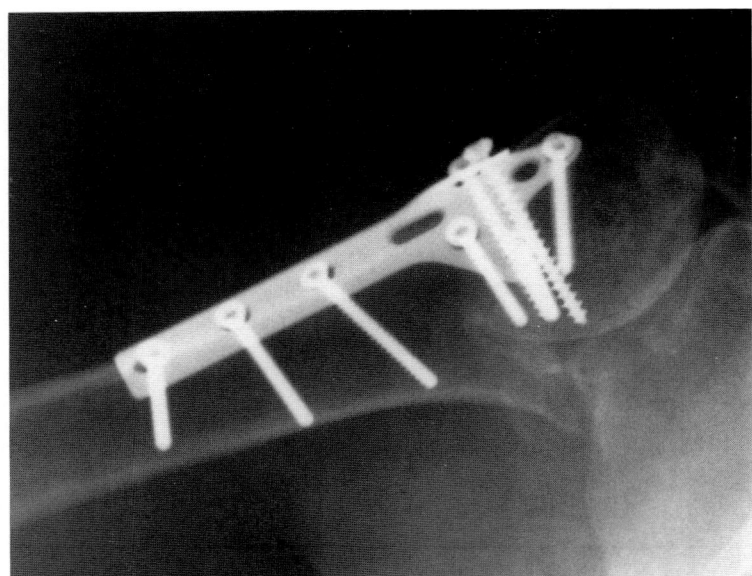

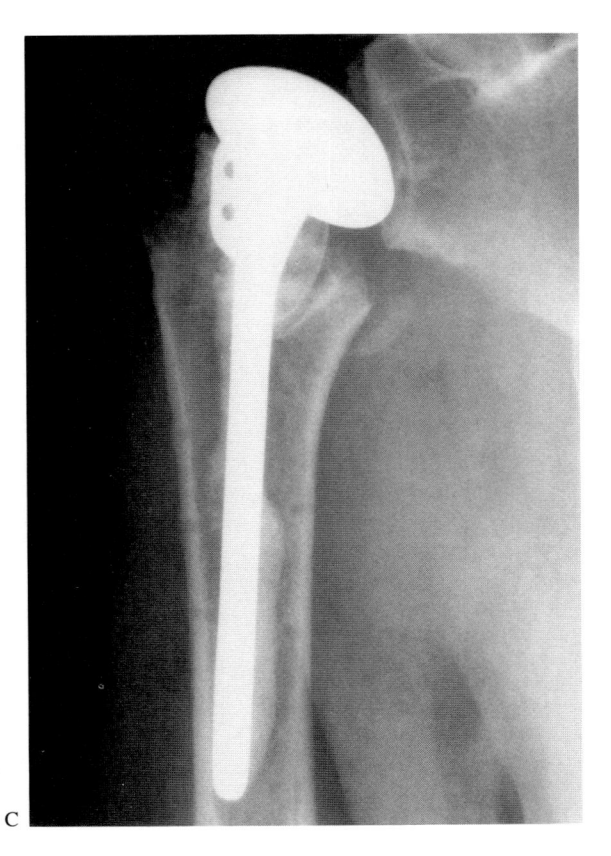

Shoulder Arthroplasty for Proximal Humeral Fractures   191

Figure 14–8. **A** and **B.** A malunion of a proximal humerus fracture after open reduction and internal fixation. The medial aspect of the shaft is articulating with the inferior aspect of the glenoid, the greater tuberosity is prominent, and the head has cystic changes. **C.** A humeral head replacement was performed with minimal bone removal. The prosthesis was placed so that it was medial to the proximal aspect of the shaft. The greater tuberosity was "excavated" so that the prosthesis could fit into and above it to prevent lateralization of the tuberosity, and to avoid impingement. An acromioplasty was also performed.

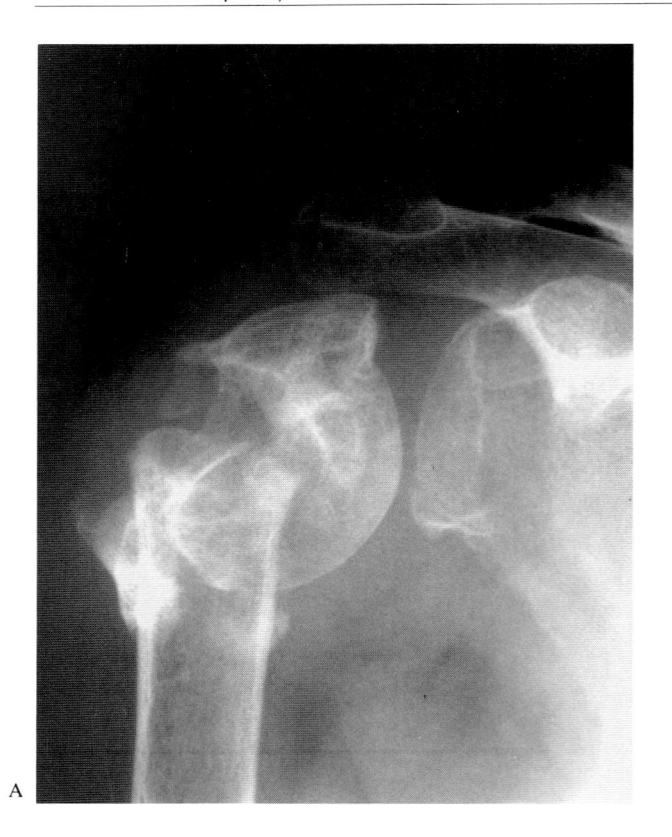

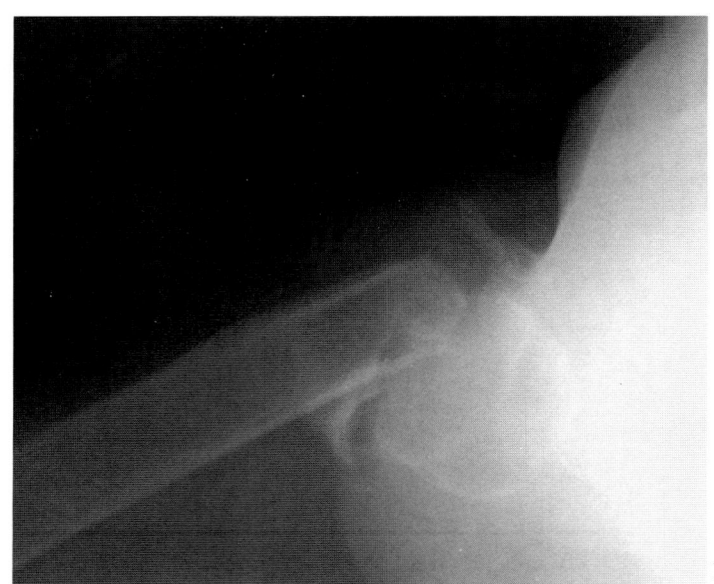

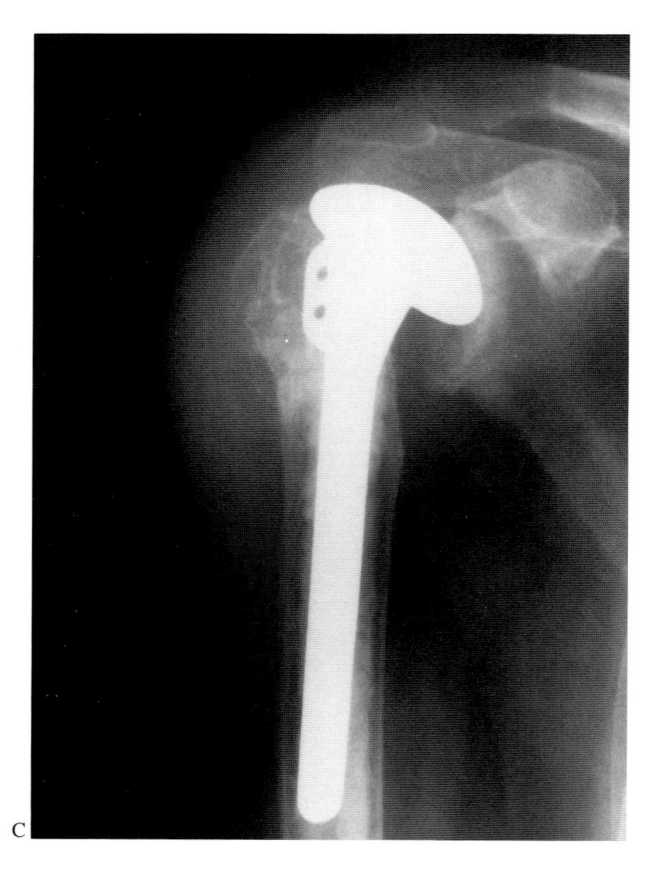

Figure 14–9. **A** and **B.** Anteroposterior and axillary views of a surgical neck nonunion, with malposition and osteopenia of the head fragment. **C.** The osteopenic, malpositioned, scarred head has been removed, but large tuberosity bone–rotator cuff segments have been maintained. The nonunion has been eliminated with the placement of a cemented prosthetic replacement. The tuberosities were reconstructed below the head and healed to the shaft. The need for immobilization, which allows an internally fixed nonunion time to heal, has been eliminated. Early passive motion was started.

ment is necessary to identify any neurologic injuries. Approximately 1 in 10 fractures will have a neurologic or vascular injury.[19]

Other complications that can occur include heterotopic ossification, which is usually mild and not a cause of poor motion; soft-tissue contracture; deep infection; glenoid erosion (not a common problem in long-term series); and prosthetic instability.[4,6,15,17,19,20,21,23,25,33]

REFERENCES

1. Bigliani LU. Fractures of the proximal humerus. In: Rockwood CA Jr, Matsen FA III, eds. *The Shoulder*. Philadelphia: WB Saunders, 1990;1:278–334.
2. Bigliani LU. Fractures of the proximal humerus. In: Rockwood CA Jr, Green DP, Bucholz RW, eds. *Fractures in Adults*. 3rd ed. Philadelphia: JB Lippincott, 1990;1:871–927.
3. Leyshon RL. Closed treatment of fractures of the proximal humerus. *Acta Orthop Scand* 1984;55:48–51.
4. Neer CS II. Displaced proximal humeral fractures, part II. Treatment of three-part and four-part displacement. *J Bone Joint Surg [Am]* 1970;52:1090–1103.
5. Neer CS II. Fractures about the shoulder. In: Rockwood CA Jr, Green DP, eds. *Fractures*. 1st ed. Philadelphia: JB Lippincott, 1984;1:585–623.
6. Svend-Hansen H. Displaced proximal humeral fractures. A review of 49 patients. *Acta Orthop Scand* 1974;45:359–364.
7. Young TB, Wallace WA. Conservative treatment of fractures and fracture-dislocations of the upper end of the humerus. *J Bone Joint Surg [Br]* 1985;67:373–377.
8. Neer CS II. Displaced proximal humeral fractures, part I. Classification and evaluation. *J Bone Joint Surg [Am]* 1970;52:1077–1089.
9. Neer CS II. Four-segment classification of displaced proximal humeral fractures. *Instr Course Lect*. 1975;24:160–168.
10. Codman EA. *The Shoulder*. Boston: Thomas Todd, 1934.
11. Kristiansen B, Christiansen SW. Proximal humeral fractures. Late results in relation to classification and treatment. *Acta Orthop Scand* 1987;58:124–127.
12. Stableforth PG. Four-part fractures of the neck of the humerus. *J Bone Joint Surg [Br]* 1984;66:104–108.
13. Paavolainen P, Bjorkenheim J-M, Slatis P, Paukka P. Operative treatment of severe proximal humeral fractures. *Acta Orthop Scand* 1983;54:374–379.
14. Yamano Y. Comminuted fractures of the proximal humerus treated with hook plate. *Arch Orthop Trauma Surg* 1986;105:359–363.
15. Neer CS II. Articular replacement for the humeral head. *J Bone Joint Surg [Am]* 1955;37:215–228.
16. Bigliani LU, McCluskey GM. Prosthetic replacement in acute fractures of the proximal humerus. *Semin Arthroplasty* 1990;1:129–137.
17. Cofield RH. Comminuted fractures of the proximal humerus. *Clin Orthop* 1988;230:49–57.
18. Frich LH, Sojbjerg JO, Sneppen O. Shoulder arthroplasty in complex acute and chronic proximal humeral fractures. *Orthopedics* 1991;14:949–954.
19. Fischer RA, Nicholson GP, McIlveen SJ, McCann PD, Flatow EL, Bigliani LU. Primary humeral head replacement for severely displaced proximal humerus fractures. *Orthop Trans* 1992;16:779.
20. Kraulis J, Hunter G. The results of prosthetic replacement in fracture-dislocations of the upper end of the humerus. *Injury* 1976;8:129–131.
21. Neer CS II, McIlveen SJ. Recent results and technique of prosthetic replacement for 4-part proximal humeral fractures. *Orthop Trans* 1986;10:475.
22. Neer CS II, McIlveen SJ. Replacement de la tete humerale avec reconstruction des tuberosities et de la coiffe dan les fractures desplacees a 4 fragments. Resultats actuals et techniques. *Rev Chir Orthop* 1988;74 (Suppl II):31–40.
23. Tanner MW, Cofield RH. Prosthetic arthroplasty for fractures and fracture-dislocations of the proximal humerus. *Clin Orthop* 1983;179:116–128.
24. Willems WJ, Lim TEA. Neer arthroplasty for humeral fractures. *Acta Orthop Scand* 1985;56:394–395.
25. Sorensen KH: Pseudarthrosis of the surgical neck of the humerus. *Acta Orthop Scand* 1964;34:132–138.
26. Bloom MH, Obata WG. Diagnosis of posterior dislocation of the shoulder with use of Velpeau axillary and angle-up roentgenographic views. *J Bone Joint Surg [Am]* 1967;49:943–949.
27. Fourrier P, Martini M. Post-traumatic avascular necrosis of the humeral head. *Int Orthop* 1977;1:187–190.
28. Gerber C, Schneeberger AG, Vinh T-S. The arterial vascularization of the humeral head. An anatomic study. *J Bone Joint Surg [Am]* 1990;72:1486–1494.
29. Sturzenegger M, Fornaro E, Jakob RP. Results of surgical treatment of multifragmented fractures of the humeral head. *Arch Orthop Trauma Surg* 1982;100:249–259.
30. Jakob RP, Kristiansen T, Mayo K, Ganz R, Muller ME. Classification and aspects of treatment of fractures of the proximal humerus. In: Bateman JE, Welsh RP, eds. *Surgery of the Shoulder*. Philadelphia: BC Decker, 1984:330–343.
31. Jakob RP, Miniaci A, Anson PS, Jaberg H, Osterwalder A, Ganz R. Four-part valgus impacted fractures of the proximal humerus. *J Bone Joint Surg [Br]* 1991;73:295–298.
32. Neer CS II, Watson KC, Stanton RJ. Recent experience in total shoulder replacement. *J Bone Joint Surg [Am]* 1982;64:319–337.
33. Marotte JH, Lord G, Bancel P. L'arthroplastie de Neer dans les fractures et fractures-luxations complexes de l'epaule: Aprops de 12 cas. *Chirurgie* 1978;104:816–821.
34. Cuomo F, Flatow EL, Miller SR, Maday MG, McIlveen SJ, Bigliani LU. Open reduction and internal fixation of 2- and 3-part proximal humerus fractures. *Orthop Trans* 1990;14:588.
35. Hawkins RJ, Bell RH, Gurr K. The three-part fracture of the proximal part of the humerus. Operative treatment. *J Bone Joint Surg [Am]* 1986;68:1410–1414.
36. Hughes M, Neer CS II. Glenohumeral joint replacement and postoperative rehabilitation. *Phys Ther* 1975;55:850–858.
37. Coventry MB, Laurnen EL. Ununited fractures of the middle and upper humerus. Special problems in treatment. *Clin Orthop* 1970;69:192–198.
38. Scheck M. Surgical treatment of nonunions of the surgical neck of the humerus. *Clin Orthop* 1982;167:255–259.
39. Bigliani LU, Flatow EL, McCluskey GM, Fischer RA. Failed prosthetic replacement for displaced proximal humerus fractures. *Orthop Trans* 1991;15:747–748.

15 Arthritis of Dislocation

John J. Brems, M.D.

The pathologic entity referred to as arthritis of dislocation was first discussed by Neer et al. in 1982.[1] They recognized that within the class of degenerative arthritis is a group of patients who had a history of surgical repair for instability. Questions arose regarding the etiology of arthritis within this subgroup. In studying those patients who had surgical repairs for instability, several factors that were thought to be responsible for the development of arthritis were identified. Samilson and Prieto[2] made similar observations and defined a condition called dislocation arthropathy of the shoulder. They found radiographic evidence of arthritis in patients who had just one dislocation and furthermore concluded that posterior instability results in a higher incidence of arthritis.

In the last few years, there have been several reports discussing probable contributing factors to the development of this condition.[3-5] It is hoped that in recognizing some of the probable iatrogenic factors related to the arthritis of dislocation, surgical techniques may be modified to minimize its incidence.

This chapter reviews those surgical factors that are probably involved in the etiology of arthritis of dislocation. In the absence of a statistically controlled population, one cannot establish a valid cause-and-effect relationship between those factors. Nevertheless, several factors that have a strong association with the development of arthritis of dislocation have been identified.

ETIOLOGY

Nonsurgical Factors

There is very little information published regarding the incidence of arthritis following glenohumeral dislocations. Rowe[6] and others discussed the complications associated with acute shoulder dislocations, such as fractures, cuff tears, nerve injuries, and recurrent instability, but little mention is made of the late complication of arthritis. Even in Samilson and Prieto's series[2] of 74 patients, only 16 developed arthritis, and 6 of those had delayed reduction of a posterior dislocation. They further found that the number of recurrent dislocations did not increase the likelihood for the development of arthritis. There was a positive correlation between patient age at the time of dislocation and the development of arthritis. The older the patient at the time of initial dislocation, the more likely the development of arthritis. There was no correlation found between the presence of a Hill-Sachs defect, glenoid rim fracture, or severity of trauma with the development of arthritis of dislocation.

It is virtually impossible to calculate and predict the incidence of arthritis developing in an unstable shoulder. Due to the fact that most patients are very young and mobile, long-term patient tracking and follow-up are nearly impossible. Furthermore, the long time interval between the traumatic incident and development of arthritis may be several decades. So many other countless minor traumatic episodes likely occur during this interval, making the cause-and-effect relationship difficult to establish.

Considering the very large numbers of people who sustain shoulder dislocations, together with the relative rarity of glenohumeral arthritis, it does not seem plausible that shoulder instability by itself is a significant risk factor for the development of arthritis. Unreduced dislocations and associated displaced articular fractures certainly will lead to arthritis, but the statistical probability for developing glenohumeral arthritis following recurrent reducible dislocations or subluxations, treated nonoperatively, remains impossible to prove but must be necessarily small. Although it is difficult to identify causative factors between glenohumeral arthritis and instability when managed nonoperatively, there are several well-identified surgical factors that strongly predispose the patient to developing arthritis of dislocation.

Surgical Factors

Understanding and treating shoulder instabilities are the most difficult of all shoulder problems. Classification of instability itself seems to become increasingly complex as we develop a more complete understanding of the mechanical, physiologic, kinematic, neurologic, and psychogenic aspects of shoulder instability. Assessment of each of these factors is critical in delivering proper and effective treatment for shoulder instability. It is the failure to address the instability in these terms that leads to inappropriate or incomplete treatment. Inappropriate or incomplete nonoperative treatment will probably not result in arthritis, but this same inappropriate or incomplete surgical treatment will lead to arthritis inevitably. Unfortunately, the arthritis of instability develops while patients are young and productive. Hence, their disability is relatively greater when compared to those who develop arthritis in later life.

FAILURE TO DIAGNOSIS DEGREE AND DIRECTION OF INSTABILITY

Assessing the direction of instability is not always as simple as one might expect. When the patient arrives at the office with a radiograph documenting an anterior dislocation, the assessment appears easy. Unfortunately, not all instabilities are traumatic or complete dislocations. Furthermore, these apparently well-documented instabilities are not always anterior, nor are they necessarily unidirectional. The athlete with the documented traumatic dislocation may have had a history of inferior or posterior subluxations that were unrecognized.

Consider the gymnast or competitive swimmer who presents with anterior shoulder pain, yet has no frank history of instability. Routine clinical examination reveals anterior apprehension; 6 weeks of rotator cuff strengthening fails to diminish the symptoms and a Bristow procedure is contemplated. A more detailed history would likely reveal a pattern of hyperlaxity with paresthesias in the involved extremity and a subjective feeling of "loose" joints, frequently with a history of chondromalacia patellae. A more thorough physical examination would likely reveal multidirectional instability with laxity evident posteriorly and inferiorly as well as anteriorly. There would likely be a dimple or sulcus sign; the asymptomatic shoulder would likely reveal a very similar painless laxity pattern with global instability (Figure 15–1). General examination would likely reveal some degree of elbow hyperextensibility, excessive laxity of the metacarpophalangeal joints, and hyperflexibility of the wrists. Any procedure designed to tighten just the front of this shoulder joint would likely result in posterior subluxation.

Often with the patient in pain, the office examination is difficult, and it may take repeated examinations on repeated visits to fully appreciate the degree and direction of the instability. Only when there is a thorough assessment of both the symptomatic and the asymptomatic shoulder, based on repeated examinations, can the proper surgical procedure be planned. Failure to diagnosis the scope and direction of the instability puts a patient at increased risk for the development of arthritis of dislocation.

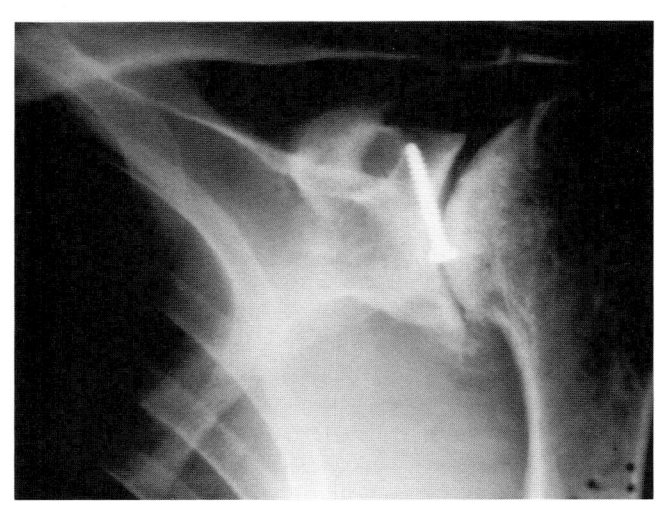

Figure 15–2. True anteroposterior view of the shoulder, showing degenerative joint changes with loss of humeral head sphericity, loss of joint space, and glenoid osteophyte formation associated with a loose screw. At arthrotomy, the head of the screw was intra-articular.

COMPLICATIONS OF METAL

Zuckerman and Matsen[7] discussed complications related to the use of screws and staples around the shoulder joint. Until their publication, little had been written regarding the problems of metal used in and around the shoulder. They reviewed a series of 37 patients, 21 of whom developed arthritis when screws were used as part of the instability repair and 14 of whom developed similar problems when staples were used. The hardware need not be placed in poor position to cause problems. Screws, staples, pins, wires, and other nonbiologic materials may fracture, fragment, or migrate,[8] which then may result in joint destruction. Intra-articular screws, staples, and bone fragments also likely lead to rapid deterioration of the joint (Figures 15–2 and 15–3).

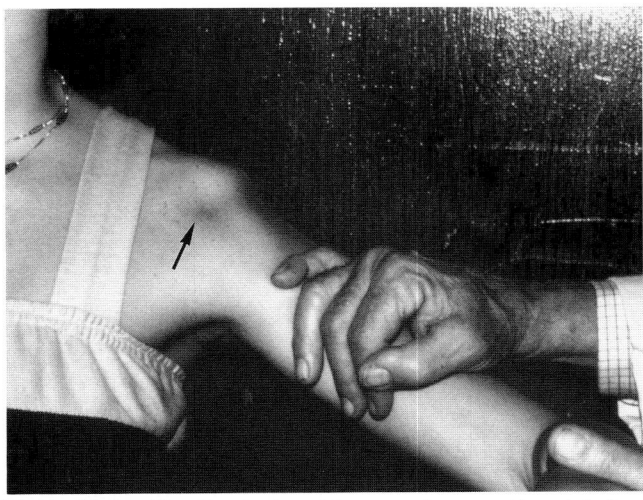

Figure 15–1. The dimple sign at the arrow is seen with an inferior stress applied to the shoulder. This degree of laxity is consistent with probable multidirectional shoulder instability.

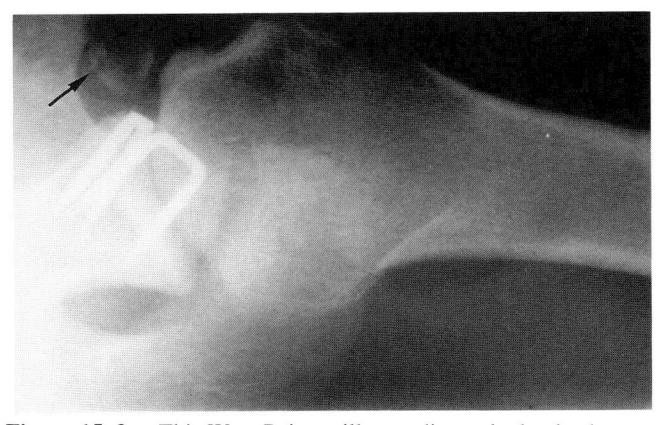

Figure 15–3. This West Point axillary radiograph clearly shows two staples within the glenohumeral joint. A loose body is present at the arrow and considerable degenerative changes are seen, with narrowing of the glenohumeral joint space.

The hardware fixation device may remain outside the joint proper, but if the shoulder remains unstable, the head may come in contact with the hardware as it dislocates. The head of the screw or staple may become impaled or impressed on the humeral head, leading to subsequent cartilage degeneration (Figure 15–4).

Although the use of staples and screws for instability repairs has been successful in many patients worldwide, injudicious use and placement can lead to rapid joint destruction. Even when properly placed intraoperatively, the potential for hardware failure, fracture, and migration always exists. Newer soft-tissue techniques, though not foolproof, seemingly eliminate this one major cause of severe joint destruction in young active people.

ONE STANDARD PROCEDURE FOR ALL

Causes of shoulder instability are indeed multifactorial and complex. Muscle, bone, ligament, and nerve are all variably involved. Added to that list are psychological factors, including volition, motivation, disability interpretation, and secondary gain. Genetic factors and recreational factors also influence clinical shoulder instability. With these many variables involved, it hardly seems reasonable to expect one or two surgical procedures alone to manage them all. In fact, most instability repairs are designed to address specific anatomic defects.

Although for surgeons it is easy and tempting to become familiar and content with one type of instability repair, the universal application of one procedure to manage all instabilities is another major factor in the development of arthritis. The Putti-Platt procedure cannot possibly help the posterior subluxating shoulder; the Bristow cannot properly treat the unstable shoulder caused by malrotation of a surgical neck fracture; the Magnuson-Stack procedure cannot possibly treat the shoulder with multidirectional instability.

The orthopaedic surgeon who treats shoulder instabilities must become familiar and confident with the array of procedures available to treat them. The procedures must be adapted to and address the specific pathology in each individual case. One cannot expect that the entire spectrum of instability can be managed with one type of "favorite" procedure.

THE WRONG SIDE

Another major surgical cause for the development of arthritis of dislocation is performing the procedure on the wrong side of the joint. Understanding the degree and direction of the instability may be difficult and requires repeated clinical examinations. Radiologic documentation of instability at the time of acute injury is uncommon, as the shoulder is often reduced before the patient arrives at the emergency room. Furthermore, many clinically unstable shoulders can subluxate and do not frankly dislocate. The office examination is difficult to perform because of patient apprehension and muscle guarding. Pain is poorly localized, the asymptomatic shoulder may have more laxity than the symptomatic one, and the patient history may offer no clue as to the direction of the instability. Hawkins and Schutte[9] discussed the use of intraoperative fluoroscopy to assist in diagnosing the direction of instability in those cases where the office examination was inconclusive. The arthroscope is an additional diagnostic tool available to the shoulder surgeon, but significant pitfalls exist (vide infra). Tightening the wrong side of the joint results in an imbalance of ligamentous forces and with time, degenerative joint disease will ensue.

If a patient has posterior laxity and sustains a traumatic anterior dislocation, anterior repairs such as a Putti-Platt, Magnuson-Stack, or Bristow procedure will likely result in the development of degenerative changes. Excessive relative tightening of the anterior structures will displace the humeral head posteriorly, resulting in joint incongruity, cartilage wear, and ultimately osteoarthritis. In the same way, a posterior glenoid osteotomy in the face of anterior laxity will likely cause further anterior instability and arthritis.

The concept of balance cannot be overemphasized. Surgical procedures for shoulder instability, regardless of type, should have the primary goals of reestablishing and rebalancing capsular tension on all sides of the joint. Hawkins and Angelo[10] discussed the association of degenerative joint disease in the shoulder resulting from imbalance and excessive tightening of tissues on one side of the joint.

INAPPROPRIATE USE OF THE ARTHROSCOPE

The arthroscope has brought tremendous advances in the management of intra-articular processes. In the shoulder, it has furthered our understanding of ligament anatomy through visualization of structures in an in vivo state; it has

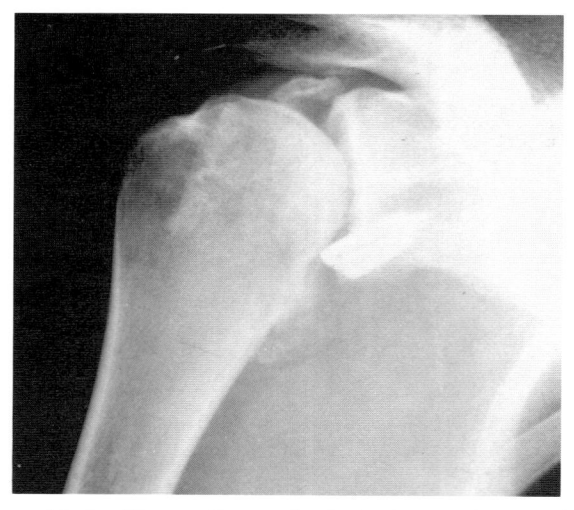

Figure 15–4. These arthroscopic staples became loose and remained intra-articular in the anterior-inferior quadrant of the glenohumeral joint, causing severe joint destruction in this 23-year-old man.

advanced our understanding of pathologic processes; and it has permitted surgical procedures to be performed with less tissue morbidity, less expense, and less patient discomfort.

But the arthroscope suffers the same failings as the scalpel when held by an inexperienced surgeon. The arthroscope may indeed be damaging when it gouges and scrapes the articular surfaces. Arthroscopic management of instability repairs can result in intra-articular staples, migration of metal, and secondary degenerative changes (Figure 15–5). Biodegradable tacks are now under development and may obviate some of these problems.

A variety of arthroscopic procedures and techniques are being developed to treat instabilities, but none afford the opportunity to balance tissues circumferentially. Some surgeons promote the arthroscopic treatment of multidirectional instability using arthroscopic sutures through one bone hole. Whether these newer techniques treat the instability remains to be seen. More importantly, long-term evaluation should be mandatory before these newer techniques are routinely performed. To date, no well-performed arthroscopic stabilization procedure has the statistical long-term success rate as the best-performed open procedure. One should remain hesitant to jump in too early and perform these nonanatomic arthroscopic instability repairs. Perhaps with the introduction of biodegradable fixation devices, arthroscopic Bankart repairs may become safe and effective without increasing the incidence of arthritis.

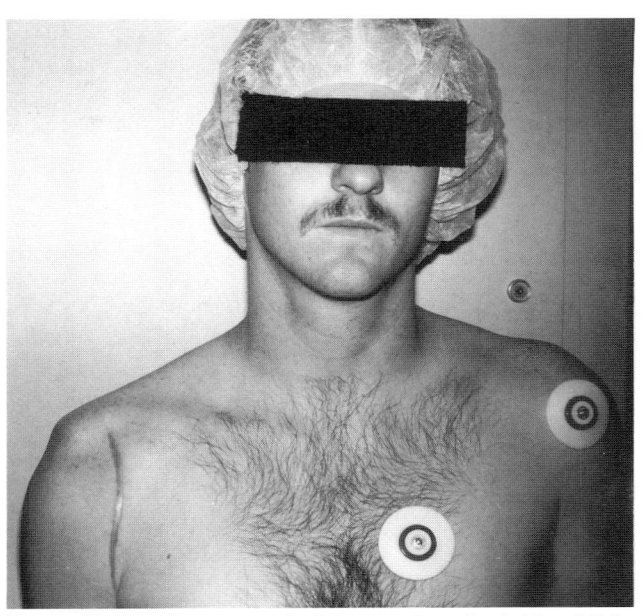

Figure 15–6. The most typical presentation of arthritis of dislocation is a young person with one or several scars around the shoulder, deltoid atrophy, and loss of joint motion from progressive arthritis.

CLINICAL PRESENTATION

The most typical clinical feature of patients with arthritis of dislocation is their young age (Figure 15–6). In two series,[1,11] the average age of patients with this disabling condition was 38 years. In each of these series, there were patients in their 20s who had such advanced arthritis that prosthetic shoulder arthroplasty was necessary. When traumatic fractures and rheumatoid arthritis were excluded, nearly all patients with glenohumeral arthritis under the age of 40 had prior repairs for instability, and all had one or more of the surgical factors identified above.

Patients present with pain that is usually associated with activity, but as motion becomes increasingly impaired, rest pain and night pain increase. Motion becomes more restricted, and the activities of daily living become more difficult with the loss of internal and external rotation. The inability to reach up the back, to pass a belt, and to reach into the back pocket becomes more and more difficult as the condition progresses. As external rotation becomes limited, patients complain of the inability to reach the back of their head and experience difficulty in dressing, particularly in placing the arm through a shirt or coat sleeve. If the patient rolls over onto the involved shoulder while sleeping, the arm is forced into adduction. When motion in this plane is restricted, pain occurs and the patient is awakened.

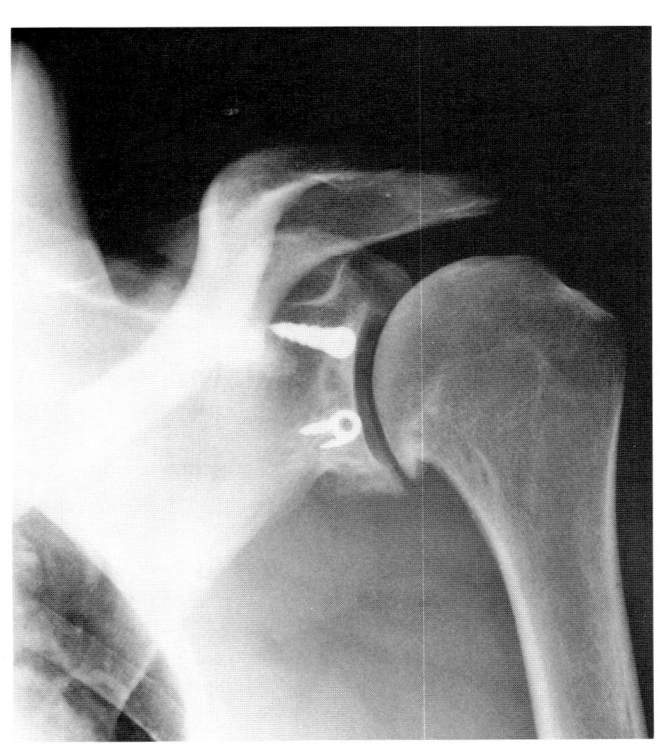

Figure 15–5. This true anteroposterior projection shows two arthroscopic staples. The inferior one shows bent prongs and the inferior tong appears loose. Early degenerative changes are seen, with osteophytes present on the inferior glenoid and projecting inferiorly on the anatomic neck of the humerus.

When obtaining a history, the physician should inquire about prior treatment. It is surprising how many patients have been treated for a frozen shoulder because a radiograph documenting arthritis was never obtained. Many patients have been through extensive physical therapy programs for their stiff joint and, not surprisingly, their pain only increased as the physical therapist tried to mobilize their arthritic shoulder joint.

The physical examination begins with observation. If appropriate, the examining physician should watch the patient undress. Considerable information concerning the limitation of motion and function can be obtained at this time. Even the type of clothing worn may provide some insight as to the extent of disability. Both shoulders must be free of all clothing material. As observation continues, the examiner views the patient not only from the front, but also from the side and back as well (Figure 15–7). This allows one to compare shoulder morphology and muscle development. Asymmetric muscle contours likely represent atrophy from muscle or nerve injury. The location of prior surgical scars, along with their length, direction, and condition, is noted.

While viewing the patient from the side in a sitting or standing position, particular note should be made regarding the relationship between the arm and the coronal plane (Figure 15–8). Often there is malposition of the arm because of a fixed anterior or posterior subluxation. This occurs when a prior surgical procedure tightened one side of the joint and pushed the humeral head in the opposite direction.

In palpating the shoulder, the examiner usually finds specific joint-line tenderness and the presence of diffuse tenderness throughout the neck and shoulder region. The neck is always examined to rule out cervical causes of shoulder pain. Limited glenohumeral motion may result in ipsilateral neck pain secondary to trapezius strain as the trapezius tries to rotate the scapula during elevation.

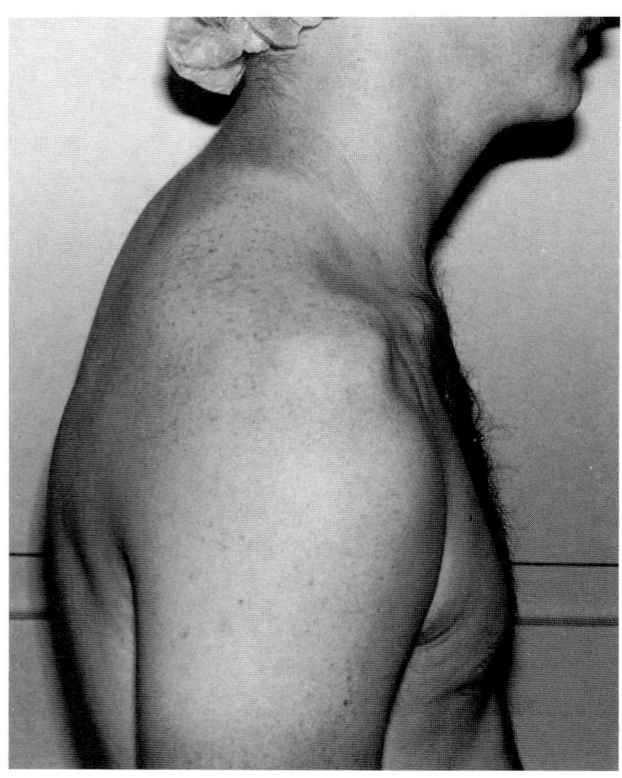

Figure 15–8. This side view of the patient seen in Figure 15–6 shows the humeral axis anterior to its anatomic position, as if the arm is in a fixed anterior subluxated position. A prior procedure left the posterior capsule excessively tight, forcing the humerus anteriorly.

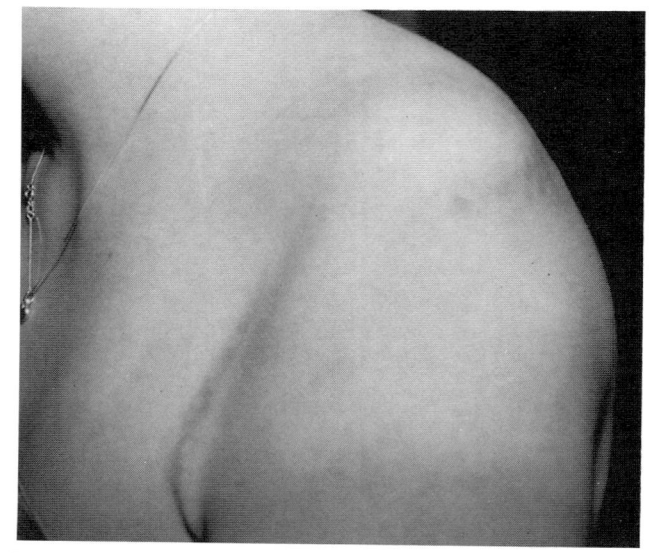

Figure 15–7. The patient must be examined from all perspectives. This side view demonstrates an anterior and posterior scar with the classic anterior muscle wasting and the prominent acromion from lateral or posterior deltoid injury.

The range of shoulder joint motion is measured and recorded. The specifics in measurement of shoulder motion are recorded elsewhere.[12] Total shoulder elevation, glenohumeral elevation, external rotation, and internal rotation all become increasingly limited as the condition progresses. Crepitus is usually perceived while the range of motion is being assessed. Often there is such severe limitation of motion that residual laxity that may have caused the condition cannot be appreciated. A strength assessment and peripheral nerve assessment complete the physical examination. In recording strength of the deltoid (anterior, middle, and posterior heads) and rotator cuff muscles, the examiner must understand how pain may influence strength. A strength assessment in the face of pain may give a false interpretation of muscle condition. Despite a careful, well-performed neurologic examination, if patients have had prior surgery and are contemplating total shoulder arthroplasty, an electromyogram, specifically of the axillary nerve and the suprascapular nerve, may also be helpful.

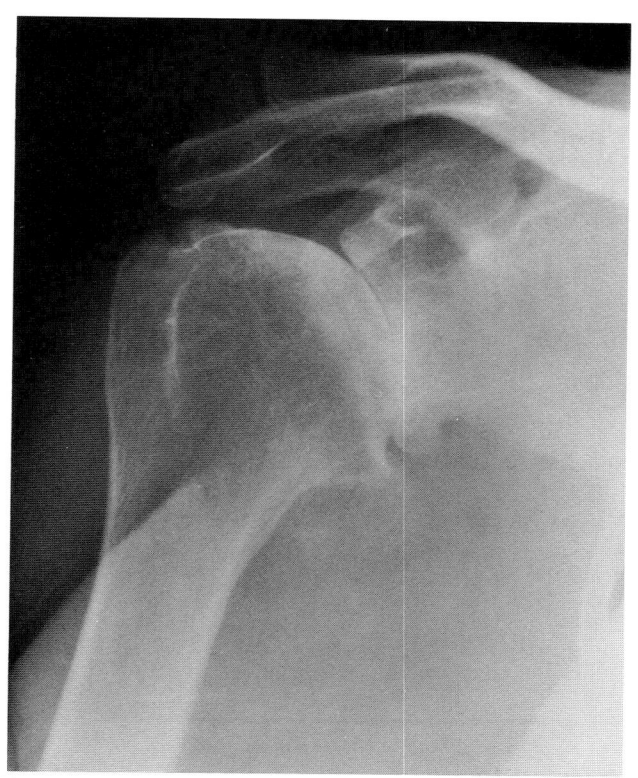

Figure 15–9. This true anteroposterior projection shows advanced osteoarthritis in this 34-year-old who had a Putti-Platt repair 6 years earlier. There is a complete loss of glenohumeral joint space, and large glenoid and humeral osteophytes. Total external rotation at that time was less than 5 degrees.

RADIOLOGIC EVALUATION

A standard shoulder series is obtained, including true anteroposterior and axillary lateral projections (Figure 15–9 and 15–10). The true anteroposterior projection shows the status of the glenohumeral joint space, the length of glenoid neck, and inferior humeral and glenoid osteophytes. Evidence of prior surgery is usually seen with the presence of hardware, bone blocks, or osteotomies. Disuse osteopenia is a characteristic feature of advanced arthritis regardless of cause and is nearly always seen.

The axillary lateral projection provides considerable information regarding the anterior-posterior relationship of the glenohumeral joint. This view also reveals evidence of prior surgery with hardware such as screws and staples. Particular information regarding a fixed malposition is best seen on this projection. Following anterior repairs with excessively tightened anterior capsular ligaments, one sees a fixed, posteriorly subluxated arthritic joint. The converse is also true regarding excessive tightening of the posterior structures resulting in a fixed, anterior subluxation. Glenohumeral joint congruity, articular cartilage thickness, wear patterns of the glenoid, and glenoid bone stock and version are best appreciated on this film.

A computerized tomography scan may provide additional information in planning a total shoulder arthroplasty.[13] The relationships of the glenohumeral joint are well seen. Glenoid orientation, neck-face angle, and bone stock assessment are possible with computerized tomographic scanning, but pitfalls exist. Despite its increasing popularity, no indications exist for magnetic resonance imaging of the shoulder with this condition.

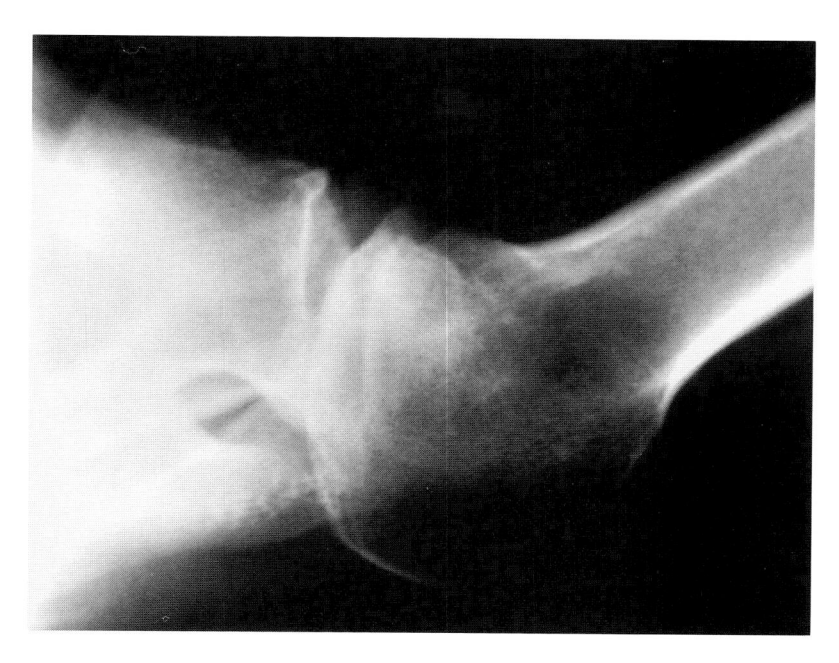

Figure 15–10. This West Point axillary projection shows advanced osteoarthritis of dislocation. Note the fixed posterior position in this patient, 7 years following a Putti-Platt procedure.

Patients who complain of neck pain as part of their clinical syndrome should have anteroposterior, lateral, and oblique views of the cervical spine obtained. If indicated, consultation with a spine surgeon is entertained.

SURGICAL CONSIDERATIONS

Despite the young age of patients with arthritis of dislocation, shoulder arthroplasty is the procedure of choice. Frequently, the arthritis involves both the humeral head and the glenoid. Consequently, total shoulder arthroplasty is indicated. If, in the judgment of the surgeon, the glenoid articular cartilage is of sufficient quantity and quality, humeral head hemiarthroplasty alone may be considered.

Although these patients are young, shoulder arthrodesis should rarely be considered as a surgical alternative in this condition. In the 1990s, shoulder arthrodesis is rarely indicated for aseptic arthritis regardless of patient age. Similarly, cheilectomy should not be considered. At best, it is only temporizing, providing no more than minimal pain relief and insignificant improvement in motion. Cheilectomy only adds one more surgical procedure, resulting in more scar and muscle injury.

Shoulder arthroplasty should be performed when the joint cartilage has been destroyed by the arthritic process. The surgeon should be cautioned that despite the young age of these patients, delaying the procedure only results in more soft-tissue contractures, muscle atrophy, and progressive glenoid bone loss. The surgical technique for shoulder arthroplasty has been well described.[14–16] Specific considerations associated with arthritis of dislocation are now discussed.

Incisions

Nearly all patients with the arthritis of dislocation have one or more surgical scars on their involved shoulder. These scars are often widened, occasionally hypertrophic, and frequently not present in the ideal location for the surgical approach to an arthroplasty. Fortunately, the vascular supply around the shoulder is abundant and skin necrosis is distinctly uncommon. For that reason, and because excellent exposure is required for shoulder arthroplasty, crossing of prior incisions, even at acute angles, can be done if necessary. The best surgical approach for shoulder arthroplasty is through the deltopectoral interval, keeping the entire deltoid origin intact. A long straight incision is used, beginning at the anterior border of the clavicle, passing over the tip of the coracoid process, and terminating over the deltoid insertion. It is unlikely that the prior surgical procedures for instability repair were performed through this type of incision. If a deltopectoral scar is present at the time of shoulder arthroplasty, then it should be excised.

Deltoid Muscle

When multiple procedures have been performed about the shoulder, the deltoid muscle likely becomes injured. Frequently, there is extensive intramuscular scarring in addition to the scar and adhesions that form between the undersurface of the deltoid and rotator cuff. Not infrequently, the anterior deltoid is severely atrophied with little recognizable muscle tissue present. Electromyographic study of the complete deltoid should then be performed prior to surgery, and too often one finds injury to the branches supplying the anterior head of this muscle.

As the surgical dissection progresses, all adhesions between the rotator cuff and deltoid should be released. A combination of sharp and blunt dissection is required to minimize muscle injury while being particularly careful to avoid injuring the axillary nerve and its branches.

A functioning anterior deltoid is critically important in forward elevation of the shoulder. Even the strongest rotator cuff with an absent or weakened anterior deltoid will result in severe dysfunction of the arm. In those patients with severe anterior deltoid loss, the lateral head may be released from the lateral acromion and advanced medially. Particular care must be given to proper reattachment of the transferred origin. An abduction pillow or brace is recommended for 6 to 8 weeks to protect the muscle repair. During this time, however, aggressive passive range-of-motion exercises are performed to minimize the inevitable adhesions that will again form within the subacromial space.

Rotator Cuff and Capsule

Most anterior instability repairs or surgical approaches for them involve the subscapularis muscle and tendon. This results in scarring and dense adhesions between the subscapularis and coracoid muscles, which must be released, always remaining cognizant that the musculocutaneous nerve is very close to the dissection field. In addition to completely releasing these adhesions, the subscapularis tendon must be lengthened to prevent loss of external rotation. Increasing external rotation is possible only with proper restoration of the physiologic tendon length.

Occasionally, a Z-plasty lengthening is required to ensure that adequate length is available at the time of rotator cuff closure (Figure 15–11). If, after the superior half of the pectoralis major tendon is released, external rotation cannot reach 40 degrees, then a subscapularis lengthening is performed as the joint is opened. Furthermore, the subscapularis becomes scarred to the base of the coracoid process and must be freed to ensure mobilization of this entire muscle-tendon unit. The coracohumeral ligament, which also becomes shortened, tight, and contracted, must be released from the coracoid process.

A similar lengthening procedure is performed on the infraspinatus muscle if it is shortened and contracted from prior posterior procedures. Additionally, an anterior tightening procedure may result in posterior subluxation and an

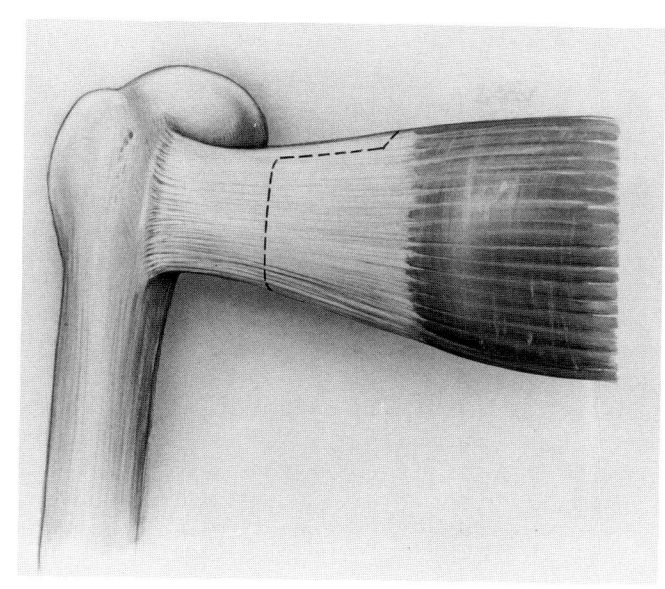

Figure 15–11. If there is considerable anterior or posterior soft-tissue contracture, the rotator cuff is opened in a Z-fashion providing increased length of the soft-tissue sleeve during joint closure.

enlarged posterior capsule. In this case, the enlarged capsule should be reefed and the joint volume diminished to prevent instability following shoulder arthroplasty. Conversely, if a prior posterior repair resulted in anterior subluxation and an enlarged anterior capsule, it too should be tightened at the time of shoulder arthroplasty.

Humerus

Humeral changes in arthritis of dislocation are nonspecific and mimic typical degenerative joint disease. There are periarticular osteophytes at the margins of the joint surface on the anatomic neck. Depending on the extent of the process, there is moderate to complete absence of articular cartilage. Humeral head sphericity is lost, and the head is variably collapsed. As in all shoulder arthroplasties, it is of paramount importance to maintain the proper tension in the myofascial sleeve of the deltoid and rotator cuff to ensure adequate postoperative function. This is accomplished by maintaining as much humeral length as possible and by positioning the humeral component above the tip of the greater tuberosity (Figure 15–12).

The version of the component must be such that the joint remains stable with internal and external rotation. This balance between stability and motion is critical if one is to achieve a successful arthroplasty with adequate functional results.

In young patients, there is usually very adequate humeral bone stock to provide component stability without requiring methylmethacrylate. If a stable press-fit that permits immediate rotational and axial stability is possible, methylmethacrylate is not needed. Conversely, if doubt exists regarding component stability, methylmethacrylate is used to achieve immediate stability and allow postoperative exercises without risk.

Glenoid

Ideally, the arthroplasty should be performed prior to significant glenoid bone loss. The forces of malposition and subluxation cause the glenoid rim to erode. Most commonly the bone loss is posterior and related to excessive tightening of the anterior capsule and rotator cuff. The anterior aspect of the glenoid exhibits similar erosive patterns with anterior subluxation of the shoulder joint. Unlike the humerus, where there is usually a large amount of bone, the normal glenoid provides minimal bone for prosthesis support and fixation. As the erosion progresses, not only are significant orientation changes occurring, but also progressive bone loss continues. Computerized tomography is valuable in determining glenoid version and may be useful in assessing bone stock available for the prosthesis.[13]

Although there is an ever-increasing variety of glenoid configurations available today, principles of glenoid replacement have not changed. These include the following:

1. Proper sizing of the component to match the surface area of the natural glenoid.
2. Optimal orientation ensuring that the component is not retroverted. Glenoid bone graft is rarely indicated but may be necessary in the face of excessive posterior bone loss. It is generally easier and better to lower the high side of the bone rather than bone graft the low side. As the glenoid surface is moved laterally, the infraspinatus and subscapularis muscles become relatively shortened.

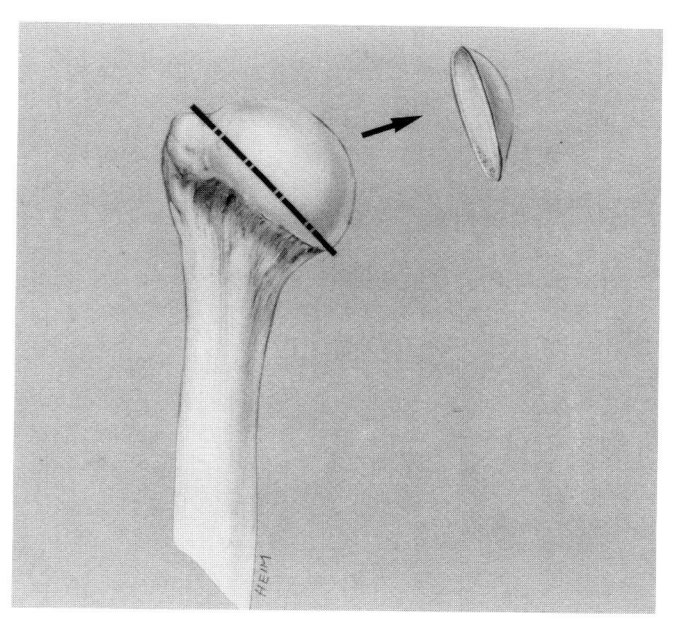

Figure 15–12. Only a small amount of humeral head is removed to be certain that the tension in the myofascial sleeve on both the rotator cuff and the deltoid is maintained. The component must sit above the greater tuberosity to ensure physiologic tension in the rotator cuff and prevent impingement.

3. Preservation of subchondral bone and contouring the glenoid face to ensure subchondral support throughout.
4. Adequate immediate fixation using either methylmethacrylate or screws.
5. Minimal intrinsic constraint of the prosthesis with the humerus to reestablish as near-normal anatomic forces as possible.

Metal-backed components may offer theoretical advantages in the glenoid, but as of yet do not have proven clinical advantages. Newer high-density polyethylenes are thought to exhibit better wear characteristics than conventional ultra-high-molecular-weight polyethylene.

Hardware

In principle, hardware in and around the shoulder joint should be removed at the time of arthroplasty. However, if staples, screws, or metal anchors are deemed to be stable, buried well within bone and not involving the articulation, they may be left in place. Considerable muscle tissues may be damaged when trying to retrieve hardware from bone. Conversely, if preoperative radiographs indicate loose hardware within bone or if the hardware is only within the soft tissues, then every effort should be made to remove it. There is considerable evidence available documenting the ability of this hardware to migrate throughout the body when placed near the shoulder joint.

REHABILITATION

Postoperative rehabilitation following shoulder arthroplasty is discussed in Chapter 7. Only specific concerns as they relate to arthroplasty in arthritis of dislocation are discussed.

The surgeon and physical therapist must carefully balance two competing concerns as the rehabilitation program is initiated and developed. First is the concern related to multiple prior surgeries and excessive dense scarring. Minimizing further scarring requires early and aggressive range-of-motion exercises. The other is concerned about joint stability. Frequently, soft tissues are lengthened on one side of the joint and tightened on the other. Relative rest of the joint is needed to allow adequate soft-tissue healing for maintenance and preservation of stability. Yet if the joint is rested too long, further scarring and contracture will occur. Satisfactory management of this balancing act requires a close interaction and relationship between the patient, physical therapist, and surgeon. Passive range-of-motion exercises should be initiated within 48 hours of surgery, placing the arm in the safe planes of motion.

If the deltoid was injured and required reconstruction or medial advancement, an abduction brace or pillow is used to relieve tension on the repair, but passive exercises in elevation and rotation still begin within 48 hours of shoulder arthroplasty. Specific modifications in the rehabilitation program may be dictated by the degree of laxity and associated intraoperative soft-tissue reconstructions. For example, if there was a large posterior pouch, one would perhaps limit supine elevation and supine forward flexion because muscle and gravitational forces would tend to pull the humeral head into the region of capsular reefing. On the other hand, elevation in the scapular plane would be permitted and strengthening of the infraspinatus may provide a buttress posteriorly.

If there was excessive anterior laxity at the time of shoulder arthroplasty, the surgeon should consider limiting passive external rotation to 40 degrees and strengthen the internal rotators to provide a further buttress against anterior instability.

Motion exercises usually continue for many months to overcome the abundant scar and contractures around the joint. Once passive motion allows elevation of 140 degrees and external rotation of 40 degrees, deltoid and rotator cuff strengthening begin. The concept of balance is important in strengthening the internal and external rotators, and neither one should be performed in excess of the other.

Postoperative Arthroplasty Activities

Patients with arthritis of dislocation who require arthroplasty are young, active, and athletic. Fortunately, the loads experienced by the shoulder joint are continuous and not of an impact nature. This physiologic and kinematic feature allows patients to return to most sporting activities without restriction. Generally, all noncollision–type activities are not only permitted, but encouraged.[17] Activities such as golf, bowling, swimming, archery, dance, and all racquet sports are permitted following total shoulder arthroplasty. Noncollision basketball, baseball, and certain weight-lifting programs are also encouraged.

Those sports that involve collisions or potential collisions are discouraged. The major activities in this category include football, hockey, rugby, and alpine skiing. Most patients return to gainful employment, not just in nonphysical occupations, but also to those duties requiring considerable physical demands.

SUMMARY

Arthritis of dislocation is a unique form of degenerative joint disease involving the shoulder. It seems that a large number of patients who develop arthritis of dislocation have had prior instability repairs. In studying large numbers of patients, several factors seem to recur. Careful, repeated examinations of both the symptomatic and the asymptomatic shoulder may uncover subtle subluxations; examination of other peripheral joints may reveal evidence of hyperlaxity and multidirectional instability. In understanding the nature, direction, and extent of instability patterns, more appropriate stabilization procedures may diminish the incidence of arthritis of dislocation. Today's techniques and the surgical management of instabilities obviate the need for hardware, which has been shown to have significant impact on the incidence of this arthritis. Surgeons should realize the potential benefits and risks of arthroscopic stabilization procedures, and only after satisfactory analyses should these procedures be done by orthopaedic surgeons at large.

When the arthritis of dislocation does develop, shoulder arthroplasty is a reasonable treatment option, despite the young age of patients. In the technique of shoulder arthroplasty for this condition, specific surgical principles must be kept in mind. Preservation of deltoid function is paramount. Restoration of muscle length and proper tensioning are critical for successful functional outcomes. Component positioning and orientation must account for any bone loss and alterations in soft-tissue tension and quality.

No shoulder arthroplasty, no matter how well performed, will be successful without adequate physician-directed rehabilitation. With a well-performed shoulder arthroplasty in a well-motivated patient, joint replacement for arthritis of dislocation should provide long-term satisfaction.

REFERENCES

1. Neer CS, Watson KC, Stanton FJ. Recent experience in total shoulder replacement. *J Bone Joint Surg [Am]* 1982;64:319–337.
2. Samilson RL, Prieto V. Dislocation arthropathy of the shoulder. *J Bone Joint Surg [Am]* 1983;65:456–460.
3. Hawkins RJ, Angelo RL. Glenohumeral arthritis: A late complication of the Putti-Platt repair. *J Bone Joint Surg [Am]* 1990;72:1193–1197.
4. Hawkins RH, Hawkins RJ. Failed anterior reconstruction for shoulder instability. *J Bone Joint Surg [Br]* 1985;67:709–714.
5. Morrey BF, Janes JM. Recurrent anterior dislocation of the shoulder: Long term follow-up of the Putti-Platt and Bankart procedures. *J Bone Joint Surg [Am]* 1976;58:252–256.
6. Rowe CR. Prognosis in dislocation of the shoulder. *J Bone Joint Surg [Am]* 1956;38:957–977.
7. Zuckerman JD, Matsen FA. Complications about the glenohumeral joint related to the use of screws and staples. *J Bone Joint Surg [Am]* 1984;66:175–180.
8. Lyons FA, Rockwood CA. Migration of the pins used in operations on the shoulder. *J Bone Joint Surg [Am]* 1990;72:1262–1267.
9. Hawkins RJ, Schutte JP. The assessment of glenohumeral translation using manual and fluoroscopic techniques. *Orthop Trans* 1988;12:727.
10. Hawkins RJ, Angelo RL. Osteoarthritis following an excessively tight Putti-Platt repair. *Orthop Trans* 1988;12:674.
11. Brems JJ. Shoulder replacement in arthritis of dislocation. *Orthop Trans* 1989;13:235.
12. Neer CS. *Shoulder Reconstruction*. Philadelphia: WB Saunders, 1990:4–10.
13. Friedman RJ, Hawthorne KB, Genez B. Evaluation of glenoid bone loss with computerized tomography for total shoulder arthroplasty. *Orthop Trans* 1991;15:749.
14. Rockwood CA. Technique of total shoulder replacement. *Instr Course Lect* 1990;39:437–447.
15. Cofield RH. Degenerative and arthritic problems of the glenohumeral joint. In: Rockwood CA, Matsen FA, eds. *The Shoulder*. Philadelphia: WB Saunders, 1990;2:718–740.
16. Brems JJ, Wilde AH. Arthroplasty principles. In: Watson MS, ed. *The Shoulder*. London: Churchill-Livingstone, 1991:459.
17. Neer CS, Brems JJ. Shoulder replacement in the athletic and active patient. In: Jackson DW, ed. *Shoulder Surgery in the Athlete*. Rockville, MD: Aspen, 1985:93–101.

16 Massive Rotator Cuff Defects and Glenohumeral Arthritis

Gerald R. Williams, Jr., M.D., and Charles A. Rockwood, Jr., M.D.

The association of degenerative arthritis of the glenohumeral joint and massive rotator cuff insufficiency is a complex problem. The average patient is in the seventh decade of life and frequently harbors contralateral rotator cuff disease that may be asymptomatic. The condition may be produced by basic calcium phosphate (BCP) crystals in the synovial fluid; it may be an apatite-associated destructive arthritis, an idiopathic arthritis, a hemorrhagic arthritis, or a severe localized rheumatoid-like process; or it may be secondary to chronic attrition of the rotator cuff.

HISTORICAL REVIEW

In 1934 E. A. Codman,[1] in his now classic text *The Shoulder: Rupture of the Supraspinatus Tendon and Other Lesions in or about the Subacromial Bursa,* described a condition known as hygroma of the subacromial bursa. He presented one patient, a 51-year-old woman, with severe destruction of the glenohumeral joint, recurrent swelling of the shoulder, cartilaginous bodies attached to the synovium, and complete absence of the rotator cuff. He believed that these changes were the final stages of a chronically neglected rotator cuff rupture.

In 1967 DeSeze[2] described "l'epaule senile hemmorrhagique" or "hemorrhagic shoulder of the elderly." Its clinical features included recurrent, spontaneous effusions of the glenohumeral joint with a bloody or blood-streaked fluid, degenerative changes of the glenohumeral joint, and radiographic evidence of chronic rotator cuff insufficiency. DeSeze[2] quoted earlier reports of Galmiche and Deshayes (1958),[3] Burman et al. (1964),[4] Banna and Hume Kendall (1964),[5] Shepard (1963),[6] and Snook (1963)[7] which dealt with spontaneous hemarthrosis of the glenohumeral joint in the elderly. Subsequent case reports of "l'epaule senile hemmorrhagique" were provided by Bauduin and Famaey[8] and Lamboley et al.[9] The report of Lamboley et al.[9] provides one of the earliest documented cases of a patient with similar findings in the knee.

In 1981, McCarty and coworkers[10-12] introduced the term "Milwaukee shoulder" to describe four women who presented with recurring large effusions, severe glenohumeral joint destruction, and massive rotator cuff defects. Their joint fluid contained active collagenases, neutral proteases, and microspheroids laden with hydroxyapatite crystals, which McCarty and colleagues postulated were active in perpetuating joint destruction. The synovium was hypertrophic, contained many pedunculated loose bodies, and exhibited findings consistent with synovial chondromatosis.

In 1982 Lequesne et al.[13] reported six cases of "l'arthropathie destructice rapide de l'epaule" ("rapid destructive arthritis of the shoulder"). All six cases were women aged 65 to 81 years with recurrent blood-streaked effusions and radiographic evidence of rotator cuff degeneration.

In 1983 Neer, Craig, and Fukuda[14,15] termed the condition of glenohumeral joint arthritis associated with rotator cuff deficiency as "cuff tear arthropathy." They described the clinical features, operative findings, and proposed mechanism of pathogenesis in 26 patients undergoing total shoulder arthroplasty for cuff tear arthropathy. They reported that they could find no description of the condition in the medical literature and concluded that cuff tear arthropathy was a newly described condition that was peculiar to the glenohumeral joint because of the unique anatomy of the rotator cuff.

In 1984 Dieppe et al.[16] described a similar problem of the shoulder, which they called apatite-associated destructive arthritis (arthropathy) or idiopathic destructive arthritis (IDA) of the shoulder.

In 1988 Campion et al.[17] reported that the clinical essence of "l'arthropathie destructice rapide de l'epaule," cuff tear arthropathy, Milwaukee shoulder, and apatite-associated destructive arthropathy was contained in DeSeze's original description of "l'epaule senile hemmorrhagique."[2]

In 1989 McCarty[18] stated that the description of the essential pathoanatomic features of the Milwaukee shoulder syndrome, cuff tear arthropathy, and apatite-associated destructive arthropathy predated even DeSeze's[2] 1967 description of "l'epaule senile hemmorrhagique." According to McCarty,[18] the relevant pathoanatomy was reported as early as the mid-19th century (1873) by Robert Adams,[19,20] who was the Regius Professor of Surgery at the University of Dublin, and his colleague, Robert Smith.[21,22] Adams[19,20] recognized two types of "chronic rheumatic arthritis"—localized and generalized. The generalized form resembled rheumatoid arthritis as we currently know it, while the localized form demonstrated morphologic characteristics identical to those found in cuff tear arthropathy or the Milwaukee shoulder. These characteristic features included degenerative changes with loss of articular cartilage and formation of marginal osteophytes, absence of the rotator cuff, presence of a large amount of fluid ("1 pint"), rupture of the long head of the biceps, effacement of the superior portion of the humeral head, erosion of the acromion and distal aspect of the clavicle, and synovial hypertrophy with frequent formation of pedunculated loose bodies.

ETIOLOGY

At this point in time we simply do not know the etiology of severe degenerative arthritis of the glenohumeral joint when associated with severe deficiency of the rotator cuff. However, from an extensive review of the literature it appears that this condition has been known since 1873. The rheumatologic literature has centered primarily on the biochemical aspects of the problem, while the orthopaedic descriptions have emphasized the importance of mechanical factors.

Rotator Cuff Tear Induced Theory

In his description of hygroma of the subacromial bursa in 1934, Codman[1] concluded by saying that he could not "state positively" what the condition was, although he was convinced that it was the late result of a neglected rupture of the rotator cuff. Codman postulated that rupture and retraction of the short rotators left the "head of the bone free under the deltoid; chronic synovitis, effusion, and slow distention of the bursa and joint followed."[1]

In 1983 Neer et al.[14] also postulated that certain chronic, massive tears would progress to a degenerated glenohumeral joint if left untreated. They cited mechanical and nutritional alterations in the rotator cuff–deficient shoulder that could result in joint destruction and disorganization. The mechanical factors included gross anteroposterior instability of the humeral head, proximal humeral migration and increased impingement wear, and rupture or dislocation of the long head of the biceps resulting in increased impingement and instability. The nutritional factors were the loss of a closed joint space and joint inactivity. They hypothesized that the loss of a closed joint space would lead to decreased pressure and leaking of synovial fluid into the subacromial space, both of which could result in poor cartilage nutrition. Joint inactivity was thought to cause structural changes in articular cartilage, changes in water and glycosaminoglycan concentration in cartilage, and disuse osteoporosis of subchondral bone.

Histologic studies performed on the 26 shoulders treated operatively revealed three basic observations: First, the humeral articular cartilage was atrophic and covered by a disorderly fibrous membrane. Second, the subchondral bone of the glenoid and the humerus was atrophic, except at points where a fixed subluxation or dislocation had resulted in point contact, which produced sclerosis. There were marginal osteophytes and the joint surfaces were denuded of cartilage. Third, the subsynovial layers of the joint contained many fragments of "articular cartilage." These changes resembled those seen in neuropathic arthropathy but were not as extensive. The authors concluded that the observed pathologic findings were secondary to abnormal trauma to the glenohumeral articular surfaces caused by marked instability present in the cuff-deficient shoulder.

It was estimated that only 4% of full-thickness rotator cuff defects will progress to cuff tear arthropathy.[14] According to Neer, this is because the tear never becomes "sufficiently large" or because the tear is subsequently sealed by bursal tissue.

All patients in Neer and colleague's[14,15] initial series complained of pain in association with external rotation weakness. Only 2 of the 26 patients could actively elevate past 90 degrees. Most patients exhibited recurrent swelling of the shoulder as a result of synovial fluid accumulation, which communicated between the glenohumeral joint and the subacromial space—the "fluid sign." The fluid was often blood-streaked and associated with ecchymosis about the shoulder in 5 patients.

Radiographic findings included proximal humeral migration; erosions of the anterior one-third of the acromion, distal aspect of the clavicle, glenoid, and coracoid process; anterior and posterior dislocations of the glenohumeral joint; osteoporosis; and subchondral collapse of the proximal humeral articular surface.[14] In all patients, arthrograms demonstrated full-thickness rotator cuff defects. Ten patients demonstrated communication of dye into the acromioclavicular joint; Craig[23] later termed this the "geyser sign." Neer postulated that the pathologic findings were caused by mechanical and nutritional alterations in the glenohumeral joint resulting from chronic unrepaired massive tears of the rotator cuff.

However, the term "cuff tear arthropathy" infers that there is a tear in the rotator cuff and the degenerative arthritis of the glenohumeral joint is secondary to the tear. In reality, the cuff is not torn but is severely degenerated and characterized by a 5 cm or larger massive defect.

Klimaitis et al.[24] in 1988 also hypothesized that mechanical disruption of the rotator cuff could be responsible for hastening the degenerative arthritis in the glenohumeral joint. They presented two cases of rapidly progressive destructive shoulder arthropathy in elderly women with generalized osteoarthropathy who had been using forearm crutches for walking. The glenohumeral joints of both women contained hydroxyapatite crystals and the clinical appearance in both cases was that of the Milwaukee shoulder or cuff tear arthropathy syndrome. The authors concluded that the progressive glenohumeral joint destruction in these two patients may have been the result of hastened rotator cuff attrition from repetitive stresses imparted by prolonged use of forearm crutches.

In 1990, Hamada et al.[25] presented long-term radiographic data on 22 shoulders with massive rotator cuff tears that were treated nonoperatively. The patients were selected using a special arthrographic technique, which in the authors' hands was 80% accurate in determining size and location of rotator cuff ruptures. The initial plain radiographs were analyzed for narrowing of the acromiohumeral interval and degenerative changes of the humeral head, tuberosities, acromion, acromioclavicular, and glenohumeral joints. Seven of the 22 shoulders had been followed for more than 8 years. In 5 of the 7 shoulders, the degenerative changes had progressed radiographically. The authors concluded that massive rotator cuff tears would progress to cuff tear arthropathy and that each step of progression would be accompanied by characteristic radiographic changes.

Alternatively, Rockwood et al.[26-29] reported that none of their patients demonstrated progressive radiographic or joint deterioration following acromioplasty and rotator cuff debridement for chronic massive irreparable rotator cuff defects. They reported follow-up data on 30 shoulders at an average of 6.6 years (range, 3 to 13 years) from the time of surgery.[29] Twenty-two of these 30 shoulders were completely free of degenerative changes. Eight shoulders had mild degenerative changes that were not progressive in nature. Among these 8 patients, there were 6 excellent and 2 good results.[29]

Levy et al.[30] reported on their experience with isolated arthroscopic acromioplasty for the treatment of full-thickness rotator cuff tears. Twenty-five patients were followed for a minimum postoperative period of 1 year. Good to excellent results were obtained in 84% of cases, and smaller tears responded better than larger tears. Ellman[31] as well as Esch et al.[32] also reported good results following isolated arthroscopic acromioplasty for full-thickness rotator cuff defects. Although the follow-up time was short, these authors did not report the development of progressive joint destruction.

The incidence of joint destruction is much lower than would be anticipated given the large numbers of patients with untreated rotator cuff tears. Pettersson[33] documented partial- or full-thickness rotator cuff defects in 13 of 27 asymptomatic live subjects ranging in age from 55 to 85 years with no history of trauma. Several cadaver studies[34-37] also documented a relatively high, age-related incidence of rotator cuff defects. McLaughlin[34] stated that over 25% of shoulders in the anatomy laboratory have a torn or degenerated cuff. Cotton and Rideout[35] documented 36 partial- or full-thickness rotator cuff defects in 106 necropsy specimens. Grant and Smith[36] studied the shoulders of 95 age-verified cadaver subjects and found that the incidence of cuff defects increased with age as follows: 0% for 17 to 46 years, 25% for 49 to 56 years, and 18% for 77 to 86 years. DePalma et al.[37] also noted an age-related incidence of rotator cuff defects of 0 to 100% of autopsy or cadaver specimens ranging in age from the fifth decade to the ninth decade of life.

It is apparent that full-thickness rotator cuff defects are compatible with good shoulder function and that the incidence of complete joint destruction is much lower than the incidence of full-thickness rotator cuff defects. Conceivably, there is a small subset of patients with full-thickness rotator cuff defects who will progress to degenerative changes in the glenohumeral joint. An alternative explanation, however, is that the destructive glenohumeral changes and massive rotator cuff defects encountered in cuff tear arthropathy are not causally related.

Crystal Induced Theory

McCarty et al.,[10-12] Dieppe et al.,[16] Schumacher et al.,[38] and others[39,40] noted the association of hydroxyapatite or BCP crystals with the severe destruction of the glenohumeral joint. McCarty et al.[10-12] performed morphologic and biochemical studies of joint fluid and synovium in patients with Milwaukee shoulder. Electron microscopic studies of the synovial fluid exhibited BCP crystals usually in the form of hydroxyapatite. Histologic studies revealed calcific foci within synovial microvilli and in the subsynovial layers. Chemical studies revealed the presence of active collagenase and neutral protease. McCarty et al.[10-12,41] hypothesized that subsynovial metaplasia resulted in calcium phosphate crystals that were then shed through the synovium into the glenohumeral joint, where they were phagocytized by synovial macrophage-type cells to form calcium phosphate microspheroids. This caused the release of active collagenase and neutral protease, which caused further "strip mining" of additional calcium phosphate crystals within the synovium as well as destruction of hyaline cartilage, the rotator cuff, and the remaining structures within the glenohumeral joint.

These[10-12] original observations pertained to four patients, three of whom had bilateral disease and one of whom had unilateral symptoms. Subsequently, Halverson et al.[42] reported 11 additional cases of Milwaukee shoulder, with involvement of the knee in 7. Synovial fluid from the knee joints also revealed BCP crystals. Isolated destructive arthritis of the hip and knee in association with BCP crystals has also been reported.[17]

Although Dieppe et al.[16,17] also documented the association between severe glenohumeral joint destruction and BCP crystals, they questioned McCarty and coworkers' theory that the process represents a crystalline-induced arthropathy. Unlike McCarty et al.,[10-12] Dieppe et al.[43-45] have been unable to document the presence of active collagenase or neutral protease in the synovial fluid of patients with Milwaukee shoulder. Furthermore, Dieppe et al.[45] reported that 30 to 50% of all joints affected with osteoarthritis contained BCP crystals. They listed three possible sources of these mineral deposits in osteoarthritis: (1) wear particles from the joint surface, (2) cartilage mineralization with or without subsequent shedding, and (3) synovial or subsynovial cartilaginous metaplasia (i.e., synovial chondromatosis). They hypothesized that crystal deposition in osteoarthritis is an opportunistic event and that the presence of crystal deposits can modify the underlying disease process.[45]

DIAGNOSIS

Chief Complaint

The primary complaints of patients with glenohumeral arthritis and massive rotator cuff deficiency are pain and loss of active shoulder motion. The pain characteristically interferes with sleep and is worse with activity. The symptoms of pain and loss of motion have usually been present for several years. The patients are typically elderly, in their seventh decade or older. The average ages of the patients in the series of Neer et al.[14] and Rockwood and Williams[46] were 69 and 72 years, respectively. There is a large bias towards the female gender as well as dominant-arm involvement. Twenty-three of the 26 patients in the Neer series[14] had some discomfort in the contralateral shoulder. Although radiographic evidence of chronic rotator cuff insufficiency was common, only 5 of these 26 patients had roentgenographic evidence of rotator cuff tear arthropathy in the contralateral shoulder.

Many patients will give a history of multiple corticosteroid injections. Although no correlation was made between severity of symptoms and history of corticosteroid injection, 6 (30%) of the 20 patients in Rockwood and Williams[46] series gave a history of multiple corticosteroid injections. One patient reported receiving between 20 and 25 steroid injections over a 3.5-year period. Neer et al.[14] reported that 16 (62%) of their 26 patients with rotator cuff tear arthropathy had received prior corticosteroid injections. However, 7 patients had not received corticosteroid injections until after the development of roentgenographic changes and only 6 had had more than three injections. Therefore, Neer et al.[14] concluded that steroid injections did not seem to be an etiologic factor in the development of rotator cuff tear arthropathy.

Physical Examination

Physical examination typically reveals atrophy of the supraspinatus and infraspinatus muscles, as well as weakness of active flexion, external rotation, and abduction. Passive arcs of motion are also limited. Only two patients in the series of Neer et al.[14] could actively elevate the shoulder above 90 degrees. In Rockwood and Williams[46] series, 6 of the 21 shoulders exhibited significant loss of external rotation. Neer et al.[14] reported that the majority of patients had significant recurrent swelling of the shoulder reminiscent of hygroma of the subacromial bursa as described by Codman in 1934.[1] The synovial fluid was often blood-streaked, and in Neer's series[14] was associated with ecchymosis around the shoulder in 5 of the 26 patients. Recurrent glenohumeral effusions were present in 3 of the 20 shoulders in Rockwood and Williams'[46] series.

Radiographic Findings

Characteristic radiographic findings include proximal humeral migration and severe erosion of the glenohumeral joint involving the glenoid, base of the coracoid process, distal end of the clavicle, and anterior aspect of the acromion.[14] Dennis et al.[47] reported acromial stress fractures associated with cuff tear arthropathy in three patients. Robert Adams[19,20] as well as Neer et al.[14] also recognized the separation of the acromion into anterior and posterior portions. However, they did not attribute this finding to trauma. Neer et al.[14] attributed this finding in 3 of their 26 patients to unfused acromial apophyses (os acrominale). Additional radiographic findings include collapse of the proximal humeral articular surface as well as anterior or posterior dislocations or subluxations.[14] If posterior glenoid erosion is suspected in association with posterior subluxation, a computerized tomographic scan of both shoulders can be helpful to compare glenoid version.

Although arthrography, magnetic resonance imaging, and ultrasonography are not necessary to make the diagnosis, they will reveal characteristic findings of chronic rotator cuff rupture. In addition, arthrography will often reveal an abnormal communication between the glenohumeral joint and the acromioclavicular joint. This geyser sign[23] can be associated with pathologic distension or pseudoganglion formation of the acromioclavicular joint.

SURGICAL MANAGEMENT

Treatment options for the patient with degenerative arthritis and an irreparable rotator cuff defect include arthrodesis,[48,49] constrained arthroplasty,[50-52] semiconstrained arthroplasty,[14,53-57] and hemiarthroplasty.[46,48,58] Arthrodesis may not be acceptable or well tolerated by the elderly population affected with this problem, particularly since the condition may be bilateral.[49] Cofield and Briggs[49] reported a series of glenohumeral arthrodeses including 12 patients in whom the indication for arthrodesis was an irreparable rotator cuff tear. Two of the 12 patients developed pseudarthroses and 6 patients required reoperation.

Constrained arthroplasties of the shoulder have been plagued with the same high rates of loosening and mechanical failure that have been reported with constrained arthroplasties of other joints.[50-52,56,59] Loosening rates as high as 25% have been reported for cemented constrained glenohumeral arthroplasties.[59] Lettin et al.[51] reviewed the results of 50 constrained Stanmore total shoulder replacements. Of the 40 patients with adequate follow-up, 10 developed glenoid loosening. Eight of these 10 patients underwent revision with another constrained arthroplasty and 1 underwent resection arthroplasty. Of the 8 patients who had a revision, 6 developed repeated loosening, necessitating eventual resection arthroplasty.

Post et al.[52] reviewed the results of constrained arthroplasty using the Michael Reese prosthesis in 102 patients. Series I and II patients were followed for an average of 10.8 years and 4 years, respectively. The 24 patients in series I experienced 4 major complications, resulting in 13 revisions. The 78 patients in series II experienced 15 major complications and 8 revisions. Of those who had not undergone revision, 20 had significant pain.

Clayton et al.[54] reported the use of a subacromial polyethylene spacer as a means of constraint against superior humeral subluxation in 7 patients with irreparable rotator cuff defects and arthritic articular surfaces. Although the authors noticed no difference between the results of the 7 patients who had received the spacer and 15 additional patients who had undergone conventional hemiarthroplasty or total shoulder arthroplasty using the Neer prosthesis, the patients with a spacer did appear to have less predictable pain relief. Five of the 7 had at least mild pain compared to only 6 of the 15. According to Neer,[56] the use of subacromial spacers has generally been discontinued.

The use of a semiconstrained prosthesis has been reported by Neer et al.[14,56,57] Amstutz et al.,[53] and Gristina et al.[55] Neer et al.[14,56,57] described optional 200% and 600% enlarged glenoid components with superior hoods to resist proximal subluxation of the humeral component in patients with rotator cuff deficiency. The 600% component was abandoned because of the interference with rotator cuff repair.[56] The DANA total shoulder, as reported by Amstutz et al.,[53] offers an optional glenoid component that has a dorsal hood to resist superior subluxation as well as extended anterior and posterior lips to prevent anterior and posterior subluxation. Gristina et al.[55] also described an optional hooded glenoid component to resist dorsal subluxation in cases of cuff insufficiency.

Experience with the hooded glenoid components is limited when compared to standard nonconstrained components. Few total shoulder arthroplasty series have tabulated the results using the semiconstrained glenoid component separately from the standard glenoid. However, Neer[56] noticed a significantly higher incidence of radiolucent lines around these semiconstrained glenoid components and believes that the likelihood of loosening is greater as a result of increased stress imparted to the bone-cement interface by the added constraint.

Biomechanical support for Neer's concerns is provided by Orr et al.[60] who reported in 1988 on a finite element analysis of the natural glenoid as well as prosthetic glenoids of various designs. Hooded glenoid components were associated with increased compressive stresses under the superior portion of the component and increased tensile stresses under the inferior part. They concluded that the abnormal stresses encountered with hooded components would result in an increased tendency for the component to tip superiorly and lead to early loosening.

Total shoulder arthroplasty using a nonconstrained prosthesis has been reported by Neer et al.[14,56,57] and others[51,53,55,61-66] to be very successful in relieving pain and improving function for a variety of pathologic conditions affecting the glenohumeral joint. They reported that the rates of humeral component radiolucent line formation and clinical loosening have been insignificant.[56,57] However, some authors[66,67] expressed concern over the durability of the cemented glenoid components because of the high incidence of complete and incomplete radiolucent lines, which have been reported to occur in 30 to 93% of cases.[56,59,64,66,68]

Neer et al.[56,57] observed that 30% of cases demonstrated a radiolucent line around the glenoid component at follow-up, but 94% were present on the initial postoperative radiograph. Neer[56] has only revised 2 of his 615 shoulder arthroplasties because of glenoid component loosening. Franklin et al.[67] reviewed all the reported series of nonconstrained total shoulder arthroplasties in the literature and found only a 3.6% rate of glenoid loosening in 766 cases, with a follow-up period ranging from 20 months to 10 years. These observations have led Neer[56] to conclude that the high incidence of glenoid radiolucent lines is a result of poor cementing technique.

Conversely, Cofield[66] expressed concern over potential glenoid component loosening. He reported significant radiolucent lines around the glenoid component in 60 of 73 total shoulder arthroplasties followed for 2 years or longer. In 8 of these cases, the glenoid was considered to be grossly loose. Migration of the component with superior tilting of the articular surface occurred in 7 of these 8 shoulders. At the time of review, 3 patients with loose glenoid components had undergone revision because of pain and the fourth was considering it. Of the remaining 52 shoulders with radiolucent lines, the lines were increasing in extent or thickness in 17 cases.

Although the overall rate of glenoid loosening for all diagnostic categories appears to be relatively low,[56,67] Franklin et al.[67] reported an association between glenoid loosening and rotator cuff deficiency with proximal humeral migration. Seven (50%) of the 14 patients in their series with rotator cuff deficiency demonstrated glenoid component loosening while none of the 16 patients with an intact cuff had a loose glenoid component. There was a direct correlation between proximal humeral migration and glenoid component loosening. They theorized that the eccentric superior loading of the glenoid component caused increased compressive stresses on the superior rim of the prosthesis, which resulted in loosening and superior tilting of the component. They referred to this phenomenon as the "rocking-horse" glenoid and credited Gristina with first recognizing that a significant shift of the prosthetic glenohumeral joint's instant center of rotation could abnormally stress the glenoid anchorage.

Arntz and Matsen[48] reviewed the results of hemiarthroplasty in 10 patients with combined glenohumeral arthritis and irreparable rotator cuff defects at an average of 37 months after surgery (range, 18 to 120 months). Preoperatively, 8 of the 10 patients had severe pain. Postoperatively, no patient had significant pain. In addition, active flexion improved from a preoperative average of 71 degrees to a postoperative mean of 110 degrees. Arntz and Matsen[48] concluded that humeral hemiarthroplasty is the procedure of choice in patients with combined glenohumeral arthritis and irreparable rotator cuff defects. They reserved arthrodesis for those patients with a combined loss of the anterior deltoid and rotator cuff, and younger patients who required substantial shoulder strength at low angles of flexion.

Other authors[54,69,70] also reported excellent pain relief following hemiarthroplasty of the glenohumeral joint. In

1974, Neer[70] reported the results of replacement arthroplasty in 48 shoulders with osteoarthritis of the glenohumeral joint. Forty-seven of the 48 shoulders were treated with hemiarthroplasty and 1 shoulder received both a humeral and a glenoid prosthesis. Of the 46 hemiarthroplasty patients with adequate follow-up, 42 had excellent pain relief. Marmor[69] reported excellent pain relief with hemiarthroplasty in 11 of 12 rheumatoid shoulders.

Alternatively, Zuckerman and Cofield[71] questioned the adequacy of pain relief obtained with hemiarthroplasty as compared to total shoulder arthroplasty. They reported the results of hemiarthroplasty in 92 patients with glenohumeral osteoarthritis and concluded that pain relief was less predictable than would have been expected following resurfacing of both the glenoid and the proximal humeral articular surface.

Lohr et al.[72] reported on 22 shoulders with cuff tear arthropathy that were replaced by hemiarthroplasty, nonconstrained total shoulder arthroplasty, or semiconstrained total shoulder arthroplasty. Hemiarthroplasty gave the poorest results for pain relief while the nonconstrained and semiconstrained devices resulted in a high incidence of radiologic and clinical loosening of the glenoid component. The authors concluded that cuff tear arthropathy remains "one of the most difficult entities to treat."

Clayton et al.[54] compared the results of total shoulder arthroplasty and hemiarthroplasty in a small group of patients at an average follow-up of 4 years and 7 months. Seven patients underwent humeral hemiarthroplasty while eight received a total shoulder arthroplasty using the Neer prosthesis. Although the numbers were small, the authors noticed no significant difference in either pain relief or function between the two groups. However, one patient developed pain 5 years following hemiarthroplasty in conjunction with significant erosion of the glenoid and acromion by the prosthesis.

Pollock et al.[58] in 1992 compared the results of total shoulder arthroplasty with humeral hemiarthroplasty in 30 shoulders with rotator cuff deficiency at an average of 41 months postoperatively. Satisfactory pain relief was obtained in 95% of the hemiarthroplasty group compared to 91% of the total shoulder arthroplasty group. Hemiarthroplasty also required a shorter operative time and hospital stay. The authors preferred hemiarthroplasty to total shoulder arthroplasty in rotator cuff–deficient shoulders.

Rockwood[46] has been performing humeral hemiarthroplasty for combined degenerative arthritis of the glenohumeral joint and irreparable full-thickness defects of the rotator cuff since 1974. Rockwood and Williams[46] reviewed the results in 21 shoulders and concluded that humeral hemiarthroplasty is the procedure of choice in this condition (Figure 16–1). They reserved arthrodesis for patients with arthritis, an irreparable rotator cuff, and a nonfunctioning deltoid muscle.

Authors' Surgical Technique for Hemiarthroplasty

Many of the patients with arthritis and rotator cuff deficiencies not only have pain with active motion, but also have poor active and passive ranges of motion and weak shoulder muscles. The authors believe that before surgery is instituted, the patient must be on a gentle program to stretch the shoulder enough to be able to get the hand to at least the overhead position. Once this has been accomplished, then the remaining cuff muscles, deltoid, and scapular stabilizers—trapezius, serratus anterior, rhomboideus major and minor, and latissimus dorsi muscles—must be strengthened. To operate and perform a hemiarthroplasty on a weak, stiff shoulder can only lead to suboptimal results.

The details of the surgical approach for shoulder arthroplasty are discussed in Chapter 6. However, certain aspects of the surgical technique, for this condition, deserve special mention.

1. As in all shoulder arthroplasty procedures, it is important to position the patient so that complete access to the anterior and superior aspects of the shoulder is possible. The top of the table should be removed and replaced with a special headrest that can be shifted off to the side of the table, such as a Crutchfield or McConnell head support. In addition, positioning should be such that the affected arm rests lateral to the edge of the table so that complete extension and adduction of the shoulder, which are required during placement of the humeral component, can be accomplished without hindrance.

2. The release of the upper half of the pectoralis major insertion can be useful for better exposure of the inferior joint and gaining some external rotation of the joint. If a severe contracture is encountered, the entire insertion of the pectoralis major may be released. Since there are other internal rotators, it is not necessary to repair the tendon.

3. Although the coracoacromial ligament is usually excised during total shoulder arthroplasty in patients with an intact rotator cuff, it should be preserved during hemiarthroplasty with a deficient cuff to act as a static restraint to anterosuperior subluxation.

4. Identification and protection of the axillary nerve are always important in shoulder arthroplasty, and perhaps more so during prosthetic replacement in patients with an insufficient cuff, since the humerus has migrated proximally and brought with it the subscapularis and the axillary nerve. After the conjoined tendon has been retracted medially, digital palpation is used to locate the axillary nerve as it courses inferiorly across the anterior surface of the subscapularis muscle. The nerve then hooks around the inferior corner of the subscapularis muscle and heads back posteriorly to exit through the quadrangular space. Inferiorly the nerve lies adjacent to the inferior joint capsule. The axillary nerve should be protected throughout the procedure, particularly when the inferior humeral capsular attachment is released.

5. Since the supraspinatus is necrotic and retracted, the superior margin of the subscapularis tendon is easily identified. Occasionally, a portion of the superior subcapularis tendon is also detached.

6. Patients with arthritis and a deficient cuff usually have osteoporosis of the proximal portion of the humerus; there-

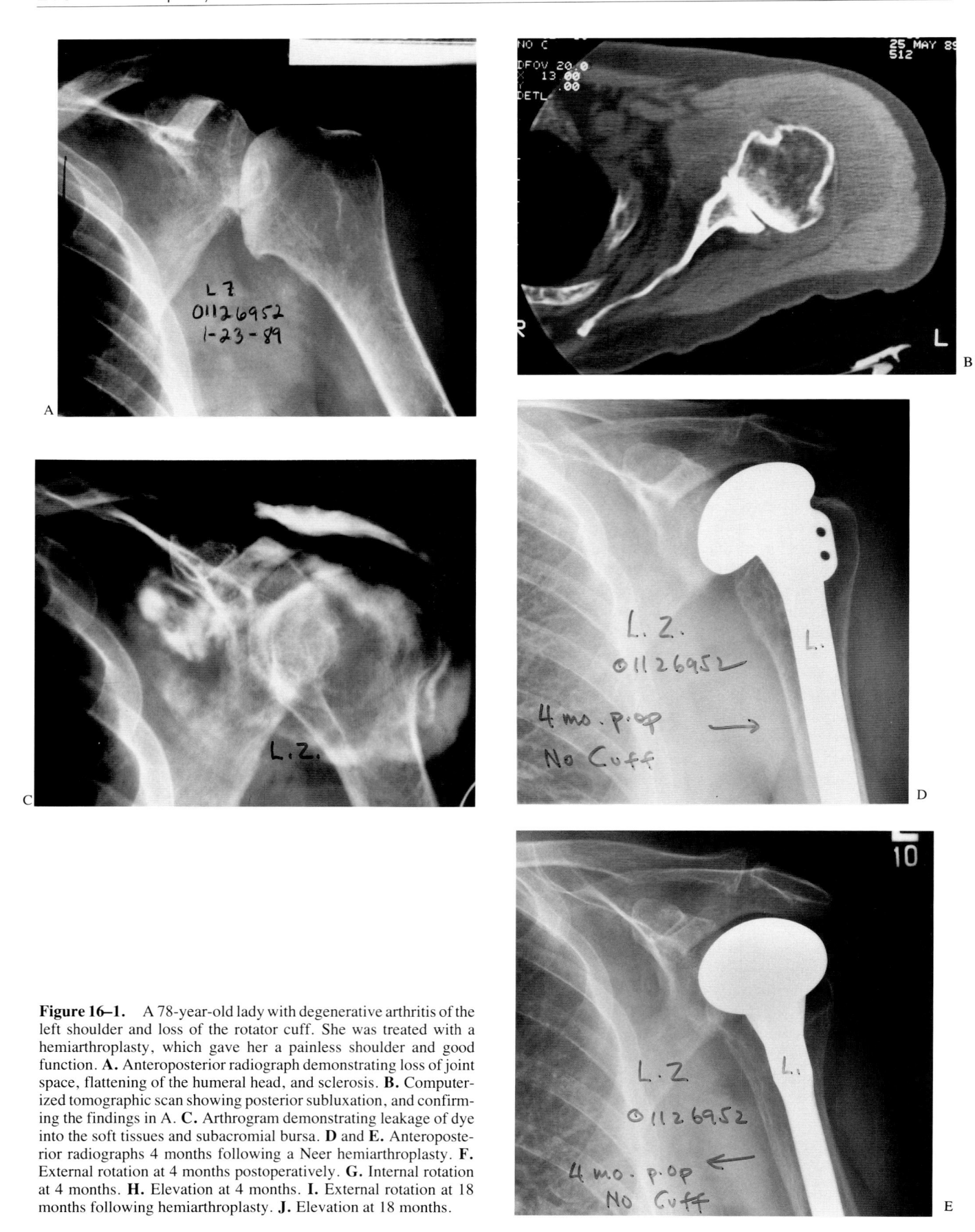

Figure 16–1. A 78-year-old lady with degenerative arthritis of the left shoulder and loss of the rotator cuff. She was treated with a hemiarthroplasty, which gave her a painless shoulder and good function. **A.** Anteroposterior radiograph demonstrating loss of joint space, flattening of the humeral head, and sclerosis. **B.** Computerized tomographic scan showing posterior subluxation, and confirming the findings in A. **C.** Arthrogram demonstrating leakage of dye into the soft tissues and subacromial bursa. **D** and **E.** Anteroposterior radiographs 4 months following a Neer hemiarthroplasty. **F.** External rotation at 4 months postoperatively. **G.** Internal rotation at 4 months. **H.** Elevation at 4 months. **I.** External rotation at 18 months following hemiarthroplasty. **J.** Elevation at 18 months.

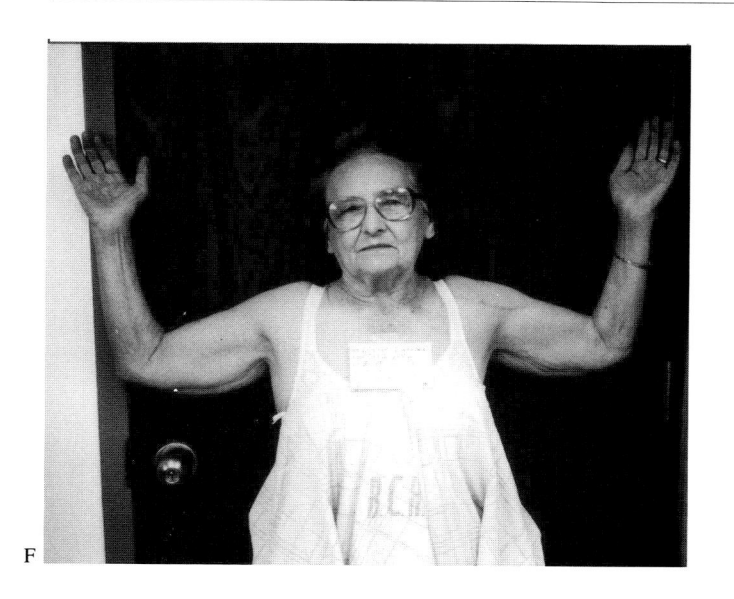

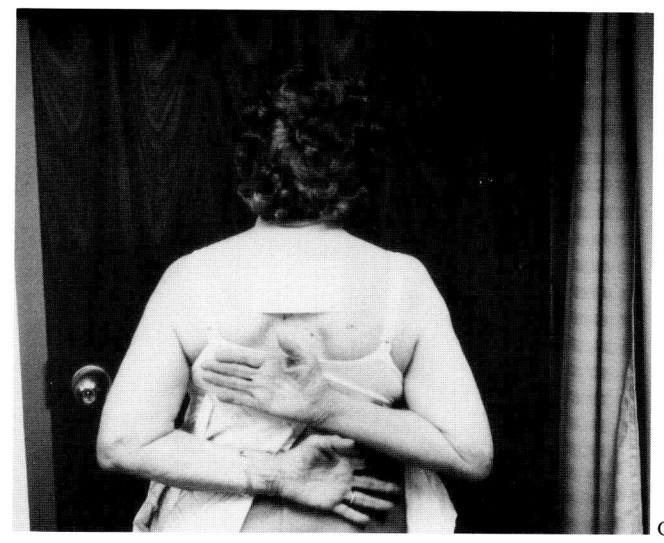

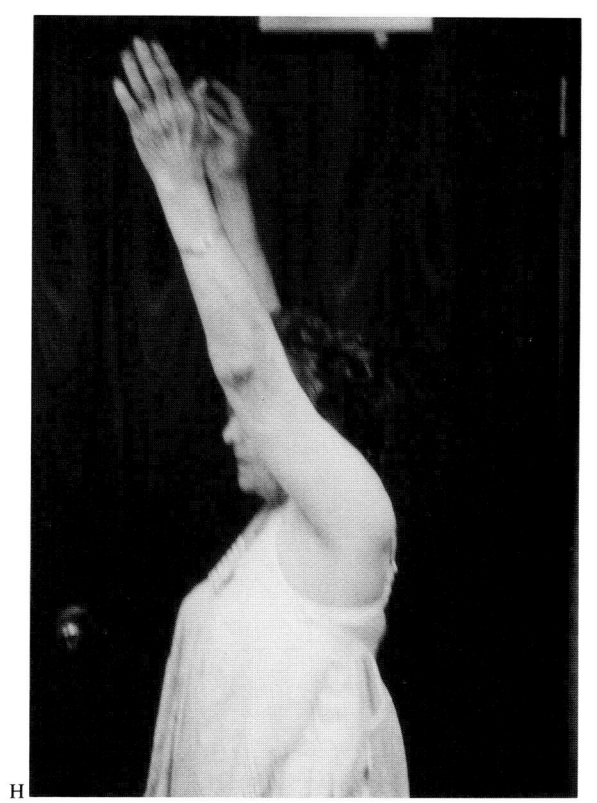

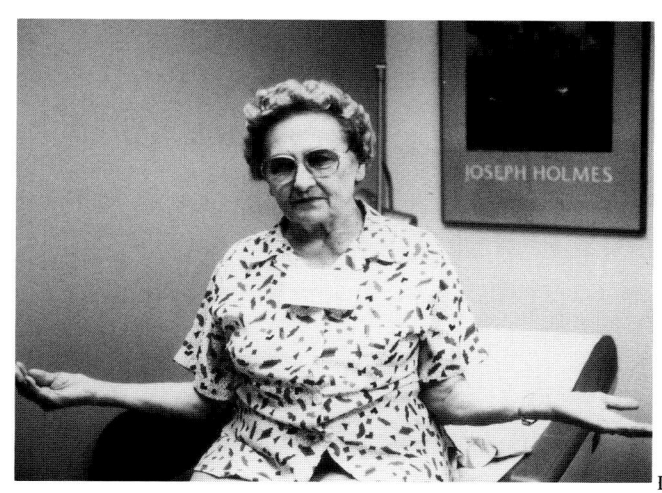

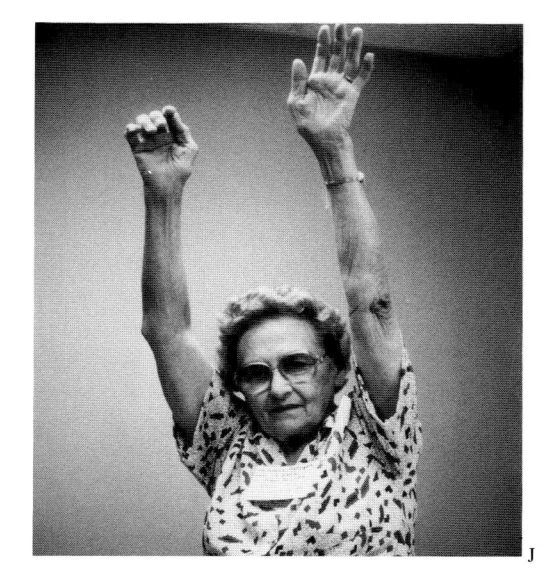

Massive Rotator Cuff Defects and Glenohumeral Arthritis 211

Figure 16-1. (Continued)

fore, excessive external rotation force should not be used to dislocate the proximal end of the humerus from the glenoid fossa. If the humerus does not dislocate easily, additional inferior and posterior capsule must be released, taking care to protect the axillary nerve.

7. With the humerus dislocated and the humeral head excised, the appropriately sized trial prosthesis should be seated within the humerus. The use of a modular prosthesis with multiple body sizes to fit and fill the proximal part of the humerus is recommended. There are multiple sizes of trial heads to balance the soft-tissue tension and obtain the best conformity of the head to the remaining glenoid fossa and inferior surface of the acromion. In many instances, because of the superior and medial migration of the proximal part of the humerus, the region of the glenoid, coracoid process, and the inferior aspect of the acromion takes on the appearance of a deep acetabulum. Remember that 30 to 35 degrees of external rotation of the arm must be obtained at the time of subscapularis tendon repair. This requires that the subscapularis muscle tendon be freed of scar and adhesions 360 degrees around its circumference, to become a free and dynamic muscle tendon unit. Humeral head size and neck length are chosen based upon the ability to repair the subscapularis. A larger humeral head component is useful in restoring the deltoid moment arm; however, a humeral head that is too large can prevent adequate external rotation when the subscapularis tendon is reattached. In Rockwood and Williams' series[46] of 21 hemiarthroplasties, 6 patients preoperatively had significant loss of external rotation. These patients underwent subscapularis lengthening in order to increase external rotation. The entire tendinous insertion was removed subperiosteally from the lesser tuberosity, and after it was freed from the surrounding soft tissues, was reattached to the cut edge of the neck of the humerus through drill holes. This lengthened the subscapularis by moving its insertion 1 to 2 cm medially. A coronal Z-lengthening of the subscapularis, which is required in more severe cases of internal rotation contracture, was not required in any of these 6 patients.

8. Severe deficiency of the subscapularis can lead to postoperative instability. Two of the patients in Rockwood and Williams' series[46] of 21 hemiarthroplasties required transfer of the upper 50% of the pectoralis major to the lesser tuberosity to prevent anterior instability of the prosthesis.

9. Cancellous bone graft from the resected humeral head can be used to fill any defects in the proximal part of the humerus. Twenty of the 21 prostheses placed in Rockwood and Williams' series[46] were not cemented. One patient required cement fixation of the prosthesis because of severe cystic formation and bone loss in the proximal end of the humerus.

10. Nine of the 21 shoulders in Rockwood and Williams' series[46] exhibited asymmetric posterior wear and erosion of the glenoid. In these 9 patients, the humeral osteotomy was made with the arm in only 0 to 15 degrees of external rotation in order to place the prosthesis in less-than-physiologic retroversion.

POSTOPERATIVE REHABILITATION

The importance of postoperative rehabilitation following hemiarthroplasty cannot be overemphasized. It is essential for the operating surgeon to take the lead in teaching and supervising the rehabilitation program. On the afternoon of surgery, the arm is passively flexed 100 degrees or as far as pain allows. On the first postoperative day, the surgeon instructs the patient in supine passive flexion exercises using the motor strength of the opposite extremity. In addition, the patient is instructed in pendulum exercises, passive external rotation exercises, and active-assisted flexion exercises using a pulley. These exercises should be performed four to six times per day.

On the second postoperative day the patient is encouraged to begin actively using the arm to assist in activities of daily living such as drinking, eating, brushing the teeth, and combing the hair. This early mobilization is made possible by secure reattachment of the subcapularis and by preservation of the entire deltoid origin.

The patient is discharged usually on the third or fourth postoperative day. Pendulum exercises, passive flexion and external rotation exercises, active-assisted flexion using an overhead pulley, and progressive active range-of-motion exercises are continued at home four to six times a day. The range of motion has usually improved enough to institute strengthening exercises using graduated rubber bands at 6 weeks postoperatively. Specific anterior deltoid–strengthening exercises are prescribed in cases of anterior deltoid weakness. Vigorous anterior deltoid rehabilitation is essential for overhead function since the rotator cuff is deficient.

RESULTS

The results of hemiarthroplasty using the above-mentioned technique have been very gratifying. The overwhelming reason that patients sought medical attention, in Rockwood and Williams' series,[46] was unremitting pain. Therefore, pain relief was the primary objective of surgery.

Pain relief was 95% successful in the series by Pollock et al.[58] and 100% in the series by Arntz and Matsen.[48] Excellent pain relief was obtained by Neer[70] in 47 of 48 patients.

In Rockwood and Williams' series of 21 cases,[46] preoperatively the pain rating was severe in 19 shoulders, moderate in 1 shoulder, and mild in 1 shoulder. Postoperatively, 87% of the patients had mild or no pain. Twelve shoulders had no pain, 6 shoulders had mild pain, and 3 shoulders had moderate pain. Of the 3 patients with moderate pain, 2 had undergone three prior attempts at rotator cuff reconstruction with allograft rotator cuff and 1 patient had suffered a denervated anterior deltoid as a result of a previously malplaced surgical incision. All 3 of these patients had severe pain preoperatively and stated that the surgery had been beneficial to significantly reduce the amount of their pain.

Active flexion in the patients in Rockwood and Williams' series[46] improved from an average preoperative value of 70 degrees (range, 0 to 180 degrees) to a postoperative average of 120 degrees (range, 15 to 180 degrees). Of the 19 patients who underwent unilateral replacement, 8 achieved flexion equal to that of the nonoperated arm, 2 achieved 25 and 45 degrees more flexion than the opposite arm, 3 achieved flexion to within 25 degrees or less of the opposite arm, and 6 did not achieve flexion to within 25 degrees of the opposite arm. Of these latter 6 patients, 3 had 90 degrees or more of active flexion.

In the six patients with significant preoperative loss of external rotation, the subscapularis advancement (as described in no. 7 of the operative details) resulted in an average gain of 30 degrees of external rotation (range, 0 to 45 degrees). There were no instances of anterior or posterior instability postoperatively. This included the nine patients with significant preoperative posterior glenoid wear in whom the prosthesis was implanted in less-than-physiologic retroversion.

SUMMARY

The condition of glenohumeral arthritis associated with massive rotator cuff deficiency in the shoulder, also known as cuff tear arthroplasty or Milwaukee shoulder, was probably first described by Adams in 1873. While the etiology remains unclear, this condition is best treated using a hemiarthroplasty procedure for pain relief.

REFERENCES

1. Codman EA. *The Shoulder: Rupture of the Supraspinatus Tendon and Other Lesions in or about the Subacromial Bursa.* Boston: Thomas Todd, 1934:478–480.
2. DeSeze M. *L'Epaule Senile Hemmorrhagique. L'Actualite Rheumatologique.* Paris: Expansion Scientifique Francaise, 1967;1.
3. Galmiche P, Deshayes P. Hemarthrose essentielle recidivante. *Rev Rhum Mal Osteoartic* 1958;25:57–58.
4. Burman M, Sutro C, Guariglia E. Spontaneous hemorrhage of bursae and joints in the elderly. *Bull Hosp Jt Dis Orthop Inst* 1964;25:217–239.
5. Banna A, Hume Kendall P. Spontaneous hemarthrosis of the shoulder joint. *Ann Phys Med* 1964;7:180–184.
6. Shepard E. Swelling of the subacromial bursa—Report of 16 cases. *Proc R Soc Med* 1963;56:162–163.
7. Snook GA. Pigmented villonodular synovitis with bony invasion—A report of 2 cases. *JAMA* 1963;184:424–425.
8. Bauduin MP, Famaey JP. A propos d'un cas de'epaule senile hemmorrhagique. *Belge Rheum Med Phys* 1969;24:135–140.
9. Lamboley C, Bataille R, Rosenberg F, et al.: L'epaule senile hemmorrhagique—A propos de nine observations. *Rhumatologie* 1977;29:323–330.
10. McCarty DJ, Halverson PB, Carrera GR, Brewer BJ, Kozin F. Milwaukee shoulder—Association of microspheroids containing hydroxyapatite crystals, active collagenase, and neutral protease with rotator cuff defects. I. Clinical aspects. *Arthritis Rheum* 1981;24:464–473.
11. Halverson PB, Cheung HS, McCarty DJ, Garancis J, Mandel N. Milwaukee shoulder—Association of microspheroids containing hydroxyapatite crystals, active collagenases, and neutral protease with rotator cuff defects. II. Synovial fluid studies. *Arthritis Rheum* 1981;24:474–483.
12. Garancis JC, Cheung HS, Halverson PB, McCarty DJ. Milwaukee shoulder—Association of microspheroids containing hydroxyapatite crystals, active collagenase, and neutral protease with rotator cuff defects. III. Morphologic and biochemical studies of an excised synovium showing chondromatosis. *Arthritis Rheum* 1981;24:484–491.
13. Lequesne M, Fallut M, Coulombe R, et al.: L'arthropathie destructive rapide de l'epaule. *Rev Rhum Mal Osteoartic* 1982;49:427–437.
14. Neer CS, Craig EV, Fukuda H. Cuff tear arthropathy. *J Bone Joint Surg [Am]* 1983;65:1232–1244.
15. Neer CS II. Cuff tears, biceps lesions and impingement. In: *Shoulder Reconstruction.* Philadelphia: WB Saunders, 1990:124–134.
16. Dieppe PA, Doherty M, MacFarlane DG, Hutton CW, Bradfield JW, Watt I. Apatite associated destructive arthritis. *Br J Rheumatol* 1984;23:84–91.
17. Campion GV, McCrae F, Alwan W, Watt I, Bradfield J, Dieppe PA. Idiopathic destructive arthritis of the shoulder. *Semin Arthritis Rheum* 1988;17:232–245.
18. McCarty DJ. Robert Adams' rheumatic arthritis of the shoulder—"Milwaukee shoulder" revisited. *J Rheumatol* 1989;16:668–670.
19. Adams R. *A Treatise of Rheumatic Arthritis of All the Joints.* 2nd ed. London: John Churchill and Sons, 1873:1–568.
20. Adams R. *Illustrations of the Effects of Rheumatic Gout or Chronic Rheumatic Arthritis on All the Articulations: With Descriptive and Explanatory Statements.* London: John Churchill and Sons, 1857:1–31.
21. Smith RW. Observations upon chronic rheumatic arthritis of the shoulder—I. *Dublin Q J Med Sci* 1853;XV:1–16.
22. Smith RW. Observations upon chronic rheumatic arthritis of the shoulder—II. *Dublin Q J Med Sci* 1853;XV:343–358.
23. Craig EV. The geyser sign and torn rotator cuff—Clinical significance and pathomechanics. *Clin Orthop* 1984;191:213–215.
24. Klimaitis A, Carroll G, Owen E. Rapidly progressive destructive arthropathy of the shoulder—A viewpoint on pathogenesis. *J Rheumatol* 1988;15:1859–1862.
25. Hamada K, Fukuda H, Mikasa M, Kobayashi Y. Roentgenographic findings in massive rotator cuff tears—A long term observation. *Clin Orthop* 1990;254:92–96.
26. Rockwood CA. Shoulder function following decompression of irreparable cuff lesions. *Orthop Trans* 1984;8:92.
27. Rockwood CA. The management of patients with massive rotator cuff defects by acromioplasty and rotator cuff debridement. *Orthop Trans* 1986;10:622.
28. Rockwood CA, Burkhead WZ. Management of patients with massive rotator cuff defects by acromioplasty and rotator cuff debridement. *Orthop Trans* 1988;12:190–191.
29. Rockwood CA, Williams GR, Burkhead WZ. Debridement of massive, degenerative lesions of the rotator cuff. *Orthop Trans* 1992;16:740.
30. Levy HJ, Gardner RD, Lemak LJ. Arthroscopic subacromial decompression in the treatment of full thickness rotator cuff tears. *Arthroscopy J Arthrosc Rel Surg* 1991;7:8–13.
31. Ellman H. Arthroscopic subacromial decompression—Analysis of one to three year results. *Arthroscopy J Arthrosc Rel Surg* 1987;3:173–181.
32. Esch JC, Ozerkis LR, Helgager JA, Kane N, Lilliott N. Arthroscopic subacromial decompression—Results according to the degree of rotator cuff tear. *Arthroscopy J Arthrosc Rel Surg* 1988;4:241–249.
33. Pettersson G. Ruptures of the tendon aponeurosis of the shoulder joint in anterior/inferior dislocation. *Acta Chir Scand Suppl* 1942;77:1–184.

34. McLaughlin HL. Rupture of the rotator cuff. *J Bone Joint Surg [Am]* 1962;44:979–983.
35. Cotton RE, Rideout DF. Tears of the humeral rotator cuff. *J Bone Joint Surg [Br]* 1964;46:314–328.
36. Grant JCB, Smith GC. Age incidence of rupture of the supraspinatus tendon. *Anat Rec* 1948;100:666.
37. DePalma AF, Gallery G, Bennett GA. Variational anatomy and degenerative lesions of the shoulder joint. *Instr Course Lect* 1949;6:255–281.
38. Schumacher HR, Miller JL, Ludvico C, Jessar RA. Erosive arthritis associated with apatite crystal deposition. *Arthritis Rheum* 1981;24:31–37.
39. Newman JH, Chavin KD, Chavin IF. Milwaukee shoulder syndrome: A new crystal induced arthritis syndrome associated with hydroxyapatite crystals—A case report. *Del Med J* 1983;55:167–169.
40. Kuchartz EJ. Zespol Milwaukee. *Wiad Lek* 1987;40:18–20.
41. Halverson PB, Garancis JC, McCarty DJ. Histopathological and ultrastructural studies of synovium in Milwaukee shoulder syndrome—A basic calcium phosphate crystal arthropathy. *Ann Rheum Dis* 1984;14:36–44.
42. Halverson PB, McCarty DJ, Cheung HSA, Ryan LM. Milwaukee shoulder syndrome—Eleven additional cases with involvement of the knee in seven (basic calcium phosphate crystal deposition disease). *Semin Arthritis Rheum* 1984;14:36–44.
43. Dieppe PA, Cawston T, Mercer E, et al. Synovial fluid collagenase in patients with destructive arthritis of the shoulder joint. *Arthritis Rheum* 1988;31:882–890.
44. Cawston TE, Dieppe PA, Mercer E, et al. Milwaukee—Synovial fluid contains no active collagenase. *Br J Rheumatol* 1987;26:311–312.
45. Dieppe PA, Watt I. Crystal deposition in osteoarthritis—An opportunistic event? *Clin Rheum Dis* 1985;11:367–392.
46. Rockwood CA, Williams GR. Gleno-humeral-acromio arthritis and severe disease: Management with hemiarthroplasty. *Orthop Trans* 1992;16:743.
47. Dennis DA, Ferlic DC, Clayton ML. Acromial stress fractures associated with cuff tear arthropathy—A report of three cases. *J Bone Joint Surg [Am]* 1986;68:937–940.
48. Arntz C, Matsen F. Irreparable tears of the musculotendinous cuff. *Orthop Trans* 1989;13:240–241.
49. Cofield RH, Briggs BT. Glenohumeral arthrodesis. *J Bone Joint Surg [Am]* 1979;61:668–677.
50. Coughlin MJ, Morris JM, West WF. The semiconstrained total shoulder arthroplasty. *J Bone Joint Surg [Am]* 1979;61:574–581.
51. Lettin AWF, Copeland SA, Scales JT. The Stanmore total shoulder replacement. *J Bone Joint Surg [Br]* 1982;64:47–51.
52. Post M, Haskell SS, Jablon M. Total shoulder replacement with a constrained prosthesis. *J Bone Joint Surg [Am]* 1983;62:327–335.
53. Amstutz HC, Thomas BJ, Kabo JM, et al. The DANA total shoulder arthroplasty. *J Bone Joint Surg [Am]* 1988;70:1174–1182.
54. Clayton ML, Ferlic DC, Jeffers PD. Prosthetic arthroplasty of the shoulder. *Clin Orthop* 1982;164:184–190.
55. Gristina AG, Roman RL, Kammire GC, Webb LX. Total shoulder replacement. *Orthop Clin North Am* 1987;18:445–453.
56. Neer CS II. Glenohumeral arthroplasty. In: *Shoulder Reconstruction*. Philadelphia: WB Saunders, 1990:143–272.
57. Neer CS II, Watson KC, Stanton FJ. Recent experience in total shoulder replacement. *J Bone Joint Surg [Am]* 1982;64:319–337.
58. Pollock RG, Deliz EB, McIlveen SJ, Flatow EL, Bigiliani L. Prosthetic replacement in rotator cuff deficient shoulders. *J Shoulder Elbow Surg* 1992;1:173–186.
59. McElwain JP, English E. The early results of porous-coated total shoulder arthroplasty. *Clin Orthop* 1987;218:217–224.
60. Orr TE, Carter DR, Schurman DJ. Stress analysis of glenoid component designs. *Clin Orthop* 1988;232:217–224.
61. Adams MA, Weiland AJ, Moore JR. Non constrained total shoulder arthroplasty. *Orthop Trans* 1986;10:232.
62. Bade HA, Warren RF, Ranawat CS, Inglis AE. Long term results of Neer total shoulder arthroplasty. In: Bateman JE, Welsh RP, eds. *Surgery of the Shoulder*. St. Louis: CV Mosby, 1984:294.
63. Barrett WP, Thornhill TS, Thomas WH, et al. Non constrained total shoulder arthroplasty for patients with polyarticular rheumatoid arthritis. *Orthop Trans* 1987;11:238.
64. Brems JJ, Wilde AH, Borden LS, Boumphrey FRS. Glenoid lucent lines. *Orthop Trans* 1986;10:231.
65. Cofield RH. Unconstrained total shoulder prosthesis. *Clin Orthop* 1983;173:97–108.
66. Cofield RH. Total shoulder arthroplasty with the Neer prosthesis. *J Bone Joint Surg [Am]* 1984;66:899–906.
67. Franklin JL, Barrett WP, Jackins SE, Matsen FA. Glenoid loosening in total shoulder arthroplasty—Association with rotator cuff deficiency. *J Arthroplasty* 1988;31:39–46.
68. Hawkins RJ, Bell RH, Jallay B. Experience with the Neer total shoulder arthroplasty—A review of 70 cases. *Orthop Trans* 1986;10:232.
69. Marmor L. Hemiarthroplasty for the rheumatoid shoulder joint. *Clin Orthop* 1977;122:201.
70. Neer CS II. Replacement arthroplasty for glenohumeral osteoarthritis. *J Bone Joint Surg [Am]* 1974;56:1–13.
71. Zuckerman JD, Cofield RH. Proximal humeral prosthetic replacement in glenohumeral arthritis. *Orthop Trans* 1986;10:231.
72. Lohr JF, Cofield RH, Uhthoff HK. Glenoid component loosening in cuff tear arthropathy. *J Bone Joint Surg [Br]* 1991;73(Suppl II):106.

17 Shoulder Arthroplasty for High-Grade Tumors

Martin M. Malawer, M.D., and Albert J. Aboulafia, M.D.

The shoulder girdle is the third most common musculoskeletal site to be affected by primary sarcomas of bone,[1,2] and the two most common primary tumors of bone involving the shoulder girdle are chondrosarcoma and osteosarcoma. The shoulder girdle is also a common site for soft-tissue sarcomas.[3]

Within the past 15 years, limb-sparing surgical procedures have brought about major advances in the management of such malignancies.[4] The management of high-grade sarcomas of bone follows not only the general techniques of arthroplasty but also the principles of oncologic surgery. This chapter describes the unique staging studies, biopsy technique, and anatomic and surgical considerations involved in the management of high-grade sarcomas involving the shoulder girdle. Emphasis is placed on reconstruction of large surgical defects of the proximal part of the humerus, the most common site of shoulder girdle sarcomas, with a custom modular shoulder arthroplasty endoprosthesis (Figure 17–1).

HISTORICAL BACKGROUND

Early reports of shoulder girdle resections were confined to cases involving resections of individual bones or portions of the scapula. The first such report appeared in 1820.[5] In it, Liston described a partial scapulectomy for an aneurysmal tumor involving the scapula. Mussey, in 1837, performed a near-total scapulectomy with resection of the clavicle in a patient with recurrent chondrosarcoma who had previously undergone a glenohumeral disarticulation.[6] The first attempts at limb-sparing surgery were for tumors of the scapula, and the first total scapulectomy was performed by Syme in 1856.[7] In 1909, De Nancrede[8] published a review of "the end results after total excision of the scapula for sarcoma," and concluded that tumors of the shoulder girdle were best treated with forequarter amputation. Attempts at tumor resection around the shoulder fell into disrepute thereafter and forequarter amputation continued to be the favored surgical treatment.

The first interscapulothoracic resection, or triple bone resection, was performed by Pranishkov in 1908 and reported by Bauman 6 years later.[9] The case involved removal of the scapula and surrounding soft tissue with resection of the head of the humerus and outer third of the clavicle. The proximal end of the humerus was attached to the remaining clavicle using metallic sutures to reconstruct a functioning shoulder joint. Between 1908 and 1913, Bauman, in conjunction with Tikhoff, performed three such operations and Bauman credited Tikhoff as the originator of the procedure. Reports of the procedure remained isolated in the Russian literature until 1928, when Linberg[10] published his now classic paper on interscapulothoracic resection for malignant tumors of the shoulder joint region. Linberg likewise credited Tikhoff as the originator of the operation, which consequently became referred to as the Tikhoff-Linberg procedure. Over the past 60 plus years, more than 80 cases of Tikhoff-Linberg resections have been reported in the literature. Most, however, have been in the form of case reports or small series.[11–19]

Historically, most shoulder resections were performed for scapular tumors or periscapular soft-tissue sarcomas; tumors of the proximal portion of the humerus were treated by amputation. Today, however, osteosarcoma of the proximal humerus is the most common indication for limb-sparing surgery for tumors about the shoulder girdle. Many advances have occurred in the surgical resection and reconstruction of such tumors. Unfortunately, most have been reported as a Tikhoff-Linberg procedure or "modified" Tikhoff-Linberg resection even though the term was never intended to refer to resection of tumors of the proximal part of the humerus.

In the early 1970s, the work of William Enneking led to new concepts and terminology in the field of orthopaedic oncology.[20] These included a better appreciation of the need to evaluate surgical margins, the relationship of the tumor to anatomic compartments (intracompartmental versus extracompartmental), the status of the glenohumeral joint (intra-articular versus extra-articular), and the extent of soft-tissue involvement. With the advent of chemotherapy for high-grade bone sarcomas in the early 1970s, Marcove[21] and Francis[11] were the first to attempt resections for high-grade sarcomas of the proximal part of the humerus. The first limb-sparing procedure for a proximal humeral bone sarcoma at the National Institutes of Health took place in 1978 in a 15-year-old girl with an osteosarcoma of the proximal humerus.

CLASSIFICATION OF SHOULDER GIRDLE RESECTIONS

In 1965, Papaioannou and Francis[22] published a classification system for resections about the scapula. The scheme was based on the extent of bone to be resected and included four

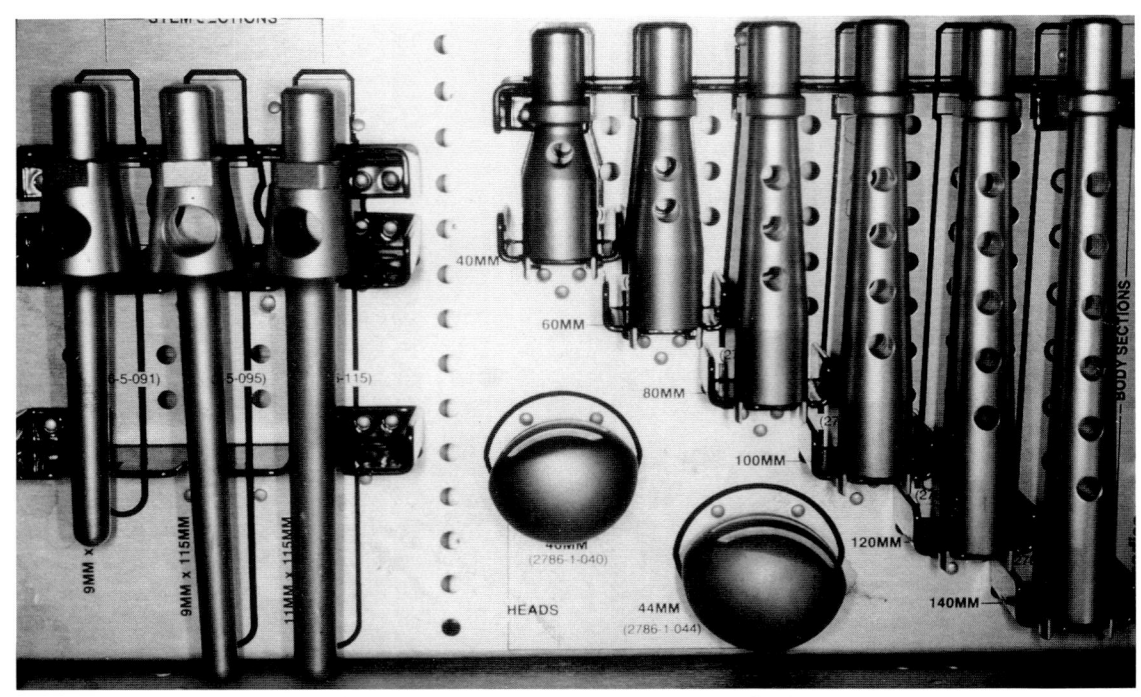

Figure 17–1. Trial components of a modular oncology system. The stem section includes 9-mm- and 11-mm-diameter stems. The body section includes 40-mm to 140-mm components in 20-mm increments.

categories: total scapulectomy, near-total scapulectomy, radical subtotal scapulectomy, and subtotal or partial scapulectomy. In an attempt to establish a classification that included all major shoulder girdle resections, Samilson et al.[23] added the classic interscapulothoracic resection (Tikhoff-Linberg) and forequarter amputation. In 1991, Malawer et al.[24] proposed a unified classification system for resections about the shoulder girdle that permits a precise description of surgical procedures and facilitates accurate comparisons and evaluation of data (Figure 17–2).

Malawer's classification scheme refers not only to bony resection but also to soft-tissue resection, and reflects concepts in orthopaedic oncology that have emerged over the past 15 years. It identifies six types of resections: Type I is an intra-articular resection of the proximal part of the humerus; type II is a partial scapular resection; type III is an intra-articular total scapulectomy; type IV is an extra-articular total scapulectomy with resection of the humeral head; type V is an extra-articular resection of the proximal part of the humerus and the glenoid; and type VI represents an extra-articular humeral and total scapular resection.

The six types of resection are further divided into subtypes A or B. Subtype A denotes an intact abductor mechanism, whereas B indicates resection of part or all of the abductor mechanism. The system further identifies the structures resected and their relationship to the glenohumeral joint. Type I, II, and III resections are always intra-articular, while type IV, V, and VI resections are always extra-articular. Types IA, IIA, and IIIA are intracompartmental resections whereas all type B resections are extracompartmental. When tumor extends into the soft tissues (extracompartmental), the abductor mechanism is almost always resected with the specimen. This is usually the case for all but the most low-grade sarcomas of bone. The abductor mechanism is usually retained in patients undergoing type I, II, or III resection, which are most frequently indicated for benign or intracompartmental low-grade lesions of the proximal humerus and scapula, respectively. Type IV, V, and VI resections, by contrast, usually entail resection of the abductors. These procedures are most often indicated for extracompartmental tumors of the scapula and proximal humerus. A marginal or wide resection can be accomplished by any of the above procedures, depending on the extent of the tumor. Thus, the type of resection indicated for a given tumor depends upon the location and stage of the tumor as described by Enneking et al.[20] (Figure 17–3).

STAGING STUDIES

Once a sarcoma of the shoulder girdle is suspected, plain radiographs should be obtained. The plain radiograph remains a valuable tool in developing a differential diagnosis, evaluating a pathologic or an impending pathologic fracture, and obtaining information relating to tumor growth and aggressiveness. Additional studies are performed to evaluate the extent of local disease and to search for distant metastasis. Staging studies should be performed prior to biopsy since postsurgical artifacts obscure detail.

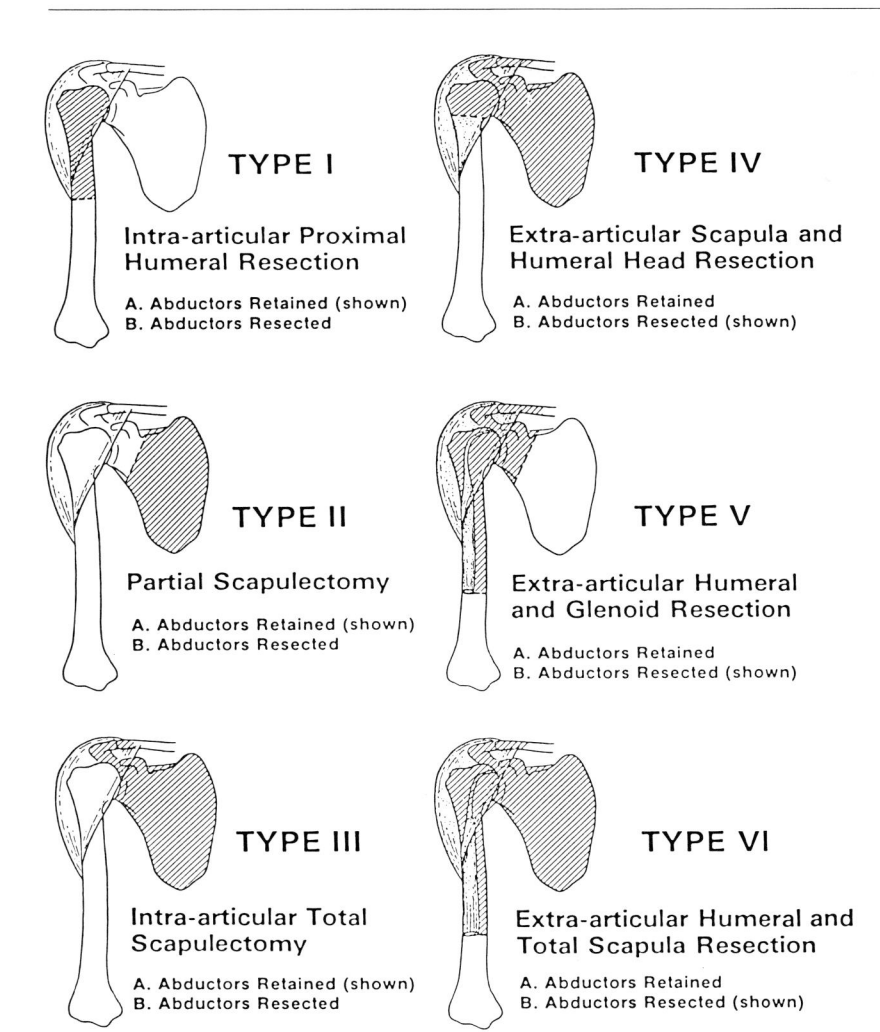

Figure 17-2. Surgical classification system for shoulder girdle resections.

- **TYPE I** — Intra-articular Proximal Humeral Resection
  - A. Abductors Retained (shown)
  - B. Abductors Resected
- **TYPE II** — Partial Scapulectomy
  - A. Abductors Retained (shown)
  - B. Abductors Resected
- **TYPE III** — Intra-articular Total Scapulectomy
  - A. Abductors Retained (shown)
  - B. Abductors Resected
- **TYPE IV** — Extra-articular Scapula and Humeral Head Resection
  - A. Abductors Retained
  - B. Abductors Resected (shown)
- **TYPE V** — Extra-articular Humeral and Glenoid Resection
  - A. Abductors Retained
  - B. Abductors Resected (shown)
- **TYPE VI** — Extra-articular Humeral and Total Scapula Resection
  - A. Abductors Retained
  - B. Abductors Resected (shown)

The local extent of extraosseous disease is best evaluated with computerized tomography (CT) or magnetic resonance imaging (MRI). MRI is more sensitive than CT in evaluating the extent of soft-tissue spread. Special attention is paid to determining chest wall and/or neurovascular involvement. Arteriography remains a valuable tool in determining vascular involvement. Displacement of the vessels is indicative of anterior extension of tumor. MRI is used to evaluate the intraosseous extent of tumor and is more sensitive and specific than a technetium bone scan for this purpose. The technetium scan, however, should be used to search for distant bony metastasis. MRI, in conjunction with the bone scan, is used to determine safe margins for resection.

Joint involvement is difficult to determine. Arthrography and arthroscopy are contraindicated because of the possibility of contaminating the surrounding musculature with tumor (Figure 17-4). A CT of the chest is performed to determine the presence of pulmonary metastases, which does not preclude resection of the primary tumor. Long-term survival and cure are possible with resection of pulmonary metastases and chemotherapy.

BIOPSY TECHNIQUE

The importance of the biopsy technique cannot be overemphasized. Inadvertent contamination of the neurovascular structures or the chest wall must be avoided when a biopsy of the scapula is performed. For tumors arising in the proximal part of the humerus, the standard deltopectoral interval should be avoided, because this approach leads to contamination of the subscapularis and pectoralis muscles, as well as the neurovascular structures by hematogenous tumor spread along the pectoral and subscapularis fascia. Should this occur, limb-sparing surgery may not be possible. All lesions of the proximal part of the humerus should be approached through the anterior third of the deltoid.

If staging studies reveal a soft-tissue mass, a true cut needle biopsy may be adequate to obtain sufficient tissue for histologic diagnosis. A needle biopsy is preferred in such a circumstance, since it causes less soft-tissue contamination. If there is not a soft-tissue mass favorable for biopsy or if inadequate tissue is obtained, a Craig needle biopsy could be performed under fluoroscopic control. Care should be taken

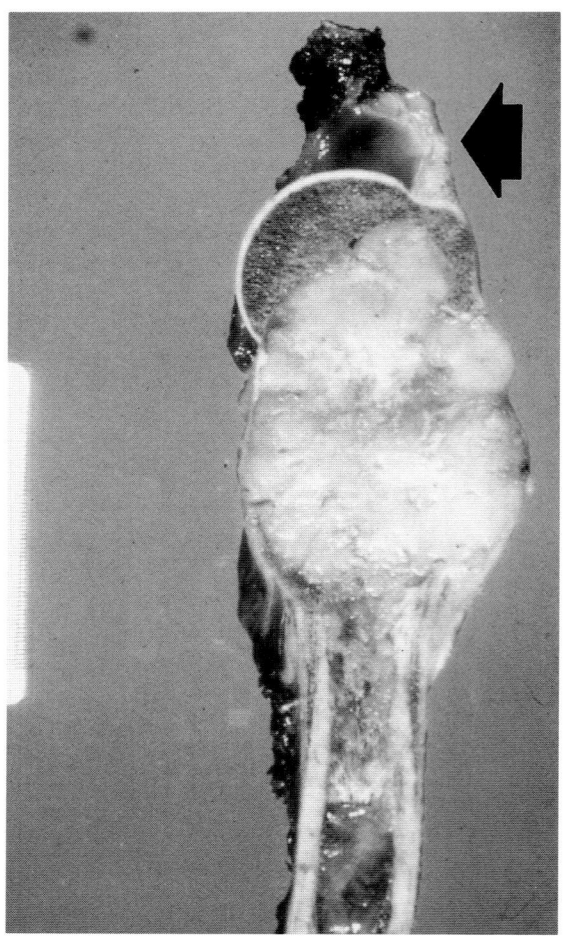

Figure 17–3. Gross specimen showing direct tumor spread along the capsule of the shoulder joint. This was a stage IIB lesion, and wide margins were obtained with a type V extra-articular resection.

not to involve the joint or the muscles of the rotator cuff. If an incisional biopsy is necessary, it should be placed in a longitudinal fashion over the anterior third of the deltoid. The bone should be plugged with methylmethacrylate or bone wax. Meticulous attention must be paid to absolute hemostasis in order to avoid local spread of tumor cells from the subsequent hematoma.

UNIQUE ANATOMIC CONSIDERATIONS

Tumors arising from the body of the scapula are initially surrounded by a cuff of soft tissue. As sarcomas enlarge, they involve the axillary vessels and the brachial plexus. Lesions originating in the neck of the scapula or glenoid expand to involve the periscapular tissue or the glenohumeral joint. Important areas to evaluate prior to attempted resection include the chest wall, axillary vessels, brachial plexus, and proximal humeral/periscapular soft tissues. Extension of large suprascapular tumors into the anterior and posterior triangles of the neck can make resection especially difficult. In such cases, consultation with surgeons from other subspecialties may be necessary. Tumors arising in the proximal part of the humerus may enlarge and present with a soft-tissue component. In many cases, the tumor breaks through cortical bone underneath the deltoid and extends medially, displacing the subscapularis and coracobrachialis muscles. The axilla must be examined carefully for contiguous tumor spread as well as for nodal involvement. A large extraosseous component of tumor may also hide in the posterior deltoid and triceps area.

SURGICAL TECHNIQUE

The surgical management of high-grade tumors of the shoulder region involves three phases: wide resection of the tumor, reconstruction of the bony defect, and soft-tissue reconstruction.

Phase 1: Wide Resection of the Tumor

Resection of high-grade shoulder tumors takes place in a logical sequential series of five steps. Each step must be performed in the correct order to prevent neurovascular injury and unnecessary contamination of tissue planes. High-grade sarcomas around the shoulder have a proclivity for

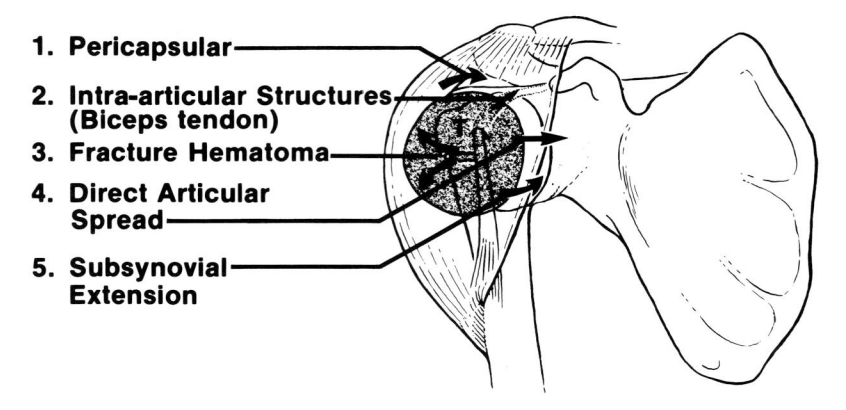

Figure 17–4. Mechanisms of local tumor spread for sarcomas of the shoulder.

1. Pericapsular
2. Intra-articular Structures (Biceps tendon)
3. Fracture Hematoma
4. Direct Articular Spread
5. Subsynovial Extension

intra-articular and extra-articular spread. Tumors originating in proximity to the shoulder joint can spread by direct capsular extension, tracking along the long head of biceps, contamination from a poorly placed biopsy, and pathologic fracture. For these reasons, intra-articular resection causes an unacceptable risk of local recurrence. For high-grade sarcomas about the shoulder, a type V extra-articular resection as described by Malawer et al.[15] is routinely performed. The resection includes en bloc extra-articular resection of the proximal end of the humerus and the glenoid as well as all or part of the deltoid, biceps, triceps, and rotator cuff.

The patient is positioned supine on the operating table and induced with general endotracheal anesthesia. A Foley catheter is placed in the bladder and intravenous antibiotic prophylaxis initiated. The patient is then placed in a lateral position. The skin is prepared from the hairline proximally to the costal margin distally, and from the midline medially to the medial border of the scapula posteriorly. The entire extremity, including the hand, is included in the preparation to allow one to move the extremity and assess distal pulses intraoperatively. Resection then begins, with each of the following five steps performed sequentially:

STEP 1: AXILLARY EXPLORATION TO DETERMINE RESECTABILITY

The incision begins over the proximal to middle third of the clavicle, extends distally over the deltopectoral groove, and continues along the medial border of the biceps muscle. The biopsy site is circumscribed by the incision and remains with the resected specimen (Figure 17–5).

The incision is carried down through the superficial fascia to identify the deep fascia of the pectoralis major and deltoid muscles. Anterior skin flaps are raised to identify the distal third of the pectoralis major and the short head of the biceps. The insertion of the pectoralis major on the humerus is identified and transected just proximal to its tendinous insertion. The axillary sheath and the coracoid process are then identified. Prior to exploration of the neurovascular bundle, the pectoralis minor, short head of the biceps, and coracobrachialis muscles are tagged and divided near their origin on the coracoid process (Figure 17–6). It is at this point that the final determination of the patient's suitability for limb-sparing surgery is made. More extensive dissection prior to this point would lead to tumor contamination of tissue that might be required for flaps in the event of a forequarter amputation.

STEP 2: NEUROVASCULAR EXPLORATION

The axillary sheath is freed of overlying fat using blunt dissection, and vessel loops are passed around the proximal and distal portions of the exposed neurovascular bundle (Figure 17–7). With gentle medial traction on the bundle, the axillary nerve and the anterior and the posterior circumflex humerus arteries are identified. All three structures are ligated and divided. If the neurovascular bundle is free of tumor, dissection for limb-sparing surgery continues. The musculocutaneous nerve is identified and preserved as long as tumor-free margins are obtained. The short and long heads of the biceps are separated by dividing the deep fascia between them distal to the tumor mass. The radial nerve is identified at the inferior border of the latissimus dorsi muscle as it passes around and behind the humerus. Using blunt dissection, the radial nerve is traced distally to free it from the humerus along the spiral groove. The ulnar nerve is identified along its distal course in a similar fashion. This is facilitated by dividing the intermuscular septum between the biceps and triceps muscles.

STEP 3: EXPOSURE OF THE NECK OF THE SCAPULA

The humerus is exposed by separating the short and long heads of the biceps. The site of the humeral osteotomy is

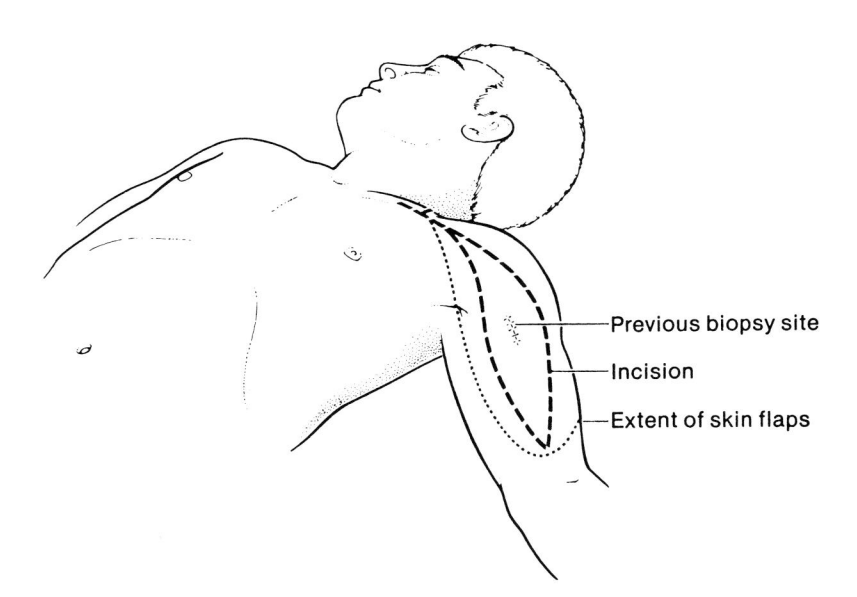

Figure 17–5. Biopsy position and incision.

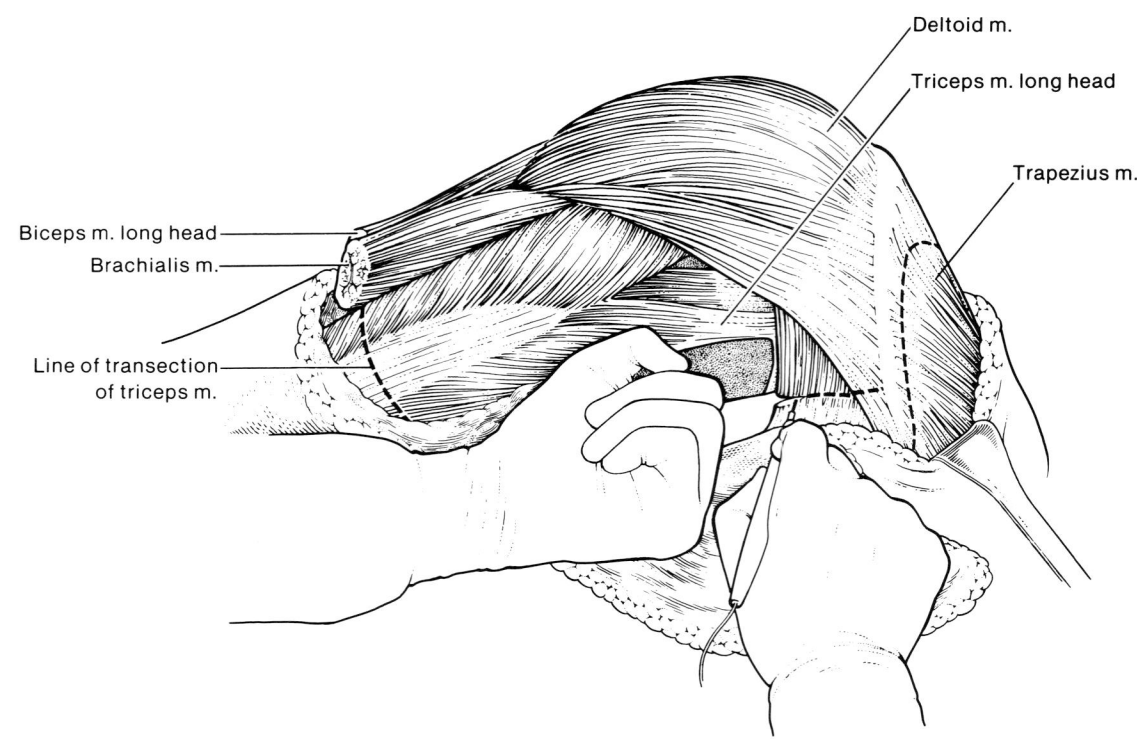

Figure 17–10. Division of the posterior musculature.

marrow from the remaining cut end of the humerus are examined microscopically to confirm tumor-free margins prior to continuing with the procedure. The specimen, which includes the biopsy site, proximal part of the humerus, shoulder joint, glenoid, upper portion of the long head of the biceps, and brachialis, is removed. The deltoid muscle covers the tumor. The insertions of the supraspinatus, infraspinatus, pectoralis major, latissimus dorsi, teres major, teres minor, and subscapularis muscles remain covering the tumor and constitute the free margins.

Phase 2: Reconstruction of the Bony Defect
Various techniques have been described for reconstruction of bony defects following proximal humeral resection for high-grade sarcomas. Allografts have been used in an effort to maintain a functional shoulder joint and preserve motion, or in combination with internal fixation to obtain an arthrodesis. Resection arthroplasty has also been used, but leaves the patient with a flail shoulder. The authors utilize a modular endoprosthesis that is custom-fitted intraoperatively (Figure 17–11). The principles of reconstruction are the same whether an endoprosthesis or an allograft is used. The functional goals of surgery are a pain-free shoulder and arm that is mobile with normal elbow and hand function.

If an endoprosthesis is chosen, the remaining medullary cavity of the humerus is prepared using a power reamer. The canal is reamed 1 to 2 mm larger than the diameter of the prosthetic stem, to allow for a cement mantle. The length of the resected specimen is measured, and a trial modular

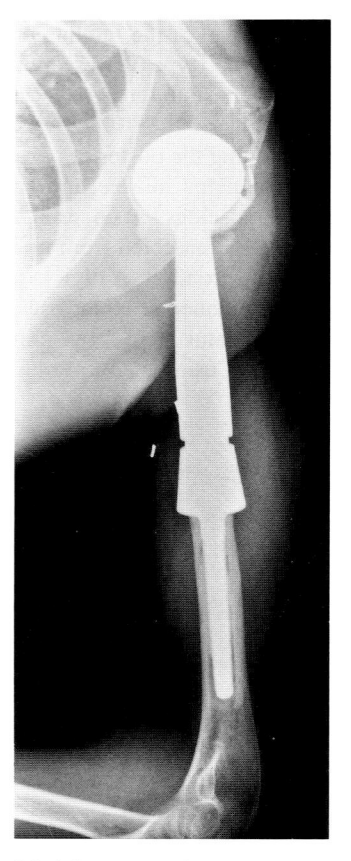

Figure 17–11. Modular prosthesis used for reconstruction of the bony defect following type V resection.

intra-articular and extra-articular spread. Tumors originating in proximity to the shoulder joint can spread by direct capsular extension, tracking along the long head of biceps, contamination from a poorly placed biopsy, and pathologic fracture. For these reasons, intra-articular resection causes an unacceptable risk of local recurrence. For high-grade sarcomas about the shoulder, a type V extra-articular resection as described by Malawer et al.[15] is routinely performed. The resection includes en bloc extra-articular resection of the proximal end of the humerus and the glenoid as well as all or part of the deltoid, biceps, triceps, and rotator cuff.

The patient is positioned supine on the operating table and induced with general endotracheal anesthesia. A Foley catheter is placed in the bladder and intravenous antibiotic prophylaxis initiated. The patient is then placed in a lateral position. The skin is prepared from the hairline proximally to the costal margin distally, and from the midline medially to the medial border of the scapula posteriorly. The entire extremity, including the hand, is included in the preparation to allow one to move the extremity and assess distal pulses intraoperatively. Resection then begins, with each of the following five steps performed sequentially:

STEP 1: AXILLARY EXPLORATION TO DETERMINE RESECTABILITY

The incision begins over the proximal to middle third of the clavicle, extends distally over the deltopectoral groove, and continues along the medial border of the biceps muscle. The biopsy site is circumscribed by the incision and remains with the resected specimen (Figure 17–5).

The incision is carried down through the superficial fascia to identify the deep fascia of the pectoralis major and deltoid muscles. Anterior skin flaps are raised to identify the distal third of the pectoralis major and the short head of the biceps. The insertion of the pectoralis major on the humerus is identified and transected just proximal to its tendinous insertion. The axillary sheath and the coracoid process are then identified. Prior to exploration of the neurovascular bundle, the pectoralis minor, short head of the biceps, and coracobrachialis muscles are tagged and divided near their origin on the coracoid process (Figure 17–6). It is at this point that the final determination of the patient's suitability for limb-sparing surgery is made. More extensive dissection prior to this point would lead to tumor contamination of tissue that might be required for flaps in the event of a forequarter amputation.

STEP 2: NEUROVASCULAR EXPLORATION

The axillary sheath is freed of overlying fat using blunt dissection, and vessel loops are passed around the proximal and distal portions of the exposed neurovascular bundle (Figure 17–7). With gentle medial traction on the bundle, the axillary nerve and the anterior and the posterior circumflex humerus arteries are identified. All three structures are ligated and divided. If the neurovascular bundle is free of tumor, dissection for limb-sparing surgery continues. The musculocutaneous nerve is identified and preserved as long as tumor-free margins are obtained. The short and long heads of the biceps are separated by dividing the deep fascia between them distal to the tumor mass. The radial nerve is identified at the inferior border of the latissimus dorsi muscle as it passes around and behind the humerus. Using blunt dissection, the radial nerve is traced distally to free it from the humerus along the spiral groove. The ulnar nerve is identified along its distal course in a similar fashion. This is facilitated by dividing the intermuscular septum between the biceps and triceps muscles.

STEP 3: EXPOSURE OF THE NECK OF THE SCAPULA

The humerus is exposed by separating the short and long heads of the biceps. The site of the humeral osteotomy is

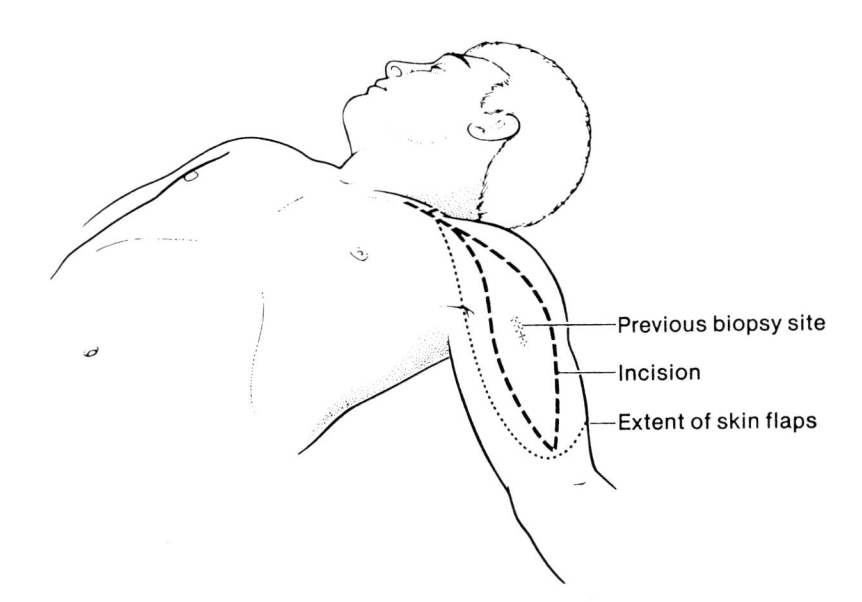

Figure 17–5. Biopsy position and incision.

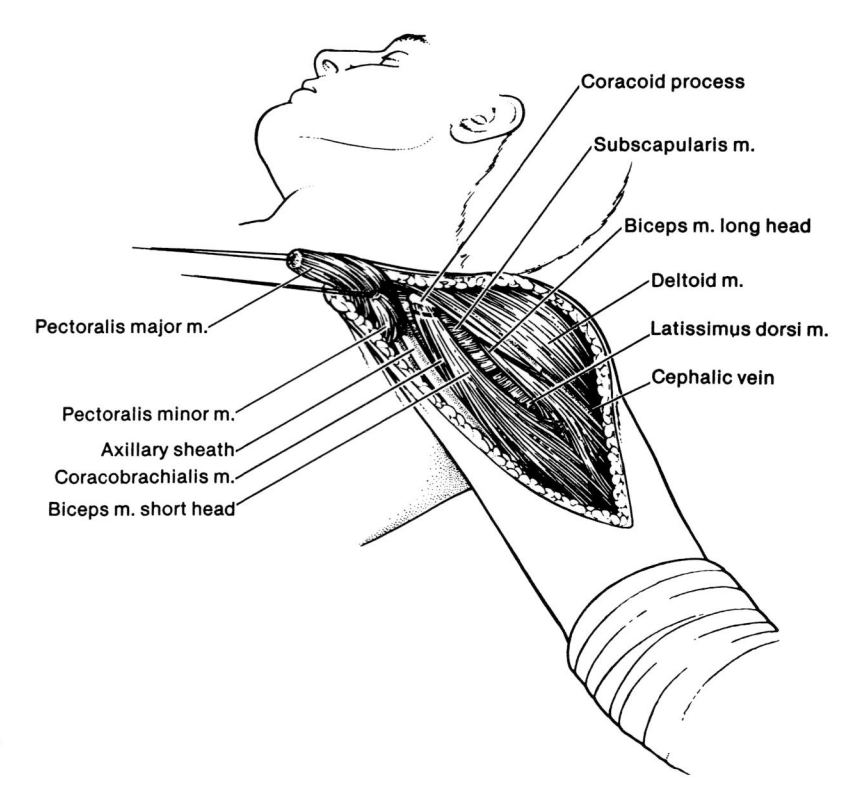

Figure 17–6. Exploration of the axilla to determine resectability.

chosen based on preoperative studies, and the long head of the biceps and the brachialis muscle are divided at this level. A small fascial incision is made along the inferior border of the latissimus dorsi, a digit is passed behind the latissimus dorsi and teres major muscles several centimeters from their insertion, and they are then transected at this level. The humerus is externally rotated to expose the subscapularis muscle, which is transected at the level of the coracoid process. Care is taken not to enter the joint space. After transection of these muscles, the anterior portion of the neck of the scapula is visualized (Figure 17–8).

STEP 4: POSTERIOR INCISION AND LATERAL SKIN FLAP

The extremity is positioned across the chest and the operating table turned away from the surgeon to allow

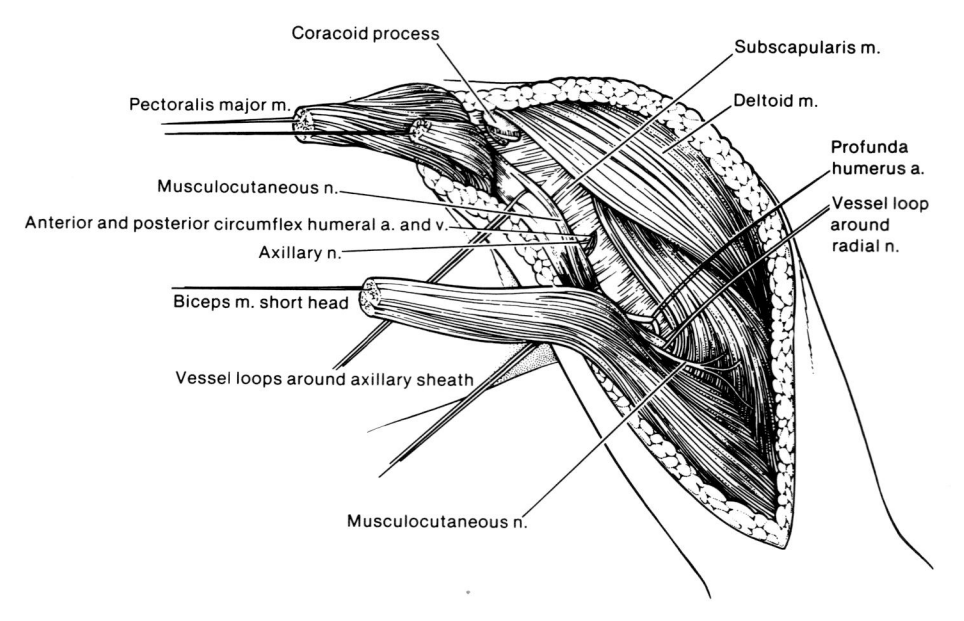

Figure 17–7. Exposure for neurovascular exploration.

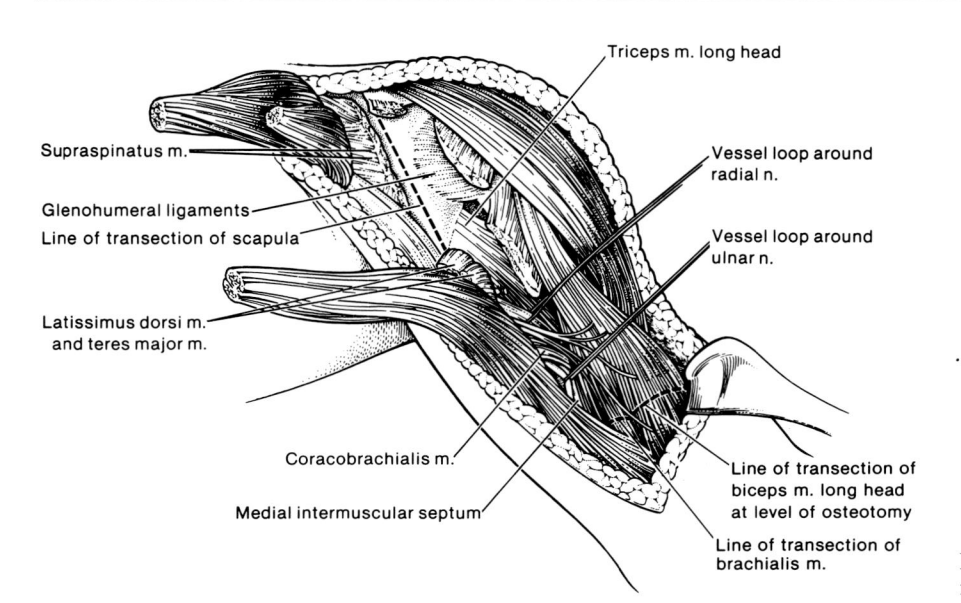

Figure 17–8. Exposure to the anterior neck of the scapula.

visualization posteriorly. The posterior incision begins anteriorly over the junction of the middle and lateral thirds of the clavicle. The incision continues posteriorly along the lateral third of the scapula to the distal edge of the scapula (Figure 17–9). The posterior skin flap is fashioned by dissecting between the anterior and the posterior incision over the deltoid muscle to the level of the midhumerus. If the entire scapula is to be removed (type VI resection), the posterior skin incision must be large enough to expose muscle over the entire scapula.

The thick fascia joining the posterior border of the deltoid muscle to the infraspinatus muscle and scapular spine is divided. The deltoid muscle is left covering the tumor mass. The trapezius muscle is transected from its insertions along the scapular spine and acromion. A digit is passed under the teres minor up to the planned scapular osteotomy site. The supraspinatus, infraspinatus, and teres minor muscles are transected under tension using electrocautery over the neck of the scapula (Figure 17–10). All transected muscles are tagged proximally. The radial and ulnar nerves are identified again and protected as the triceps muscles are transected at the level of the humeral osteotomy.

STEP 5: CLAVICULAR, SCAPULAR, AND HUMERAL OSTEOTOMIES

The clavicle is divided at the junction of the proximal and middle one-third level. The scapula is divided through its surgical neck, medial to the coracoid process. If the entire scapula is to be resected, the incision extends to the medial border of the scapula. The rhomboids, levator scapulae, and trapezius muscles are divided near their insertions on the scapula. The teres major, teres minor, supraspinatus, infraspinatus, and subscapularis muscles need not be divided if a complete scapular resection is performed.

The humerus is transected at the level determined preoperatively using an oscillating saw. Frozen sections of the

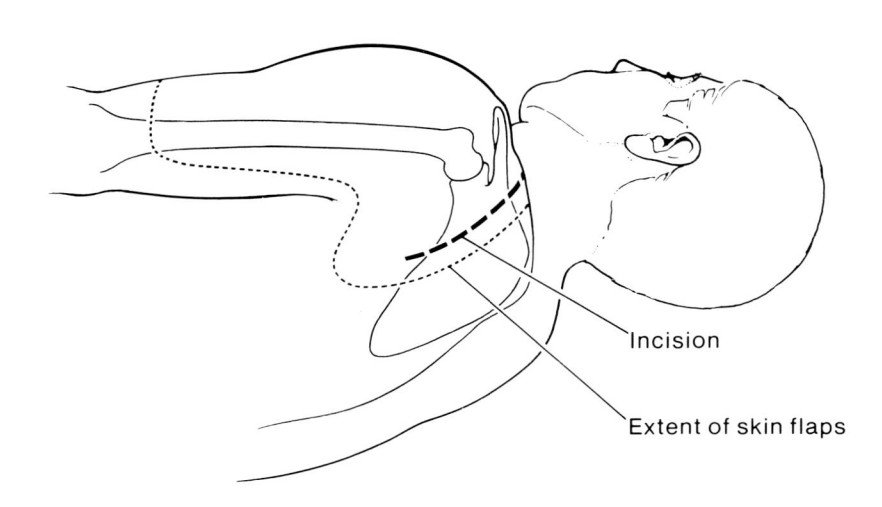

Figure 17–9. Posterior incision and lateral skin flap.

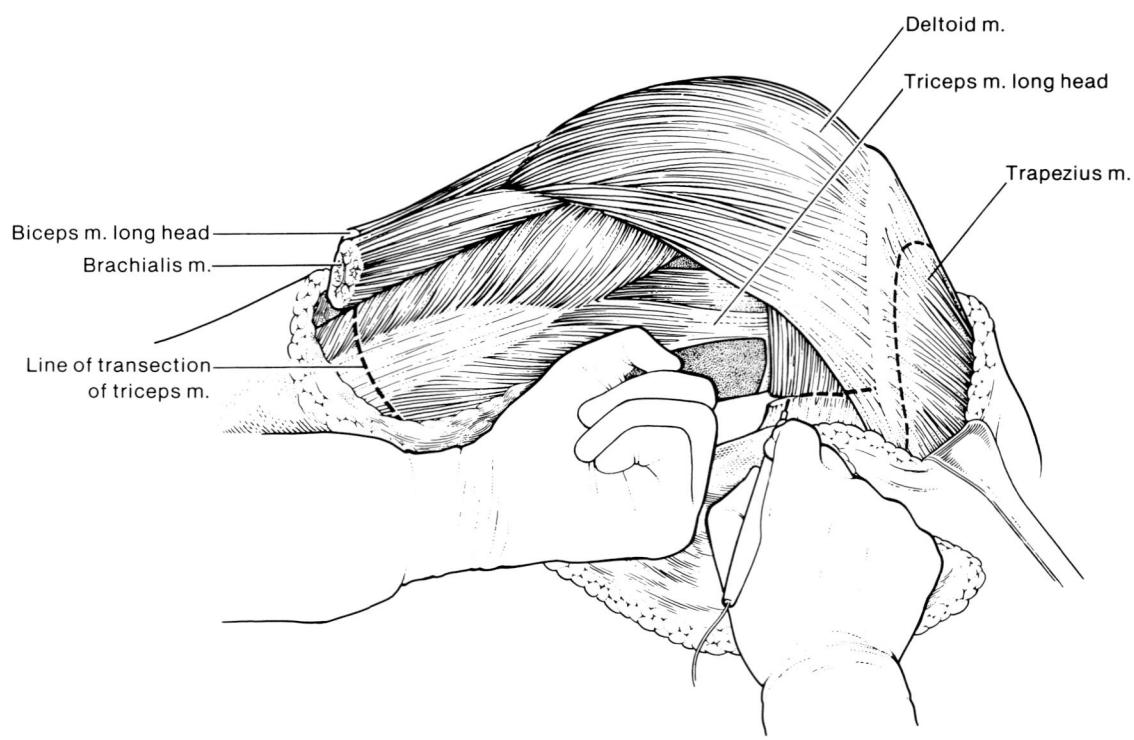

Figure 17–10. Division of the posterior musculature.

marrow from the remaining cut end of the humerus are examined microscopically to confirm tumor-free margins prior to continuing with the procedure. The specimen, which includes the biopsy site, proximal part of the humerus, shoulder joint, glenoid, upper portion of the long head of the biceps, and brachialis, is removed. The deltoid muscle covers the tumor. The insertions of the supraspinatus, infraspinatus, pectoralis major, latissimus dorsi, teres major, teres minor, and subscapularis muscles remain covering the tumor and constitute the free margins.

Phase 2: Reconstruction of the Bony Defect

Various techniques have been described for reconstruction of bony defects following proximal humeral resection for high-grade sarcomas. Allografts have been used in an effort to maintain a functional shoulder joint and preserve motion, or in combination with internal fixation to obtain an arthrodesis. Resection arthroplasty has also been used, but leaves the patient with a flail shoulder. The authors utilize a modular endoprosthesis that is custom-fitted intraoperatively (Figure 17–11). The principles of reconstruction are the same whether an endoprosthesis or an allograft is used. The functional goals of surgery are a pain-free shoulder and arm that is mobile with normal elbow and hand function.

If an endoprosthesis is chosen, the remaining medullary cavity of the humerus is prepared using a power reamer. The canal is reamed 1 to 2 mm larger than the diameter of the prosthetic stem, to allow for a cement mantle. The length of the resected specimen is measured, and a trial modular

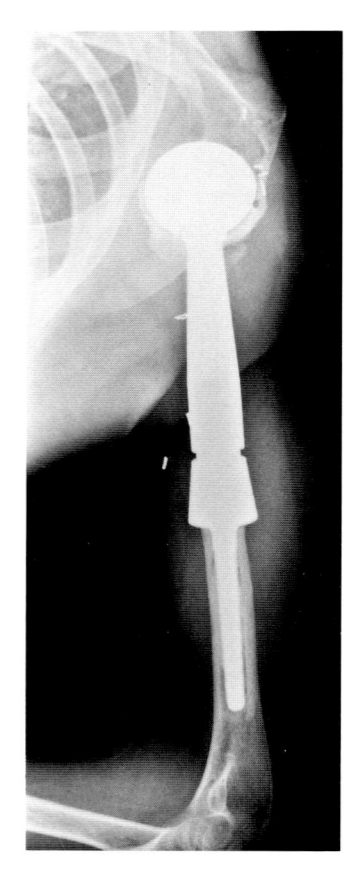

Figure 17–11. Modular prosthesis used for reconstruction of the bony defect following type V resection.

prosthesis is used to approximate its length. Appropriate length of the prosthesis is determined by appreciating the amount of soft-tissue tension in the biceps muscle during trial reduction. The brachial artery is palpated to make certain that it is not under tension. If the prosthesis is too long, arterial flow to the extremity may be compromised; if it is too short, elbow flexion motor strength will be weakened due to inappropriate tension of the biceps muscle.

A modular endoprosthesis, which can be custom-fitted during surgery, is helpful in balancing these two factors, and the authors now routinely utilize this device. Once the optimal length of the prosthesis has been determined, it is assembled and cemented into the medullary canal with polymethylmethacrylate using standard cementing technique. The head of the prosthesis is positioned in 45 degrees of retroversion with respect to the transected portion of the scapula while the arm is in neutral rotation. The radial nerve is positioned anterior to the prosthesis so that it does not become trapped between the prosthesis and muscle during soft-tissue closure and reconstruction. The head of the prosthesis is placed under the remaining portion of the subscapularis muscle on the anterior portion of the neck of the scapula (Figure 17–12).

Phase 3: Soft-Tissue Reconstruction

Multiple muscle transfers are used to protect the neurovascular bundle and to prevent the prosthesis from lying subcutaneously. Two drill holes are made through the scapula at the level of the spine, the lateral border of the scapula, and the distal portion of the remaining clavicle. To provide horizontal stability for the prosthesis, 3-mm Dacron tapes are passed through holes in the head of the prosthesis into the scapula and tied. Another Dacron tape is passed through the drill holes in the distal portion of the clavicle into the holes in the head of the prosthesis, and secured to provide vertical stability. As a result of these measures, static suspension of the prosthesis from the clavicle and scapula is obtained (Figure 17–13).

The pectoralis minor muscle is sutured to the subscapularis muscle and over the neurovascular bundle to prevent the bundle from being compressed against the prosthesis. The pectoralis major muscle is closed over the prosthesis to the cut edge of the scapula and secured by Dacron tape through drill holes. Next, the trapezius, supraspinatus, infraspinatus, and teres minor muscles are secured to the superior and lateral borders of the transected pectoralis major. The teres major and latissimus dorsi muscles are secured to the inferior border of pectoralis major. The proximal cut edge of the short head of the biceps is secured under appropriate tension to the remaining clavicle. The long head of the biceps and the brachialis muscle are tenodesed to the short head of the biceps muscle to provide additional strength for elbow flexion. The remaining triceps muscle is secured anteriorly along the lateral border of the biceps to cover the lower and lateral portions of the prosthesis.

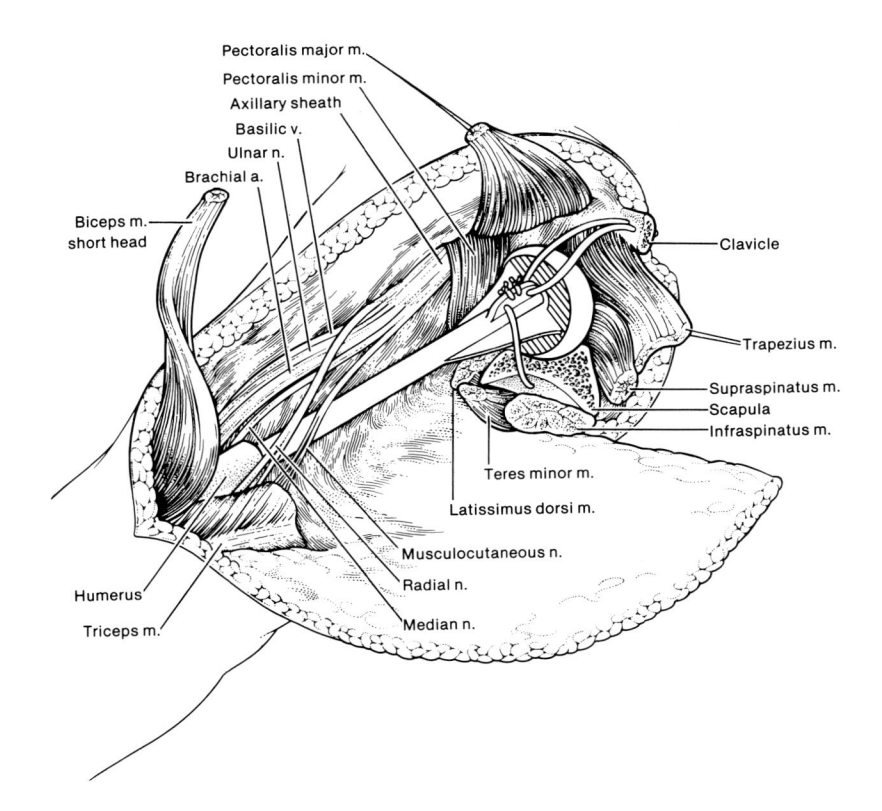

Figure 17–12. The prosthesis is assembled and secured in place.

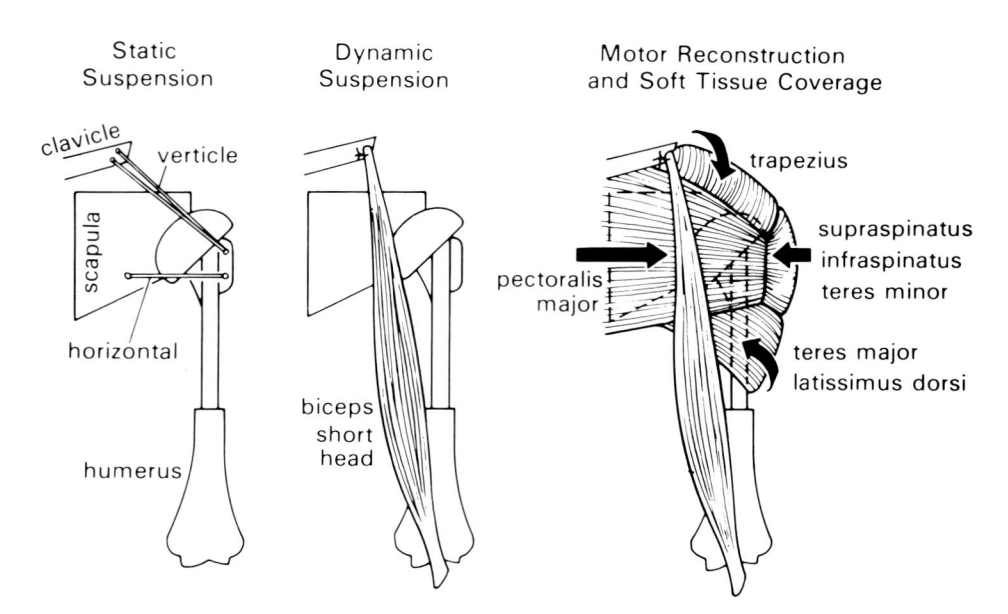

Figure 17–13. Stability of the prosthesis is obtained through static and dynamic tension.

POSTOPERATIVE MANAGEMENT AND EXPECTED FUNCTION

The extremity is kept in a shoulder immobilizer for 2 weeks, and the patient is instructed to avoid elbow extension. Active elbow flexion is encouraged within the first few days of surgery. The patient can sit in a chair within 3 days following surgery, and is ambulatory by the fourth postoperative day. Chemotherapy is delayed, usually 2 to 4 weeks, until the wound is healed. Hand function remains undisturbed following resections for tumors around the shoulder girdle. Elbow flexion strength is diminished but adequate for participating in activities of daily living and carrying objects weighing up to 30 lb (Figure 17–14). Muscle transfers, as outlined above, and appropriate tension are of critical importance in optimizing functional results. The shoulder girdle remains stable and pain-free but abduction is limited to between 10 and 30 degrees. Patients are given a self-directed therapy program consisting of Codman's exercises and passive range-of-motion exercises assisted by the contralateral extremity.

DISCUSSION

This chapter reviews the unique considerations of limb-sparing surgery for high-grade sarcomas of the shoulder girdle and describes the role of shoulder arthroplasty. Emphasis is placed on lesions arising in the proximal part of the humerus, the most common site of malignant tumor involvement for the shoulder girdle. Seventy shoulder girdle resections for high-grade sarcomas involving this site have been performed to date, and 25 have been type V resections. Of the 70 resections performed, revision has been required in

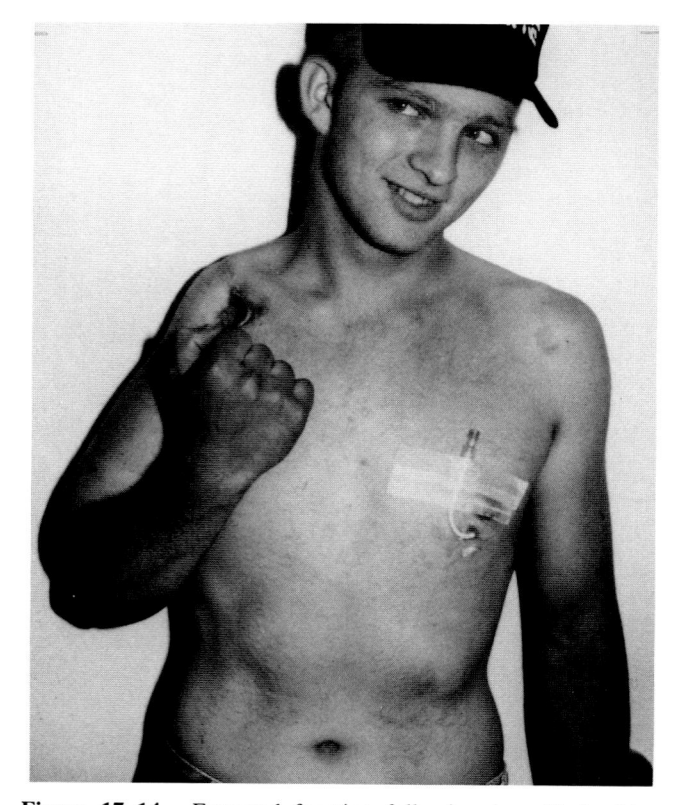

Figure 17–14. Expected function following type V shoulder resection. Hand function is undisturbed with active elbow flexion of 120 degrees.

only 2 cases. There have been two local recurrences. One was treated by local excision; the other with a forequarter amputation.

REFERENCES

1. Dahlin DC. *Bone Tumors: General Aspects and Data on 6,221 Cases*. 3rd ed. Springfield: Charles C Thomas, 1978.
2. Dahlin DC, Coventry MB. Osteosarcoma, a study of 600 cases. *J Bone Joint Surg [Am]* 1967;49:101–110.
3. Rosenberg SA, Suit FD, Baker LH. Sarcomas of soft tissue. In: DeVita VT, Hellman S, Rosenberg SA, eds. *Cancer: Principles and Practice of Oncology*. 2nd ed. Philadelphia: JB Lippincott, 1985:1243–1293.
4. Enneking WF. *Musculoskeletal Tumor Surgery*. New York: Churchill-Livingstone, 1983;1:355–410.
5. Liston R. Ossified aneurysmal tumor of the subscapular artery. *Ediul Med J* 1820;16:66–70.
6. Mussey RD. Removal by dissection of the entire shoulder blade and collar bone. *Am J Med Sci* 1837;21:390–394.
7. Syme J. *Excision of the Scapula*. Monograph. Edinburgh: Edmonston and Douglas, 1864.
8. De Nancrede CBG. The original results after total excision of the scapula for sarcoma. *Ann Surg* 1909;30:1–223.
9. Bauman PK. Resection of the upper extremity in the region of the shoulder joint. *Khirurg Arkh Velyaminova* 1914;30:145–149.
10. Linberg BE. Interscapulo-thoracic resection for malignant tumors of the shoulder joint region. *J Bone Joint Surg* 1928;10:344–349.
11. Francis KC, Worchester JN. Radical resection for tumors of the shoulder with preservation of a functional extremity. *J Bone Joint Surg [Am]* 1962;44:1423–1430.
12. Guerra A, Capanna R, Biagini R, et al. Extra-articular resection of the shoulder (Tikhoff-Linberg). *Ital J Orthop Traumatol* 1985;11:151–157.
13. Janecki CJ, Nelson CL. En bloc resection of the shoulder girdle: Technique and indications—Report of a case. *J Bone Joint Surg [Am]* 1972;54:1754–1758.
14. Malawer MM. Surgical technique and results of limb-sparing surgery for high grade bone sarcomas of the knee and shoulder: Analysis of 33 consecutive cases. *Orthopedics* 1985;8:597–607.
15. Malawer MM, Meller I, Dunham WK. Shoulder girdle resections for bone and soft tissue tumors: Analysis of 38 patients and presentation of a unified classification system. In: Yamamuro T, ed. *International Symposium on Limb-Salvage in Musculoskeletal Oncology*. New York: Springer-Verlag, 1988:519–530.
16. Malawer MM, Sugarbaker PJ, Lambert PT, et al. The Tikhoff-Linberg procedure: Report of ten patients and presentation of a modified technique for tumors of the proximal humerus. *Surgery* 1985;97:518–528.
17. Marcove RC, Lewis MM, Huvos AG. En bloc upper humeral interscapulothoracic resection. The Tikhoff-Linberg procedure. *Clin Orthop* 1977;124:219–228.
18. Pack GT, Baldwin JC. The Tikhoff-Linberg resection of shoulder girdle. Case report. *Surgery* 1955;38:751–757.
19. Pack GT, Crampton RS. The Tikhoff-Linberg resection of the shoulder girdle. *Clin Orthop* 1961;19:148–161.
20. Enneking WF, Spanier SS, Goodman MA. A system for the surgical staging of musculoskeletal sarcoma. *Clin Orthop* 1980;153:106.
21. Marcove RC. Neoplasms of the shoulder girdle. *Orthop Clin North Am* 1975;6:541–552.
22. Papaioannou AN, Francis KC. Scapulectomy for the treatment of primary malignant tumors of the scapula. *Clin Orthop* 1965;41:125–132.
23. Samilson RL, Morris JM, Thompson RW. Tumors of the scapula. A review of the literature and an analysis of 31 cases. *Clin Orthop* 1968;58:105–115.
24. Malawer MM, Meller I, Dunham WK. A new surgical classification system for shoulder-girdle resections: Analysis of 38 patients. *Clin Orthop* 1991;267:33–43.

only 2 cases. There have been two local recurrences. One was treated by local excision; the other with a forequarter amputation.

REFERENCES

1. Dahlin DC. *Bone Tumors: General Aspects and Data on 6,221 Cases*. 3rd ed. Springfield: Charles C Thomas, 1978.
2. Dahlin DC, Coventry MB. Osteosarcoma, a study of 600 cases. *J Bone Joint Surg [Am]* 1967;49:101–110.
3. Rosenberg SA, Suit FD, Baker LH. Sarcomas of soft tissue. In: DeVita VT, Hellman S, Rosenberg SA, eds. *Cancer: Principles and Practice of Oncology*. 2nd ed. Philadelphia: JB Lippincott, 1985:1243–1293.
4. Enneking WF. *Musculoskeletal Tumor Surgery*. New York: Churchill-Livingstone, 1983;1:355–410.
5. Liston R. Ossified aneurysmal tumor of the subscapular artery. *Ediul Med J* 1820;16:66–70.
6. Mussey RD. Removal by dissection of the entire shoulder blade and collar bone. *Am J Med Sci* 1837;21:390–394.
7. Syme J. *Excision of the Scapula*. Monograph. Edinburgh: Edmonston and Douglas, 1864.
8. De Nancrede CBG. The original results after total excision of the scapula for sarcoma. *Ann Surg* 1909;30:1–223.
9. Bauman PK. Resection of the upper extremity in the region of the shoulder joint. *Khirurg Arkh Velyaminova* 1914;30:145–149.
10. Linberg BE. Interscapulo-thoracic resection for malignant tumors of the shoulder joint region. *J Bone Joint Surg* 1928;10:344–349.
11. Francis KC, Worchester JN. Radical resection for tumors of the shoulder with preservation of a functional extremity. *J Bone Joint Surg [Am]* 1962;44:1423–1430.
12. Guerra A, Capanna R, Biagini R, et al. Extra-articular resection of the shoulder (Tikhoff-Linberg). *Ital J Orthop Traumatol* 1985;11:151–157.
13. Janecki CJ, Nelson CL. En bloc resection of the shoulder girdle: Technique and indications—Report of a case. *J Bone Joint Surg [Am]* 1972;54:1754–1758.
14. Malawer MM. Surgical technique and results of limb-sparing surgery for high grade bone sarcomas of the knee and shoulder: Analysis of 33 consecutive cases. *Orthopedics* 1985;8:597–607.
15. Malawer MM, Meller I, Dunham WK. Shoulder girdle resections for bone and soft tissue tumors: Analysis of 38 patients and presentation of a unified classification system. In: Yamamuro T, ed. *International Symposium on Limb-Salvage in Musculoskeletal Oncology*. New York: Springer-Verlag, 1988:519–530.
16. Malawer MM, Sugarbaker PJ, Lambert PT, et al. The Tikhoff-Linberg procedure: Report of ten patients and presentation of a modified technique for tumors of the proximal humerus. *Surgery* 1985;97:518–528.
17. Marcove RC, Lewis MM, Huvos AG. En bloc upper humeral interscapulothoracic resection. The Tikhoff-Linberg procedure. *Clin Orthop* 1977;124:219–228.
18. Pack GT, Baldwin JC. The Tikhoff-Linberg resection of shoulder girdle. Case report. *Surgery* 1955;38:751–757.
19. Pack GT, Crampton RS. The Tikhoff-Linberg resection of the shoulder girdle. *Clin Orthop* 1961;19:148–161.
20. Enneking WF, Spanier SS, Goodman MA. A system for the surgical staging of musculoskeletal sarcoma. *Clin Orthop* 1980;153:106.
21. Marcove RC. Neoplasms of the shoulder girdle. *Orthop Clin North Am* 1975;6:541–552.
22. Papaioannou AN, Francis KC. Scapulectomy for the treatment of primary malignant tumors of the scapula. *Clin Orthop* 1965;41:125–132.
23. Samilson RL, Morris JM, Thompson RW. Tumors of the scapula. A review of the literature and an analysis of 31 cases. *Clin Orthop* 1968;58:105–115.
24. Malawer MM, Meller I, Dunham WK. A new surgical classification system for shoulder-girdle resections: Analysis of 38 patients. *Clin Orthop* 1991;267:33–43.

SECTION V

Results and Survivorship of Total Shoulder Arthroplasty

18 Long-Term Results of Total Shoulder Arthroplasty

John D. Henry, M.D., and Thomas S. Thornhill, M.D.

Total shoulder arthroplasty is a well-established and widely accepted method of treatment for a variety of shoulder disorders. Numerous reviews detailing the successful results of the procedure have been published. Unfortunately, lack of uniformity in methods of reporting results makes comparison of different studies and analysis of some variables at times difficult. Ideally, reported results should include information regarding component fixation methods, pain relief, patient satisfaction, range of motion, strength, stability, functional improvement, complications, reoperations, revisions, and radiographic results. The American Shoulder and Elbow Surgeons have proposed a standardized form that facilitates uniformity and completeness in evaluating results.

The reported experience in the literature suggests that good to excellent results following total shoulder arthroplasty using contemporary techniques can be expected in most situations. This chapter presents the clinical, radiographic, and survivorship results of nonconstrained, semiconstrained, and constrained total shoulder arthroplasty systems.

NONCONSTRAINED TOTAL SHOULDER ARTHROPLASTY

The most commonly used and widely reported type of nonconstrained total shoulder system is the Neer design. This prosthesis is a resurfacing or anatomic design that replaces the humeral and glenoid articular surfaces. The surface geometry of the prosthetic humeral head and that of the glenoid component conform to the radius of curvature of the natural glenohumeral articular surface. Stability is provided by the integrity of the rotator cuff and adjacent soft tissues. The humeral component may be cemented or applied with a press-fit and is available in two head thicknesses as well as a variety of stem lengths and widths. The glenoid component features a keel for anchoring the component in the scapular neck, and is available in either a standard polyethylene or metal-backed polyethylene design. Both glenoid components are secured with methylmethacrylate, and recently a metal-backed version with porous coating and screw fixation was introduced. In recent years other designs have emerged and provide modularity, a wider range of head sizes, and a greater variety of stem diameters.

Clinical Results

The results of 860 nonconstrained Neer II total shoulder arthroplasties obtained from 12 reported series are summarized in Table 18–1.[1–12] The preoperative diagnostic categories are primarily rheumatoid arthritis, osteoarthritis, and posttraumatic arthritis. Average follow-up ranges from 2.3 to 5.6 years. Choice of component fixation is variable, but the majority of earlier series utilized cemented standard polyethylene glenoid components.

Satisfactory pain relief is consistently achieved and maintained in 82 to 93% of patients at the latest follow-up. Patient satisfaction with the results of surgery is also encouragingly high (89 to 97%). Improvement in range of motion is variable and dependent on diagnostic category. Average gains in active forward elevation range from 12 to 60 degrees and average gains in external rotation range from 13 to 29 degrees for all diagnostic categories combined. The key determinants of increased range of motion, as shown by Cofield,[2] are the diagnosis and closely associated status of the rotator cuff and shoulder capsule. Patients with rheumatoid arthritis who have greater soft-tissue disease and bony deficiency typically achieve a return of range of motion that is one-half to two-thirds of normal. Patients with osteoarthritis and less soft-tissue pathology, however, may expect a return of motion that is three-fourths or four-fifths of normal. In Cofield's study,[2] the range of motion in active abduction for all patients increased from an average of 76 degrees preoperatively to 120 degrees postoperatively. Those patients with a normal rotator cuff had an increase in active abduction to 143 degrees postoperatively.

Functional improvement is reported from series to series using a variety of different evaluation guidelines, making comparison among studies difficult. Neer[1] suggested two systems for grading results: a full exercise program and a limited goals rehabilitation program. Patients in the full exercise program were graded excellent, satisfactory, or unsatisfactory. Patients who had a massive deficiency of bone or muscle were placed in a limited goals category and were graded either successful or unsuccessful. The purpose of the limited goals program was to ensure stability in patients whose structural integrity of the rotator cuff and shoulder capsule was deficient. In this situation, aggressive physical therapy to obtain full motion or strength is undesirable, since it places stability at risk.

In the full exercise program, an excellent result was

Table 18–1. Clinical Results of Neer II Total Shoulder Arthroplasty (860 Procedures)

AUTHOR(S)	NO. OF SHOULDERS	AVERAGE FOLLOW-UP (y) (RANGE)	DIAGNOSIS	PAIN RELIEF	PATIENT SATISFACTION	AVERAGE ACTIVE FORWARD ELEVATION (AND POSTOP. GAIN) (DEGREES)	AVERAGE EXTERNAL ROTATION (AND POSTOP. GAIN) (DEGREES)
Neer et al.,[1] 1982	194	3.1 (2.0–8.3)	Mixed				
Cofield,[2] 1984	73	3.8 (2.0–6.5)	Mixed	92%	92%	120 (+44)	48 (26)
Bade et al.,[3] 1984	38	4.5 (2.0–7.3)	Mixed	93%		118 (+50)	
Wilde et al.,[4] 1984	38	3.0 (0.7–2.4)	Mixed	92%			
Kelly et al.,[5] 1987	40	3.0 (1.0–5.5)	RA	88%	97%	75 (+20)	40 (29)
Barrett et al.,[6] 1987	50	3.5 (2.0–7.5)	Mixed	88%	94%	100 (+29)	54 (23)
Frich et al.,[7] 1988	50	2.3 (1.0–3.5)	Mixed	92%		58–78 (+12–30)	17–21 (13–19)
Brenner et al.,[8] 1989	37	5.6 (2.0–10.8)	Mixed	82%	90%	115 (+37)	41 (24)
Hawkins et al.,[9] 1989	70	3.3 (2.0–8.6)	Mixed	91%		131 (+60)	36 (18)
McCoy et al.,[10] 1989	29	3.0 (1.0–7.3)	RA	93%		76 (+15)	
Weiss et al.,[11] 1990	33	4.9 (3–10)	Mixed	93%		96 (+47)	
Henry et al.,[12] 1992	208	5.3 (2.0–15.8)	Mixed	90%	89%	97 (+38)	36 (23)

RA = rheumatoid arthritis.

defined as having the following: Patient was enthusiastic about the operation, had no significant pain, and used the shoulder fully; muscle strength was near-normal; active elevation of the arm was within 35 degrees of the normal side; and internal and external rotation was within 90 percent of the normal side. In a satisfactory result, the following were present: Patient was satisfied with the operation, had pain only occasionally or aching with changes in the weather, had good daily shoulder function from the top of the head and below, had a minimum of 30 percent of normal motor strength, and had 90 to 135 degrees of elevation and rotation to 50 percent of the normal side. An unsatisfactory result meant that these criteria were not met. Patients in the limited goals program were graded successful if they were able to achieve 90 degrees of elevation and 20 degrees of external rotation, had satisfactory pain relief, and maintained shoulder stability. Approximately 23% of the total number of patients in the series fell into the limited goals category and of these, 95% were rated successful and 5% unsuccessful. Approximately 67% of patients in the full exercise program achieved an excellent clinical rating while 19% were rated satisfactory and 14% were rated unsatisfactory. When analyzed by diagnostic category, 90% of patients with osteoarthritis had excellent and 7.5%, satisfactory results. However, 65% of patients with rheumatoid arthritis had excellent; 28%, satisfactory; and 7%, unsatisfactory results.

Other authors have reported functional results following total shoulder arthroplasty by grading the patient's ability to perform specific activities of daily living. Henry et al.[12] reported the functional results of 208 Neer total shoulder arthroplasties at 2.0 to 15.8 years of follow-up. Functional assessment was based on a 36-point system and scored with a 4-point maximum in each of nine activities of daily living and included the ability to use the back pocket, attend to perineal care, wash the opposite axilla, eat with a utensil, comb hair, carry 10 to 15 lb with the arm at the side, use the hand with the arm at shoulder level, use the hand over the head, and sleep on the operated side.

The average preoperative score of all shoulders was 9.5 and this improved to 25.3 postoperatively. Patients with osteoarthritis showed the most improvement, from an average preoperative score of 11.7 to an average postoperative score of 32.9, while scores for patients with rheumatoid arthritis improved from 7.1 preoperatively to 24.6 postoperatively.

The activities of daily living with which patients consistently had the most difficulty in performing were the ability to carry 10 to 15 lb with the arm at the side and use of the hand overhead. Barrett et al.[6] in a similar study evaluated patients' ability to perform five activities of daily living. Preoperatively only 14% of the shoulders could be used to perform all five activities satisfactorily, while 78% could do so after surgery. Kelly et al.[5] assessed the functional ability of 41 total shoulder arthroplasties by grading nine activities of daily living. Each activity of daily living scored 4 points for a maximum of 36 possible points. Preoperatively the mean score was 16 and postoperatively was improved to 30. No patient's functional ability deteriorated after surgery, despite the fact that function was frequently affected by disease and other upper extremity joints.

Several authors have reported results of various other nonconstrained total shoulder arthroplasty systems. The clinical and radiographic results parallel those of the Neer design. Gristina et al.[13] reported the results of 109 spherical total shoulder arthroplasties at an average follow-up of 3.2 years. The pain relief was 90%. Patient satisfaction was 94% and active forward elevation was 108 degrees on average. Approximately two-thirds of the glenoids had radiolucent lines but only four cases of glenoid loosening were reported.

Radiographic Results

Analysis of sequential radiographs looking for changes at the prosthetic-bone or bone-cement interface, subsidence, and proximal migration provides important information regarding the fixation stability and success of a total shoulder arthroplasty. The reported radiographic results of 12 large series of Neer nonconstrained total shoulder arthroplasties are summarized in Table 18–2.[1-12] Most of the series report radiolucent lines at the glenoid bone-cement interface; these vary in frequency from 30 to 93%, depending on the series. The clinical relevance of these glenoid radiolucent lines is a source of disagreement among various authors. Many of these radiolucent lines are noticed on immediate postoperative radiographs and do not progress, possibly related to the surgical cementing technique.

Fortunately, the revision rates for symptomatic glenoid loosening are low. Aliabadi et al.,[14] in a radiographic study of 98 nonconstrained total shoulder arthroplasties, were unable to demonstrate a correlation between the presence of radiolucent lines about the glenoid and pain relief, range of motion, motor strength, or functional improvement. However, some authors have reported progression of radiolucencies in both width and length over sequential radiographs. While component migration and tilt clearly signify loosening of the glenoid, radiolucent lines measuring 2 mm or more in width, those that completely surround the component and involve all of the bone-cement interface or show progression are also particularly worrisome. Several authors have also reported that radiolucent lines in the region of the keel are of great concern, as the keel itself serves as an important anchor for the prosthesis in the scapular neck.

The addition of metal backing to the glenoid component does not appear to have influenced the frequency of radiolucent lines. Henry et al.[12] reported the occurrence of radiolucent lines around the glenoid in 90 (82%) of 110 shoulders with cemented all-polyethylene glenoids and in 29 (81%) of 36 arthroplasties with cemented metal-backed glenoids.

The incidence of humeral radiolucent lines is much less than that of glenoid radiolucent lines and ranges from 1 to 44% in the 12 reported series. Clinically, symptomatic humeral loosening rates have also remained low. Rates of humeral component subsidence have varied between 7 and 20%, with press-fit humeral components having a slightly higher incidence of subsidence. Rates of proximal migration following total shoulder arthroplasty have been reported in 22 and 28% of patients.[11,12]

Survivorship

Unless a major complication occurs, good to excellent results may be anticipated following a nonconstrained Neer total shoulder arthroplasty. The complications of 860 Neer total shoulder replacements reported in 12 series are summarized in Table 18–3.[1-12] The most common complications are glenoid component loosening (2.4%), instability (2.2%), and rotator cuff tear (2.6%). Humeral loosening, infection, impingement, nerve palsy, and heterotopic ossification are less common. A total of 129 complications in 860 procedures yields an overall complication rate of 15%.

In these 12 series reporting the results of 860 Neer total shoulder arthroplasties, 67 major reoperations (7.8%) have been necessary. The most common indications for reoperation have been glenoid loosening and rotator cuff tearing. Thirty-five (4.1%) of these operations, as shown in Table 18–4, have involved revision of one or both components. In 25 (71%) of the 35 revisions the component was able to be replaced. However, in 10 (29%) of the 35 revisions, the loose component was removed and could not be replaced, most commonly due to the loss of significant glenoid bone stock to support another glenoid component.

In 1984, Cofield[15] analyzed 176 consecutive Neer total shoulder arthroplasties done at the Mayo Clinic, to determine the frequency of reoperation. At the time of follow-up, eight major reoperations (4.5%) had been required. Application of Kaplan-Meier survivorship analysis techniques predicted a failure rate (need for reoperation) of 9.6% percent at 5 years of follow-up. In 1991,[16] after continued analysis of results,

Table 18–2. Radiographic Results of Neer II Total Shoulder Arthroplasty

AUTHOR(S)	NO. OF SHOULDERS	AVERAGE FOLLOW-UP (y)	RADIOLUCENT LINES (%)	
			Glenoid	Humeral
Neer et al.,[1] 1982	194	3.1	30	1
Cofield,[2] 1984	73	3.8	80	32
Bade et al.,[3] 1984	38	4.5	67	26
Wilde et al.,[4] 1984	38	3.0	93	
Kelly et al.,[5] 1987	40	3.0	83	24
Barrett et al.,[6] 1987	50	3.5	74	8
Frich et al.,[7] 1988	50	2.3		
Brenner et al.,[8] 1989	37	5.6	58	4
Hawkins et al.,[9] 1989	70	3.3	"Nearly all"	24
McCoy et al.,[10] 1989	29	3.0	86	31
Weiss et al.,[11] 1990	33	4.9	36	13
Henry et al.,[12] 1992	208	5.3	78	44

Table 18-3. Complications of Neer II Total Shoulder Arthroplasty

AUTHOR(S)	NO. OF SHOULDERS	GLENOID LOOSENING	HUMERAL LOOSENING	INFECTION	INSTABILITY	ROTATOR CUFF TEAR	IMPINGEMENT	HUMERUS FRACTURE		NERVE PALSY	HETEROTOPIC OSSIFICATION	OTHER
								Intraoperative	Late			
Neer et al.,[1] 1982	194			1	6	5	1	1		1		8
Cofield,[2] 1984	73	3				5				1		6
Bade et al.,[3] 1984	38	1	2			5	2					
Wilde et al.,[4] 1984	38			1	2		2	1			1	1
Kelly et al.,[5] 1987	40					2						1
Barrett et al.,[6] 1987	50	4			1	1	1	2		1		
Frich et al.,[7] 1988	50	3			1				1	1		1
Brenner et al.,[8] 1989	37	2	1		1	2			1			3
Hawkins et al.,[9] 1989	70	2			1	2		2		1		2
McCoy et al.,[10] 1989	29							2				
Weiss et al.,[11] 1990	33			1	1			5				
Henry et al.,[12] 1992	208	5	5	1	6		6	8	7	5	1	22
Totals	860	21	8	4	19	22	6	8	7	5	1	22
Percentage		2.4	0.9	0.5	2.2	2.6	0.7	0.9	0.8	0.6	0.1	2.6

Table 18-4. Reoperations/Revisions of Neer Total Shoulder Arthroplasty

AUTHOR(S)	NO. OF SHOULDERS	REVISIONS Component(s) Replaced	REVISIONS Component(s) Removed	OTHER REOPERATIONS
Neer et al.,[1] 1982	194	3	3	6
Cofield,[2] 1984	73	3		2
Bade et al.,[3] 1984	38	1		1
Wilde et al.,[4] 1984	38	1	1	3
Kelly et al.,[5] 1987	40		1	2
Barrett et al.,[6] 1987	50	1	3	3
Frich et al.,[7] 1988	50	1		
Brenner et al.,[8] 1989	37	1	1	
Hawkins et al.,[9] 1989	70	2	1	3
McCoy et al.,[10] 1989	28			
Weiss et al.,[11] 1990	33			
Henry et al.,[12] 1992	208	12		12
Totals	860	25	10	32
Percentages		2.9	1.2	3.7

the original projection was not proved to be true. The need for revision surgery remained under 5%.

Brenner et al.[8] reported the results of 37 Neer total shoulder arthroplasties followed for a minimum of 2 years, also using survivorship analysis methods. Failure was defined as the need for revision or the onset of patient dissatisfaction. After 11 years, a survivorship of 71% was predicted for the Neer prostheses.

SEMICONSTRAINED AND CONSTRAINED TOTAL SHOULDER ARTHROPLASTY

During the early stages in the development of total shoulder arthroplasty, a number of constrained or ball-and-socket–type prosthetic systems were utilized. The inherent stability afforded in a constrained design was an attractive feature in situations of rotator cuff and capsular deficiency. The results and complications of several of the more commonly used systems are summarized in Tables 18–5 and 18–6.[17-22] Pain relief was usually satisfactory but range of motion was more limited in comparison to the results from nonconstrained systems. Unfortunately, the frequency of major complications including symptomatic glenoid loosening, component fatigue failure, and dislocations were dramatically higher than that of nonconstrained systems and resulted in a higher number of reoperations and revisions. The indications for the use of a constrained system by today's standards are limited in most authors' opinions.

Semiconstrained total shoulder designs using a hooded glenoid component were developed as alternatives to completely constrained systems in dealing with soft-tissue defi-

Table 18-5. Clinical Results of Semiconstrained and Constrained Total Shoulder Arthroplasties

AUTHOR(S)	TYPE OF PROSTHESIS	NO. OF SHOULDERS	AVERAGE FOLLOW-UP (y) (RANGE)	PAIN RELIEF	AVERAGE FORWARD ELEVATION (GAIN) (DEGREES)	AVERAGE EXTERNAL ROTATION (GAIN) (DEGREES)
Semiconstrained						
Faludi and Weiland,[17] 1983	English-MacNab	13	3.7	Most	75 (+39)	25 (+15)
McElwain and English,[18] 1987	English-MacNab	13	3.1 (1.0–5.5)	85%	84 (+27)	
Amstutz et al.,[19] 1988	DANA	10	3.5	100%	85 (+35)	50 (−10)
Constrained						
Coughlin et al.,[20] 1979	Stanmore	16	2.6 (2.0–4.4)	50% (complete)	94 (+34)	
Post et al.,[21] 1980	Michael Reese	28	(1.3–6.0)	96%		
Lettin et al.,[22] 1982	Stanmore	40		90%	75 (+20)	

Table 18–6. Complications, Revisions, and Reoperations of Semiconstrained and Constrained Total Shoulder Arthroplasties

AUTHOR(S)	NO. OF SHOULDERS	COMPONENT FAILURE	GLENOID LOOSENING	HUMERAL LOOSENING	INFECTION	INSTABILITY	FRACTURE	OTHER	REVISION Component Replaced	REVISION Component Removed	OTHER REOPERATIONS
Semiconstrained											
Faludi and Weiland,[16] 1982	13					1	2				
McElwain and English,[17] 1987	13	3	1	1	1	1	1		1		
Amstutz et al.,[18] 1988	10		1					1	2		
Constrained											
Coughlin et al.,[19] 1979	16		1		1	1		1	1	1	1
Post et al.,[20] 1980	28	8		1	1	5			8	1	4
Lettin et al.,[21] 1982	40		10		1	3			8	9	1

ciencies commonly found in patients undergoing shoulder arthroplasty. The results and complications of several reported series are presented in Tables 18–5 and 18–6. Pain relief once again was satisfactory in the absence of complications. Improvements in range of motion were disappointing, and the frequency of complications and number of revisions and reoperations remained higher than that of nonconstrained systems.

Amstutz et al.[19] reported the results of 46 DANA total shoulder procedures at 3.5-year follow-up. Pain relief was 91%, average postoperative elevation was 85 degrees, and average external rotation was 50 degrees. Approximately 95% of the glenoids had radiolucent lines.

SUMMARY

The results reviewed in this chapter validate the efficacy of total shoulder arthroplasty in the treatment of a variety of types of glenohumeral arthritis. Total shoulder arthroplasty has evolved over the past two decades to a point now that it is one of the most successful total joint arthroplasty procedures. Predictable and consistent pain relief, restoration of function for activities of daily living, and improved range of motion are reported in most of the nonconstrained design series. Long-term studies are beginning to show lasting successful results, with the functional and pain scores not deteriorating over time. The most worrisome problem encountered thus far has been the high incidence of radiolucent lines about the glenoid component. Future advances in total shoulder arthroplasty surgery are likely to focus on improving glenoid component fixation through advances in prosthetic design and improvements in soft-tissue reconstruction and balancing techniques to avoid increased stresses at the bone-prosthesis interface.

REFERENCES

1. Neer CS, Watson KC, Stanton FJ. Recent experience in total shoulder replacement. *J Bone Joint Surg [Am]* 1982;64:319–337.
2. Cofield RH. Total shoulder arthroplasty with the Neer prosthesis. *J Bone Joint Surg [Am]* 1984;66:899–906.
3. Bade HA, Warren RF, Ranawat CS, Inglis AE: Long term results of Neer total shoulder replacement. In: Batemen JE, Welsh RP, eds. *Surgery of the Shoulder*. St. Louis: CV Mosby, 1984:294–302.
4. Wilde AH, Borden LS, Brems JJ. Experience with the Neer total shoulder replacement. In: Batemen JE, Welsh RP, eds. *Surgery of the Shoulder*. St. Louis: CV Mosby, 1984:224–228.
5. Kelly IG, Foster RS, Fisher WD. Neer total shoulder replacement in rheumatoid arthritis. *J Bone Joint Surg [Br]* 1987;69:723–726.
6. Barrett WP, Franklin JL, Jackins SE, et al. Total shoulder arthroplasty. *J Bone Joint Surg [Am]* 1987;69:865–872.
7. Frich LH, Moller BN, Sneppen O. Shoulder arthroplasty with the Neer Mark-II prosthesis. *Arch Orthop Trauma Surg* 1988;107:110–113.
8. Brenner BC, Ferlic DL, Clayton ML, Dennis DA. Survivorship of unconstrained total shoulder arthroplasty. *J Bone Joint Surg [Am]* 1989;71:1289–1296.
9. Hawkins RJ, Bell RH, Jallay B. Total shoulder arthroplasty. *Clin Orthop* 1989;242:188–194.
10. McCoy SR, Warren RF, Bade HA, et al. Total shoulder arthroplasty in rheumatoid arthritis. *J Arthroplasty* 1989;4:105–113.
11. Weiss APC, Adams MA, Moore JR, Weiland AJ. Unconstrained shoulder arthroplasty: A five year average follow up study. *Clin Orthop* 1990;257:86–90.
12. Henry JD, Thomas WH, Thornhill TS, et al. Total shoulder arthroplasty using the Neer unconstrained implant: Long term results. Abstracts of the 59th Annual Meeting of the American Academy of Orthopaedic Surgeons; Washington, D.C., February 25, 1992, pg. 224.
13. Gristina AG, Romano RL, Kammire GC, Webb LX. Total shoulder replacement. *Orthop Clin North Am* 1987;18:445–453.
14. Aliabadi P, Weissman BN, Thornhill TS, Nikpoor N, Sosman JL. Evaluation of a nonconstrained total shoulder prosthesis. *Am J Radiol* 1988;151:1169–1172.
15. Cofield RH. Unconstrained total shoulder prostheses. *Clin Orthop* 1983;173:97–108.
16. Cofield RH. Revision. In: Morrey BF, ed. *Joint Replacement Arthroplasty*. New York: Churchill-Livingstone, 1991:455–456.
17. Faludi DD, Weiland AJ. Cementless total shoulder arthroplasty: Preliminary experience with thirteen cases. *Orthopedics* 1983;6:431–437.
18. McElwain JP, English E. The early results of porous-coated total shoulder arthroplasty. *Clin Orthop* 1987;218:217–224.
19. Amstutz HC, Thomas BJ, Kabo JM, et al.: The DANA total shoulder arthroplasty. *J Bone Joint Surg [Am]* 1988;70:1174–1182.
20. Couglin MJ, Morris JM, West WF. The semiconstrained total shoulder arthroplasty. *J Bone Joint Surg [Am]* 1979;61:574–581.
21. Post M, Haskell SS, Jablon M. Total shoulder replacement with a constrained prosthesis. *J Bone Joint Surg [Am]* 1980;62:327–335.
22. Lettin AWF, Copeland SA, Scales JT. The Stanmore total shoulder replacement. *J Bone Joint Surg [Br]* 1982;64:47–51.

19 Revision Shoulder Arthroplasty

Steve A. Petersen, M.D., and Richard J. Hawkins, M.D.

Due to the success of shoulder joint replacement surgery, experience with revision shoulder arthroplasty has been limited. The incidence of revision arthroplasty surgery has been related to the initial procedure performed, ranging from 4.6% for humeral hemiarthroplasties to 24.7% for constrained total shoulder designs.[1]

Advancements in the technique of shoulder arthroplasty have favored nonconstrained designs.[2] Survivorship of a nonconstrained Neer total shoulder arthroplasty has been estimated at 90.4% at 5 years and 71% at 11 years.[3,4] The incidence of component revision for nonconstrained implants has been reported to be between 0 and 13%.[5-16] It is expected that late complications will continue to appear after longer follow-up, with an increase in the number of reoperations required for this otherwise successful procedure.

A myriad of etiologies have been defined as the cause of shoulder arthroplasty failure. Soft-tissue injury, muscle damage, bone loss, and extensive scar formation often compromise the success of revision surgery by limiting shoulder function.[2] While experience with revision shoulder arthroplasty remains limited, various principles guiding treatment can be utilized from revision arthroplasty surgery performed in other anatomic areas, and from difficult primary shoulder arthroplasties.[17,18] Due to the complexity in evaluating and treating a failed shoulder arthroplasty, it is of paramount importance to carefully define the problem or problems resulting in its failure and become familiar with the multiple options available in managing each of these problems.[19]

Revision shoulder arthroplasty has been recognized as the most technically difficult of any category of shoulder arthroplasty.[2] The purpose of this chapter is to define the reasons for shoulder arthroplasty failure, outline the preoperative evaluation, and describe the surgical principles necessary to affect the best treatment.

PATHOGENESIS OF FAILED SHOULDER ARTHROPLASTY

The pathogenesis of failed shoulder arthroplasty is intimately related to the original shoulder disorder and the type of shoulder arthroplasty that was performed for its treatment. Neer and Kirby[2] identified the common causes for failure of both humeral head replacement and nonconstrained total shoulder arthroplasty as deltoid scarring and detachment, anterior capsular shortening with scarring of the subscapularis musculature, adhesions and impingement of the rotator cuff, a prominent or retracted greater tuberosity, loss of humeral length, and uneven glenoid wear resulting in centralization or abnormal version of the glenoid component. Causes of failure for constrained shoulder arthroplasty include mechanical failure from the loss of osseous fixation, bending or breakage of the implant, and loss of the external rotators. Glenoid loosening, glenohumeral instability, and painful joint stiffness have also resulted in the revision of constrained designs.[1] It has been observed that patient cooperation during postoperative rehabilitation also plays an important role in the success of the primary arthroplasty.[14]

The causes for failed shoulder arthroplasty have been recently reviewed by several authors. Boyd et al.[8] reported shoulder arthroplasty failure occurring in 8 of 313 total shoulder arthroplasties and 8 of 123 hemiarthroplasties performed between 1974 and 1988, representing failure rates of 2.6% and 6.5%, respectively. They noted that loosening of the glenoid component in total shoulder arthroplasty and surface erosion of the glenoid after humeral head replacement were the most common causes for failure. Of interest, 11 of 18 shoulders failed within 18 months, suggesting that attention to surgical technique might avoid complications that led to early failure.

Cofield[1] reported on the Mayo Clinic experience in revision shoulder arthroplasty, with 56 nonconstrained total shoulder arthroplasties and 27 humeral hemiarthroplasties revised from 1976 to 1989. Glenoid arthritis was noted to be the most common cause for reoperation for failed humeral hemiarthroplasty, occurring in 13 (48%) of 27 shoulders. Rotator cuff deficiency and tuberosity problems, instability, and humeral component loosening were identified as other common causes for failure. Glenoid component loosening, instability, rotator cuff deficiency, humeral component loosening, and displaced or deformed high-density polyethylene components were common causes of failure for total shoulder arthroplasty. Others included infection, fracture, ectopic bone, nerve laceration, hematoma, and component malposition. Multiple causes for humeral head and total arthroplasty failure were often recognized.

Recent reports have documented the experience with failed humeral hemiarthroplasties.[20,21] In a series of 21 patients (27 shoulders) initially treated with a humeral hemiarthroplasty for proximal humeral fractures, Bigliani et al.[20] discovered multiple causes of failure occurring in 68% of the patients, with displacement or malposition of the greater tuberosity (59%) and component malposition (42%) the most common modes of failure. Aseptic loosening of uncemented components (25%), dislocation (21%), glenoid erosion (17%), nerve injury (25%), ectopic bone (13%), and deep sepsis (8%) were also commonly identified causes of failure. Interestingly, patient noncompliance with postoperative rehabilitation was again recognized as an important cause of hemiarthroplasty failure.

In a series of 64 patients who had a humeral hemiarthroplasty performed for a variety of indications, Bonutti and Hawkins[21] noted a 17% revision rate. Glenoid arthritis (54%), rotator cuff deficiency (46%), and instability (38%) were commonly observed at revision surgery, with glenoid arthritic changes most severe in patients with glenohumeral instability (Figure 19-1). Rotator cuff deficiency associated with a massive cuff tear seemed to portend a particularly poor prognosis. Revision surgery was required within 1 year after the initial procedure in 6 of 13 patients.

PREOPERATIVE EVALUATION FOR FAILED SHOULDER ARTHROPLASTY

In order to evaluate a failed shoulder arthroplasty, an organized workup is essential. Included in the evaluation are an accurate history, thorough physical examination, radiographic investigations, and adjunctive laboratory studies that may include white blood cell count with differential, erythrocyte sedimentation rate, electrodiagnostic testing, aspiration arthrogram, and radioisotopic imaging techniques. Shoulder arthroscopy is an ancillary diagnostic procedure that can also assist in the evaluation of occult glenoid component loosening.[22]

History

Important historical data include the shoulder condition resulting in the initial shoulder arthroplasty, the type of primary arthroplasty performed, and the initial postoperative rehabilitation accomplished. Significant medical or psychological disabilities that could interfere with the necessary postoperative cooperation or previous neurologic complications are additional historical data that are necessary for the planning and success of a revision procedure.

Historical information has been shown to be helpful in the diagnosis of component loosening. Bonutti and Hawkins[22] observed a history of initial pain-free motion with the delayed onset of progressive shoulder pain and a diminishing range of motion in patients with documented glenoid loosening. Humeral loosening is often accompanied by night pain and weakness in external rotation and forward elevation, otherwise suggesting rotator cuff deficiency.

Physical Examination

Excessive soft-tissue scarring or detachment, passive and active ranges of motion, the presence and direction of glenohumeral instability, assessment of rotator cuff integrity, and a comprehensive neurovascular examination need to be addressed during the physical examination. It has been noted that a painful clunk during forward elevation of the shoulder is highly suggestive of glenoid component loosening.[22]

Radiographic Evaluation

Radiographic examination is necessary for the interpretation of implant integrity, position, stability, and the identification of osseous deficiencies or radiolucencies involving the arthroplasty components. A standard radiographic series should include true anteroposterior views in internal and external rotation of the glenohumeral joint, scapular lateral view, and an axillary view of the shoulder. If additional information is required of the acromioclavicular joint and subacromial arch, additional views may include an anteroposterior view of the acromioclavicular joint and a supraspinatus outlet view. Biplanar, trispiral tomography is often helpful for evaluating glenoid or humeral bone loss, and fluoroscopically positioned spot views may help to identify radiolucent lines at the bone-implant interfaces.

Currently there are no established radiographic criteria for diagnosing loosening of the components. It may be assumed, however, that a change in component position is consistent with a definite diagnosis of component loosening, and that complete radiolucent lines more than 2 mm in width surrounding either the glenoid or the humeral component are

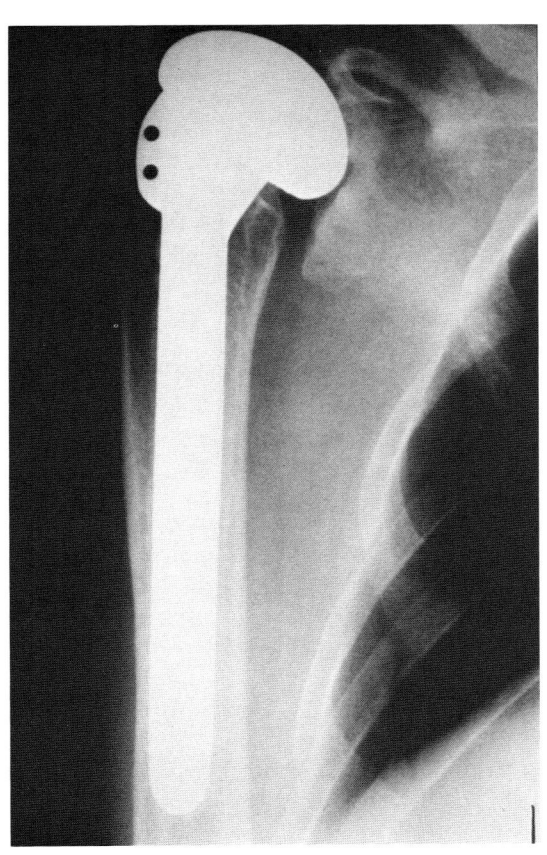

Figure 19-1. Failed humeral hemiarthroplasty with painful glenoid arthritis requiring revision to total shoulder arthroplasty.

associated with possible loosening of the component. Despite these criteria, Boyd et al.[8] found that of five humeral and seven glenoid components grossly loose at surgery, radiographic loosening was suspected on only four occasions.

Adjunctive Laboratory Studies

While a normal white blood cell count and differential commonly are present in the face of low-grade sepsis, continued elevation of the sedimentation rate may be a reliable indicator of infection in the presence of joint replacement. It has been demonstrated that a sedimentation rate that remains higher than 40 mm/hr after the first postoperative year suggests the presence of infection in total hip arthroplasty and it may be reasonable to assume that this is similar for other joint arthroplasties as well.[23] Joint aspiration with or without arthrography is an important adjunct in the workup of a painful joint arthroplasty and has been found to be successful in identifying infection approximately 70% of the time.[24] Further workup to detect infection may require the use of technetium and indium imaging techniques, and when performed in sequence have been accurate in diagnosing total joint sepsis.[25] In select situations, magnetic resonance imaging combined with radionuclide scanning is effective in defining deep sepsis and its associated soft-tissue extension.[26]

Electrodiagnostic testing should include electromyography and nerve conduction velocity studies and may prove helpful in selected cases when the history and physical examination suggest previous neurologic injury. This information is also helpful in evaluating unusual pain patterns or confusing findings that may exist as part of the patient's history or physical examination.

Diagnostic Arthroscopy

Arthroscopic evaluation of the glenoid component is a useful adjunct in the diagnosis of loosening.[22] Routine arthroscopic approaches can be used to examine a total shoulder arthroplasty and specifically address the problem of glenoid loosening. Visualization can be accomplished via a standard posterior approach, with a probe introduced through an anterior portal functioning as a lever underneath the glenoid component. If it is obvious that the probe can move or shift the glenoid component, loosening is confirmed.

While shoulder arthroscopy could also be utilized to assess the status of the rotator cuff, obtain biopsy specimens to rule out infection, and evaluate suspected malposition of the glenoid component, this technique is currently indicated for patients with a history suggestive of glenoid loosening who have equivocal radiographic findings. Unfortunately, arthroscopic evaluation has been found to be of no value in investigating humeral component loosening, as there is often dense scar surrounding the proximal bone-prosthesis interface.

PRINCIPLES OF REVISION SHOULDER ARTHROPLASTY

Pain relief, followed by restoration of motion, stability, and strength of the glenohumeral joint, remains the goals of primary and revision surgery. These goals are often compromised by extensive soft-tissue scarring or deficiencies and bone loss that remain unique to revision shoulder reconstruction. A paucity of literature exists evaluating the surgical experience and clinical follow-up for revision shoulder arthroplasty. Neer's series[2] remains the largest patient follow-up study to date, suggesting that while 85% of the patients have satisfactory pain relief and function for the activities of daily living, only 10 of 34 patients are able to rehabilitate towards near-normal function. Many of Neer's patients were only considered capable of limited rehabilitation goals because of significant predisposing soft-tissue or bony deficiencies.

While Boyd et al.[8] demonstrated satisfactory pain relief in 13 (81%) of 16 patients with a revised total shoulder arthroplasty or humeral hemiarthroplasty after a 24- to 84-month follow-up, others[20,21] had less optimistic results after revision of humeral hemiarthroplasties. Of 14 shoulders revised for a failed humeral arthroplasty, Bigliani et al.[20] rated 0 excellent, 9 good, 3 fair, and 2 poor results. All hemiarthroplasties had been initially performed for the treatment of proximal humeral fractures and the failures were commonly related to avoidable technical errors. Bonutti and Hawkins[22] noted variable results after revision of a failed humeral hemiarthroplasty, with only 7 (54%) of 13 patients satisfied with their revision surgery and 4 patients requiring additional revision surgeries.

While scar tissue, muscle deficiencies, neurologic injury, and bone loss will alter the success of revision arthroplasty and dictate modifications in rehabilitation, attention to surgical principles in handling these problems allows for more predictable results. Such principles are founded in the merits of careful soft-tissue dissection, release of soft-tissue contractures, adequate mobilization of muscle-tendon units, and careful attention to component positioning in the presence of bone defects or preexisting glenohumeral instability.

General Considerations

It is preferable to utilize previous skin incisions if possible, entering through a deltopectoral exposure, and preserving the origin of the deltoid on most occasions. The repair of a large rotator cuff tear may necessitate partial detachment of the deltoid origin, requiring meticulous repair of the deltoid origin with stable attachment through bone to the acromion and clavicle whenever possible. Complete lysis of scar tissue in the subacromial and subdeltoid regions and release of the coracohumeral ligament at the coracoid base are important maneuvers for the management of scarred tissues and the restoration of soft-tissue tension.

Component removal is often challenging, with attention

particularly focused on the extraction of all methylmethacrylate, especially in the presence of deep sepsis. Methylmethacrylate removal may prove to be extremely difficult when confronting humeral component loosening, and the use of cement removal instruments and high-powered drills is often helpful. Ultrasound equipment for cement removal has exceptional promise and is a safe and reproducible technique that does not alter the host bone.[27]

The use of modular humeral components may avoid having to remove a well-fixed humeral component for glenoid reconstruction, and affords the additional advantage of optimal soft-tissue tensioning by selecting the appropriate head size and neck length.[28] Removal of a nonmodular humeral component may be facilitated by the use of specialized extraction equipment.[29] When the revision arthroplasty has been completed, motion, stability, and the integrity of the soft tissues are assessed and an appropriate postoperative rehabilitation program is instituted.

Soft-Tissue Contractures and Deficiencies

Limited motion is often a frequent occurrence associated with a failed shoulder arthroplasty, and release of scar tissue, restoration of a detached deltoid origin, and repair of rotator cuff tears all allow for the best results in an otherwise compromised situation. Restoration of the glenohumeral joint line during the revision procedure is difficult, although necessary for balancing the soft tissues and restoring glenohumeral kinematics.[18]

Contractures of the anterior shoulder joint often necessitate a coronal Z-plasty with lengthening of the subscapularis and anterior capsule, and is generally indicated for external rotation of less than 30 degrees. If the anterior tissues are atrophic, a Z-lengthening may be difficult to perform and in that instance, an extralabral, anterior capsular release at its glenoid insertion has been successful (Figure 19–2).[30] Additional lengthening of the anterior structures can also occur after partial elevation of the subscapularis from its fossa, and reattachment of the subscapularis tendon medial to the lesser tuberosity. Similarly, posterior and inferior capsular contractures limiting internal rotation or overhead motion, respectively, can be accomplished with capsular releases at their glenoid insertion.

Rotator cuff deficiency is often associated with anterior or superior instability of the shoulder. Repairable rotator cuff tears are secured into an osseous trough after mobilization of healthy cuff tissue with occasional added transposition of subscapularis and/or infraspinatus tendons. Extreme thinning of the rotator cuff tissue is often noted in patients with an inflammatory arthropathy or excessive scarring from previous surgery.[2,15,18,19] On those occasions, it is important to maintain the osseous integrity of the subacromial outlet, avoiding anterior acromioplasty, distal clavicle resection, and coracoacromial ligament excision. Preserving the coracoacromial arch helps to capture the humeral head from further superior migration, and provides a fulcrum for glenohumeral motion. When rotator cuff tears cannot be repaired, it is prudent to consider reconstruction of the shoulder with a humeral hemiarthroplasty, avoiding the insertion of a glenoid component.[31] Humeral hemiarthroplasty avoids possible glenoid component loosening that can result from eccentric loading and rocking of the component.[32] In using a hemiarthroplasty for this situation, it is critical to select a humeral head size that achieves adequate tensioning of the soft tissues without excessive crowding of the posterior capsule while preserving the coracoacromial arch.[31]

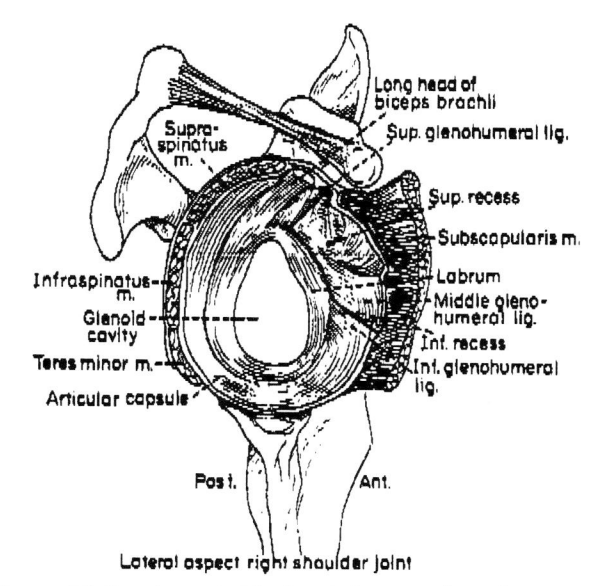

Figure 19–2. An extralabral anterior capsular release can be performed to release anterior contractures and restore external rotation. (Reproduced with permission from Cofield.[30])

Glenohumeral Instability

The treatment of glenohumeral instability for failed shoulder arthroplasties is challenging. Superior instability has been addressed above in the discussion of rotator cuff deficiencies. Anterior or posterior instability is usually the result of (1) soft-tissue contracture opposite the direction of instability, (2) insufficiency of the soft tissues in the direction of the instability, or (3) malposition of the humeral or glenoid components (Figure 19–3). Surgical reconstruction generally requires removal of the components to allow for changes in their version, thereby restoring stability and balancing the soft tissues (Table 19–1).[30] Inferior instability in association with failed arthroplasty may be associated with a loss of height of the proximal part of the humerus. Using the tension of the supraspinatus as a guide, the humeral component can be placed proud in the humeral shaft, usually requiring methylmethacrylate fixation and bone grafting. Persistent inferior instability may require postoperative casting to provide stability through scar formation, but this is at the expense of deltoid muscle weakness.[14]

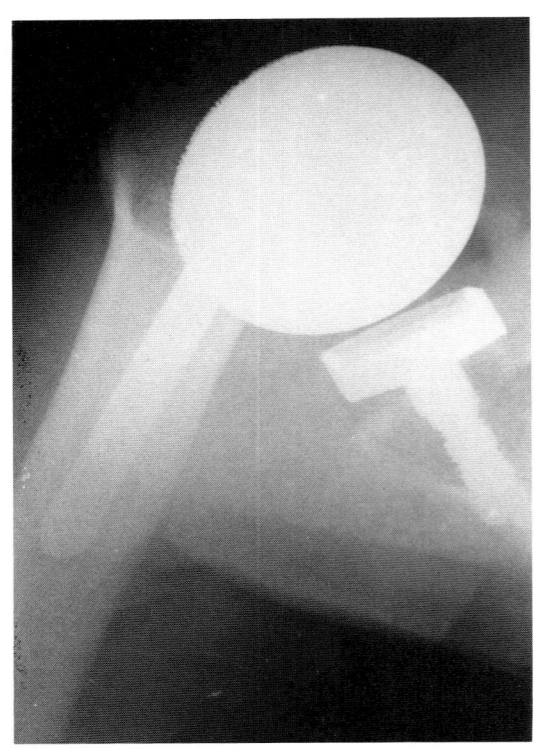

Figure 19-3. Malpositioned glenoid component resulting in excessive anteversion and anterior instability that required revision arthroplasty.

Component Loosening and Bone Deficiencies

GLENOID

Glenoid component loosening and glenoid arthritis are common causes of failure for total shoulder arthroplasty and humeral hemiarthroplasty, respectively.[1,8,21] Osseous deficiencies involving the glenoid are also common and further compromise reconstruction and component fixation.[2,33,34]

Glenoid bone deficiencies can be described as peripheral, central, or complex (peripheral and central), and because of limited glenoid bone stock, pose a significant reconstructive challenge. Complex deficiencies will often preclude placement of the glenoid component despite heroic attempts at reconstructive bone grafting. On these occasions, a hemiarthroplasty may offer the best treatment option. Bone grafting of a severely deficient glenoid utilizing autogenous iliac crest bone graft may be considered at the time of humeral hemiarthroplasty, permitting later glenoid reconstruction if the bone graft incorporates.[19] Resection of the glenoid component without glenoid component replacement has been reported sporadically, with reasonable results.[6,19,22]

Peripheral glenoid bone loss can often be treated by (1) glenoid preparation with concentric spherical reaming, (2) autogenous bone graft reconstruction, (3) asymmetric surface preparation with the use of an augmented or custom component, or (4) removing bone from the "proud" glenoid rim to match the deficient side.[33-35] Altered version of the humeral component is necessary on most occasions to accommodate whatever glenoid reconstruction is performed. Collins et al.[35] showed that concentric spherical glenoid reaming increases the stability of the component and permits component stabilization even if the posterior third of the glenoid is deficient. Friedman et al.[36] demonstrated that bone grafting for posterior glenoid deficiencies should be considered if there is more than 15 degrees of glenoid retroversion.

Halsey and Norris[33] and Neer and Morrison[34] showed success with glenoid reconstruction utilizing autogenous bone graft. It has been advocated by Neer and Kirby[2] that a metal-backed component have at least 80% contact with the underlying glenoid and an all-polyethylene component should have complete bony contact to avoid warp and failure of the component. Fixation of the glenoid component for revision surgery has been traditionally achieved with methylmethacrylate. However, the use of uncemented designs may have an application in these situations.[37] Regardless of glenoid preparation for peripheral deficiencies, the practice of restoring glenoid neck length with excess methylmethacrylate should be discouraged.

Central bone deficiencies, if severe, require a humeral hemiarthroplasty without glenoid component insertion. Less severe central glenoid bone deficiencies can usually be treated with a bone graft or concentric glenoid reaming and glenoid component insertion. As medialization of the glenoid increases, fixture of the glenoid component becomes difficult, if not impossible. Extreme central glenoid deficiencies treated with a hemiarthroplasty may be augmented with autogenous bone graft in the hope that graft incorporation would allow glenoid reconstruction at a future date.[19]

Table 19-1. Techniques for Treating Shoulder Instability*

Posterior instability
Lengthen contracted subcapularis and anterior capsule
Preserve inferior glenohumeral ligament complex
Remove less humeral bone
Decrease retrotorsion
Use thicker component(s)
Eliminate glenoid retroversion
Repair subcapularis securely
Anterior instability
Lengthen contracted posterior capsule
Preserve inferior glenohumeral ligament complex
Remove less humeral bone
Increase retrotorsion
Avoid glenoid anteversion
Repair subcapularis securely
Inferior instability
Preserve or restore humeral length
Tension supraspinatus and superior capsule
Use thicker component(s)

*Reproduced with permission from Cofield.[30]

HUMERUS

Humeral deficiencies associated with failed arthroplasty may be classified as metaphyseal, diaphyseal, or combined. Metaphyseal or combined deficiencies are often associated with the tenuous fixation of the rotator cuff attachments, resulting in considerable disability. It is important to restore humeral height, which allows for improved tension of the rotator cuff and deltoid musculature.[2] A scanogram of the contralateral humerus can serve as a template, providing the necessary measurements required for restoring humeral length. The increased humeral height is accomplished by placing the humeral component "proud" in the shaft, fixing it distally with methylmethacrylate, securing the tuberosities to the humeral shaft, and providing bone graft as necessary.

Combined metaphyseal and diaphyseal or large diaphyseal defects may require the use of a large allograft replacement or a custom humeral prosthetic component with or without autogenous bone grafting. While uncemented humeral component fixation has proved very successful in primary shoulder replacements, there is evidence that humeral hemiarthroplasty revision should employ cement fixation in most instances (Figure 19–4).[22] Recent advances in press-fit anatomic modular humeral stem systems may have a role in the uncemented fixation of a revised humeral component.

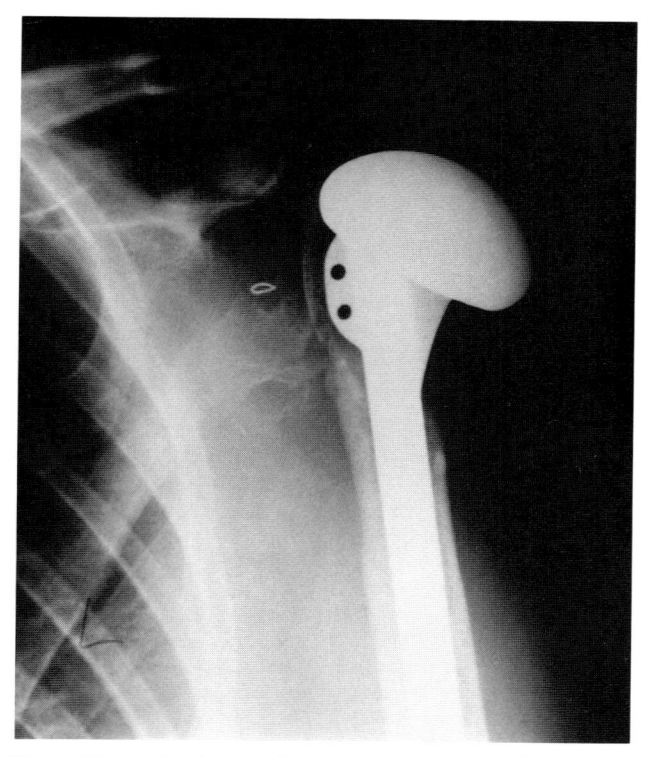

Figure 19–4. Inadequate fixation of an uncemented component resulting in mechanical loosening of a hemiarthroplasty. Note excessive malrotation of the humeral component.

Humeral Fractures

Humeral fractures after shoulder arthroplasty can occasionally result in clinical failure necessitating surgical revision. Bonutti and Hawkins[38] favor aggressive treatment of these injuries with rigid fixation provided by a long-stem humeral component, autogenous bone grafting, and the use of cerclage if necessary (Figure 19–5). Similarly, Norris and McElheny[29] noted success with the use of a long-stem humeral head prosthesis for diaphyseal fractures associated with revision arthroplasty. These fractures can occur intraoperatively, and are often associated with osteopenia, aggressive humeral reaming, malunion of the upper humerus or tuberosity fragments, and soft-tissue contractures requiring manipulation. While a press-fit can be achieved, it is not recommended unless the metaphysis is intact, providing secure rotational control. Indications for a long-stem humeral head component include diaphyseal penetration with prior prosthetic replacement, postoperative diaphyseal fracture at the prosthetic tip, and an intraoperative diaphyseal fracture during prosthetic humeral revision. New modular long-stem designs may allow the additional advantage of managing soft-tissue tension through the selection of different humeral neck lengths.

Infection

Deep sepsis associated with shoulder arthroplasty is uncommon, approximating 0.4% for the Neer design and 2.2% for constrained designs.[39] Management of infected tissues requires removal of all components and methylmethacrylate, with primary or delayed exchange of the implants. Prolonged antibiotic use is necessary, with bacterial sensitivity to the antibiotic established and bactericidal levels determined. Experience would suggest that a minimum of 28 days on intravenous antibiotics after component extraction is necessary to eradicate deep sepsis associated with joint arthroplasty. Primary arthroplasty exchange should be cautiously reserved for non–glycocalyx-producing, gram-positive organisms, based on the experience of infections around total hip arthroplasties.[24] While revision techniques remain an attractive solution to this difficult problem, resection arthroplasty is an option when faced with osteomyelitis requiring extensive acute debridement or deltoid dysfunction.[19,40]

SUMMARY

Recognition of the problems associated with a failed shoulder arthroplasty is necessary for successful revision surgery. The common findings of excessive scar, muscular weakness, and osseous deficiencies involving the humerus and glenoid contribute to extremely complex revisions and necessitate a carefully designed and monitored postoperative rehabilitation program. Revision to a nonconstrained prosthetic design is favored, and while pain relief is often predictable after revision surgery, residual function is often compromised by the preoperative condition of the soft tissues.

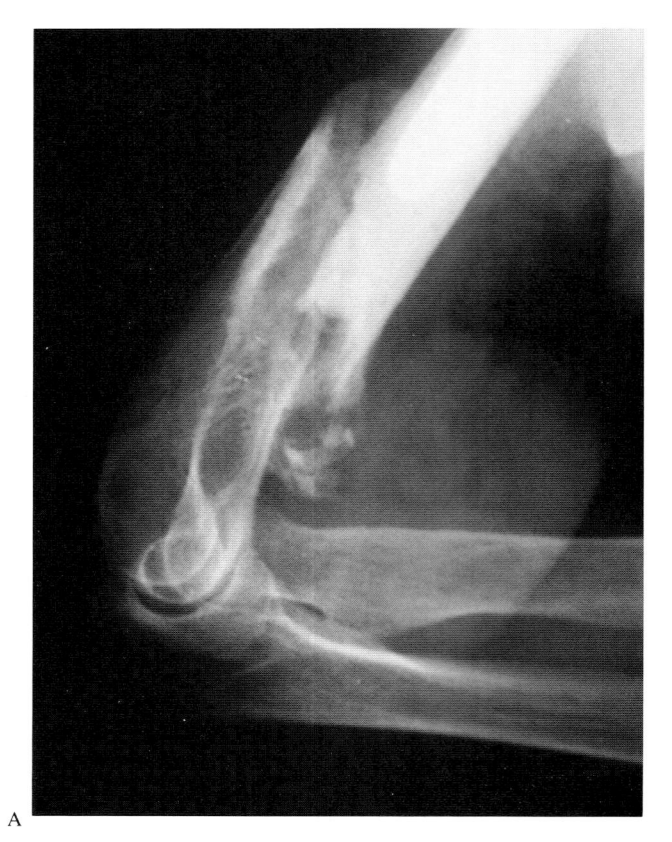

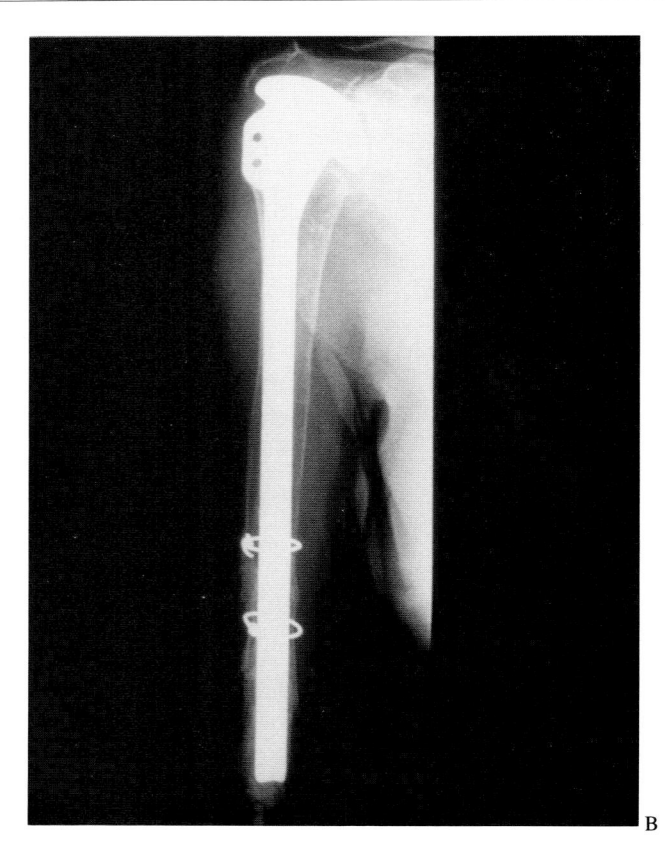

Figure 19–5. **A.** Fractured humerus distal to the tip of a humeral prosthesis. **B.** Reconstruction with a long-stem humeral component, cerclage fixation, and bone grafting.

Numerous reconstructive techniques are available for the release of soft-tissue contractures and restoration of soft-tissue and osseous deficiencies. Critical to the success of an arthroplasty is the status of the rotator cuff, and if it is found to be deficient, limited function and unpredictable pain relief can result. Component revision is often necessary for component loosening or when treating glenohumeral instability. Glenoid component insertion is not advised in the presence of massive rotator cuff tearing or extreme glenoid bony deficiency. Revision of a humeral arthroplasty may be most predictably treated with secure fixation afforded by methylmethacrylate. Deep infection is best treated with either thorough acute debridement, complete cement removal, secondary component exchange and antibiotics, or a resection arthroplasty.

The complexity of revision shoulder arthroplasty remains a supreme challenge for the experienced shoulder surgeon.[22] The difficulty of this surgery can often be matched by unpredictable patient cooperation during the postoperative rehabilitation program. Identifying the sources of failure and understanding the principles of surgical management are necessary for the successful revision of a failed arthroplasty. It is mandatory that the indications and technique of a primary shoulder arthroplasty are optimal, thus preserving the integrity of the soft tissues and osseous structures and minimizing revision surgery.

REFERENCES

1. Cofield RH. Section IV: The shoulder/revision. In Morrey BF, Cooney WP III, eds. *Joint Replacement Arthroplasty*. New York: Churchill-Livingstone, 1991:455–466.
2. Neer CS II, Kirby RM. Revision of humeral head and total shoulder arthroplasties. *Clin Orthop* 1982;170:189–195.
3. Cofield RH. Unconstrained total shoulder prosthesis. *Clin Orthop* 1983;173:97–108.
4. Brenner BC, Ferlic DC, Clayton ML, Dennis DA. Survivorship of unconstrained total shoulder arthroplasty. *J Bone Joint Surg [Am]* 1989;71:1289–1296.
5. Amstutz HC, Thomas BJ, Kabo M, et al. The DANA total shoulder arthroplasty. *J Bone Joint Surg [Am]* 1988;70:1174–1182.
6. Barrett WP, Franklin JL, Jackins SE, Wyss CR, Matsen FA III. Total shoulder arthroplasty. *J Bone Joint Surg [Am]* 1987;69:865–872.
7. Barrett WP, Thornhill TS, Thomas WH, et al. Nonconstrained total shoulder arthroplasty in patients with polyarticular rheumatoid arthritis. *J Arthroplasty* 1989;4:91–96.
8. Boyd AD, Thomas WH, Sledge CB, Thornhill TS. Failed shoulder arthroplasty. *Orthop Trans* 1990;14:255.
9. Cofield RH. Total shoulder arthroplasty with the Neer prosthesis. *J Bone Joint Surg [Am]* 1984;66:899–906.
10. Cruess RL. Shoulder resurfacing according to the method of Neer. *J Bone Joint Surg [Br]* 1980;62:116.
11. Gristina AG, Romano RL, Kammire GC, et al. Total shoulder replacement. *Orthop Clin North Am* 1987;18:445–453.
12. Hawkins RJ, Bell RH, Jallay B. Total shoulder arthroplasty. *Clin Orthop* 1989;242:188–194.

13. McCoy SR, Warren RF, Bade HA, et al. Total shoulder arthroplasty in rheumatoid arthritis. *J Arthroplasty* 1989;4:105–113.
14. Neer CS II, Watson KC, Stanton FJ. Recent experience in total shoulder replacement. *J Bone Joint Surg [Am]* 1982;64:319–337.
15. Swanson AB, Swanson de Groot G, Sattel AB, et al. Bipolar implant shoulder arthroplasty. *Clin Orthop* 1989;249:227–247.
16. Wilde AH, Borden LS, Brems JJ. Experience with the Neer total shoulder replacement. In: Bateman JF, Welsh RP, eds. *Surgery of the Shoulder*. Philadelphia: BC Decker, 1984:224–228.
17. Boyd AD, Aliabadi P, Thornhill TS. Postoperative proximal migration in total shoulder arthroplasty. *J Arthroplasty* 1991;6:31–37.
18. Figgie HE, Inglis AE, Goldberg VM, et al. An analysis of factors affecting the long-term results of total shoulder arthroplasty in inflammatory arthritis. *J Arthroplasty* 1988;3:123–130.
19. Cofield RH, Edgerton BC. Total shoulder arthroplasty complications and revision surgery. *Instr Course Lect* 1990;39:449–462.
20. Bigliani LU, Flatow EL, McCluskey GM, Fischer RA. Failed prosthetic replacement for displaced proximal humerus fractures. *Orthop Trans* 1991;15:747–748.
21. Bonutti PM, Hawkins RJ. Revision hemiarthroplasty of the shoulder arthroplasty. *Orthop Trans* 1990;14:598.
22. Bonutti PM, Hawkins RJ. Component loosening in unconstrained shoulder arthroplasty. *Semin Arthroplasty* 1990;1:124–128.
23. Corey DC, Albright JA. Current concepts review: Clinical significance of the erythrocyte sedimentation rate in orthopaedic surgery. *J Bone Joint Surg [Am]* 1987;69:148–151.
24. McDonald DJ, Fitzgerald RH Jr, Ilstrup DM. Two-stage reconstruction of a total hip arthroplasty because of infection. *J Bone Joint Surg [Am]* 1988;71:828–834.
25. Wukich DK, Abreu SH, Callaghan JJ, et al. Diagnosis of infection by preoperative scintigraphy with indium-labeled white blood cells. *J Bone Joint Surg [Am]* 1987;69:1353–1360.
26. Petersen SA, Berquist TH, Fitzgerald RH Jr, Brown ML. Applications of magnetic resonance imaging in musculoskeletal sepsis. *Orthop Trans* 1987;11:580–581.
27. Callaghan JJ, Elder S, Stranne SK, et al. Facilitation of cement removal with ultrasonically drive tools: Evaluation of the effects on whole bone strength in a canine model. *Orthop Trans* 1991;15:536.
28. Shaffer BS, Giordano CP, Zuckerman JD. Revision of a loose glenoid component facilitated by a modular humeral component: A technical note. *J Arthroplasty* 1990;5:S79–S81.
29. Norris TR, McElheny E. The role of long-stem humeral head prosthesis in treatment of complex humeral fractures and in revision arthroplasty. *Semin Arthroplasty* 1990;1:138–150.
30. Cofield RH. Integral surgical maneuvers in prosthetic shoulder arthroplasty. *Semin Arthroplasty* 1990;1:112–123.
31. Arntz CT, Matsen FA III, Jackins S. Surgical management of complex irreparable rotator cuff deficiency. *J Arthroplasty* 1991;6:363–370.
32. Franklin JL, Barrett WP, Jackins SE, Matsen FA III. Glenoid loosening in total shoulder arthroplasty. *J Arthroplasty* 1988;3:39–46.
33. Halsey RE, Norris TR. Bone grafts for glenoid deficiency in total shoulder replacement. *Orthop Trans* 1990;14:254.
34. Neer CS II, Morrison DS. Glenoid bone grafting in total shoulder arthroplasty. *J Bone Joint Surg [Am]* 1988;70:1154–1162.
35. Collins D, Tencer A, Sidles J, Matsen FA III. Edge displacement and deformation of glenoid components in response to eccentric loading. The effect of preparation of the glenoid bone. *J Bone Joint Surg [Am]* 1992;74:501–507.
36. Friedman RJ, Hawthorne K, Genez BM. Evaluation of glenoid bone loss with computerized tomography for total shoulder arthroplasty. *Orthop Trans* 1991;15:749.
37. Cofield RH, Daly PJ. Total shoulder arthroplasty with a tissue-ingrowth glenoid component. *J Shoulder Elbow Surg* 1992;1:77–85.
38. Bonutti PM, Hawkins RJ. Fracture of the humeral shaft associated with total replacement arthroplasty of the shoulder. A case report. *J Bone Joint Surg [Am]* 1992;74:617–618.
39. Cofield RH. Section IV: The shoulder/results and complications. In: Morrey BF, Cooney WP III, eds. *Joint Replacement Arthroplasty*. New York: Churchill-Livingstone, 1991:437–453.
40. Rockwood CA, Craviotto DF, Williams GF. Resection arthroplasty as a salvage procedure for a failed shoulder prosthesis. *Orthop Trans* 1991;15:45.

20 Complications Following Shoulder Arthroplasty

James F. Silliman, M.D., and Richard J. Hawkins, M.D.

Total shoulder arthroplasty is in its infancy when compared to total hip and total knee arthroplasty. Prosthetic humeral head replacement for degenerative joint disease and complex fractures began in 1951.[1] Total shoulder arthroplasty was introduced in the early 1970's, expanding the indication to those shoulders that had glenoid abnormalities. Initially, the design of shoulder arthroplasty components incorporated constraint. As the use of the prosthetic replacement was expanding, early investigations reported on the use of a variety of components in varied patient populations. It became obvious that patients who presented with normal soft tissues, adequate bone composition, and no previous surgery about their glenohumeral joint had a better outcome and fewer complications. Reports that followed gave only brief descriptions of complications while focusing on results, and this trend has continued to date.

Studies have been published on hemiarthroplasty, constrained total shoulder arthroplasty, and nonconstrained total shoulder arthroplasty. Unfortunately, no standardization of reporting has been available and complications are often unreported. Also, it is difficult to categorize the patient populations and results. Some authors only reported on those complications that required revision surgery, while others considered a complication to be any occurrence that adversely affects the outcome. Few long-term studies on total shoulder arthroplasty are available for review, and therefore time-dependent complications such as loosening or breakage of components are not well documented.

Each patient should be individualized in relation to the indication for total shoulder arthroplasty, and the risks and benefits of surgery should be discussed in detail. The purpose of this chapter is to present the reported complications of total shoulder arthroplasty, to allow for a discussion of the possible surgical risks with each particular patient. The authors have taken the approach that a complication is anything adversely affecting the outcome of the surgery and does not necessarily lead to revision surgery. Component types are separated so that hemiarthroplasty, constrained total shoulder arthroplasty, and nonconstrained arthroplasty can be discussed individually. Patient populations are separated so that those series that include a majority of rheumatoid patients (51% or greater) are distinguished from those that do not. Unfortunately, the literature is not detailed enough or consistent in its review to allow for isolation of other presenting pathologies, such as rotator cuff tears or replacements in traumatic injuries of the glenohumeral joint.

HEMIARTHROPLASTY

Hemiarthroplasty of the shoulder was popularized in the 1950s for the surgical treatment of advanced degenerative arthritis or complex fractures of the shoulder. Seven series of hemiarthroplasty are reviewed in Table 20-1, with six reporting complications.[2-8]

Engelbrecht and Heinert's series[7] dealt with hemiarthroplasties and nonconstrained and semiconstrained total shoulder arthroplasties, and their patients are therefore not included with the other 6 series. Engelbrecht and Hardinge actually reverted back to hemiarthroplasty during their series, due to the high glenoid loosening rate with total shoulder arthroplasty (51%). In the last 6 years of their series on hemiarthroplasty, no revisions were required. The reported incidence of complications in 209 patients is presented in Table 20-2.

Superior migration of the component was the only complication reported to have an incidence greater than 1%, and this did not necessarily lead to revision or significantly affect the clinical outcome at follow-up. Also of note is that only one case of humeral loosening was reported; however, many authors commented on asymptomatic humeral radiolucent lines (Figure 20-1). As with other series, the follow-up is relatively short. Other less common complications, reviewed in Table 20-1, include tuberosity nonunion, postoperative fracture, and malposition of the humeral prosthesis due to inadequate bone resection at the time of initial component insertion (Figures 20-2 and 20-3).

NONCONSTRAINED TOTAL SHOULDER ARTHROPLASTY IN NONRHEUMATOID PATIENTS

Many authors now consider nonconstrained total shoulder arthroplasty to be the gold standard for degenerative changes in the shoulder that affect both the humeral articular surface and the glenoid cavity. Eight series were reviewed here, for a total patient count of 590, and are detailed in Table 20-3.[1,6,9-14]

The components varied between series. Copeland[13] presented a series of uncemented components with a short follow-up of 10 months. It should be noted that many of these series actually included rheumatoid patients, but the vast majority of patients in each series were nonrheumatoid. As

Table 20–1. Review of Hemiarthroplasty*

	SWANSON ET AL.[2] 33/35	NEER[3] (1974) 47/48	JONSSON ET AL.[4] 26	REDFERN 19/22	COFIELD[6] 72/78	ENGELBRECHT AND HEINERT[7] 144/150	MARMOR[8]† 10/12
Hemiarthroplasty	Bipolar	98%	(Cup 26) Mitab	Neer	Neer 70	70	
Constrained							
Nonconstrained		2%				80	
% Rheumatoid	57	0	100	100		0	100
% Revision						18	
Average follow-up	63 mo	6 y		?	3 y	4 y‡	4.5 y
Glenoid loosening						51% (32)	
Component instability	2.9% (1)	2.1% (1)				11.2% (17)	
Humeral loosening			3.8% (1)			0.66% (1)	
Superior migration	2.9% (1)		27% (7)			7.9% (12)	
Rotator cuff tear							
Infections	2.9% (1)					1.3% (2)	
Axillary nerve injury							
Intraoperative fracture					1.3% (1)		
Broken component							
Tuberosity nonunion							
Postoperative fracture	2.9% (1)						
Other	Subacromial impingement (1) AC arthritis (1)		Subacromial impingement (1)	Superficial wound (1)	Brachial plexus palsy (1)	Ossification (4)	

*The numbers below authors' names represent the number of patients in the series/the number of shoulders in the series.
†Marmor[8] did not report complications.
‡TSA Follow-up for total shoulder arthroplasty only.
AC = acromioclavicular.

Table 20–2. Complications of Hemiarthroplasty

	209 SHOULDERS
Superior migration	3.8% (8)
Component instability	1.0% (2)

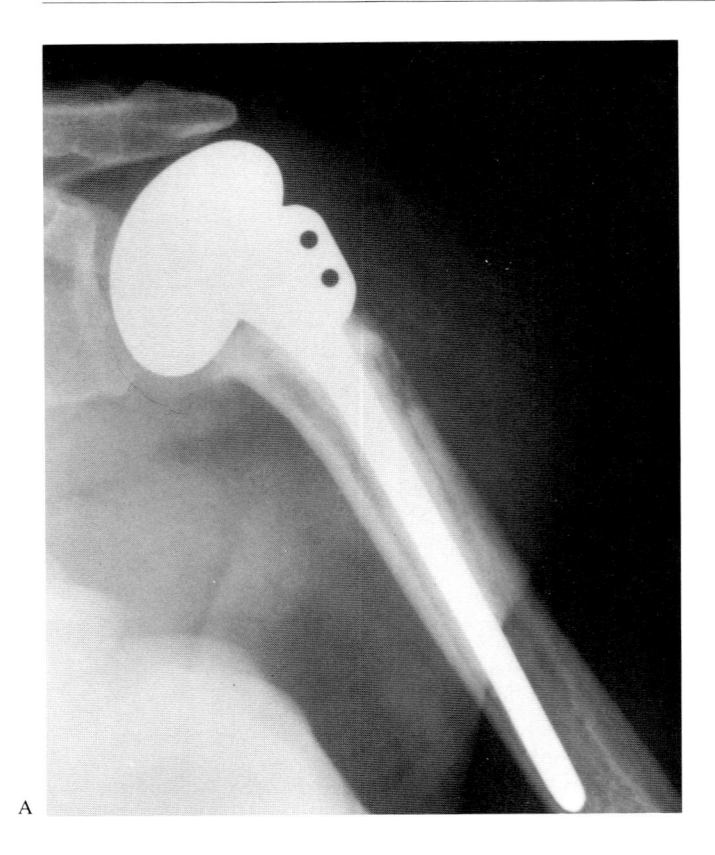

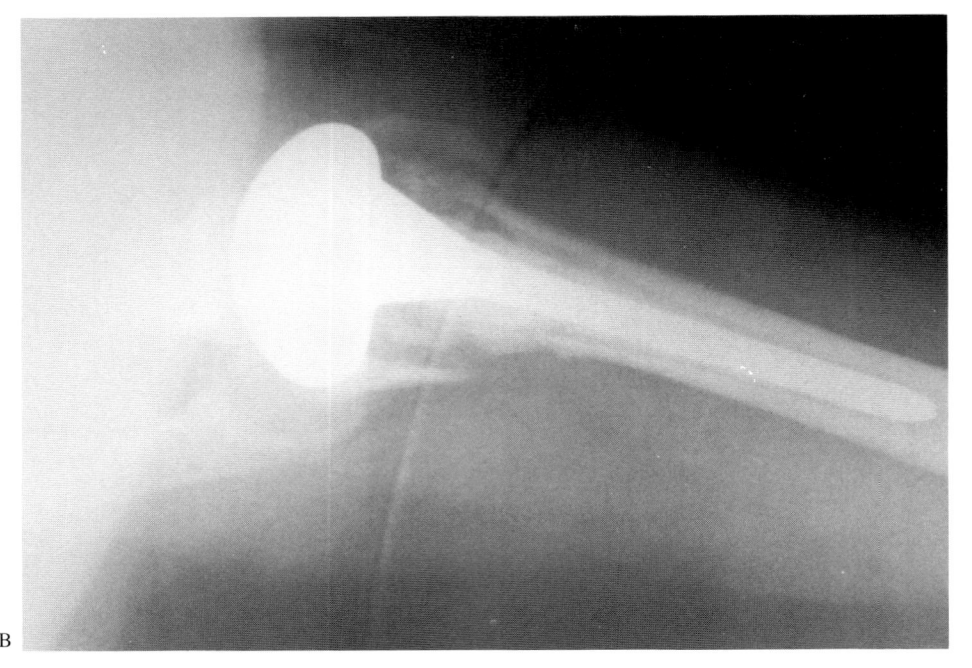

Figure 20–1. A and B. Anteroposterior and axillary radiographs, respectively, of a cemented hemiarthroplasty showing radiolucencies around the humeral component.

Table 20–11. Other Series Reviewed*

	AMSTUTZ ET AL.[33] 56	NEER AND KIRBY[34]† 36/40	CLAYTON ET AL.[35] 22	FRIEDMAN AND EWALD[36] 31/35	PRITCHETT AND CLARK[37] (FOR CHRONIC DISLOCATION)
Hemiarthroplasty			32%	3 Neer	4 Neer
Constrained	10 Hooded	Minority			
Nonconstrained	46 DANA	Majority	68% Neer	30 Neer 2 Mono	3 Neer
% Rheumatoid	32	100	64	100	0
% Revision				(All had ipsilateral elbow arthroplasty)	
Average follow-up	42 mo	42 mo	4.6 y	78 mo	2.2 y
Glenoid loosening	(65% RLL) 3.6% (2)			(37% RLL)	(80% RLL) 3.6% (2)
Component instability	5.6% (3)		4.5% (1)		1.8% (1)
Humeral loosening	(23% RLL)				
Superior migration	35.7% (20)				3.6% (2)
Rotator cuff tear					
Infections	1.8% (1)				
Axillary nerve injury					1.8% (1)
Intraoperative fracture					5.4% (3)
Broken component					
Nonunion tubercle osteotomy					
Postoperative fracture	1.8% (1)				
Other					

*The numbers below authors' names represent the number of patients in the series/the number of shoulders in the series.
†Complications were not reported by Neer and Kirby.[34]
RLL = radiolucent lines.

SUMMARY

Hemiarthroplasty and total shoulder arthroplasty have been used over the last several decades to provide pain relief and functional improvement in those patients who were debilitated from pathology about the glenohumeral joint. Custom prostheses and total shoulder arthroplasty have also been used to replace aspects of the glenohumeral joint involved in benign and malignant lesions about the shoulder.[38–40] Significant variables exist in the method of reporting results, components used, patient selection, and follow-up in each reviewed series. Methods of reporting results are often inconsistent, and many authors report complications only as they relate to rates of revision, while others report complications as they relate to rates of occurrence or radiographic parameters. These inconsistent methods make it very difficult to analyze the exact occurrence of various complications.

Some articles and series actually focused on specific complications. For example, Sneppen et al.[41] detailed ectopic ossification after total shoulder arthroplasty, and determined that a significant number of their patients undergoing Neer total shoulder arthroplasty were found to have heterotopic bone (40% of cases evaluated at 1 year). Boyd et al.[27] focused on the presence of proximal migration of the humeral component and its relationship to the outcome of total shoulder arthroplasty in a large series (Figure 20–5). They found no statistical difference in evaluating those patients who did and those who did not develop superior migration in their final outcome analysis. No direct correlation was found between superior migration and rotator cuff tearing. It was concluded that superior migration actually represented a multifactorial etiology and did not necessarily adversely affect the outcome of a shoulder arthroplasty or require a constrained prosthesis at surgery.

Glenoid loosening and component instability appear to be the most frequent complications requiring revision surgery (Figure 20–6). The rate of glenoid loosening varied in this review from 2.7% in nonconstrained total shoulder arthroplasties for the nonrheumatoid arthritis population, to 10.4% in constrained total shoulder arthroplasties performed for rheumatoid arthritis (Table 20–12). Component instability ranged from 1% in the hemiarthroplasty population to 10.2% for the constrained arthroplasties in the nonrheumatoid arthritis patient. Often, both of these complications are affected by the surgical technique and uncontrollable patient factors. Glenoid component loosening may be a major problem in the future, requiring revision surgery.

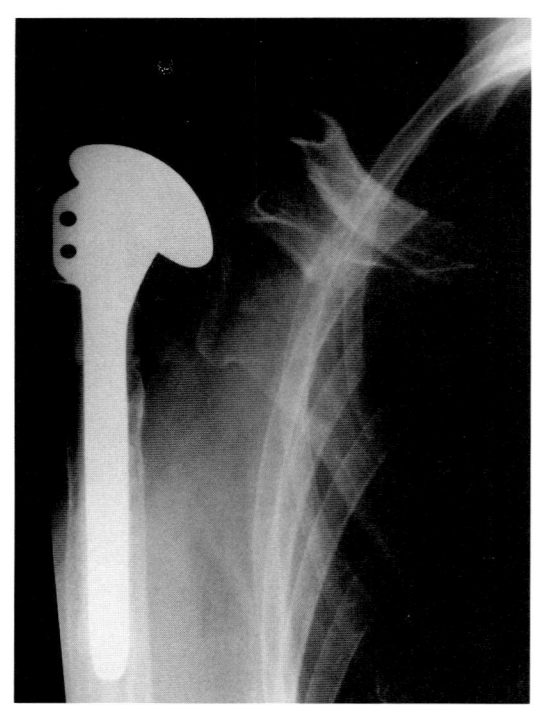

Figure 20–5. Proximal migration of the humeral component.

Table 20–12. Summary of Common Complications in Total Shoulder Arthroplasty

	SUPERIOR MIGRATION	GLENOID LOOSENING	COMPONENT INSTABILITY
Nonconstrained/ nonrheumatoid	0.7%	2.7%	3.5%
Nonconstrained/ rheumatoid	9.0%	4.2%	1.6%
Hemiarthroplasty	3.8%	0.0%	1.0%
Constrained/ nonrheumatoid	0.0%	6.3%	10.2%
Constrained/ rheumatoid	0.0%	10.4%	5.2%

Another interesting note in this review of a large patient group is that serious perioperative complications such as axillary nerve injury and infection are relatively rare. Infections ranged from approximately 2% for constrained shoulder arthroplasty to 1% or less for nonconstrained components and hemiarthroplasty. Significant brachial plexus palsy, axillary nerve palsy, or musculocutaneous nerve injuries occurred in less than 1% of cases, and most authors reported that these were transient injuries that went on to resolve with time.

It is apparent that in order to understand the complications and long-term survivorship of shoulder arthroplasty, there

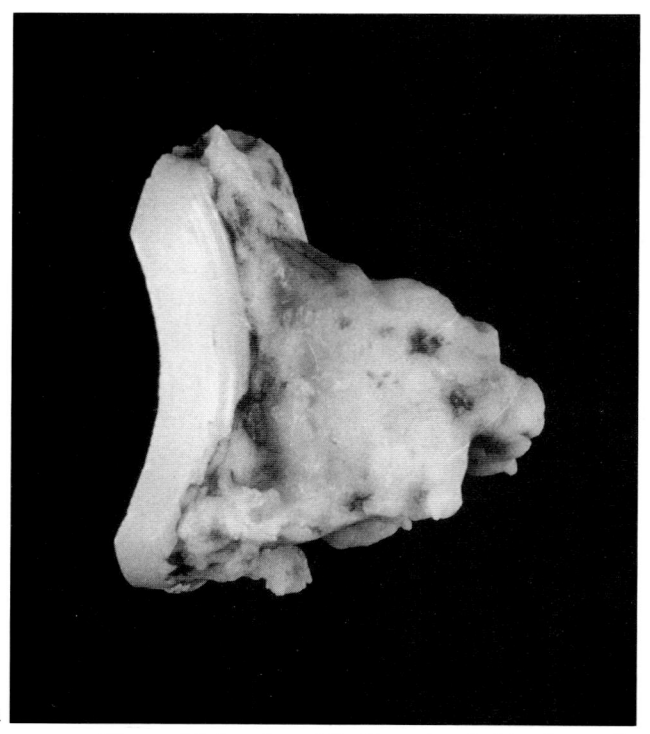

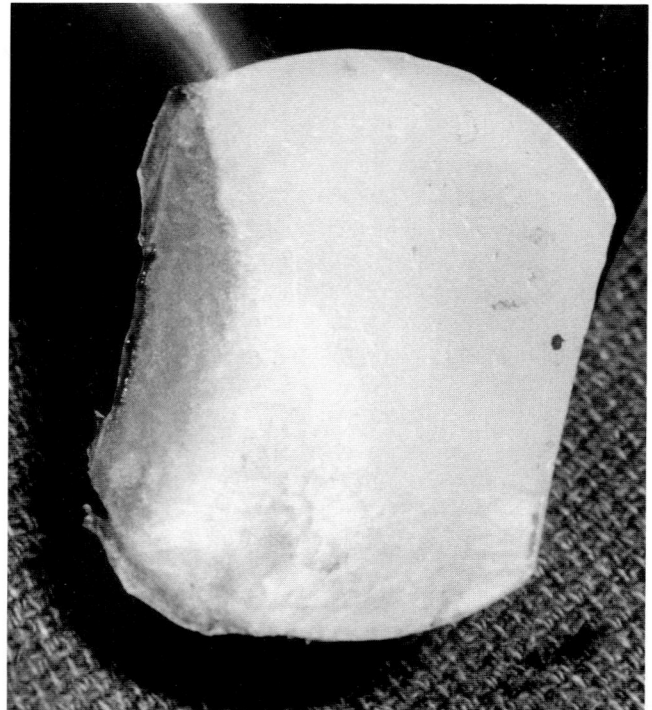

Figure 20–6. A and B. Frontal and side views of a failed cemented glenoid component demonstrating eccentric polyethylene wear.

must be more consistent reporting and greater detail, which presently are not available.

REFERENCES

1. Neer CS II, Watson KC, Stanton FJ. Recent experience in total shoulder replacement. *J Bone Joint Surg [Am]* 1982;64:319–337.
2. Swanson AB, et al. Bipolar implant shoulder arthroplasty. Long-term results. *Clin Orthop* 1989;249:227–247.
3. Neer CS II. Replacement arthroplasty for glenohumeral osteoarthritis. *J Bone Joint Surg [Am]* 1974;56:1–13.
4. Jonsson E, Egund N, Kelly I, et al. Cup arthroplasty of the rheumatoid shoulder. *Acta Orthop Scand* 1986;57:542–546.
5. Redfern TR, Hardinge K. Hemiarthroplasty for the rheumatoid shoulder. In: Post M, Morrey BF, Hawkins RJ, eds. Surgery of the Shoulder. St. Louis: Mosby-Year Book, 1990:270–272.
6. Cofield RH. Total shoulder arthroplasty: Associated disease of the rotator cuff, results, and complications. In: Bateman JE, Welsh RP, eds. *Surgery of the Shoulder*. Philadelphia: BC Decker, 1984:229–233.
7. Engelbrecht E, Heinert K. More than ten years' experience with unconstrained shoulder replacement. In: Kolbel R, Helbig B, Blauth W, eds. *Shoulder Replacement*. 1987:85–91.
8. Marmor L. Hemiarthroplasty for the rheumatoid shoulder joint. *Clin Orthop* 1977;122:201–203.
9. Gristina AG, Romano RL, et al. Total shoulder replacement. *Orthop Clin North Am* 1987;18:445–453.
10. Brenner BC, Ferlic DC, et al. Survivorship of unconstrained total shoulder arthroplasty. *J Bone Joint Surg [Am]* 1989;71:1289–1296.
11. Fleega BA. Experience with Neer II total and hemiarthroplasty of the shoulder. In Post M, Morry BF, Hawkins RJ, eds. *Surgery of the Shoulder*. St. Louis: Mosby-Year Book, 1990:302–304.
12. Barrett WP, Franklin JL, Jackins SE, et al. Total shoulder arthroplasty. *J Bone Joint Surg [Am]* 1987;69:865–872.
13. Copeland S. Cementless total shoulder replacement. In: Post M, Morrey BF, Hawkins RJ, eds. *Surgery of the Shoulder*. St. Louis: Mosby-Year Book, 1990:289–293.
14. Warren RF, Ranawat CS, Inglis AE. Total shoulder replacement indications and results of the Neer nonconstrained prosthesis. In: Inglis AE, ed. *American Academy of Orthopaedic Surgeons Symposium on Total Joint Replacement of the Upper Extremity*. St Louis: CV Mosby, 1982:56–67.
15. Lettin AW, Copeland SA, Scales JT. The Stanmore total shoulder replacement. *J Bone Joint Surg [Br]* 1982;64:47–51.
16. Laurence M. Replacement arthroplasty of the rotator cuff deficient shoulder. *J Bone Joint Surg [Br]* 1991;73:916–919.
17. Pahle JA, Kvarnes L. Shoulder replacement arthroplasty. *Ann Chir Gynaecol Suppl* 1985;198:85–89.
18. Bodey WN, Yeoman PM. Prosthetic arthroplasty of the shoulder. *Acta Orthop Scand* 1983;54:900–903.
19. Thomas BJ, Amstutz HC, Cracchiolo A. Shoulder arthroplasty for rheumatoid arthritis. *Clin Orthop* 1991;265:125–128.
20. Kelly IG, Foster RS, Fisher WD. Neer total shoulder replacement in rheumatoid arthritis. *J Bone Joint Surg [Br]* 1987;69:723–726.
21. Friedman RJ, Thornhill TS, et al. Non-constrained total shoulder replacement in patients who have rheumatoid arthritis and class-IV function. *J Bone Joint Surg [Am]* 1989;71:494–498.
22. Roper BA, Patterson JMH, Day WH. The Roper-Day total shoulder replacement. *J Bone Joint Surg [Br]* 1990;72:694–697.
23. Hawkins RJ, Bell RH, Jallay B. Total shoulder arthroplasty. *Clin Orthop* 1989;242:188–194.
24. Averill RM, Sledge CB, Thomas WH. Neer total shoulder arthroplasty. *Orthop Trans* 1980;4:287.
25. Figgie MP, Inglis AE, Figgie H, et al. Custom total shoulder arthroplasty for inflammatory arthritis. In: Post M, Morrey BF, Hawkins RJ, eds. *Surgery of the Shoulder*. St. Louis: Mosby-Year Book, 1990:285–288.
26. Kelly IG. Shoulder replacement in rheumatoid arthritis. In: Post M, Morrey BF, Hawkins RJ, eds. *Surgery of the Shoulder*. St. Louis: Mosby-Year Book, 1990:305–307.
27. Boyd AD, Aliabadi P, Thornhill TS. Postoperative proximal migration in total shoulder arthroplasty. *J Arthroplasty* 1991;6:31–37.
28. Wilde AH, Borden LS, Brems JJ. Experience with the Neer total shoulder replacement. In: Bateman JE, Welsh RP, eds. *Surgery of the Shoulder*. Philadelphia: BC Decker, 1984:224–228.
29. Post M, Jablon M. Constrained total shoulder arthroplasty. *Clin Orthop* 1983;173:109–116.
30. Post M. Constrained arthroplasty of the shoulder. *Orthop Clin North Am* 1987;18:455–462.
31. Coughlin MJ, Morris JM, et al. The semiconstrained total shoulder arthroplasty. *J Bone Joint Surg [Am]* 1979;61:574–581.
32. McElwain JP, English E. The early results of porous-coated total shoulder arthroplasty. *Clin Orthop* 1987;218:217–224.
33. Amstutz HC, Thomas BJ, et al. The DANA total shoulder arthroplasty. *J Bone Joint Surg [Am]* 1988;70:1174–1181.
34. Neer CS II, Kirby RM. Revision of humeral head and total shoulder arthroplasties. *Clin Orthop* 1982;170:189–195.
35. Clayton ML, Ferlic DC, Jeffers PD. Prosthetic arthroplasties of the shoulder. *Clin Orthop* 1982;164:184–191.
36. Friedman RJ, Ewald FC. Arthroplasty of the ipsilateral shoulder and elbow in patients who have rheumatoid arthritis. *J Bone Joint Surg [Am]* 1987;69:661–666.
37. Pritchett JW, Clark JM. Prosthetic replacement for chronic unreduced dislocations of the shoulder. *Clin Orthop* 1987;216:89–93.
38. Riebel G, Webster DA. Proximal humeral replacement for tumor. *Orthopedics* 1989;12:833–836.
39. Fielding JW, Morley DC. Hemi-replacement arthroplasty of the proximal humerus. A case report. *Clin Orthop* 1984;184:180–182.
40. Heck DA, Chao EY, et al. Titanium fibermetal segmental replacement prosthesis. *Clin Orthop* 1986;204:266–285.
41. Sneppen O, Kjaersgaard-Anderson P, Frich LH, Sojbjerg JO. Ectopic ossification after total shoulder arthroplasty: A study on 75 Neer total shoulder replacements. In: Post M, Morrey BF, Hawkins RJ, eds. *Surgery of the Shoulder*. St. Louis: Mosby-Year Book, 1990:298–301.

21 The Unstable Shoulder Arthroplasty

Bruce H. Moeckel, M.D., Russell F. Warren, M.D., David M. Dines, M.D., and David W. Altchek, M.D.

Total shoulder arthroplasty has proved to be a successful and durable procedure.[1-3] In general, the results have paralleled those achieved after other joint replacements. Pain relief can be predictably achieved in 90 to 95% of patients.[4] Active range of motion usually approximates two-thirds of normal after a rehabilitation program. However, these results depend largely on the preoperative range of motion, the diagnosis leading to the arthroplasty, and the status of the rotator cuff.[4]

Instability after prosthetic replacement is a recognized complication in many joints, including the hip, knee, and elbow. It is no surprise that instability can occur after shoulder arthroplasty where bony constraint is minimal compared to other joints. There has been limited discussion in the literature concerning the etiology and management of the unstable shoulder after arthroplasty. The incidence of instability has been reported to range from 0 to 18.2% in nonconstrained implants, with an average of 2.7%.[4] Paradoxically, the incidence in constrained implants has been reported to range from 6 to 16.7%, with an average of 9.4%.[4] Dislocation is the major form of instability with constrained implants, and usually this requires surgical treatment.

This discussion focuses on the problem of instability after a nonconstrained shoulder arthroplasty. A classification scheme based on the pathologic anatomy is presented. A literature review including the authors' personal series is used to illustrate the problem. The chapter concludes with a discussion of the treatment alternatives, along with a special emphasis on preventing this difficult problem.

CLASSIFICATION AND PATHOLOGIC ANATOMY

Instability after a nonconstrained shoulder arthroplasty can be classified based on the pathologic displacement of the humeral head on the glenoid. By identifying the direction of displacement, the possible causes can be determined and the treatment options elucidated. These directions include superior, inferior, anterior, and posterior. Instability after shoulder arthroplasty can be seen as a continuum ranging from subluxation to frank dislocation. The term "subluxation" is used when pathologic displacement has occurred but some contact remains between the humeral and glenoid prosthetic surfaces. "Dislocation" refers to those cases where no contact remains. Finally, it is possible that the pathologic displacement is a combination of the above vectors; therefore, the individual components will need to be identified to determine the treatment options.

Superior Instability

Superior displacement is the most common direction of instability and is usually related to rotator cuff failure or dysfunction. One of the rotator cuff functions is to stabilize the humeral head against the glenoid and resist the upward shear forces of the deltoid. When this is lost, the action of the deltoid will exert a superior shear, allowing the prosthetic humeral head to shift in a superior direction. Other less likely causes of superior displacement relate to not restoring the normal anatomic relationship between the scapula and the humerus. These can include implantation of the humeral component in a proud position, thereby lengthening the humerus, and malposition of the glenoid component, either tilted or implanted too inferiorly on the scapula. Both of these situations disturb the relationship between the scapula and the humerus and could, by themselves or in combination with rotator cuff failure, lead to superior displacement.

Inferior Instability

Inferior subluxation is most commonly attributed to not restoring the proper humeral length. This is most problematic when performing a hemiarthroplasty for three- and four-part fractures of the proximal part of the humerus where the normal landmarks might not be available.[5,6] Other causes include axillary neuropathy or other conditions that weaken the deltoid and are usually in the form of a subluxation since some contact remains between the prosthetic humeral head and glenoid surfaces.

Anterior Instability

Anterior instability can be seen as a subluxation or frank dislocation (Figure 21–1). Instability in this plane relates to a combination of soft-tissue imbalance and component malposition. The anterior soft-tissue restraints include the capsule with its associated glenohumeral ligaments and the subscapularis tendon. The situation in a shoulder arthroplasty is similar to the pathologic anatomy involved in shoulder instability. However, the capsule assumes less of an individual role and acts in concert with the subscapularis to provide passive anterior stabilization. The subscapularis serves as an internal rotator of the humerus, but the shoulder has an abundance of internal rotators consisting of the teres major, pectoralis major, and the latissimus dorsi. The posterior

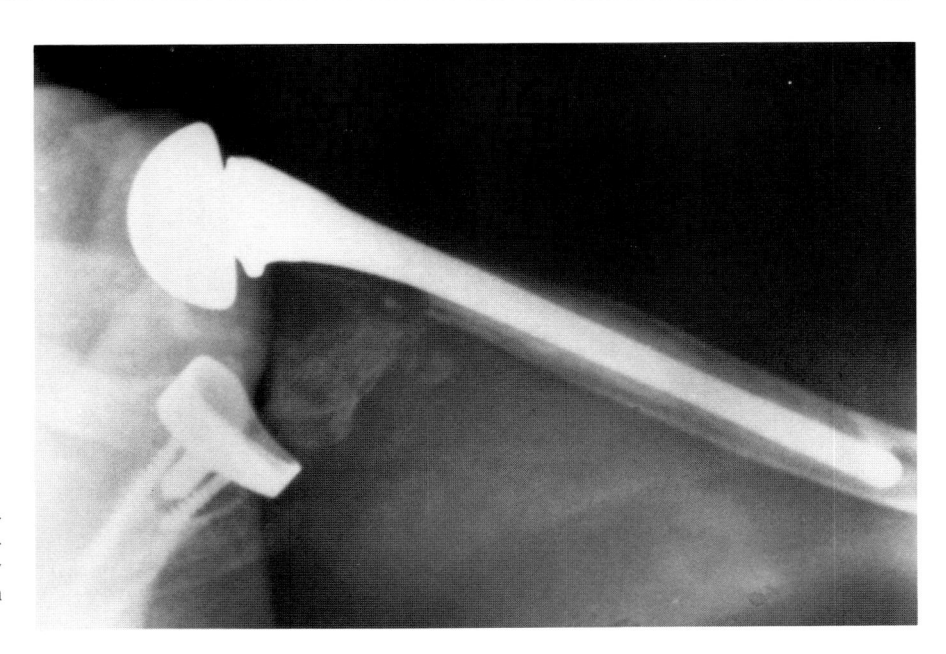

Figure 21–1. An axillary radiograph illustrating an anterior dislocation of a total shoulder arthroplasty joint. A fracture has occurred with the dislocation.

restraints are also important when discussing anterior instability, as they need to be balanced so the humeral head is not forced in the opposite direction. This is analogous to the situation following shoulder stabilizations where overtightening in one direction can lead to instability in the opposite. The posterior restraints include the posterior capsule and posterior rotator cuff tendons of the infraspinatus and teres minor. These muscles also function as external rotators as well as stabilizers of the humeral head to restrict the shear of the deltoid. All of these structures can be involved, leading to soft-tissue imbalance and subsequent instability.

Component positioning is the other major variable that affects the stability of the prosthetic glenohumeral joint. Excessive humeral or glenoid anteversion can also result in postoperative anterior instability. The version of the prosthetic components works in concert with the soft tissues and neither should be considered in isolation.

Posterior Instability

Posterior instability is the final direction to be considered. Once again, stability depends on the relationship between the soft tissues and the prosthetic components. The same soft tissues as those in the discussion on anterior instability must be balanced with a special emphasis on the subscapularis. Adequate length of this muscle-tendon unit plays a critical role in preventing posterior subluxation and dislocation by not forcing the humeral head in that direction.

Component positioning again plays a role. Excessive retroversion of either the humeral or the glenoid component can lead to posterior subluxation or dislocation. The version of the glenoid component can be especially problematic. Retroversion of the glenoid component in cases of posterior glenoid erosion is a leading cause of posterior subluxation and dislocation.

LITERATURE REVIEW

Various authors in describing their series of shoulder arthroplasties have noted problems with stability[1–23] (Table 21–1). Neer initially described his results using a vitallium hemiarthroplasty for osteoarthritis in 48 cases.[21] He described 3 cases of recurrent dislocation and 2 cases of transient subluxation. The transient subluxations resolved with muscle-strengthening exercises, while no treatment for the recurrent dislocations was indicated. One of these dislocations was in a polio patient, which was likely a contributing factor.

The larger series of Neer et al.[22] of 194 shoulder replacements noted 2 cases of anterior dislocation and 2 cases of posterior dislocation, all of which occurred within the first 3 weeks postoperatively. These were all treated with closed reduction and immobilization. This was successful in 3 of the shoulders, but the fourth developed persistent posterior subluxation after a posterior dislocation. This was attributed to a retroverted glenoid component that was not revised because the patient was satisfied with the result. Neer et al.[22] also described 2 cases of inferior subluxation, 2 instances of anterior subluxation, and 5 shoulders that developed superior subluxation. The inferior subluxation was attributed to not restoring the correct humeral length. This was treated with a plaster shoulder spica for 8 weeks but the deltoid remained weak. The 2 cases of anterior subluxation were revised because the humeral component was felt to be excessively anteverted. The superior subluxations that occurred were late findings related to traumatic disruption of the rotator cuff tendons. These were surgically corrected in 2 of the cases.

Barrett et al.[2] reported the results of 50 shoulder arthroplasties and noted 1 case of posterior subluxation and 4 shoulders that developed superior subluxation. The posterior subluxation resolved with vigorous physical therapy and the

Table 21–1. Instability Following Nonconstrained Total Shoulder Arthroplasty

AUTHOR(S)	NO. OF SHOULDERS	ANTERIOR	POSTERIOR	INFERIOR	SUPERIOR	UNCLASSIFIED
Amstutz et al. (1981)[7]	11	1			8	
Amstutz et al. (1988)[1]	56				30	3
Barrett et al. (1989)[8]	140				5	2
Barrett et al. (1987)[2]	50		1		4	
Bell and Gschwend (1986)[9]	28		1			
Brenner et al. (1989)[10]	51		1		4	
Cofield (1984)[11]	73				5	
Cofield (1983)[12]	176					3
Faludi and Weiland (1983)[13]	13	1				
Figgie et al. (1988)[14]	50	1				
Frich et al. (1988)[15]	50			1		
Hawkins et al. (1989)[16]	70		1		2	
Kay and Amstutz (1988)[17]	15				12	1
Kelly et al. (1987)[18]	42				17	
McCoy et al. (1989)[19]	29				2	
McElwain and English (1987)[20]	13					1
Neer (1974)[21]	48			2		3
Neer et al. (1982)[22]	194	4	3	2	5	
Swanson et al. (1989)[23]	35	1			35	
Total	1144	8	7	5	129	13
Percentages		0.7	0.6	0.4	11	1

superior subluxations were treated with rotator cuff strengthening in all cases followed by surgical repair in one.

Amstutz et al.[1] described their results with 56 DANA shoulder arthroplasties; there was 1 case of dislocation and 2 cases of subluxation which they treated with a hooded glenoid component. They also described a method to classify superior subluxation based on the degree of displacement. They noted 10 shoulders with 1 to 10 mm of superior subluxation and 20 shoulders with more than 10 mm of superior subluxation.

AUTHORS' SERIES

Because of the relative deficiency in the literature concerning the unstable shoulder arthroplasty and its various treatment modalities, the authors[24] undertook a study of the problem. They identified 14 patients who developed postoperative anterior or posterior instability after a nonconstrained shoulder arthroplasty. These patients were identified from a review of 250 patients who underwent a shoulder arthroplasty at the Hospital for Special Surgery from January 1, 1984 to December 31, 1989.

Anterior instability was identified in 10 patients and posterior instability in 4. There were 12 women and 2 men with an average age of 64 years (range, 48 to 79 years). Various diagnoses led to the initial shoulder arthroplasty and included osteoarthritis, posttraumatic osteoarthritis, inflammatory arthritis, cuff tear arthropathy, and failed hemiarthroplasty.

The anterior instability in all 10 patients was caused by a rupture of the repaired subscapularis tendon. In 9 patients, the surgical management consisted of mobilization and repair of the disrupted tendon. Nonabsorbable sutures were used in all cases and Mersilene tape was used to reinforce the repair in 6 shoulders. In the shoulders where a modular humeral prosthesis was employed, this feature was utilized to downsize the humeral head component in 4 cases. Stability was achieved in 5 of the 9 shoulders with an average external rotation of 15 degrees and an average forward elevation of 98 degrees.

Four patients failed and presented with recurrent instability. Three were reconstructed with a static stabilizer consisting of an Achilles tendon allograft. The bony portion of the allograft was secured to the glenoid neck with a lag screw and washer. The tendon was anchored to the lesser tuberosity with a lag screw and a soft-tissue washer (Figures 21–2 and 21–3). To correctly tension the graft, the arm was positioned in 60 degrees of abduction and 30 degrees of external rotation (Figure 21–4). A custom modular humeral head with increased retroversion was combined with the allograft in one case. This technique successfully reconstructed the anterior restraints in all three cases. Radiographs revealed reduction of the glenohumeral joint.

The posterior instability had various etiologies. Two patients had soft-tissue imbalance that led to symptomatic posterior subluxation. At revision, the lax posterior capsule

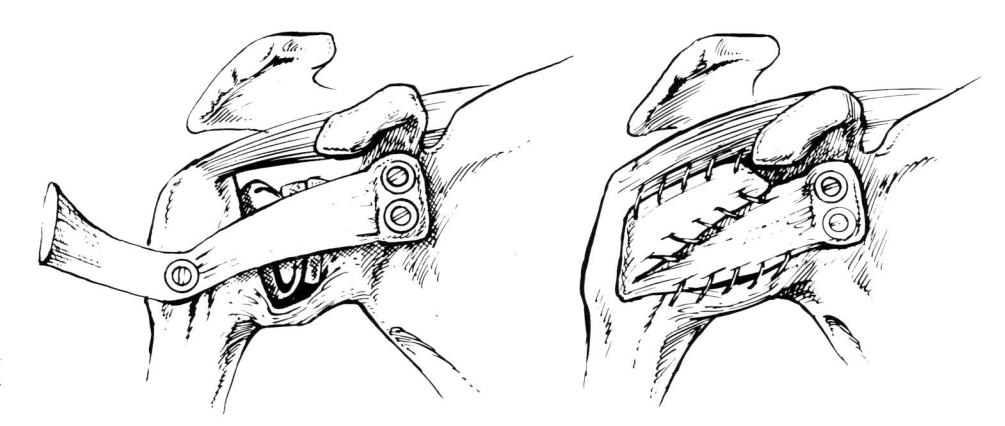

Figure 21–2. The Achilles tendon allograft is secured to the glenoid neck and humeral head.

and tight anterior structures were rebalanced. Another patient suffered a locked posterior dislocation due to an excessively retroverted humeral component. This was treated with open reduction and spica immobilization. The last patient had prior anterior shoulder stabilizations and an eroded posterior glenoid, which went unrecognized and resulted in a retroverted glenoid component (Figure 21–5). This caused posterior subluxation and required revision with a posterior bone graft (Figure 21–6). One of the four patients, a paraplegic, developed recurrent posterior instability that required re-revision and ultimately a resection arthroplasty. The other three patients had an average external rotation of 42 degrees with 120 degrees of forward elevation.

EVALUATION AND TREATMENT

The etiology of instability after shoulder arthroplasty relates to soft-tissue imbalance and/or component malposition. Since there is limited constraint built into the components, stability depends on soft-tissue balance. If the soft tissues around the shoulder are too loose, then instability may occur. If the soft tissues are too tight, instability will also occur through one of two mechanisms. The first is tendon rupture at the site of a soft-tissue repair as the patient attempts to obtain more motion than is allowed. The second is that overtightening can force the humeral head in the opposite direction and lead to instability. This highlights the importance of assessing the range of motion in the operating room. The early postoperative rehabilitation must stay within the limits defined at surgery to allow for soft-tissue healing.

During the preoperative planning, it is essential to review the axillary radiograph to determine whether bony erosion has occurred leading to abnormal glenoid version, and to assess the position of the humeral head on the glenoid. Galinat and Howell[25] pointed out that the posterior border of the scapula provides a useful landmark as it should be nearly perpendicular to the glenoid face. The humeral head should be centered on the glenoid, reflecting the soft-tissue balance around the shoulder. If good-quality axillary radiographs cannot be obtained, computerized tomographic or magnetic resonance imaging scans combined with three-dimensional analysis may provide the needed information to assist in the preoperative planning (Figure 21–7).

Once postoperative instability is suspected, a systematic evaluation is begun. This involves a thorough history, physical examination, and radiographic evaluation. The history centers on the particulars of the initial arthroplasty with attention directed at the range of motion achieved intraoperatively and postoperatively. Whether the patient noted an "event" associated with the postoperative rehabilitation becomes important and the therapist can often provide

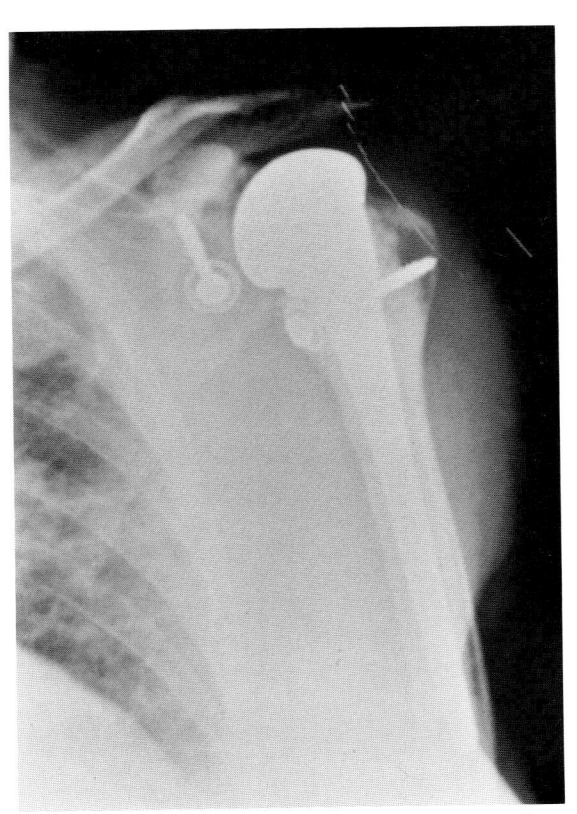

Figure 21–3. A radiograph demonstrating the allograft reconstructing the anterior restraints.

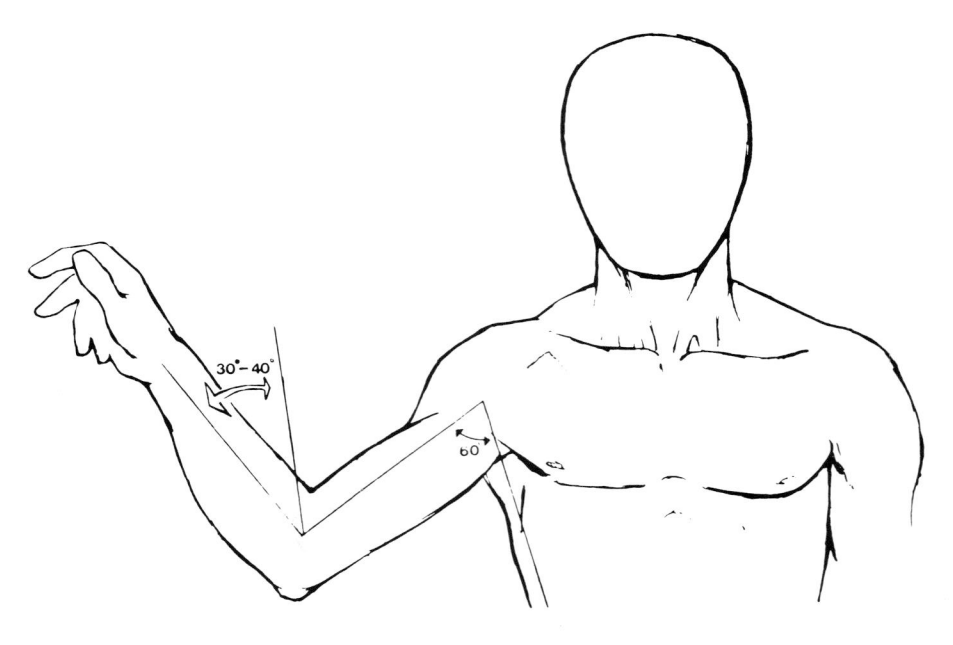

Figure 21–4. An illustration of the arm position during reconstruction to establish the correct tensioning in the graft.

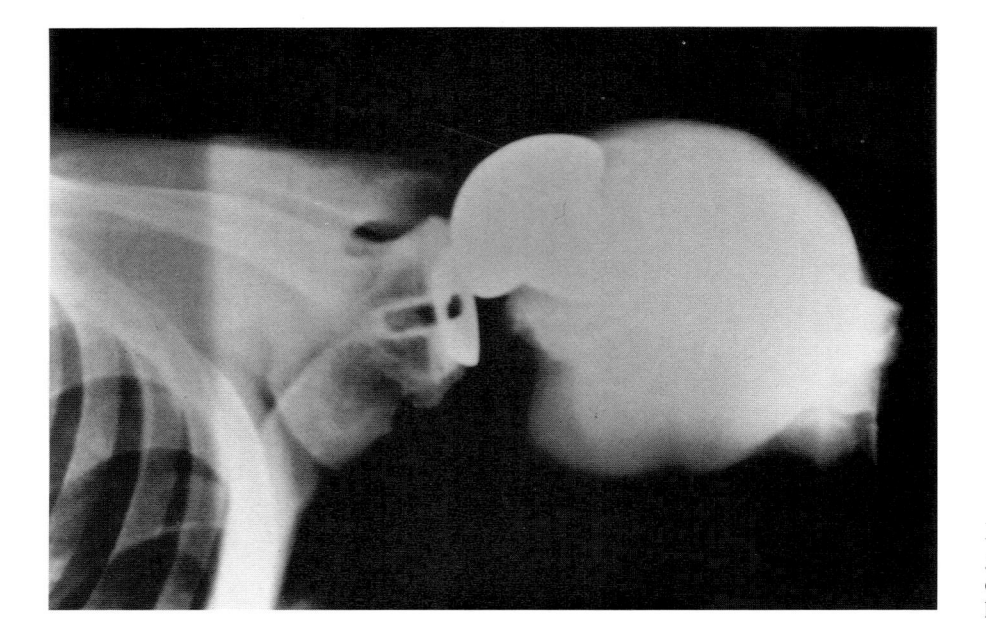

Figure 21–5. An axillary radiograph revealing a retroverted glenoid component with resulting posterior humeral subluxation.

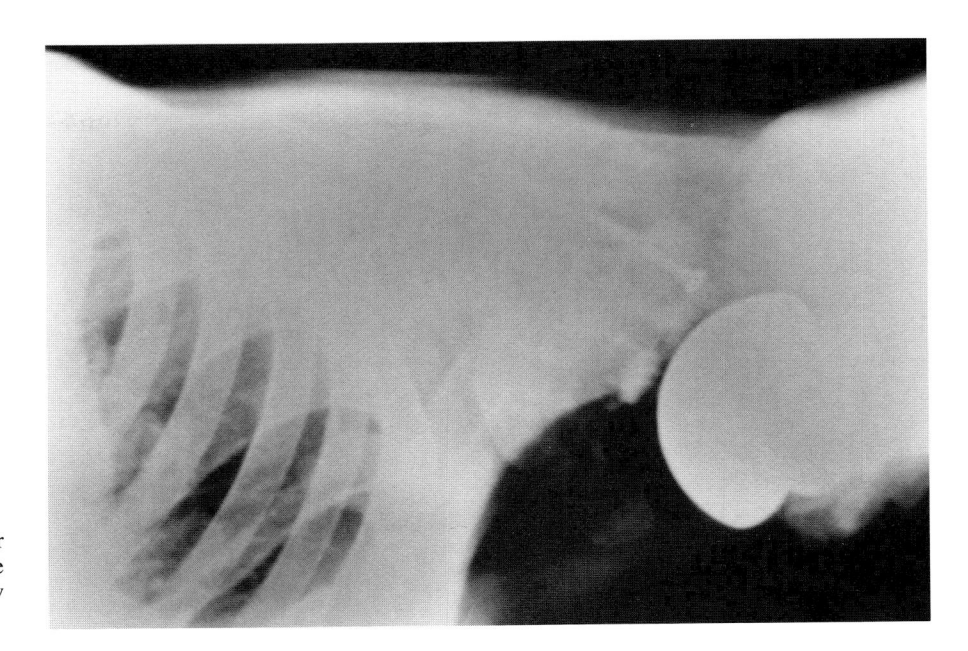

Figure 21–6. A radiograph after glenoid revision with posterior bone grafting. The humeral head is now centered on the glenoid face.

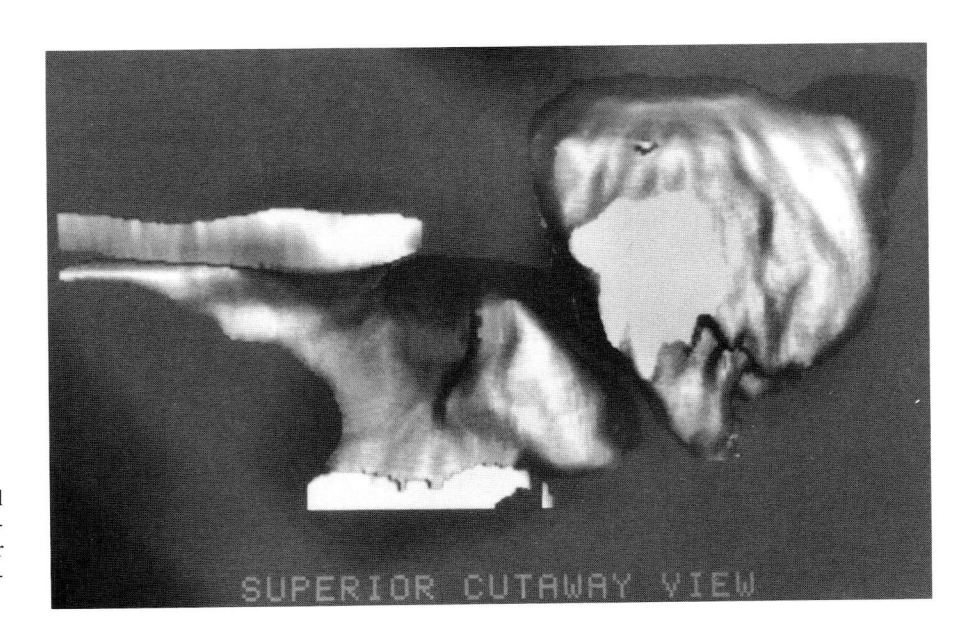

Figure 21–7. A three-dimensional magnetic resonance image reconstruction of a shoulder with posterior glenoid erosion and posterior subluxation of the humeral head.

this information. The physical examination centers on active and passive range of motion. The passive range of motion offers clues concerning the presence of contractures around the prosthetic glenohumeral joint as well as the direction of the instability. This discussion applies to the instances of painful subluxations, as dislocations usually present in a more obvious fashion.

Radiographic analysis begins with the plain radiographs including true anteroposterior, scapular Y, and axillary views. These should be closely inspected to determine the relative position of the humeral head to the prosthetic glenoid surface, and the position of the prosthetic components in relation to the host bone. The relative version of the glenoid component can be ascertained from the axillary view. The height of the glenoid component as compared to the scapula and the true glenoid must also be determined. Finally, the tilt of the glenoid component is illustrated on the true anteroposterior projection of the shoulder.

The radiographic analysis is also applied to the humeral component. The relationship between the prosthetic head and the greater tuberosity can be used to determine the position of the component. If the greater tuberosity is not available, a radiograph of the opposite arm will serve to determine if the length of the humerus has been restored. The version of the humeral component can be inferred from the physical examination. Radiographic techniques that have recently been described can determine the version of the humeral component from plain films,[26] and may be helpful if the version becomes an issue.

Additional radiographic modalities such as computerized tomographic or magnetic resonance imaging scans might serve a role in the future. However, they are presently limited by the scatter produced from the prosthetic components.

Anterior Instability

In general, the primary etiology of anterior instability is a disruption of the repaired subscapularis tendon from the early postoperative rehabilitation exceeding the allowable amount of external rotation. At present, to avoid this the authors attempt to achieve 30 to 40 degrees of external rotation at the time of the subscapularis repair. In addition, if the anterior tissues are inadequate, Mersilene tape is used to reinforce the repair. If using a modular design, overtensioning the soft tissues can occur if an excessively large head component is inserted. To avoid this, the shoulder is tested with a trial head component in place. On average, one should be able to displace the head posteriorly and anteriorly 50% of the glenoid width. Inferiorly, it should be able to translate 5 to 10 mm, with the head never being below the center of the glenoid. After the final components are implanted, the ultimate range of motion must be assessed in the operating room, and this provides guidelines for the postoperative rehabilitation.

The nonoperative treatment of anterior instability is not successful in managing this problem. The surgical management of postoperative anterior instability secondary to subscapularis rupture should include mobilization and repair of the tendon. If a modular prosthesis is in place, changing the head size can be used to adjust the soft-tissue tension. Custom humeral heads enable the surgeon to modify humeral version without stem revision. The importance of the subscapularis repair cannot be overemphasized, as it is much more difficult to repair a ruptured subscapularis tendon.[4]

For cases of recurrent instability where the subscapularis is insufficient, augmentation is recommended. A new technique has been described whereby an Achilles tendon allograft is utilized to replace the incompetent subscupularis and anterior capsule. This technique has proved successful in the limited number of patients in whom it was used.

The treatment of the soft tissues as illustrated above depends on first determining that the prosthetic components are in their proper orientation. The components work in unison with the soft tissues to maintain stability. If there is excessive anteversion involving either the humeral or the glenoid component, the soft tissues will be unable to resist the anteriorly directed forces. Therefore, if malpositioning of the component is involved, this must be corrected at the time of revision surgery. Modular prostheses offer another method to deal with this problem by enabling the surgeon to modify humeral version without stem revision.[9] Custom modular humeral heads have been designed to decrease the amount of humeral anteversion, increase the humeral head retroversion, and help resist the tendency towards anterior subluxation.

Posterior Instability

The etiology of posterior instability is multifactorial and often relates to the preoperative diagnosis. Typically this involves the patient with osteoarthritis and associated posterior glenoid erosion. The preoperative axillary view and computerized tomographic scan must be carefully inspected to determine the presence of posterior glenoid erosion, which if unrecognized can result in a retroverted glenoid component (Figure 21–8).[27] Once recognized, bone grafting the glenoid (Figure 21–9), anterior glenoid osteotomy, or inserting custom glenoid components (Figure 21–10) can be combined with decreasing the amount of humeral retroversion to prevent posterior instability. The combined amount of retroversion in both components should be 40 degrees.[28,29] Therefore, if the glenoid is in a more retroverted position, the surgeon should decrease the retroversion in the humeral stem.

Anterior soft-tissue contractures combined with posterior capsular laxity can also lead to posterior instability. The subscapularis often has a fixed contracture that must be lengthened at the time of revision. The axillary view is helpful in these instances because it can demonstrate the position of the humeral head relative to the glenoid face. This requires soft-tissue rebalancing, often in combination with decreasing the amount of humeral and/or glenoid retrover-

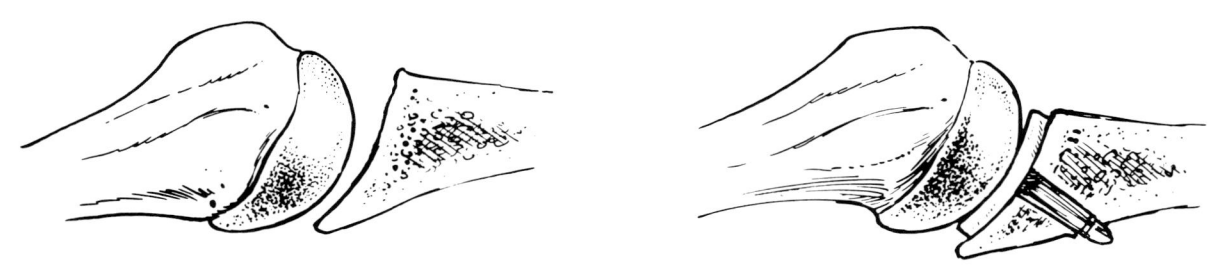

Figure 21-8. An illustration demonstrating posterior erosion of the glenoid leading to a retroverted glenoid component.

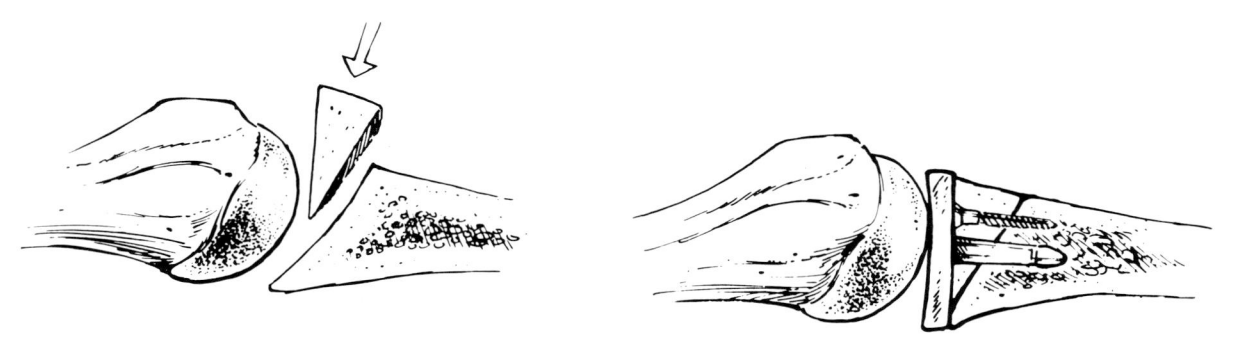

Figure 21-9. Bone grafting the posterior aspect of the glenoid to correct for posterior glenoid erosion.

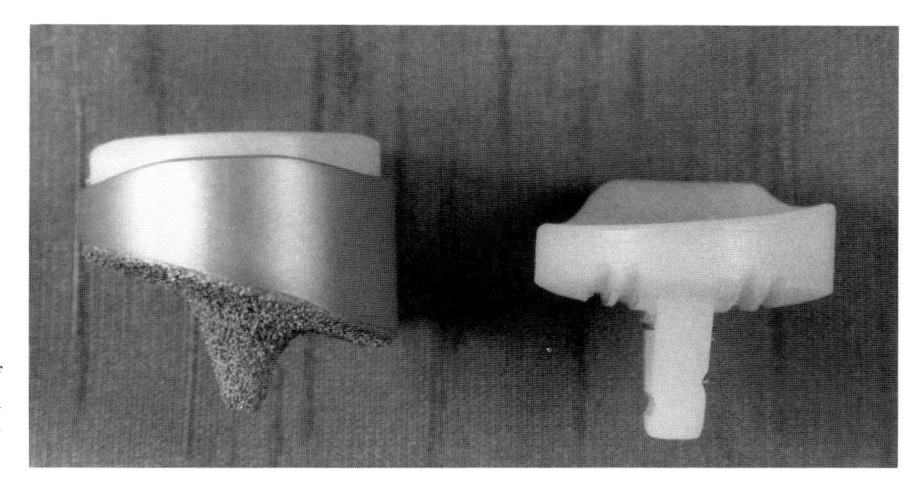

Figure 21-10. Two examples of custom glenoid components with posterior augmentation that may be utilized for posterior glenoid deficiency.

sion to maintain stability. Another cause of posterior instability involves excessive humeral retroversion. This should be decreased with component revision, or in the case of a modular prosthesis, custom modular humeral heads with decreased retroversion built into the head component can be used.

The management of the patient with posterior instability should involve an analysis of the etiology, which will lead to the available treatment options. The modular prosthesis adds to these options especially when component version becomes an issue. Access to the glenoid is facilitated by removing the modular head and humeral version can be modified without stem revision.[30]

Superior Instability

Superior subluxation is most commonly attributed to rotator cuff dysfunction. There has been a large variation in the incidence reported by various authors. Amstutz et al.[1] described a 52% incidence of some degree of subluxation after total shoulder arthroplasty. Most other authors usually noted a much lower incidence of superior subluxation or postoperative traumatic rotator cuff tears. Patient management should be based on the treatment of rotator cuff tears in general. Often these patients develop an impingement-like syndrome that will respond to physical therapy, nonsteroidal anti-inflammatory medication, and injections. When their function is severely impaired, the rotator cuff will need to be repaired.

This is one of the most common complications seen after shoulder arthroplasty, with most patients responding to conservative management.[28] The rates of glenoid loosening have been described as both increased with rotator cuff tears[2] and not related to the quality of the rotator cuff tissue.[19] In patients with massive loss of rotator cuff tissue precluding an adequate repair, the glenoid component should not be used, and a hemiarthroplasty with a large humeral head should be considered. This appears to be a better option than total shoulder arthroplasty in dealing with cuff tear arthropathy. In patients with a repairable rotator cuff, total shoulder arthroplasty is indicated.

If a patient who underwent prior total shoulder arthroplasty presents with loosening of the glenoid and a large unrepairable rotator cuff tear, then removal of the glenoid and conversion to a hemiarthroplasty is probably the best course of action. In performing the hemiarthroplasty, soft-tissue stability anteriorly and posteriorly is required to prevent subluxation. This may be difficult with extensive rotator cuff tears but generally adequate tissue remains. Otherwise, transfers of autogenous tissue like the pectoralis major or an allograft may be considered. A modified postoperative rehabilitation follows with a limited goals approach as described by Neer, et al.[22] Hooded glenoid components have not proved successful.[28]

The other less common cause of superior subluxation involves component positioning. If the glenoid is placed too low or the humeral head is placed too high, superior subluxation can result and would require component revision in symptomatic cases.

Inferior Instability

Inferior subluxation immediately after shoulder arthroplasty is a common occurrence. This is caused by muscle weakness or possibly the loss of negative intraarticular pressure. This usually resolves with a return of deltoid muscle tone. Long-term inferior instability has been the least frequently reported instability complication after total shoulder arthroplasty. The most common etiology relates to component malposition. Restoring humeral length is most problematic when treating conditions that distort the anatomy around the proximal aspect of the humerus. These include fractures and revision surgery. The greater tuberosity provides a commonly used landmark to guide placement of the humeral component, as the head should extend just above the level of the greater tuberosity. After a fracture of the proximal part of the humerus, the tuberosities are often distorted. This mandates that component placement be assessed by inserting a trial in the shaft followed by tensioning the arm inferiorly. In this situation, the humeral prosthesis is positioned such that the superior aspect of the head is in the upper third of the glenoid with inferior traction. The humeral component is cemented to ensure the proper positioniong. A glenoid prosthesis that is placed too high on the scapula may cause the same problem. The coracoid can serve as a guide in those instances of glenoid distortion.[29]

The treatment for inferior instability caused by muscle weakness would be physical therapy to strengthen the muscles. This has been described in the literature, with mixed results.[22] If component malposition is implicated, then revision surgery becomes necessary to restore deltoid length.

SUMMARY

Instability after shoulder replacement is a difficult problem to treat successfully. Prevention by proper component positioning and soft-tissue balancing is far superior than any type of revision procedure. The necessary postoperative rehabilitation should include a physical therapy program that respects the range of motion obtained in the operating room. Salvage methods for symptomatic instabilities include reconstruction of the soft-tissue envelope, revision of components, and possibly allografts to replace soft-tissue deficiencies.

REFERENCES

1. Amstutz HC, Thomas BJ, Kabo M, Jinnah RH, Dorey FJ. The DANA total shoulder arthroplasty. *J Bone Joint Surg [Am]* 1988;70:1174–1182.
2. Barrett WP, Franklin JL, Jackins SE, Wyss CR, Matsen FA III. Total shoulder arthroplasty. *J Bone Joint Surg [Am]* 1987;69:865–872.
3. Cofield RH. Total shoulder arthroplasty with the Neer prosthesis. *J Bone Joint Surg [Am]* 1984;66:899–906.
4. Cofield RH, Edgerton BC. Total shoulder arthroplasty: Complications and revision surgery. *Instr Course Lect* 1990;39:449–462.
5. Moeckel BH, Dines DM, Warren RF, Altchek DW. Modular hemiarthroplasty for fractures of the proximal humerus. *J Bone Joint Surg,* 1992;74A:884–889.
6. Dines DM, Altchek DW. Hemiarthroplasty techniques for proximal humerus fractures. *Comp Orthop* 1991;Jan/Feb:25–31.
7. Amstutz HC, Sew Hoy AL, Clarke IC. UCLA anatomic total shoulder arthroplasty. *Clin Orthop* 1981;155:7–20.
8. Barrett WP, Thornhill TS, Thomas WH, Gebhart EM, Sledge CB. Nonconstrained total shoulder arthroplasty in patients with polyarticular rheumatoid arthritis. *J Arthroplasty* 1989;4:91–96.
9. Bell SN, Gschwend N. Clinical experience with total arthroplasty and hemiarthroplasty of the shoulder using the Neer prosthesis. *Int Orthop* 1986;10:217–222.
10. Brenner BC, Ferlic DC, Clayton ML, Dennis DA. Survivorship of unconstrained total shoulder arthroplasty. *J Bone Joint Surg [Am]* 1989;71:1289–1296.
11. Cofield RH. Total shoulder arthroplasty with the Neer prosthesis. *J Bone Joint Surg [Am]* 1984;66:899–906.
12. Cofield RH. Unconstrained total shoulder prostheses. *Clin Orthop* 1983;173:97–108.
13. Faludi DD, Weiland AJ. Cementless total shoulder arthroplasty: Preliminary experience with thirteen cases. *Orthopedics* 1983;6:431–437.
14. Figgie HE, Inglis AE, Goldberg VM, Ranawat CS, Figgie MP, Wile JM. An analysis of factors affecting the long-term results

of total shoulder arthroplasty in inflammatory arthritis. *J Arthroplasty* 1988;3:123–130.
15. Frich LH, Moller BN, Sneppen O. Shoulder arthroplasty with the Neer Mark-II prosthesis. *Arch Orthop Trauma Surg* 1988;107:110–113.
16. Hawkins RJ, Bell RH, Jallay B. Total shoulder arthroplasty. *Clin Orthop* 1989;242:188–194.
17. Kay SP, Amstutz HC. Shoulder hemiarthroplasty at UCLA. *Clin Orthop* 1988;228:42–48.
18. Kelly IG, Foster RS, Fisher WD. Neer total shoulder replacement in rheumatoid arthritis. *J Bone Joint Surg [Br]* 1987;69:723–726.
19. McCoy SR, Warren RF, Bade HA III, Ranawat CS, Inglis AE. Total shoulder arthroplasty in rheumatoid arthritis. *J Arthroplasty* 1989;4:105–113.
20. McElwain JP, English E. The early results of porous-coated total shoulder arthroplasty. *Clin Orthop* 1987;218:217–224.
21. Neer CS II. Replacement arthroplasty for glenohumeral osteoarthritis. *J Bone Joint Surg [Am]* 1974;56:1–13.
22. Neer CS II, Watson KC, Stanton FJ. Recent experience in total shoulder replacement. *J Bone Joint Surg [Am]* 1982;64:319–337.
23. Swanson AB, de Groot Swanson G, Sattel AB, Cendo RD, Hynes D, Jar-Ning W. Bipolar implant shoulder arthroplasty. Long-term results. *Clin Orthop* 1989;249:227–247.
24. Moeckel BH, Altchek DW, Warren RF, Wickiweicz TL, Dines DM. The management of the unstable shoulder arthroplasty. *Orthop Trans.* 1991;15:748.
25. Galinat BJ, Howell SM. The glenohumeral joint. *Orthop Trans* 1988;12:143.
26. Frich LH, Moller BN. Retroversion of the humeral prosthesis in shoulder arthroplasty. *J Arthroplasty* 1989;4:277–280.
27. Friedman RJ, Hawthorne K, Genez B. Evaluation of glenoid bone loss with computerized tomography for total shoulder arthroplasty. *Orthop Trans* 1991;15:749.
28. Cofield RH. Degenerative and arthritic problems of the glenohumeral joint. In: Rockwood CA, Matsen FA, eds. *The Shoulder*. Philadelphia: WB Saunders, 1990:678–749.
29. Neer CS II. Glenohumeral arthroplasty. In: Neer CS II, ed. *Shoulder Reconstruction*. Philadelphia: WB Saunders, 1990:143–272.
30. Shaffer BS, Giordano CP, Zuckerman JD. Revision of a loose glenoid component facilitated by a modular humeral component. *J Arthroplasty* 1990;5:S79–S81.

SECTION VI

Current Trends in Total Shoulder Arthroplasty

22 Bipolar Shoulder Arthroplasty

Alfred B. Swanson, M.D., and Genevieve de Groot Swanson, M.D.

The painful shoulder presenting as an isolated symptom in an otherwise healthy patient receives appropriate attention because of the patient's complaints and the severe loss of function frequently due to inflammation and impingement. In osteoarthritis, the symptoms of pain and loss of motion are chronic complaints; the symptoms often do not respond to conservative treatment and are not always treated satisfactorily. In the rheumatoid arthritis patient, whose functional activity has been restricted by multiple-joint involvement, shoulder disabilities are frequently ignored by both the patient and the physician. Although decreased range of motion results in loss of functional activity through limitation of hand placement in space, the patient will usually not complain unless experiencing severe crepitation or instability. A variety of surgical procedures have been developed for the joints of the hand, wrist, elbow, and lower extremity, but the surgical treatment of the arthritic shoulder has received less attention until more recently.

ANATOMIC CONSIDERATIONS

Restoration of glenohumeral function is difficult to achieve because of the unique and complex anatomy about the shoulder girdle and the dependency of active motion on the integrity of the musculotendinous and ligamentous units. The shoulder girdle could be described as having five joints: the glenohumeral joint, scapulothoracic joint, sternoclavicular joint, acromioclavicular joint, and subdeltoid joint, which is not a true anatomic joint but has two musculotendinous surfaces moving against each other.

The function of the scapulothoracic joint, although not frequently involved in the arthritic process, depends on the integrity of the surrounding muscles and a stable glenohumeral joint to add motion to the upper extremity. Dysfunction of the acromioclavicular joint can limit shoulder motion through pain, incongruity, and instability. Resection of this commonly involved joint should be considered in reconstructive procedures. The glenohumeral joint, a true ball-and-socket articulation, derives its stability, movement, and normal function not so much from the joint surfaces as from an exquisite interplay of motor tendon units, proper tension of the ligamentous and capsular structures, and nonrestrictive gliding planes.

Superior subluxation of the humeral head is well recognized in patients with injuries to the rotator cuff and may also result from excessive contraction of the long muscles across a disorganized joint. The vertical shearing action of the deltoid muscle, which lifts the humeral head in relation to the glenoid surface, is normally combined with the horizontal forces of the rotator cuff muscles, especially the supraspinatus, to create a coupling compressive force that keeps the humeral head level with the glenoid cavity (Figure 22–1).[1] The subdeltoid bursa forms a cleavage between the deltoid muscle and the underlying periarticular rotator cuff muscles. Adhesions in this area will restrict gliding and therefore abduction, where the greater tuberosity is pulled superiorly and medially by the action of the supraspinatus muscle to allow the humeral head to slip under the coracoacromial arch. This mechanism is extremely important in the pathomechanics of the arthritic shoulder.

IMPLANT DESIGN CONSIDERATIONS

The basic concepts for shoulder arthroplasty implant design require engineering, anatomic and physiologic considerations, as well as evaluation of implant materials and the patient's needs. An efficient implant procedure for the shoulder joint should simplify the joint's mechanism, because the complexity of the normal mechanisms are difficult to accurately reproduce.

The implants or prostheses used in shoulder reconstruction can be classified as:

1. Hemiarthroplasty, which replaces the head of the humerus with an intramedullary stemmed implant such as reported by Neer.[2] This is especially useful in patients following a fracture-dislocation of the proximal part of the humerus.
2. Total joint replacement, which includes four basic types.
    A. Nonconstrained, which has a humeral prosthesis articulating with a glenoid component, and both are fixed to bone.[3–6] This implant results in a satisfactory outcome if the musculotendinous units are intact or reconstructible. However, glenoid fixation has been a problem, particularly in the presence of inadequate bone stock as seen with rheumatoid arthritis, and loosening at the bone-cement interface can occur. The nonconstrained implants also do not address the problem of superior subluxation of the humeral head.
    B. Bipolar or bicentric, which has interlocked humeral and glenoid components, but the glenoid component is not fixed to bone.[7–10]
    C. Semiconstrained, which has a conforming component for the glenoid.[11,12]

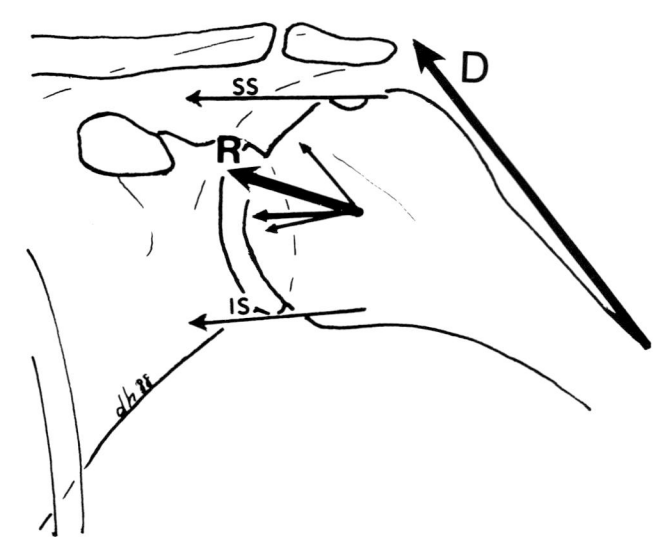

Figure 22–1. The vertical shearing action of the deltoid muscle combines with the transverse forces generated by a normal rotator cuff to create a force couple passing through the glenoid surface. Loss of rotator cuff function results in vertical subluxation due to the unopposed deltoid effect. D = deltoid vector; SS = supraspinatus vector; IS = infraspinatus vector; R = resultant forces. (Reproduced with permission from Swanson et al.[10])

D. Constrained, which has interlocked humeral and glenoid components that are also fixed to bone.[13–15] This could theoretically compensate for altered shoulder mechanics as seen with a torn rotator cuff; however, increased stresses at the bone-cement interface and a high early failure rate limit the indications of this procedure to a small number of cases.

BIPOLAR SHOULDER IMPLANT

History, Development, and Concept

A research project to develop implants for arthroplasty of the upper extremity joints was initiated in 1962.[7] At that time, it was noted that most arthritic patients who have lost shoulder abduction and external rotation had a tendency towards vertical or superior displacement of the humeral head, which frequently caused impingement of the superior portion of the humeral head and the greater tuberosity against the acromion and the coracoacromial ligament. In the past, corrective procedures to decrease the symptoms of impingement included resection of the acromion and the coracoacromial ligament, yet some believe that the coracoacromial arch should be preserved to maintain the head position underneath it for the prosthetic head contacts not only the glenohumeral joint, but also the coracoacromial arch. A humeral sphere of a larger diameter than normal could achieve this goal by decreasing the coupling action forces necessary to maintain the contact of the joint surfaces at the glenohumeral joint. The leverage to move a large humeral head implant would then be effected primarily by the strong deltoid muscle, and secondarily by the weaker rotator cuff muscles.

The theoretic advantages provided by a large humeral head implant include (1) smooth concentric total contact for the entire shoulder joint cavity, including the coracoacromial arch and the glenoid fossa; (2) reduction of force concentration over any one contact area and therefore decreased resistance to movement; (3) longer moment arm between the fulcrum (joint contact point) and the muscle insertion, increasing efficiency of the muscle pull; and (4) prevention of the greater tuberosity from impinging against the acromion. In 1965, a one-piece intramedullary stemmed silicone implant and an intramedullary stemmed metal implant with interchangeable snap-fit silicone heads were designed and tested in the authors' department.[7] These initial designs, although providing good pain relief, were abandoned due to inadequate motion and durability.

Definition

The concept of a bipolar shoulder arthroplasty was developed in 1975. The bipolar, or bicentric implant has a self-contained ball-and-socket component that allows motion between a distal extremity and a proximal part through two moving interfaces. In a ball-and-socket joint, such as the shoulder or hip, motion can be obtained between the cup of a prosthetic device, which moves within the "socket" (glenoid or acetabulum), and an intramedullary stemmed ball that articulates with a polyethylene bearing within that cup. This type of interposition arthroplasty is similar in concept to the Smith-Peterson cup arthroplasty, where motion occurs between the reshaped head of the femur and the inner surface of the metal cup, and between the cup's outer surface and the acetabulum.[16] This bipolar motion concept was applied to hip endoprostheses by Giliberty, Bateman, and Monk in 1974.[17,18]

The bipolar implant has a metal humeral component, and an articulating snap-fit glenoid resurfacing cup made of plastic and metal. The titanium humeral component consists of a stem, collar, neck, and ball and is supplied in two neck lengths (22 and 29 mm). The stem measures 10.16 cm in length and is tapered distally and grooved to enhance cement fixation (Figure 22–2). The 22-mm head diameter allows use of bipolar hip cups for greater sizing potential. The cup component, available in 14 outer diameters, consists of a cobalt chrome alloy shell and an ultra-high-molecular-weight polyethylene liner, which is mechanically locked inside the shell through mating ridges on the concave side of the metal shell and convex surface of the plastic cup. The spherical head of the humeral component articulates with the concave polyethylene liner.

Advantages

The bipolar shoulder arthroplasty provides the following advantages:

1. Provides new joint surfaces.

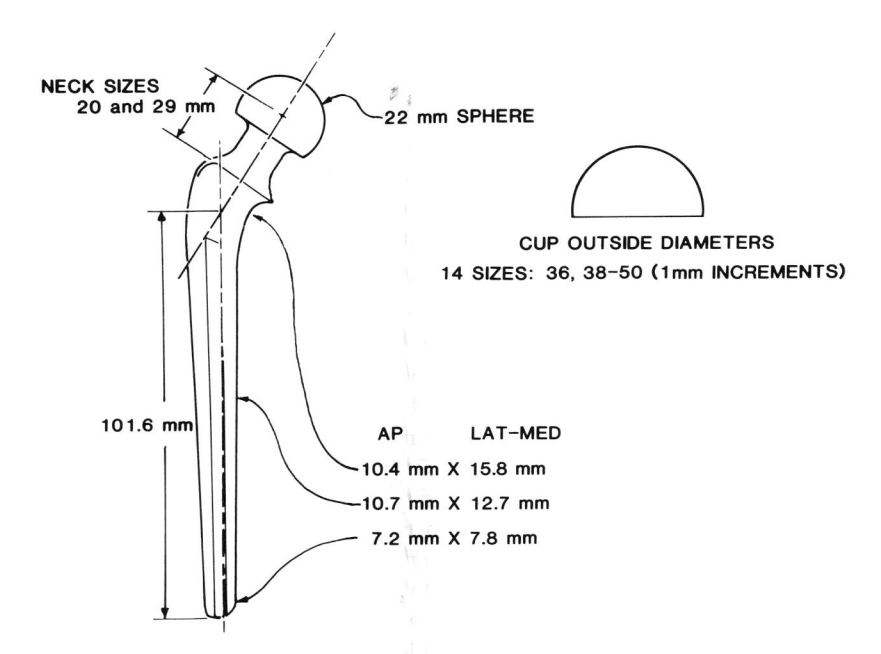

Figure 22–2. The glenoid cups are available in 14 diameters; the sphere of the humeral ball is 22 mm; two neck lengths are available. (Reproduced with permission from Swanson et al.[10])

2. Allows concentric total contact for the shoulder cavity, including the coracoacromial arch and the glenoid.
3. Acts as a spacer and prevents abutment of the greater tuberosity against the acromion, and moves the center of rotation away from the coracoacromial arch.
4. Allows the cup to align itself in the glenoid, similar to a universal joint.
5. Requires no fixation of the glenoid component.
6. Decreases the wear between the implant, glenoid, and coracoacromial arch because motion occurs both at the glenoid–outer cup interface and ball–inner cup interface. The coefficient of friction is least between the metal ball and polyethylene liner of the metal cup, so that motion will selectively occur at this interface, as demonstrated in cinefluoroscopic studies of postoperative patients.
7. Potentially increases the range of motion because of the two separate moving joint interfaces. In cases of superior subluxation, the potential for erosive acromial changes is decreased.
8. Dampens stress concentrations, and minimizes wear changes on the implant and surrounding tissues.
9. Provides stability by design of the glenoid component and its fit into the shoulder socket and surrounding soft-tissue envelope. This stability allows motion to occur within the glenohumeral implant and at the scapulothoracic joint.
10. Utilizes a standard anterior surgical approach and a straightforward procedure and soft-tissue closure.
11. Can be used as a salvage method for the failed total shoulder arthroplasty.

SURGICAL PROCEDURE

Indications

The bipolar shoulder arthroplasty is indicated for reconstruction of a severely painful, disabling arthritic shoulder, with evidence of joint destruction, incongruity, and/or subluxation. The procedure can be of particular benefit in cases with loss of rotator cuff function, in rheumatoid arthritis with severe destruction of the humeral head and/or glenoid cavity, in advanced pathology secondary to degenerative or post-traumatic arthritis, and for revision of a failed total shoulder arthroplasty. Superior subluxation of the humeral head is commonly seen in these conditions and may preclude the use of a hemiarthroplasty or nonconstrained total shoulder arthroplasty. In cases where the glenoid bone stock is inadequate, the Neer-type total shoulder arthroplasty should not be used unless bone grafting of the glenoid is done at the time of glenoid component insertion.

The use of a bipolar shoulder arthroplasty is contraindicated in presence of active or past sepsis in the shoulder, inadequate skin, inadequate bone or soft-tissue structures, poor neuromuscular function, and an uncooperative patient. Familiarity with shoulder reconstruction and rehabilitation procedures is essential in performing successful shoulder implant arthroplasty. Considerations for anterior capsular reinforcement and reconstruction of the rotator cuff should be made in the surgical planning. All patients should have a medical review and clearance and be informed about the expectations of surgery, the immediate postoperative course, and the rehabilitation program. The meticulous program used for any total joint arthroplasty is applied, with special emphasis to prevent infection through the use of perioperative prophylactic antibiotics and a laminar airflow apparatus in the operating room. General endotracheal or regional anesthesia can be used.

Technique

The patient is placed in a semireclining position close to the edge of the table. The surgical drapes are applied to allow exposure of the entire extremity for ease of manipulation as required. A deltopectoral incision, 10 to 12 cm in length, is directed downward from the level of the acromioclavicular joint, over the coracoid process, and along the anterior medial aspect of the arm (Figure 22–3A). The deltoid is separated from the pectoralis and retracted laterally to expose the coracoid process (Figure 22–3B). The anterior attachment of the deltoid muscle to the clavicle is usually preserved because of its importance for active flexion movements. The cephalic vein is identified between the deltoid and pectoralis major muscles and is occasionally ligated. The coracoid is divided with an osteotome just distal to the insertion of the pectoralis minor. The tip of the coracoid process with its attached coracobrachialis and short head of biceps origins is carefully retracted downward, protecting the neurovascular structures (Figure 22–3C,D).

If the acromioclavicular joint is involved, the cutaneous incision is extended superiorly to expose and excise the lateral end of the clavicle. With the arm in internal rotation, the deltoid muscle is retracted laterally and the subacromial bursa is identified and removed if abnormal. As the arm is externally rotated, the insertion of the subscapularis tendon to the lesser tuberosity is identified. Bleeding points are controlled. The subscapularis tendon and the shoulder joint capsule are incised longitudinally 1 cm from the bicipital groove and reflected medially (Figure 22–3E). The shoulder joint is identified, and with the position of the extremity controlled by an assistant, a synovectomy is performed as necessary for exposure. The long head of the biceps is released from its origin on the superior rim of the glenoid and dissected distally to gain enough tendon length as necessary for anterior capsular reconstruction.

The head of the humerus is dislocated into the wound by careful passive external rotation, adduction, extension, and vertical lifting of the arm. The humeral surface is usually irregular and destroyed. The portion of the humerus covered with cartilage is excised with power saws or osteotomes, taking care to avoid injury to the remaining bone stock (Figure 22–3F). It is best to preserve the greater tuberosity. However, with superior subluxation or an adduction contracture, more bone should be removed to obtain a joint space adequate for good motion. In this case, the greater tuberosity with its attached rotator cuff muscles and capsule is detached from the humerus with an osteotome, and preserved (Figure 22–3F,G). The axillary nerves and vessels are carefully protected.

Following adequate humeral head resection, the synovectomy is completed and osteophytes on the glenoid or humerus are excised. The intramedullary canal of the humerus is inspected and prepared to receive the stem of an appropriately sized implant. The center of the implant head should be placed in 30 degrees of retroversion and be well seated against this aspect of the humeral neck (Figure 22–3H). A reference mark is made on the humerus with a small rongeur. The degree of retroversion is determined by the implant's relationship to the bicipital groove and the lesser tuberosity, which face anteriorly, and by the alignment of the transverse axis between the epicondyles of the humerus. With the proper-size implant in place, passive range of motion is carried out. Enough bone should be removed to allow 90 degrees of elevation and 45 degrees of external rotation. The implant may require from 30 to 60 degrees of retroversion to be stable when external rotation is applied. Trial implants of various head sizes, and regular and long neck sizes are used to obtain a proper concentric fit of the implant head in the shoulder joint cavity, and to ensure proper neck length and avoid impingement of the proximal end of the humerus in the joint. It is important at this time to verify that there is adequate anterior capsule available for repair.

If the greater tuberosity with its muscular and capsular attachments has been detached, it is reattached to the humerus with no. 2 Dacron sutures passed through two drill holes made approximately 2 cm from the lateral end of the humerus and in the tuberosity (Figure 22–3G). The sutures are woven through the rotator cuff muscles before being passed through the tuberosity and humeral shaft and are tied inside the canal. The reattachment level can be advanced distally and slightly anteriorly to facilitate the closure of the anterior capsule. Two sutures may also be placed through drill holes in the anterior surface of the proximal shaft to reattach the capsule and subscapularis tendon (Figure 22–3I). The fit of the implant is tested again at this time.

The wound is thoroughly irrigated with saline and triple-antibiotic solution before cementing the humeral component. A canal plug made of silicone or from the resected humeral head is placed 2 cm beyond the tip of the implant to prevent distal flow of the cement and obtain improved canal filling by injecting the methylmethacrylate under pressure. The intramedullary stem of the implant is fixed within the humeral canal in the appropriate amount of retroversion with methylmethacrylate. After it has hardened, the implant head is reduced into the glenoid cavity, and the arm is taken through a range of motion to verify stability of the implant.

With the arm in neutral rotation, the medial capsule and subscapularis tendon are reinserted at their previous attachments with the no. 2 Dacron sutures (Figure 22–3 I,J). The capsulorrhaphy is reinforced by interweaving the long head of the biceps tendon (Figure 22–3K). The shoulder is taken through its range of motion to verify stability and appropriate tension of the soft-tissue closure. The coracoid is reattached either to the coracoacromial ligament or to its original anatomic position, using heavy sutures placed through drill holes. In certain cases, the coracoid process may be reattached at the anterior rim of the glenoid, after the technique of Bristow, to prevent tendencies for anterior dislocation

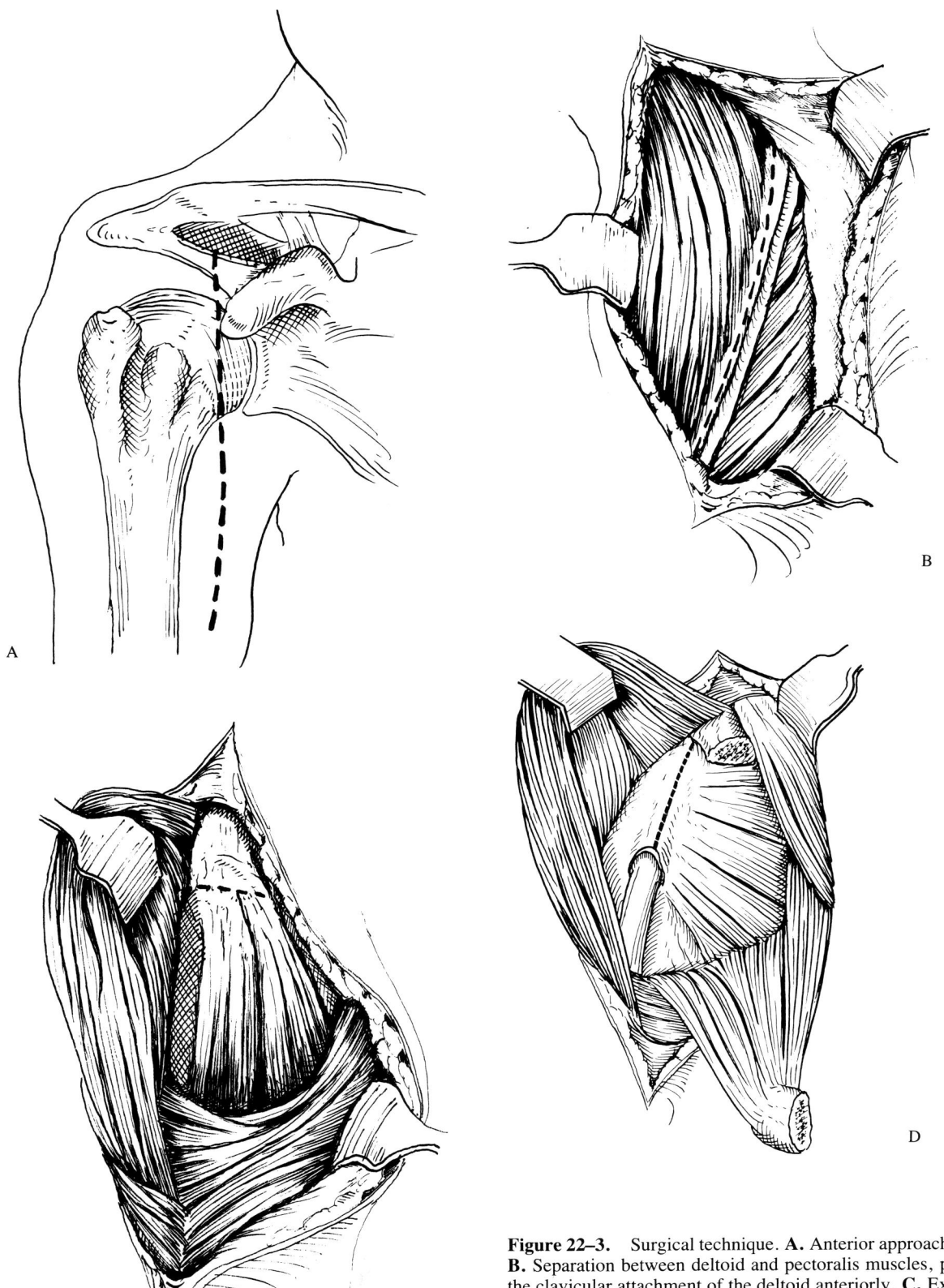

Figure 22–3. Surgical technique. **A.** Anterior approach incision. **B.** Separation between deltoid and pectoralis muscles, preserving the clavicular attachment of the deltoid anteriorly. **C.** Exposure of the coracoid. **D.** Retraction of the coracoid tip with attached musculature to expose the anterior aspect of the shoulder and the long head of the biceps tendon. (Figure continued on next page.)

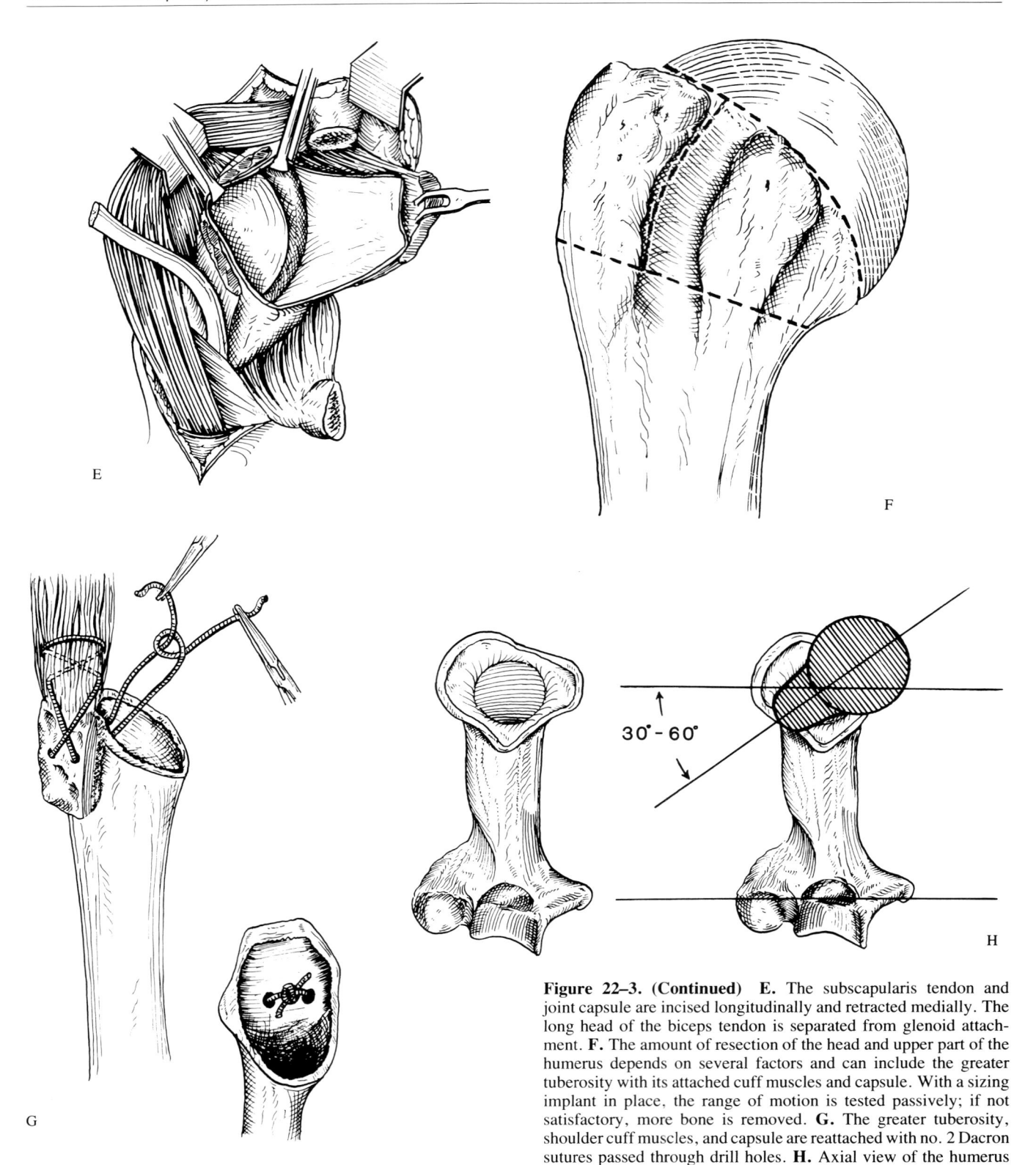

Figure 22–3. (Continued) E. The subscapularis tendon and joint capsule are incised longitudinally and retracted medially. The long head of the biceps tendon is separated from glenoid attachment. **F.** The amount of resection of the head and upper part of the humerus depends on several factors and can include the greater tuberosity with its attached cuff muscles and capsule. With a sizing implant in place, the range of motion is tested passively; if not satisfactory, more bone is removed. **G.** The greater tuberosity, shoulder cuff muscles, and capsule are reattached with no. 2 Dacron sutures passed through drill holes. **H.** Axial view of the humerus demonstrates the retroversion in which the implant is positioned relative to the transcondylar axis. This is usually 30 degrees.

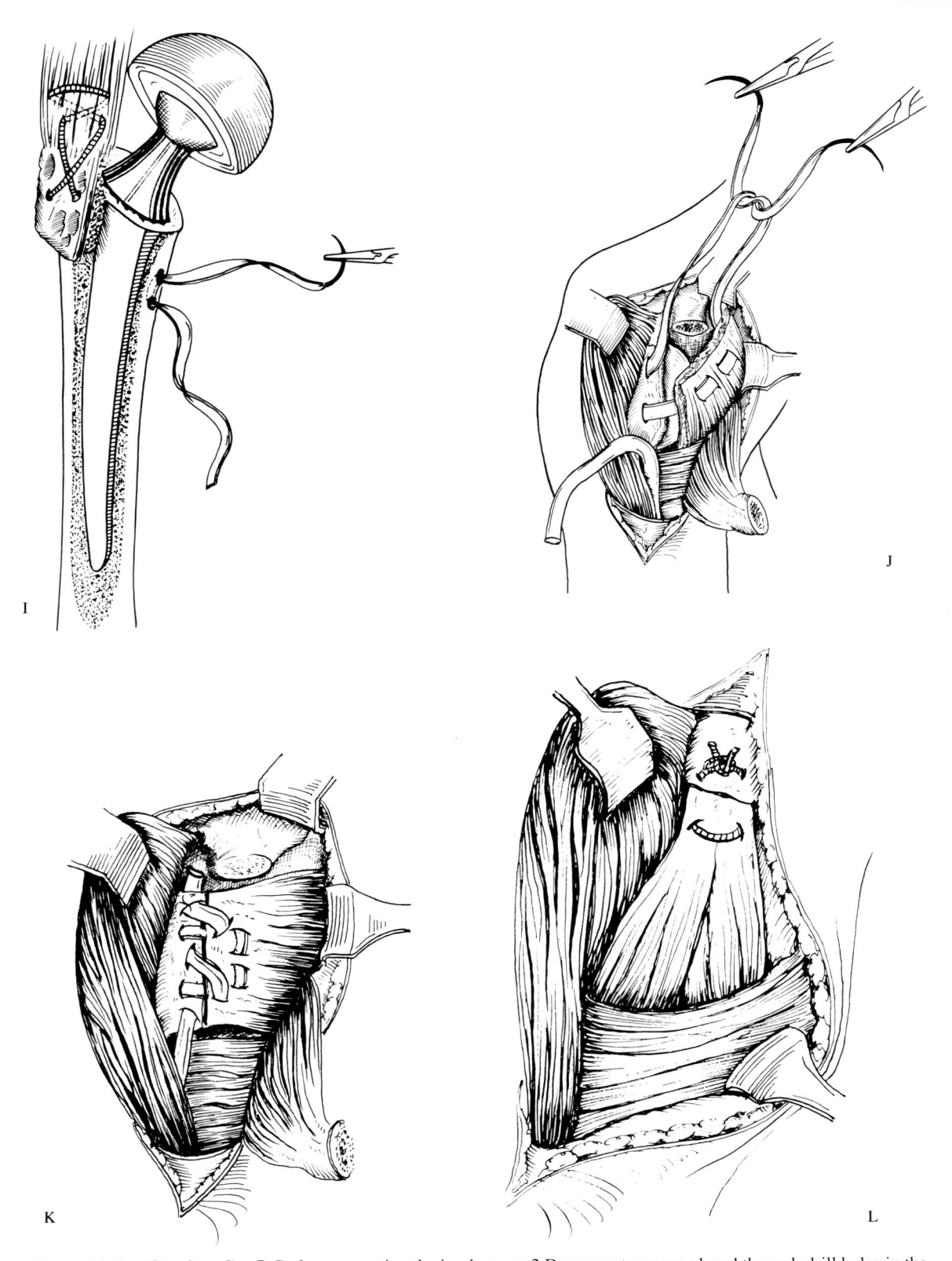

Figure 22–3. (Continued) **I.** Before cementing the implant, no 2 Dacron sutures are placed through drill holes in the anterior surface of the proximal shaft for later closure of the capsule and subscapularis tendon. A bone graft or silicone plug is placed 2 cm beyond the implant tip to prevent distal flow of cement, which is injected under pressure. **J.** Anterior capsule and subscapularis muscle closure with no. 2 Dacron sutures. **K.** The long head of the biceps tendon is interwoven to reinforce anterior closure. Closure is completed with heavy absorbable sutures and tested for implant stability. **L.** Reattachment of the coracoid process with heavy sutures passed through drill holes. (Reproduced with permission from Swanson.[8])

(Figure 22–3L). The deltoid and pectoral muscles and the subcutaneous tissues are reapproximated with absorbable sutures. The skin is closed over a rubber drain or suction apparatus. A conforming dressing is placed, and the extremity is held in a Velpeau-type dressing or sling and swathe.

Postoperative Care

The immediate postoperative care following shoulder arthroplasty requires protection of the anterior capsular incision and the reattached shoulder rotator cuff or deltoid muscles. Surgical variables may alter the postoperative plan and require further use of a Velpeau dressing, shoulder spica cast, or an abduction brace. In typical cases, the extremity is positioned to avoid humeral abduction, to maintain some humeral flexion, and to restrict motion with a sling and swathe dressing. When supine, the humerus should rest at the side on a foam wedge pillow placed under the arm to support the shoulder in 20 degrees of forward flexion and the forearm is placed across the chest. This position has been satisfactory for patient comfort and protection of the surgical repair. The patient is encouraged to relax the muscles, avoiding tension in the neck, upper back, and shoulder, and usually does not exercise the extremity until 3 to 5 days following surgery.

The exercise program is started with passive forward flexion and carried out in a supine position for 5 minute periods, 8 to 10 times daily, and the elbow can be extended with the palm up (Figure 22–4A). During this period, the patient may ambulate with the arm placed in an appropriate sling to maintain the described position. During the first 6 weeks, it is imperative that the patient avoids active flexion or abduction, or leaning on the operated extremity during activities of daily living. Excessive external rotation may disrupt the operative repair of the anterior shoulder.

At 1 week postoperatively, circumduction exercises are carried out in pronation and supination while wearing the sling, which may be removed at meal time to allow limited hand activity. Three weeks postoperatively, the sling is usually discarded and the arm may hang naturally at the side. The circumduction exercises are continued, enlarging the circles (Figure 22–4B). Flexion exercises are now done in a standing position and are guided through a passive range of motion with the nonoperated hand. Guarded passive external rotation to 20 degrees is started in a supine position (Figure 22–4C). At 4 weeks, active extension and internal rotation exercises are carried out in a standing position (Figure 22–4D, E). At 5 weeks, horizontal external rotation is added according to the patient's tolerance, and passive pulley exercises are introduced (Figure 22–4F). At 6 weeks, progressive resistive isometric exercises in forward flexion and internal and external rotation are initiated. The opposite hand may be used to provide resistance (Figure 22–4G). If the greater tuberosity is intact, abduction exercises may also be started. If there has been osteotomy and reattachment of the greater tuberosity, active abduction of the shoulder is started at 12 weeks. At this time, the patient is expected to achieve 70% of the normal range of shoulder flexion and external rotation.

Application of moist or dry heat may be beneficial prior to the exercise sessions, followed by pendulum and pulley exercises for relaxation, gradually progressing to more difficult motions. If a greater range of motion is desired, the active exercises of forward flexion, external rotation, and flexion with abduction can be done more vigorously. Patients are encouraged to continue daily exercises for up to 1 year postoperatively to maintain the range of motion and to develop additional strength. The physical therapy program and the willingness of the patient to follow the prescribed exercises for muscle strengthening are very important to the success of the procedure.

RESULTS

The bipolar shoulder arthroplasty has been used by the senior author in 60 shoulders of 54 patients (6 bilateral) since November 1976. Outcome studies with a minimum of 2-year follow-up were available for 44 shoulders. Sixteen shoulders were not included because the follow-up was less than 2 years, due to a recent arthroplasty (9 cases), death from unrelated causes (4 cases), and revision procedures (3 cases). The 40 patients (44 shoulders) were followed from 24 to 164 months after bipolar shoulder implant arthroplasty, with an average of 71 months. There were 21 patients with rheumatoid arthritis (4 bilateral cases), 14 patients with osteoarthritis, and 5 with posttraumatic arthritis. The series included 30 women and 10 men with a mean age of 63 years (range, 30 to 84 years). The bipolar shoulder arthroplasty was carried out according to the technique described. Associated procedures included coracoid osteotomy or transfer, rotator cuff reconstruction, greater tuberosity transfer, resection of the distal part of the clavicle, and capsular reinforcement with the long head of the biceps tendon.

Evaluation Methods

The clinical evaluation included assessment of pain, ability to perform activities of daily living, and measurements of shoulder motion. A shoulder score was devised based on the point system described in Table 22–1. A maximum of 10 points was allocated for each clinical category evaluated. The sum of points obtained in each category represents the patient's shoulder score, which can be classified as excellent (28 to 30 points), good (23 to 27.9 points), fair (18 to 22.9), and poor (less than 18 points).

The number of points given to each unit of shoulder motion was based on the relative value contributed to shoulder function as follows: abduction 20%, adduction 10%, flexion 40%, extension 10%, internal rotation 10%, and external rotation 10%. The scoring assigned for various positions on the arc of motion was based on shoulder impairment evaluation curves, which relate not only to the degrees of lost motion, but also more importantly to the location of the loss in the arc of motion.[19]

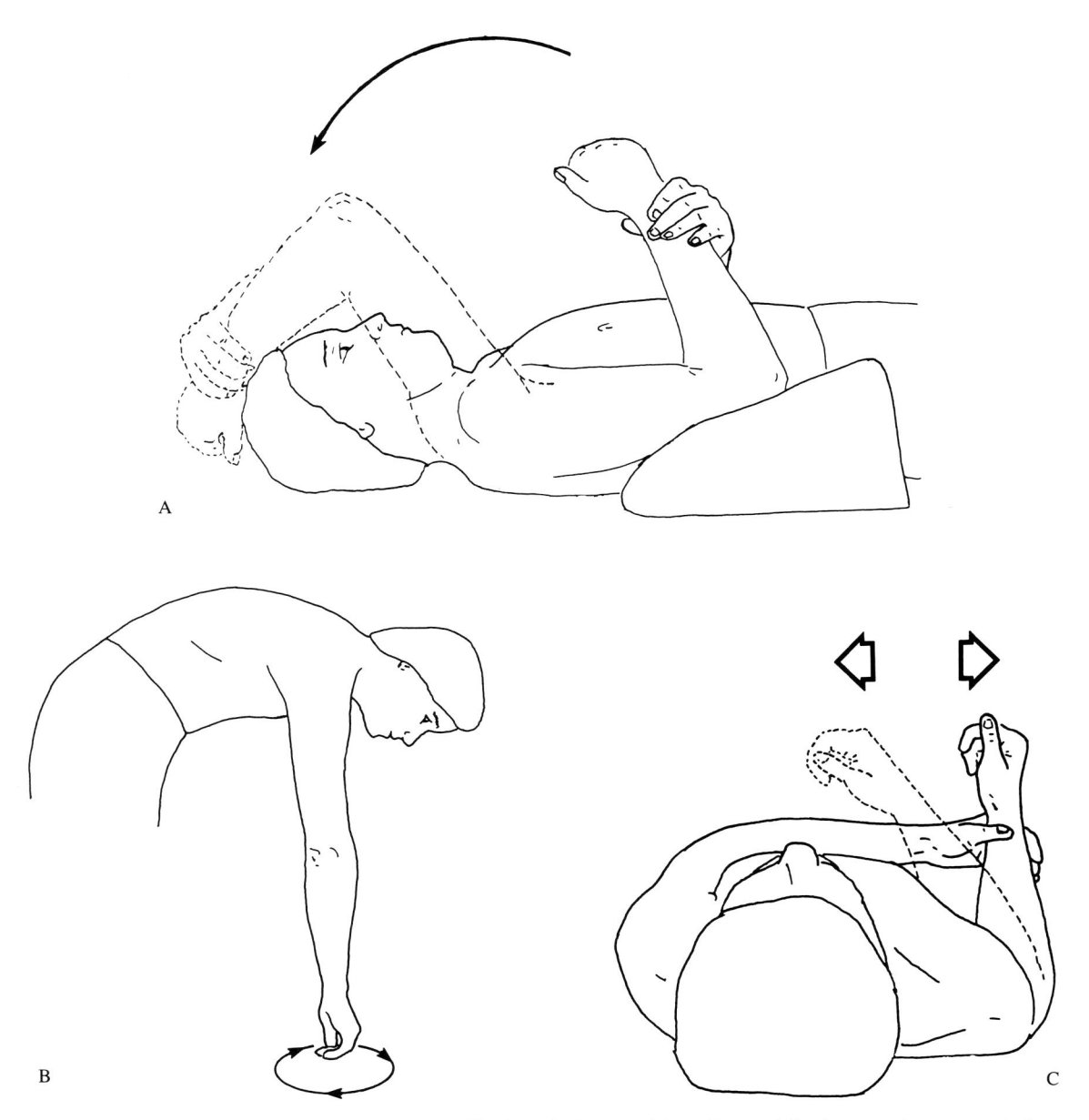

Figure 22–4. Total shoulder postoperative rehabilitation. **A.** Four to 5 days: Forward flexion exercises are carried out in a supine position. Note positioning of the wedge pillow. **B.** One week: Circumduction exercises are carried out with the forearm in pronation (shown) and then in supination. **C.** Two weeks: Guarded passive external rotation exercises to 20 degrees are started in the supine position. (Figure continued on next page.)

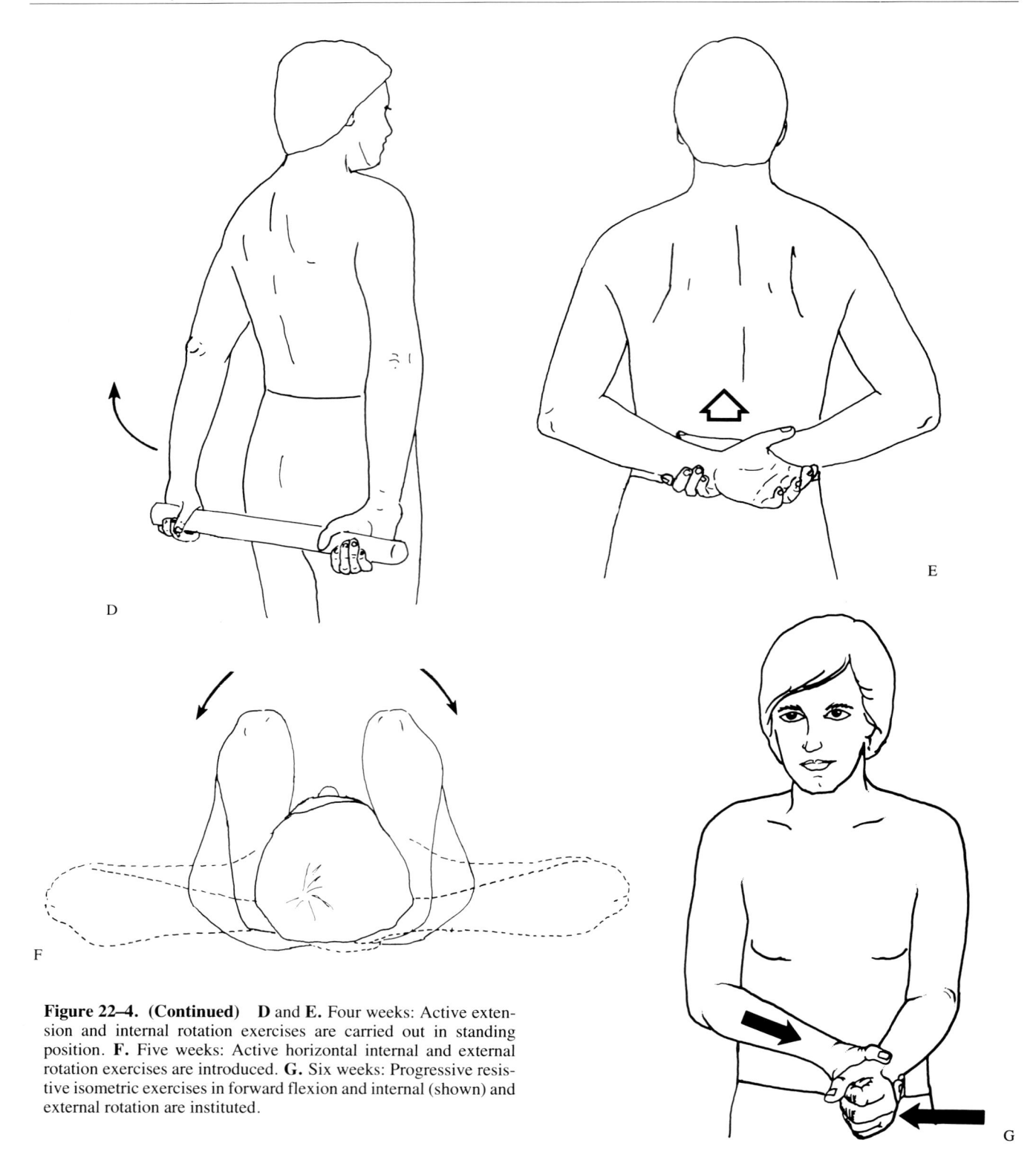

Figure 22–4. (Continued) **D** and **E.** Four weeks: Active extension and internal rotation exercises are carried out in standing position. **F.** Five weeks: Active horizontal internal and external rotation exercises are introduced. **G.** Six weeks: Progressive resistive isometric exercises in forward flexion and internal (shown) and external rotation are instituted.

Table 22–1. Shoulder Score System

	ROM Score (10 points)			Pain Score (10 points)	
	ROM (DEGREES)	POINTS		DEGREE	POINTS
Abduction (2 points)	0–19	0.8		Pain-free	10
	20–39	1.2		Minimal pain after heavy work	8
	40–89	1.4		Pain with daily activity	6
	90–129	1.6		Pain with shoulder motion	4
	130–149	1.8		Pain at rest	0
	150–180	2.0			
Adduction (1 point)	0–9	0.8			
	10–39	0.9			
	40–50	1.0		ADL Score (10 Points)	
Flexion (4 points)	0–9	1.2		ACTIVITY	POINTS
	10–19	2.0		Independent, normal activities	10
	20–49	2.6		Slight restrictions for heavy work overhead	8
	50–89	3.0			
	90–129	3.4		Most ADL	6
	130–159	3.6		Light activities only, assistance for some ADL	4
	160–180	4.0			
Extension (1 point)	0–29	0.9		Inability to use shoulder for function	0
	30–50	1.0			
Internal rotation (1 point)	0–19	0.9			
	20–49	0.7			
	50–69	0.8			
	70–79	0.9		Shoulder Score (30 points)	
	80–90	1.0		Poor	<18.0
External rotation (1 point)	0–19	0.8		Fair	18–22.9
	20–59	0.9		Good	23–27.9
	60–90	1.0		Excellent	28–30.0

ROM = range of motion; ADL = activities of daily living

The radiologic evaluation included standard anteroposterior, axillary, and lateral views. A cinefluoroscopy was done in a few cases to evaluate the dynamics of motion. A method for measuring the superior subluxation of the humeral head was devised, based on the relationship between the center of the humeral head component and the center point of the glenoid as identified on the preoperative anteroposterior radiographs (Figure 22–5). Measurements of superior subluxation, cup position in relation to the glenoid and acromion, and studies of the bone-cement interface in the humerus were carried out[20] (Figure 22–6).

Pain

Severe pain at rest or on minimal shoulder motion was reported by all patients before surgery. Twenty-three patients had complete pain relief, 18 patients experienced minimal pain after heavy activity, and 3 patients continued to experience some pain with activities of daily living (Table 22–2, Figure 22–7).

Activity Level

All patients reported improved shoulder function and ability to perform activities of daily living. Five patients were restored to independent normal activity, 30 patients had some restrictions with heavy work and overhead activity, and 9 patients could perform most activities of daily living but had some restrictions for more strenuous activities (Table 22–2, Figure 22–8).

Motion

The functional range of motion obtained after surgery was most encouraging. The average ranges of motion were 73 degrees of abduction (range, 30 to 120 degrees), 24 degrees of adduction (range, 0 to 45 degrees), 42 degrees of extension (range, 15 to 50 degrees), 82 degrees of flexion (range, 30 to 150 degrees), 79 degrees of internal rotation (range, 30 to 90 degrees), and 31 degrees of external rotation (range, 0 to 80 degrees) (Table 22–2).

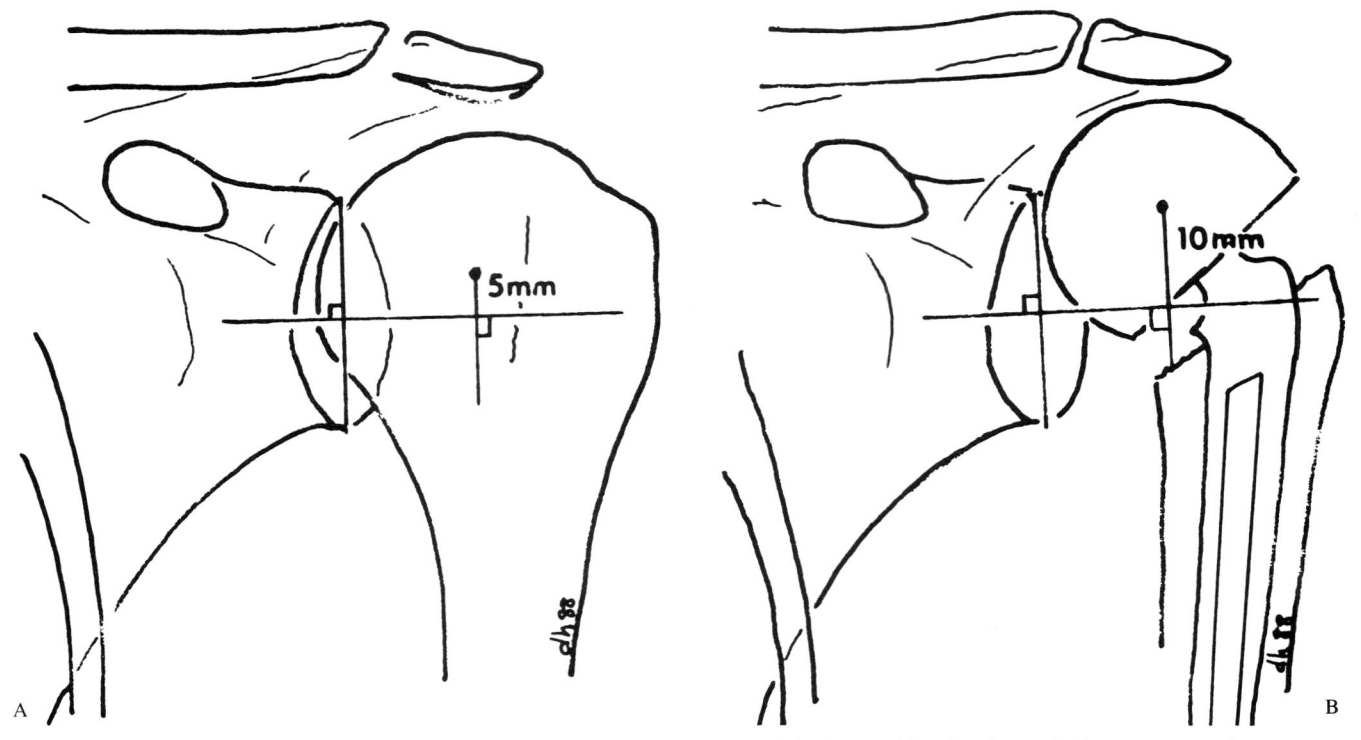

Figure 22–5. Radiographic measurements of vertical subluxation of the humeral head and prosthetic component. **A.** The center of the glenoid is identified as the midpoint between the superior and inferior bony edges of the articular surface. Position of the center of the humeral head measured in relation to a horizontal line through the glenoid center. A preoperative example of a 5-mm vertical subluxation of the humeral head is shown. **B.** Postoperatively, the position of the center of the humeral component is measured in relation to the preoperative glenoid midpoint by superimposing postoperative and preoperative radiographs. A 10-mm vertical subluxation of the implant is shown in this example. (Reproduced with permission from Swanson et al.[10])

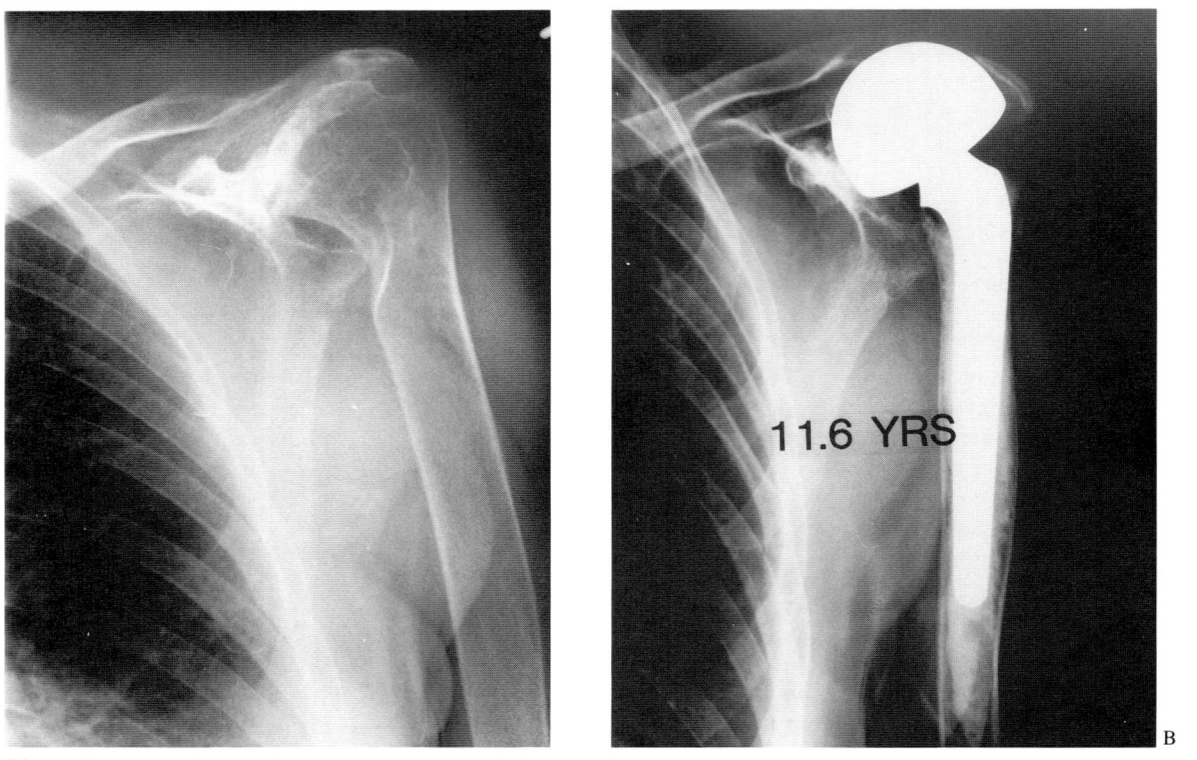

Figure 22–6. **A.** Preoperative radiograph of the left shoulder of a 56-year-old woman with rheumatoid arthritis, showing vertical subluxation of the humeral head and loss of glenoid bone stock. **B.** Radiograph made 11.6 years after bipolar shoulder arthroplasty shows good bone tolerance for the implant. Note the vertical subluxation of the humeral component. (Reproduced with permission from Swanson et al.[10])

Table 22-2. Postoperative Results for 44 Shoulders with 24 to 164 Months of Follow-up (Average, 71 Months)

DIAGNOSIS	NO. OF SHOULDERS	PAIN SCORE	ADL SCORE	ABDUCTION (DEGREES)	ADDUCTION (DEGREES)	EXTENSION (DEGREES)	FLEXION (DEGREES)	INTERNAL ROTATION (DEGREES)	EXTERNAL ROTATION (DEGREES)	SHOULDER SCORE
RA	25	9	7.5	63	24	39	78	76	34	24.6
OA	14	8.8	7.8	76	21	46	81	83	26	24.8
PTOA	5	9	9.5	85	27	47	102	80	23	27.1
Average	44	8.9	7.8	73	24	42	82	79	31	24.8

ADL = activities of daily living; RA = rheumatoid arthritis; OA = osteoarthritis; PTOA = post-traumatic osteoarthritis.

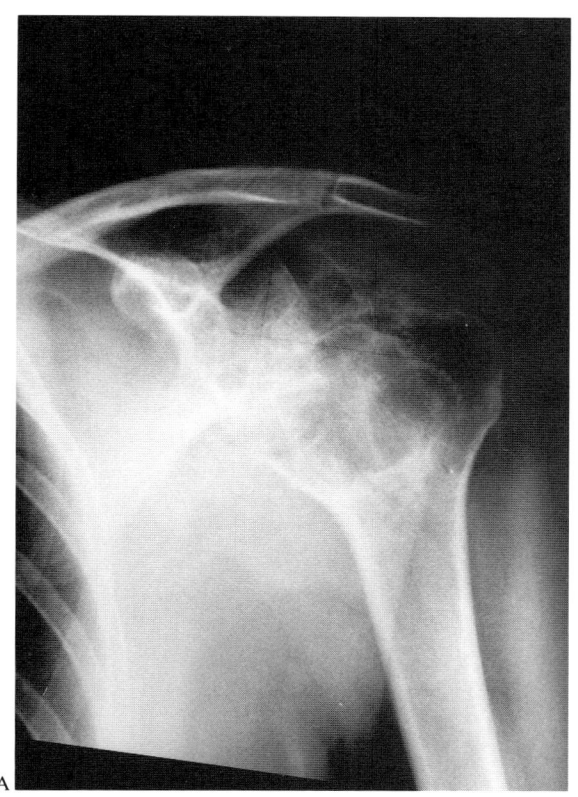

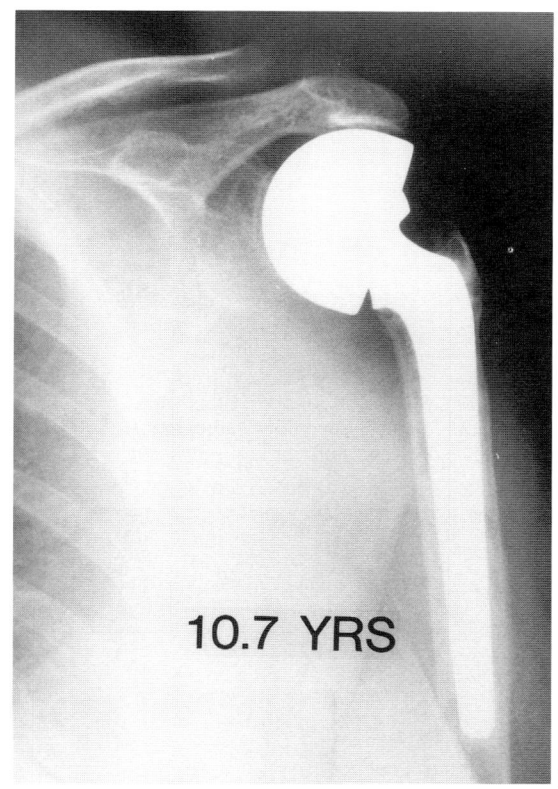

Figure 22-7. A. Preoperative radiograph showing the severe destruction of the humeral head and glenohumeral articulation in a 49-year-old woman with posttraumatic osteonecrosis of the humeral head and acromioclavicular joint arthritis. B. Radiograph made 10.7 years postoperatively showing the well-tolerated bipolar shoulder arthroplasty. Note resection of the distal end of the clavicle. She remains pain-free with an excellent functional result. (Reproduced with permission from Swanson et al.[10])

Shoulder Scores

The average postoperative shoulder scores were 8.9 points for pain, 7.8 points for performance of activities, and 8.1 points for motion, for a total of 24.8 points.

Radiographic Evaluation

The superior displacement of the humeral head preoperatively and of the bipolar component postoperatively was measured in a previous study of 39 shoulders.[10] The vertical difference between the center of the glenoid and the center of the humeral head averaged 3.3 mm preoperatively (Figure 22-6, Table 22-3). The preoperative radiograph was used as a template to measure the movement of the humeral bipolar component in relation to the glenoid. Serial measurements showed a progressive superior shift of the prosthetic head, which averaged 8.7 mm 24 months after surgery (Table 22-3). It is felt that this may have resulted from continued imbalance of the deltoid and rotator cuff muscle actions. The advantage of the bipolar shoulder arthroplasty is that even if the outer bipolar cup abuts the acromion, motion may still take place between the inner cup and the head of the prosthesis.

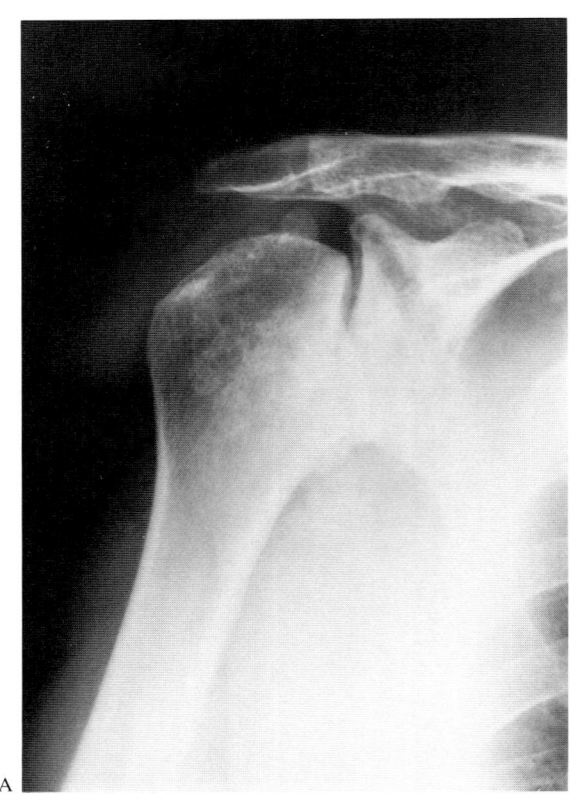

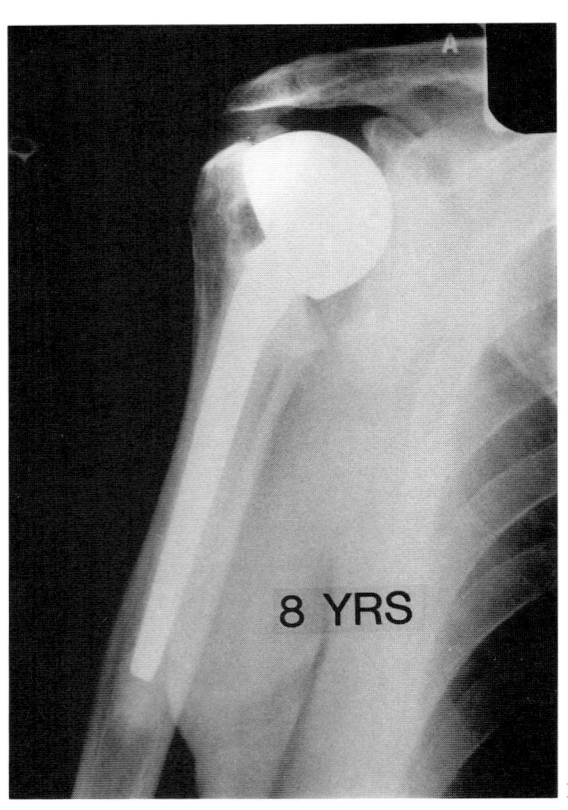

Figure 22–8. **A.** Preoperative radiograph of a 66-year-old man 7 years after sustaining a humeral head fracture. **B.** Radiograph made 8 years postoperatively shows good bone tolerance and implant placement. The patient is pain-free and has excellent shoulder function. (Reproduced with permission from Swanson et al.[10])

Table 22–3. Vertical Displacement of the Humeral or Prosthetic Head in Relation to the Glenoid Surface Preoperatively and Postoperatively*

DIAGNOSIS	HUMERAL HEAD PREOPERATIVE (mm)	PROSTHETIC HEAD POSTOPERATIVE MEASUREMENTS			
		1–2 Months (mm)	3–12 Months (mm)	13–24 Months (mm)	24 Months (mm)
RA (n = 19)†	3.5	1.9	5.0	10.0	10.0
OA (n = 20)	3.0	1.8	3.1	4.2	6.1
Average	3.3	1.8	4.4	8.7	8.7

*Reproduced with permission from Swanson et al.[10]
†One case of early postoperative subluxation excluded from measurements.
RA = rheumatoid arthritis; OA = osteoarthritis

Complications and Revisions

An anterior subcoracoid subluxation of the implant occurred 1 week after surgery in a rheumatoid arthritis patient. A closed reduction was refused and it was decided to follow the patient closely. After 11 years and 3 months, the patient continued to present with a functional shoulder and minimal pain after work and had 65 degrees of abduction, 25 degrees of adduction, 50 degrees of extension, 60 degrees of flexion, 90 degrees of internal rotation, and 30 degrees of external rotation. In a cineradiographic evaluation, most of the motion appeared to occur between the metal cup and the polyethylene liner. There was no evidence of erosive changes and no neurovascular compromise.

One patient with posttraumatic arthritis showed progression of acromioclavicular arthritis, which required a resection arthroplasty 4 years postoperatively. She continued to present with excellent pain-free motion 9 years and 8 months after revision surgery. Routine resection of the distal end of

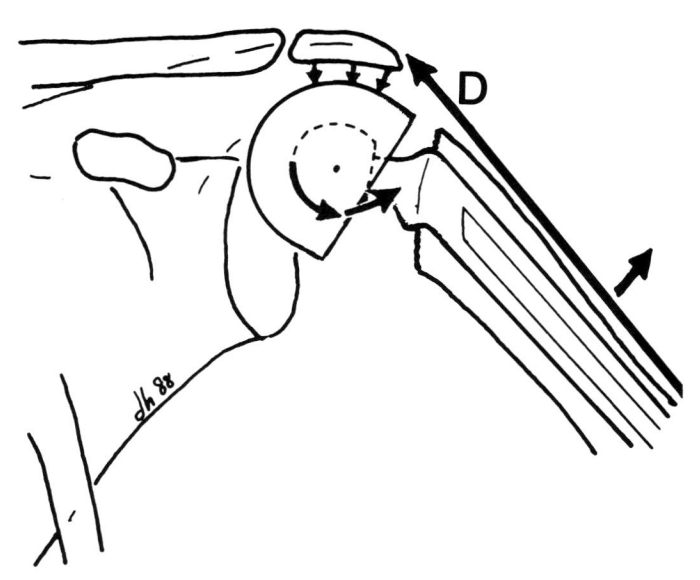

Figure 22–9. If vertical subluxation occurs, the advantage of the bipolar implant with its larger head, unfixed cup, and inner low-friction interface is the distribution of the deltoid shearing forces over a wider area of the acromion, thereby reducing the potential for erosive changes in this area. (Reproduced with permission from Swanson et al.[10])

the clavicle is now recommended in cases with radiographic evidence of acromioclavicular joint arthritis.

Excision of a bony overgrowth at the proximal end of the humerus was carried out approximately 1 year after bipolar shoulder arthroplasty in two cases who had had an excision of the humeral head for a severely comminuted fracture. Both cases continued to present with excellent results 21 months and 27 months after the revision procedure. Replacement of a long neck implant with a short neck implant and a larger head was carried out 3 years and 9 months after the initial surgery in a patient with osteoarthritis who had impingement of the coracoacromial arch due to improper selection of implant size. At the time of writing, the patient had a pain-free functional shoulder.

The bipolar implant was removed and not replaced in one patient with severe rheumatoid arthritis who developed an infection secondary to *Peptococcus* 22 months after shoulder arthroplasty. Another patient, who underwent bipolar shoulder arthroplasty 2 years after resection of the humeral head for a severely comminuted fracture, developed a persistent draining sinus tract. Four months after reconstruction, the sinus tract was excised, and the cup component and Dacron tapes (no longer used) were removed. The cultures were negative and there was no evidence of humeral component loosening. Four years later, he continued to present with a fair functional result.

Radiographically, there have been no lytic lesions or cement loosening around the humeral stem in 60 shoulders reconstructed with the bipolar implant to date.

DISCUSSION

If the natural relationships of the humeral head and the glenoid are maintained, resurfacing of both areas can provide predictable results as shown by Neer and others.[4,6] If the force couple action of the rotator cuff muscles to hold the humeral head into the glenoid during abduction is lost, the unopposed pull of the deltoid muscle will result in superior migration of the head. With severe cases, this results in impingement of the humeral head against the coracoacromial arch. It is possible that long-standing abutment of a metal humeral head against the coracoacromial arch could result in bony erosion.

The use of a larger headed implant for replacement of the humeral head moves the center of axis of rotation laterally and therefore improves the abduction forces of the deltoid muscle. The bipolar shoulder arthroplasty has an inner bearing within the glenoid cup component that allows motion to occur even when the implant abuts against the coracoacromial arch. The larger headed implant and the bipolar implant concept distribute the forces over a larger surface area and therefore decrease the load per unit area and the potential for erosive changes of the acromion (Figure 22–9). The use of the bipolar shoulder arthroplasty has a special indication in patients presenting with superior subluxation of the humerus secondary to rheumatoid arthritis or to rotator cuff deficiency. This procedure can also be used for revision surgery of a failed total shoulder arthroplasty.

REFERENCES

1. Elftman H. Biomechanics of muscle with particular application to studies of gaits. *J Bone Joint Surg [Am]* 1966;48:364.
2. Neer CS II. Articular replacement for the humeral head. *J Bone Joint Surg [Am]* 1955;37:215–228.
3. Amstutz HC, Sew Hoy AL, Clarke IC. UCLA anatomical total shoulder arthroplasty. *Clin Orthop* 1981;155:7–20.
4. Cofield RH. Total shoulder arthroplasty with the Neer prosthesis. *J Bone Joint Surg [Am]* 1984;66:899–906.
5. Hughes M, Neer CS II. Glenohumeral joint replacement and postoperative rehabilitation. *Phys Ther* 1975;55:850–858.
6. Neer CS II, Watson KC, Stanton RJ. Recent experience in total shoulder replacement. *J Bone Joint Surg [Am]* 1982;64:319–337.
7. Swanson AB. *Flexible Implant Resection Arthroplasty in the Hand and Extremities*. St. Louis: CV Mosby, 1973.
8. Swanson AB. Bipolar implant shoulder arthroplasty. In: Bateman J, Welsh PR, eds. *Surgery of the Shoulder*. Toronto: BC Decker, 1984:211–223.
9. Swanson AB, de Groot Swanson G, Maupin BK, Wei JN, Khalil MA. Bipolar shoulder implant arthroplasty. *Orthopedics* 1986;9:343–351.
10. Swanson AB, de Groot Swanson G, Sattel AB, Cendo RD, Hynes D, Jar-Ning W. Bipolar shoulder implant arthroplasty—Long-term results. *Clin Orthop* 1989;249:227–247.
11. Coughlin MJ, Morris JM, West WF. The semiconstrained total shoulder arthroplasty. *J Bone Joint Surg [Am]* 1979;61:574–581.
12. Macnab I. Total shoulder replacement. *J Bone Joint Surg [Br]* 1977;59:257.

13. Lettin AWF, Scales JT. Total replacement arthroplasty of the shoulder in rheumatoid arthritis. *J Bone Joint Surg [Br]* 1973;55:217.
14. Post M, Haskell SS, Jablon M. Total shoulder replacement with a constrained prosthesis. *J Bone Joint Surg [Am]* 1980;62:327–335.
15. Gristina AG, Webb LX. The trispherical shoulder prosthesis. *Orthop Trans* 1984;8:88.
16. Smith-Peterson MN. Arthroplasty of the hip: New method. *J Bone Joint Surg* 1939;21:269–288.
17. Giliberty RP. A new concept of a bipolar prosthesis. *Orthop Rev* 1974;3:40–45.
18. Bateman JE. Single-assembly total hip prosthesis—Preliminary report. *Orthop Dig* 1974;2:15–22.
19. Swanson AB, de Groot Swanson G. Impairment evaluation in the upper extremity. In: *Guides to the Evaluation of Permanent Impairment*. 3rd ed. (revised). Chicago: American Medical Association, 1990:14–55.
20. Brems JJ, Wilde AH, Borden LS, Boumphrey FRS. Glenoid lucent lines. *Orthop Trans* 1986;10:231.

23 Cementless Shoulder Arthroplasty

Wayne Z. Burkhead, M.D.

Cementless fixation for shoulder arthroplasty is not a new concept. Venable and Stuck's finding that chrome cobalt was indeed an electrically neutral metal opened the door for long-term implantation of metallic prostheses.[1] In addition to the constraint issues that have evolved in shoulder arthroplasty, another central issue facing surgeons has been long-term fixation of the prosthesis to bone.

CEMENT FIXATION

Self-curing polymethylmethacrylate (PMMA) was initially used in dental sciences[2] and subsequently applied to orthopaedics by Sir John Charnley.[3-5] Its material characteristics of quick curing and low modulus of elasticity made it an ideal material to serve as a grout or filler between bone and prosthesis. The predictable, early excellent results in total hip arthroplasty from the use of this bone cement, together with the use of ultra-high-molecular-weight polyethylene as a joint-bearing surface, led Neer and others to design humeral and glenoid components fixed with PMMA.

As follow-up time increased, some arthroplasty patients, primarily those with hip arthroplasties, complained of increasing pain associated with progressive radiolucent lines, osteolysis, prosthesis movement, and occasionally fracture of the cement mantle.[6-10] Macrophages were consistently seen by Charnley[5] at the bone-cement junction. Chambers[11] found strong evidence that the macrophage and osteoclast are the same cell type, and were responsible for bone resorption. This phenomenon of progressive osteolysis became known as "cement disease."[12] This concept led to an explosion of interest in porous coated and press-fit technology. It is now recognized that the same problem, progressive radiolucent lines and osteolysis, occurs with cementless designs, sometimes even when well fixed,, and that many of these problems are related to polyethylene and metallic wear debris and not the cement itself.[13-20] This led to the term "cementless disease."

LOOSENING IN TOTAL SHOULDER ARTHROPLASTY

The incidence of clinically significant loosening of either component in cemented total shoulder arthroplasty is less than that of total hip arthroplasty: 2.6% for the glenoid and 0.34% for the humerus at an average of 3.5 years. Cofield,[21] extrapolating these data out, felt that the incidence of clinically significant glenoid loosening would be roughly 5% at 5 years. However, other authors[22] found increased loosening, up to 51% in certain nonconstrained prosthetic designs. Shift in position of the glenoid component was observed in 20% of patients in Barrett's series[23] and in 15% of patients in Cofield's series,[24,25] using the Neer total shoulder arthroplasty in rotator cuff–deficient shoulders.

In the early 1970s, thermal necrosis of bone from PMMA was thought to be a contributor to glenoid loosening, along with a toxic reaction and cement shrinkage. These have largely been discounted now as significant factors in arthroplasty component loosening. Though radiolucent lines may be seen immediately postoperatively in some patients with shoulder arthroplasty, radiolucent lines have been shown to develop over time.[23,26,27] The clinical significance and etiology of radiolucent lines are still somewhat controversial. However, the increase in these lines is thought to be the result of stimulated macrophages.[28] Exactly what stimulates the macrophage, motion, cell death, or foreign body reaction is unclear, but is it most likely a combination of all three. In the shoulder, mechanical factors appear to greatly influence glenoid loosening, as seen with constrained devices that apply greater stress to the bone-cement interface, leading to more dramatic loosening. Patients with abnormal biomechanics resulting from an absent rotator cuff will have higher glenoid loosening rates because of eccentric stress and strain.[29]

While it appears that most glenoid components loosen because of mechanical factors, a detailed analysis of failed cemented glenoid fibrous membranes does not exist, such as one described for cemented acetabular components in total hip arthroplasty. Schlamzried et al.[30] found that a circumferential progressive resorption of bone immediately adjacent to the cement mantle occurred, fueled by small particles of high-density polyethylene migrating along the bone-cement interface, and that bone resorption occurs as a result of a macrophage inflammatory response to the particulate polyethylene. These authors believe that the mechanism of late aseptic loosening of the cemented acetabular component was therefore biologic in nature and not mechanical. It is most likely that the mechanism of component loosening in total shoulder arthroplasty is, like most pathologic processes, multifactorial.

IMPROVING CEMENTED FIXATION

In situations where the use of bone cement cannot be avoided, the longevity of cemented implants can be increased. The mechanical strength of the cement-prosthesis interface is known to depend on two mechanisms: mechanical interlock and specific adhesion. Mechanical interlock can be influenced by porous coating the prosthesis to improve fixation of the cement to the prosthesis and by careful preparation of the cancellous bone surface and pressurization of cement.[31] Specific adhesion can be enhanced by pretreatment of the implant or precoating the implant with a thin layer of PMMA.[32] The mechanical characteristics of the acrylic can be improved by centrifugation.[33,34]

FEATURES OF BIOLOGIC FIXATION

Over the last 20 years, research has been aimed at providing an active biologic interface between the prosthesis and bone, as well as a permanent bonding of material to bone. The achievement of a stable implant-bone composite, the interface of which is capable of remodeling, is influenced by a number of factors: pore size, implant movement, materials, and apposition.[35]

Pore sizes in the range of 100 to 500 μm show the most consistent and rapid bone ingrowth, thereby providing a microinterlock. Pore sizes less than 50 μm do not allow enough space for ingrowth to occur. Larger pores allow bone ingrowth but it takes longer for the pores to fill, and increasing the size beyond 1 mm increases the tendency for fibrous tissue rather than bony formation.[36-40] A macrointerlock, however, has been used for years in shoulder arthroplasty surgery and occurs even in the Neer II design (Figure 23–1).

Motion of the prosthesis relative to the bone will prevent bone ingrowth and make it more likely that fibrous tissue will form. Therefore, cementless designs for the shoulder must achieve an immediate interference fit to avoid implant movement. Because early range of motion is so important, Neer (personal communication, 1990) has discouraged the use of porous coated implants for fear of compromising motion. However, the author has not found that active and passive range of motion of the shoulder places excessive stress on the implant site to preclude bony ingrowth.

Bone ingrowth has been demonstrated with porous forms of cobalt chrome alloys, titanium and its alloys, carbon materials, oxide ceramics, polysulfone, polyethylene, and even PMMA.[39-50] Close apposition of the implant to bone is necessary for immediate fixation as well as complete bone ingrowth. Gaps between the porous surface and bone can be eliminated with the use of bone grafting.[51]

Fixation strength is dependent on not only the type of attachment, but also the type of bone to which the implant is attached. The interface shear strength of fully ingrown metal implants to cortical bone can exceed 1 ton/in^2.[35] Cancellous bone ingrowth, because of its more porous nature, results in lower fixation strengths. The absolute interface strength necessary for a successful shoulder arthroplasty has not been established. Clinical experience with an ingrowth prosthesis

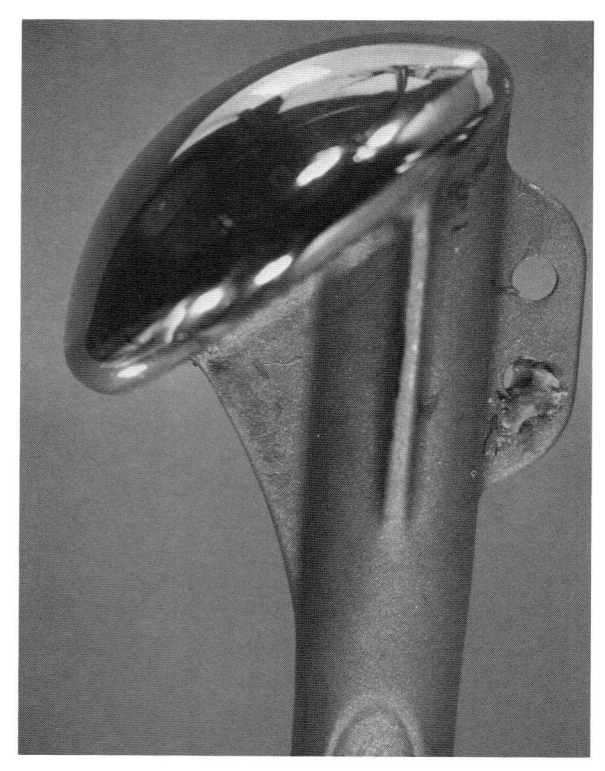

Figure 23–1. Neer prostheses showing macrointerlock with bone ingrown through the inferior suture hole.

suggests that cancellous bone ingrowth is satisfactory and can withstand the forces seen in the adult shoulder.

In an effort to stimulate the ingrowth process into porous coated implants, bioactive ceramics such as tricalcium phosphate and hydroxyapatite have been utilized (Figure 23–2). Geesink et al.[52,53] found that cortical bone-implant sheer strength was increased by a factor of three with hydroxyapatite-coated implants over simple bone ingrowth with a microinterlock. The types of implant surfaces available for biologic fixation include (1) three-dimensional porous coating, generally with beads or wires applied under high-temperature sintering or diffusion bonding processes; and (2) limited porosity surfaces, including plasma spray coating in which a molten powder is sprayed through a nozzle onto the implant substrate, and rough texturing, which occurs when the surface of the implant is grit-blasted. Newer techniques include grit-blasting with hydroxyapatite, which leaves the hydroxyapatite coating on the rough surface. These prostheses are fixed, not by a microinterlock, but by osteo-integration or ongrowth-type fixation. Grooves and slots have also been used to promote biologic fixation.[54-56]

The use of polyethylene without cement was popularized by Freeman.[57] He found that two flanged pegs, similar to the ones adopted in Copeland's design for the shoulder (Figure 22–3), allowed fixation of the tibial component without cement. The rationale is that the fins interlock and cancellous bone debris impacts within the pegs themselves. While the initial results in the tibia were encouraging, a large number of

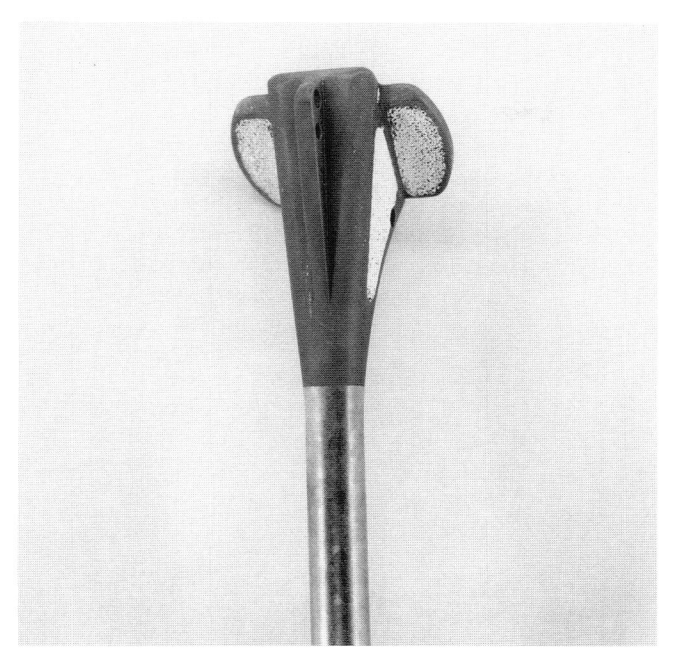

Figure 23–2. Hydroxyapatite-sprayed, porous coated, pure cancellous structured titanium humeral implant. (Select Shoulder, Intermedics Orthopedics, Austin, Texas.)

revisions have been performed in one institution, showing fibrous tissue only occurring in the pegs (Hoffmann AA, personal communication, 1992). Copeland (personal communication, 1992) subsequently changed his design. The theoretic disadvantage of this system is abrasion of the polyethylene, by the bone with which it is in direct contact, creating wear particles leading to macrophage stimulation and osteolysis.

AGE OF PATIENT

Although cementless fixation of implants was initially designed for younger patients,[58] Collier et al.[59] found that patients as old as 87 years, even in whom osteoporosis was present, responded to porous coated components in the same way that younger patients did, and that bony ingrowth did occur.

TIME TO STABLE FIXATION

While an earlier report of bone ingrowth into porous coatings showed that some ingrowth occurred at 4 weeks,[59] subsequent studies have shown that no significant bone ingrowth occurs at 4 weeks.[60] At 3 months, woven bone was just beginning to penetrate into the porous coating. Seven-month retrievals showed approximately 16% bone ingrowth into the available porous coating. At 19 months the bone appears more lamellar, containing some cement lines, and the lacunae are elliptical with morphologic signs of mature bone. The percent bone ingrowth increased over the next several years. Retrieval at 4 years and 5 months showed 80% bone ingrowth into the available porous coating.[60] The previous study that had demonstrated bone ingrowth within 4 weeks analyzed implants with protruding porous coatings and it is likely that the coatings were advanced into the bone on impaction of the implant during surgery.

REMODELING

The two major challenges associated with the success or failure of porous ingrowth systems are (1) achieving bone ingrowth, and (2) avoiding adverse bone remodeling or stress shielding after ingrowth is achieved. In order to address the

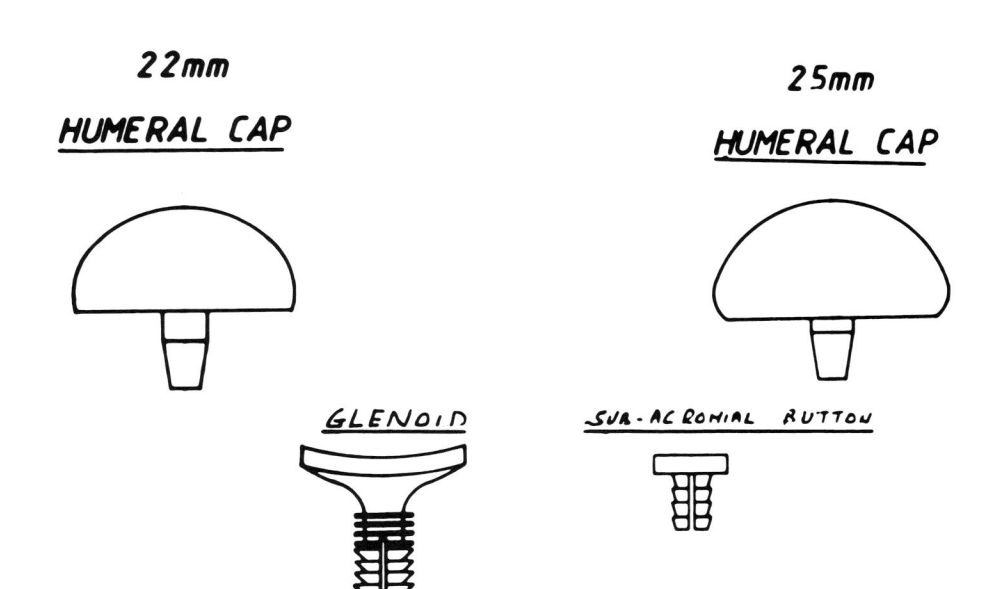

Figure 23–3. Mark I Copeland shoulder prosthesis, showing glenoid with polyethylene peg, similar to Freeman's design for the knee. Designed to be used without bone cement. (Reproduced with permission from Copeland.[73])

second challenge, an effort to define the amount of porous coating needed to simulate the stress distribution of the normal humerus has been made. Orr and Carter[61] developed a finite element model of the proximal part of the humerus (Figure 23-4). They found that a flat humeral head at a 45-degree angle to the shaft with porous coating on the undersurface came closest to the normal stress distribution for the normal humerus. The model in which the stem was fully porous coated led to marked stress shielding (Figure 23-5).

CLINICAL RESULTS WITH CEMENTLESS FIXATION OF TOTAL SHOULDER ARTHROPLASTY

If Neer was the father of cementless fixation of the humeral component, then Kessel[62,63] (Figure 23-6) could be considered the father of cementless scapular fixation. His concerns over the use of bone cement and the exothermic reaction with its effect on the fragile glenoid vault, described in his book, led him to the development of screw-in fixation for the

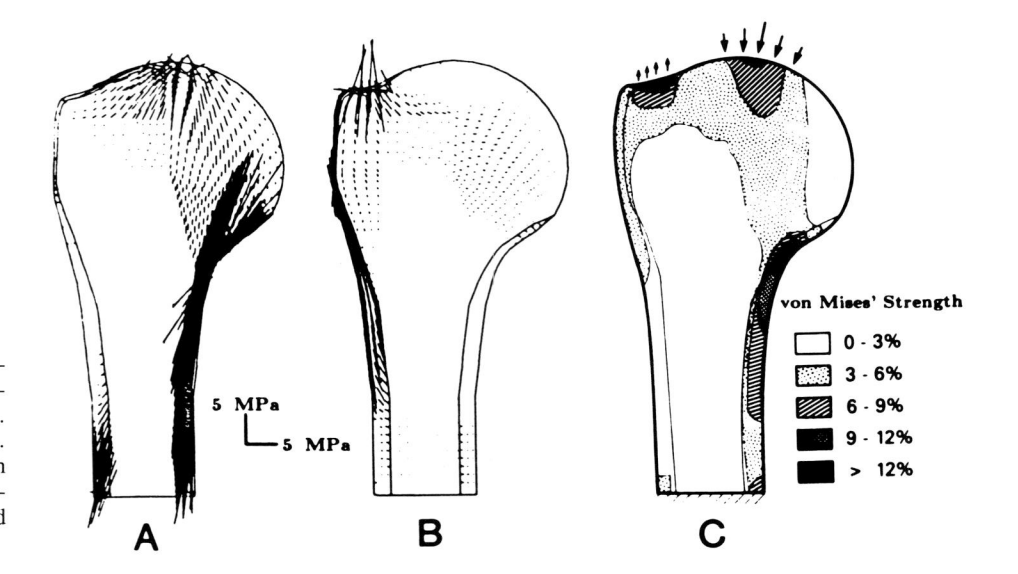

Figure 23-4. Finite element analysis—distribution for the normal humerus, equivalent-thickness model. **A.** Principle compression stresses. **B.** Principle tension stresses. **C.** Von Mize's strength contours. (Reproduced with permission from Orr and Carter.[61])

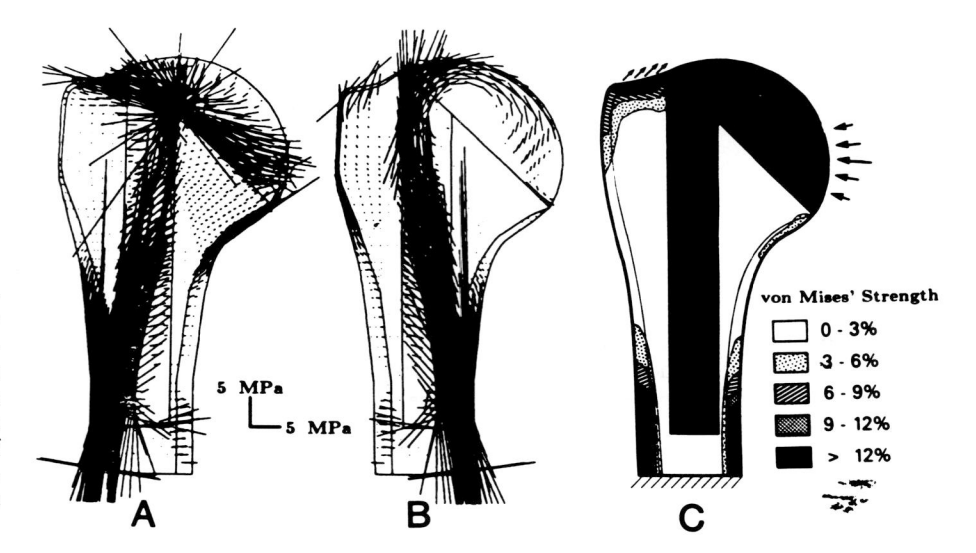

Figure 23-5. Finite element analysis stress distribution for the fully porous coated proximal humeral replacement. **A.** Principle compression stresses. **B.** Principle tension stresses. **C.** Von Mize's strength contours. Note absence of loading of the proximal part of the humerus. (Reproduced with permission from Orr and Carter.[60])

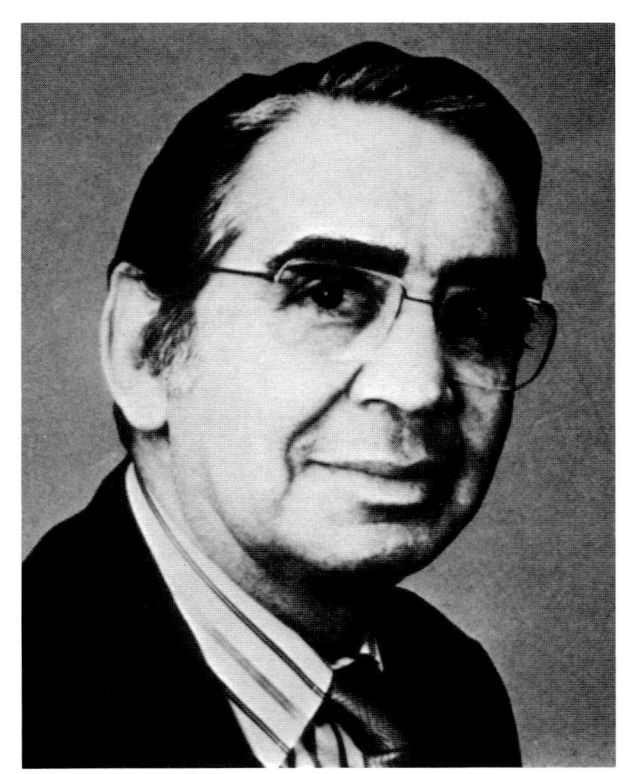

Figure 23–6. Professor Lippman Kessel, Royal National Orthopedic Hospital, London, England.

scapula, which was first used in 1973 (Figure 23–7). The insertion track for his lag screw was directed into the cancellous bone of the glenoid at an angle 20 degrees anteverted to the plane of the scapula. This was designed to make full use of the limited space and length of the glenoid vault.

Thirty-one shoulder arthroplasties reported on in 1982[63] resulted in pain relief in 28, improved function in 19, restoration of mobility in 19, and patient satisfaction in 25 shoulders. Complications were related primarily to the coupling between the screw-in glenoid component and the polyethylene cemented socket on the humeral side.

Wallensten et al.,[64] utilizing Kessel's prosthesis, however, had six failures, with three loosened glenoid components. Radiographic analysis in Wallensten's series showed that all patients eventually developed radiolucent zones around the scapular component. In 18 of the original 23 shoulders, this was visible as early as 6 months after surgery.[64] While the forces across the glenohumeral joint in the constrained Kessel device were too much for central screw fixation, this same type of cementless fixation has been incorporated in newer designs such as those developed by Bayley (Figures 23–8 and 23–9), who reported very encouraging early results with this prosthesis.[65]

McElwain and English[66] reported on the early results of porous coated total shoulder arthroplasty. The English-McNab component (Figure 23–10) was introduced into a limited clinical trial in 1976. The glenoid component, as well as the humeral component, was fully porous coated, and came with medium and long acromial pins and screws to anchor the component for short-term stability while tissue ingrowth occurred. An ultra-high-molecular-weight polyethylene bearing glenoid surface snapped into the metal glenoid component.

Clinical and radiographic results were available in only 13 of 21 patients. Radiographs (Figure 23–11) of this fully porous coated stem showed resorption of the proximal medial cortex in 9, prosthetic subsidence in 7, new bone formation in 7, and prosthetic shift in 1. A radiopaque line, extending the whole length of the prosthesis, was seen in 1 patient. A similar line was seen in a second patient surrounding the lower one-third and tip of the prosthesis only. Both patients with radiopaque lines were asymptomatic. These lines were similar in appearance to those described by Pilliar et al.,[46] who considered them to be hypertrophic cancellous bone separated from the implant by a thin layer of fibrous tissue. Bone remodeling around the glenoid component, predominantly on the superior and inferior surfaces, was identified in 5 patients. One patient had a clinically loose glenoid. The radiopaque lines seen on the humeral diaphysis were not seen on the glenoid side. Areas of radiolucency were noted around a number of screws. Faludi and Weiland[67] reported similar results in 13 patients with only 75 degrees of active abduction after implantation of the English-McNab prosthesis.

Cofield[68,69] reported his preliminary experience with bone-ingrowth total shoulder arthroplasty (Figure 23–12), performed between 1983 and 1985. A Neer-type humeral design has a cobalt chrome beaded undersurface, and the glenoid is porous coated as well. The porous surface does not extend into the stem of either the humerus or the glenoid. The porous coating is 1-mm deep, with an average pore diameter of 250 μm and porosity of 30%. A central peg is supplemented with two self-tapping screws.

A preliminary report in 1986[68] revealed that four glenoid high-density polyethylene glenoid inserts became dislodged and had to be replaced. No clinical loosening occurred in either the cemented (group I—17 patients) or uncemented (group II—21 patients) groups. Longer-term follow-up (51 months) of the uncemented glenoid component in 32 total shoulder arthroplasties is now available (Figure 23–13).[70] Ninety-six percent had little or no pain. Mean abduction was 145 degrees; external rotation, 59 degrees; and internal rotation to the T12 level. Three glenoid components had probable loosening radiographically, and 8 shoulder arthroplasty components had some degree of instability. A higher incidence of glenoid dissociation and loosening was reported with unstable arthroplasties. Of 31 shoulders, 16 (52%) had no radiolucencies. Loose beads were identified in 12 shoulders. In a more recent study between press-fit and porous coated humeral components, half of the press-fit components had radiographic evidence of loosening, whereas only 3% of

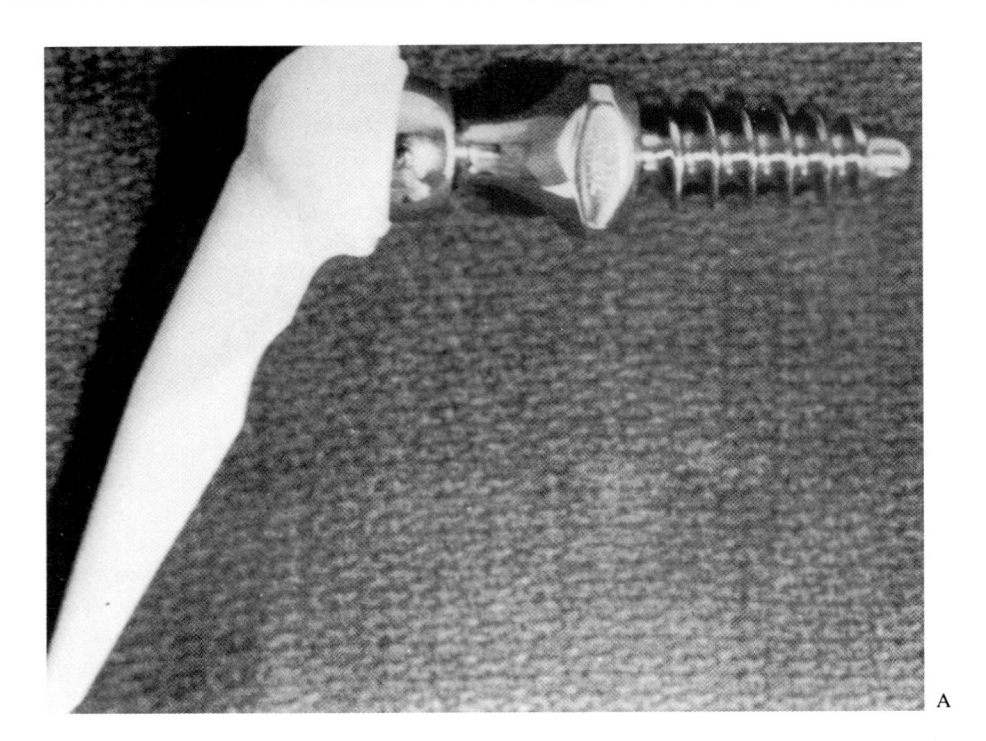

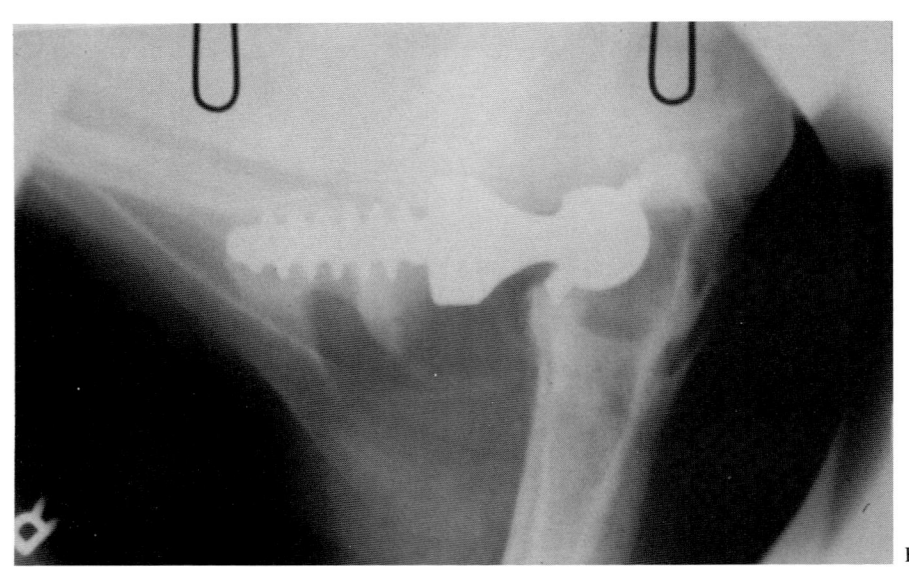

Figure 23-7. A. Kessel total shoulder prosthesis showing polyethylene humeral component and screw-in scapular component with reverse ball-and-socket configuration. (Reproduced with permission from Kessel and Bayley.[63]) **B.** Cementless scapular fixation by Kessel showing absence of lucent lines at 3-year follow-up examination. Note the anteverted position of the screw to maximize bony contact with central screw fixation.

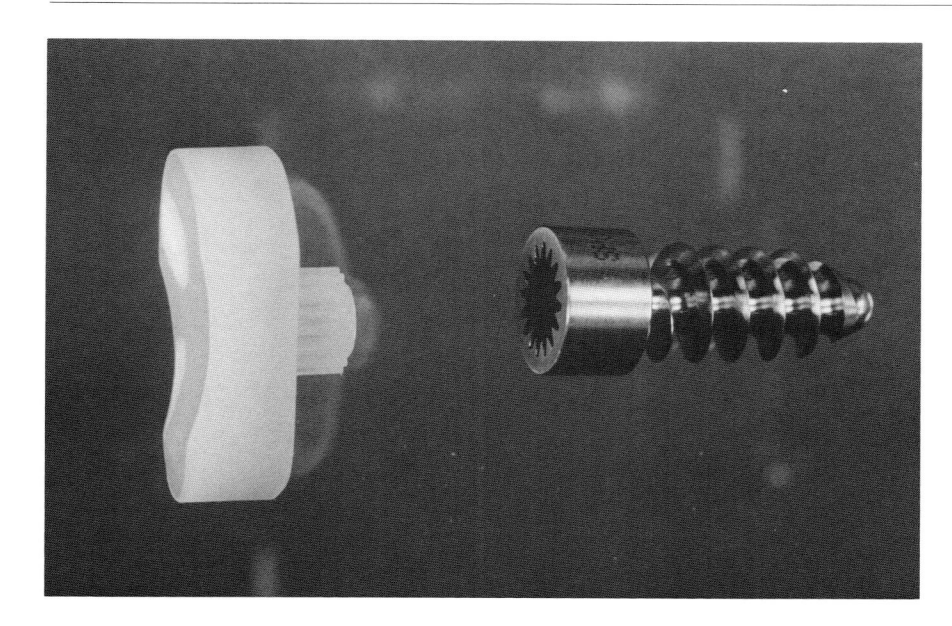

Figure 23–8. Bayley design for nonconstrained total shoulder arthroplasty based on Kessel's central screw design. (Photograph courtesy of J.I.L. Bayley.)

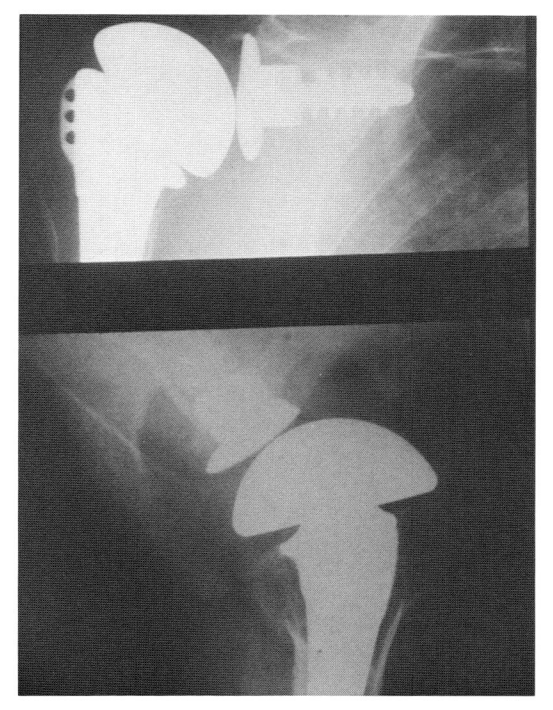

Figure 23–9. Radiographic evaluation of Bayley total shoulder arthroplasty. (Photograph courtesy of J.I.L. Bayley.)

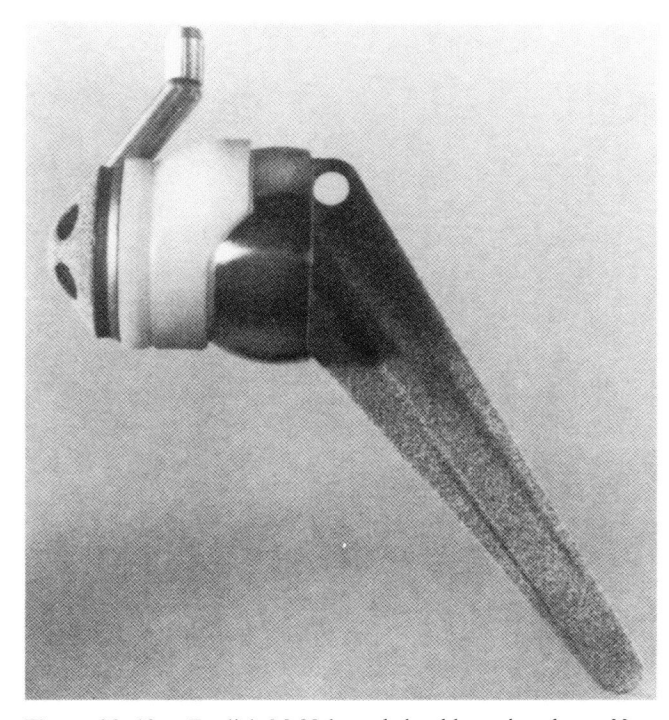

Figure 23–10. English-McNab total shoulder arthroplasty. Note the fully porous coated humeral stem. (Reproduced with permission from Faludi and Weiland.[67])

288   Arthroplasty of the Shoulder

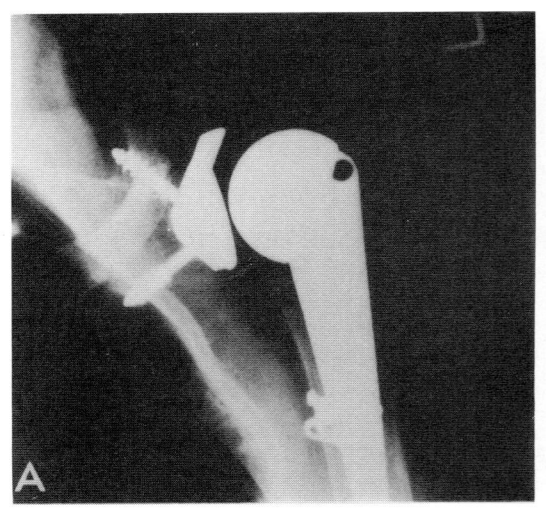

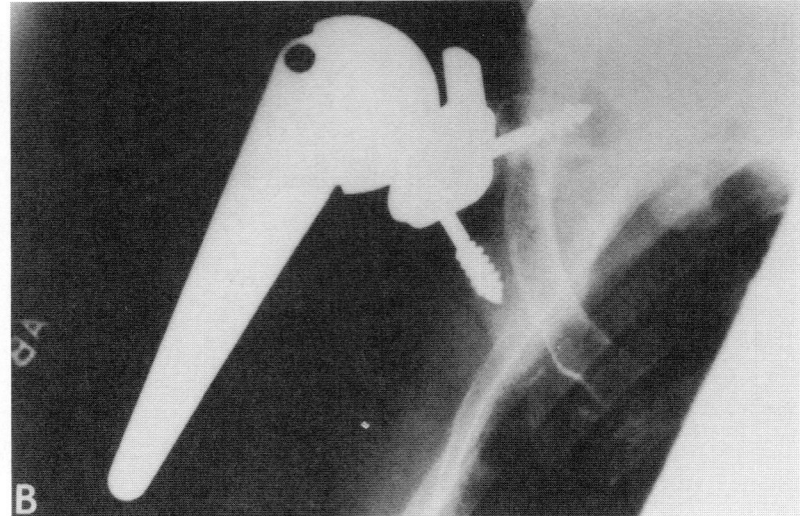

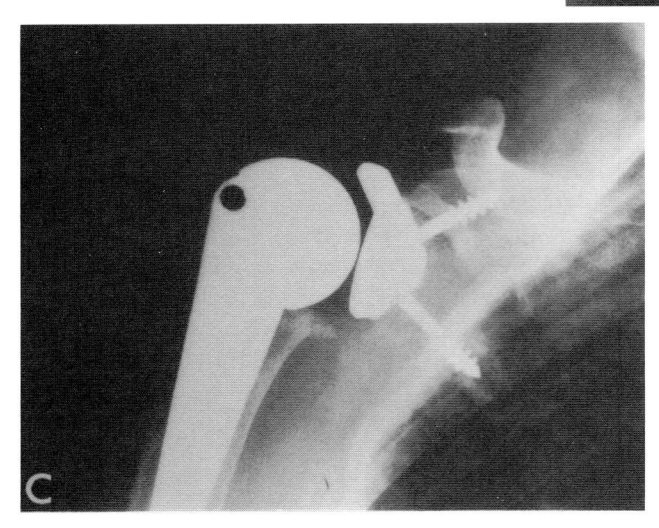

Figure 23–11. **A–C.** English-McNab total shoulder. Note the marked stress shielding in the follow-up radiographs.

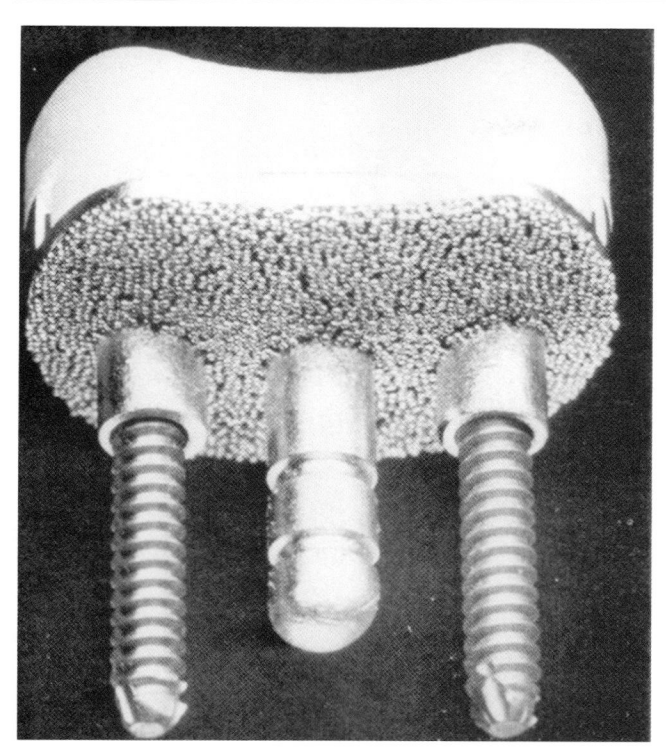

Figure 23–12. Cofield glenoid. Note the beaded cobalt chrome undersurface with screws for fixation.

stems with porous coating on the undersurfaces of the head had progressive radiolucent zones or subsidence.[71]

A design for cementless fixation of the shoulder has been developed by Copeland.[72] The initial prosthesis involved a high-density polyethylene interference fit peg on the glenoid side and a surface replacement–type humeral component with a central locating peg. In the first 10 arthroplasties, a fixation screw was used to hold the humeral prosthesis down onto the head and act as a derotation device.[72] Subsequently, the glenoid prosthesis has been modified to a polyethylene component that is now metal-backed with a central fluted taper fit peg secured by impaction and press-fitting. The humeral component is still a hollow metal cap, but made of cobalt chrome. The screw has been discontinued and the central peg is now of the fluted taper fit design (Figure 23–14). Forty-six arthroplasties have been done in 45 patients. All felt they were better after the operation and improved in functional assessment. Progressive lucencies around the glenoid component occurred in 2 patients with the Mark I high-density polyethylene components. A total of 6 patients have had sinkage of the prosthesis. There have been no progressive lucencies around the Mark II metal peg design (Copeland S, personal communication, 1992).

A simple nonconstrained shoulder replacement has been developed by Roper and Day (Figure 23–15),[73] and is designed for use with or without PMMA. It has a minimally constrained glenoid with a peg similar to that described by Freeman.[57] The humeral prosthesis is mounted on a matt-finished stem. Detailed radiographic evaluation was not included, but loosening "has not so far been a major problem, even in cases with marked erosion of the glenoid. The finned peg continues to provide good fixation."[73]

Rockwood has press-fit the Neer II prosthesis for many years, with satisfactory results. Preliminary results with the Global Shoulder System arthroplasty utilizing a press-fit on the humeral side are encouraging (Rockwood CA, personal communication, 1992). Press-fitting of the humeral component in a total shoulder arthroplasty, however, does not always ensure long-term success (Figure 23–16). Cofield[71] noted approximately a 50% incidence of radiographic loosening with press-fit Neer II components.

Worland (personal communication, 1992) implanted 56 biangular stems without PMMA (Figure 23–17). The titanium humeral stem is plasma sprayed and comes in five sizes between 9.5 and 12.5 mm. Three proximal fins achieve rotational stability. Thirty-five cases were followed for an average of 18 months, without evidence of loosening or subsidence.

Dines (personal communication, 1992) used the biomodular shoulder in a group of 20 patients treated after chronic changes secondary to proximal humeral fractures. Eight had uncemented humeral components and 6 patients underwent total shoulder arthroplasty. Only 1 of these 6 had a porous glenoid component. There was no evidence of loosening in any of the eight press-fit humeral components, either clinically or radiographically. No lucent lines or component migration were noted about the humeral component in any of these patients up to 1 1/2 years postoperatively. On the glenoid side, 1 patient was followed for 2 years, with radiographic evidence of bone ingrowth. There were no lucent lines or bone resorption noted on sequential radiographs, and clinically this patient had a good result.

AUTHOR'S PREFERRED TECHNIQUE OF CEMENTLESS SHOULDER ARTHROPLASTY

In an effort to secure long-term fixation of the humeral component in total shoulder arthroplasty, and create a millieu that is favorable to tuberosity healing in the treatment of four-part fractures, the author began research in 1985 directed towards developing a cementless shoulder arthroplasty (Figure 23–18). The humeral implant (Figure 23–18A) has porous coating to transmit stress to the proximal end of the humerus on the undersurface of the collar, as well as in the proximal one-third. This is done to achieve maximum cancellous ingrowth in the metaphysis and allow for ingrowth of the tuberosity fragments in the treatment of four-part fractures (Figure 23–19). The humeral stem is made of titanium alloy, and the ingrowth substrate is a cancellous structured commercially pure titanium (Figure 23–20). It is trapezoidal in shape proximally to provide a secure interference fit similar to that found in the Zweymuller hip.[74] A slightly exaggerated medial radius furthers the

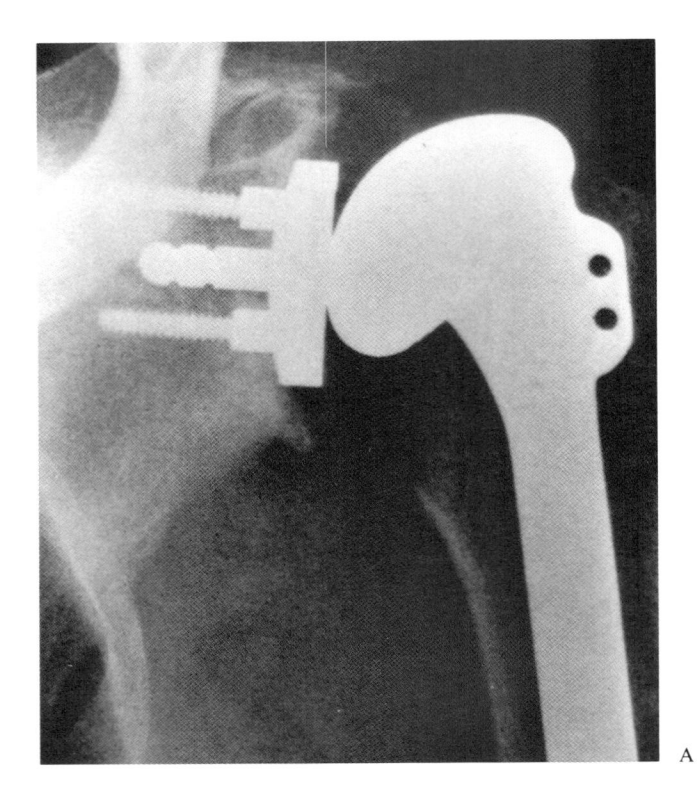

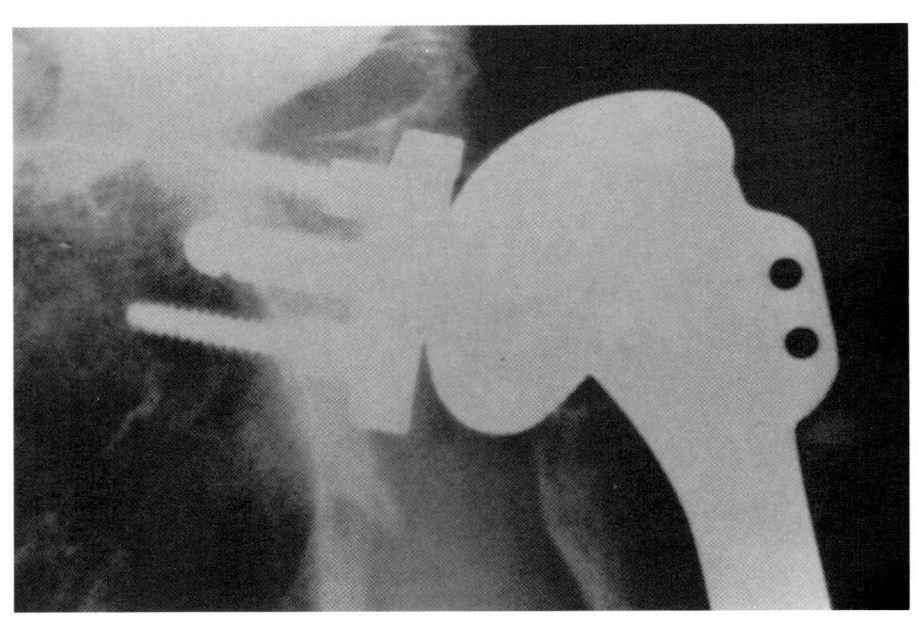

Figure 23-13. A. Cofield ingrowth glenoid component, with a beaded porous surface, smooth stem and two-screw fixation. Immediate postoperative appearance. **B.** Radiographic evaluation of porous coated glenoid surface, 51 months postoperatively. (Reproduced with permission from Cofield and Daly.[70])

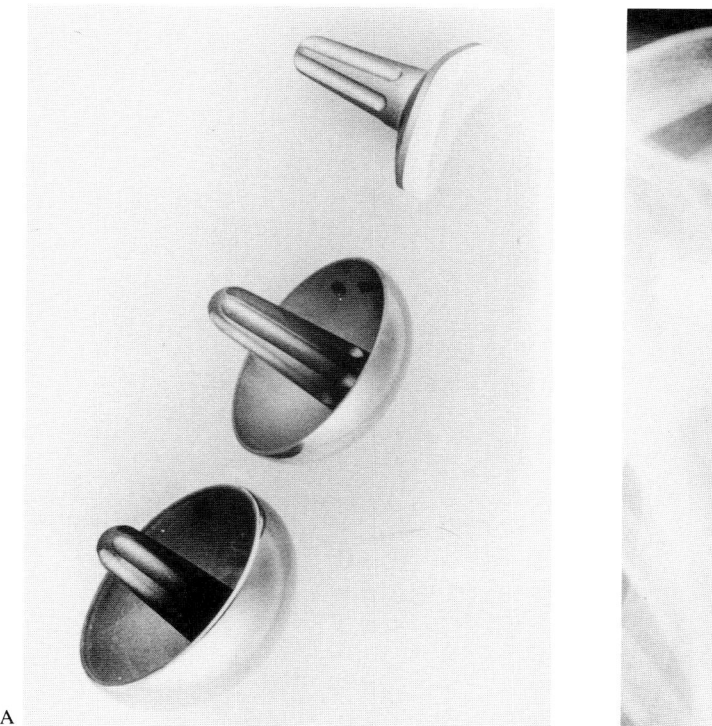

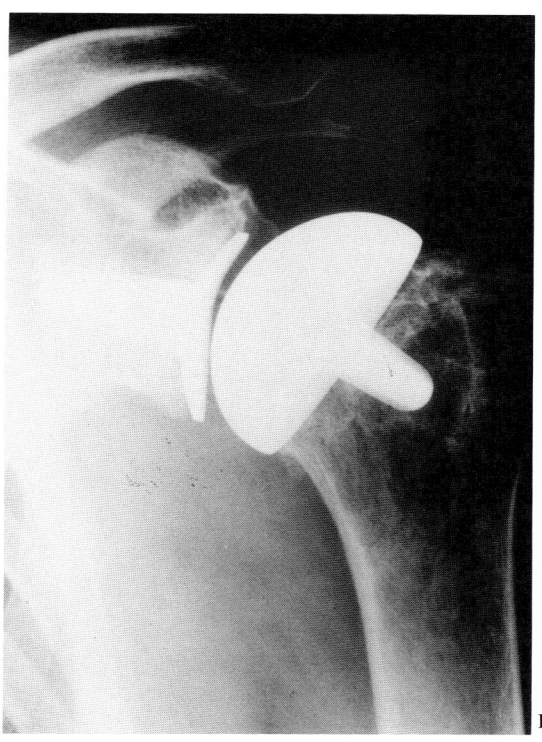

Figure 23–14. **A.** Copeland Mark II component. Note the fluted stems on the glenoid and humeral components. **B.** Anteroposterior radiograph of Copeland Mark II components in a rheumatoid arthritis patient. (Photographs courtesy of Mr. Steve Copeland, Royal Berkshire Hospital, Reading, England.)

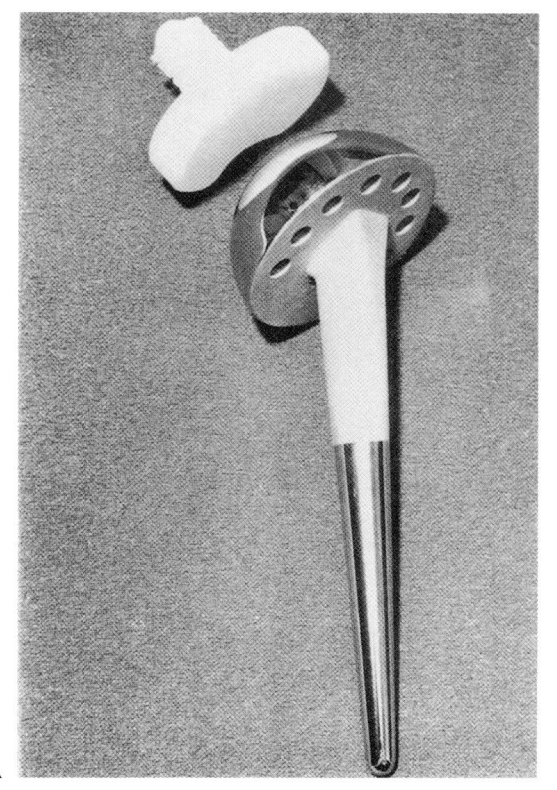

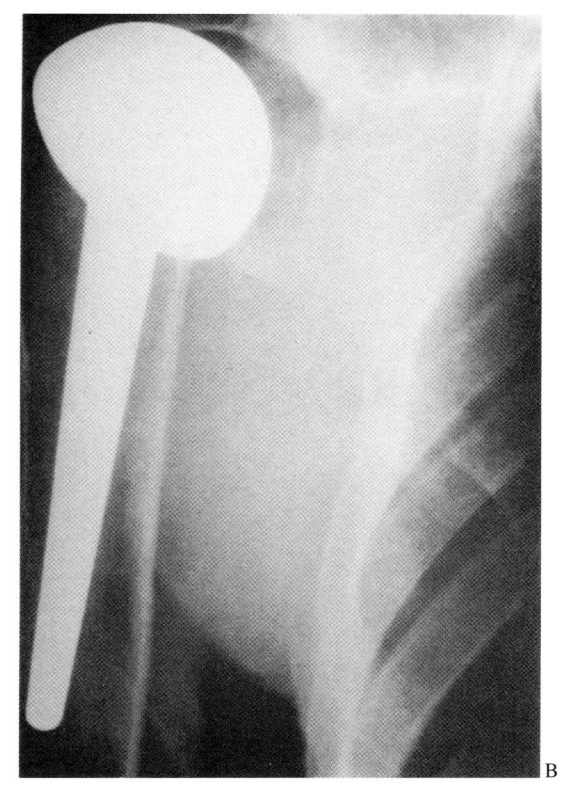

Figure 23–15. **A.** The Roper-Day prosthesis. (Reproduced with permission from Roper et al.[73]) **B.** Radiograph of Roper-Day prosthesis in situ.

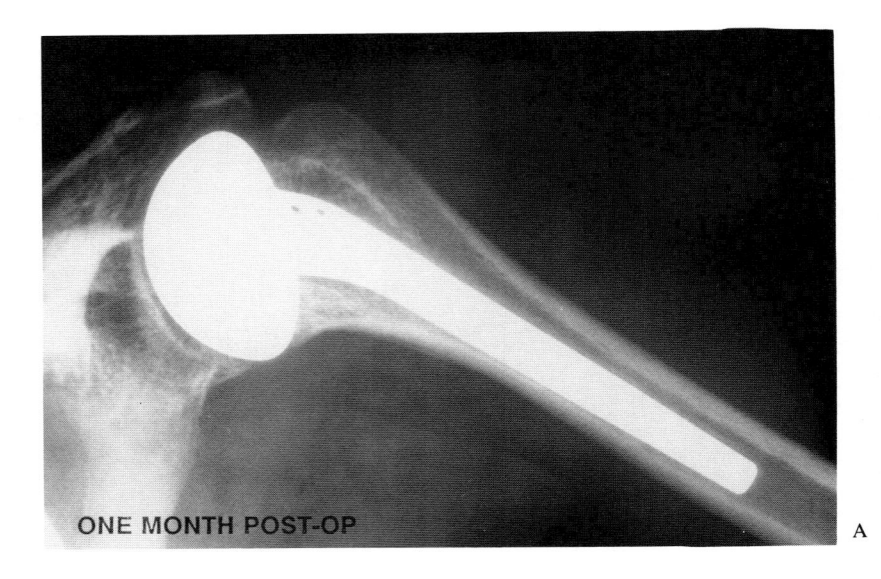

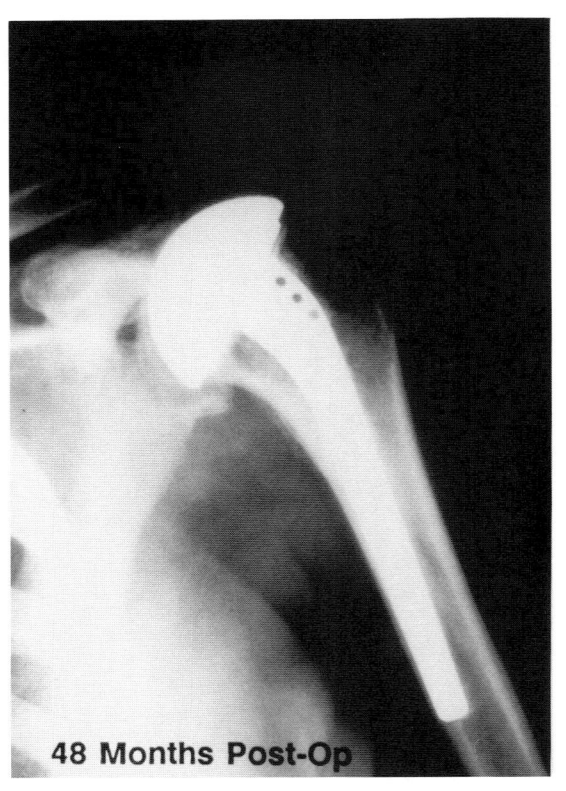

Figure 23–16. A. Radiograph 1 month after hemiarthroplasty for osteonecrosis of the left shoulder, utilizing New Jersey hemiarthroplasty (DePuy). **B.** Forty-eight months postoperatively, the patient's stem has migrated into a varus position and is nearly penetrating the cortex.

Cementless Shoulder Arthroplasty 293

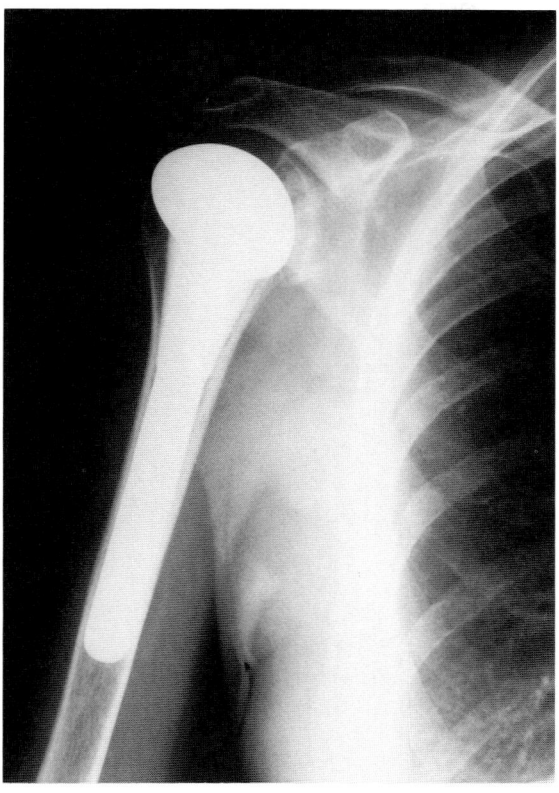

Figure 23–17. Radiographic evaluation of biangular total shoulder prosthesis. (Photograph courtesy of Richard Worland, MD, Richmond, VA.)

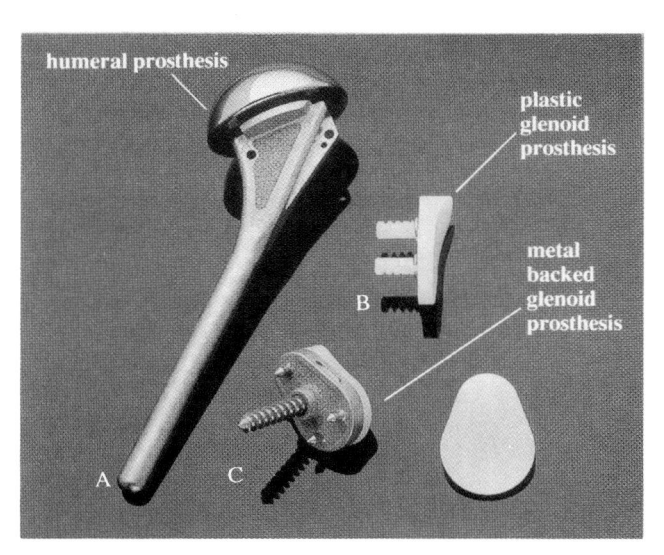

Figure 23–18. The Select Shoulder System, circa 1988. **A.** Humeral implant. Note the porous coating on undersurface and proximal body of stem. **B.** UHMWP glenoid implant with two pegs. **C.** Porous coated, metal-backed glenoid design utilizing three pegs for long-term stability, bone graft application, and a long 6.5-mm, fully threaded titanium screw. The polyethylene component snapped into the metal backing. The snap-fit features are the weakest link in any polyethylene metal-backed component composite.

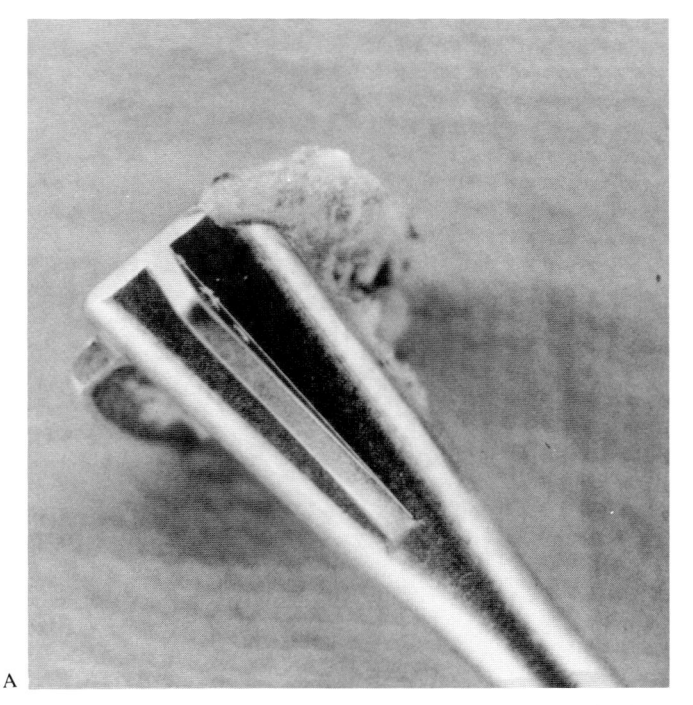

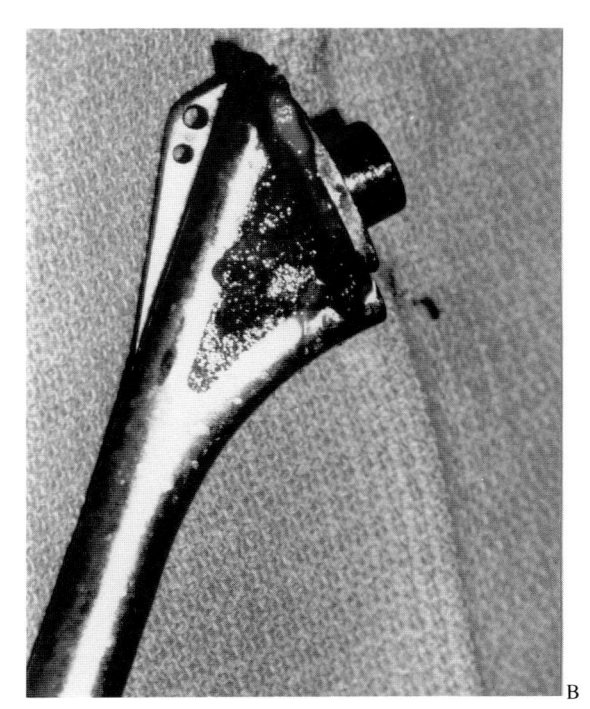

Figure 23–19. **A.** Retrieved specimen from the proximal part of the humerus in a patient with chronic instability following total shoulder arthroplasty. Note the bulk of the bone ingrowth occurs underneath the collar. **B.** Anteroposterior view of humeral ingrowth in retrieved specimen.

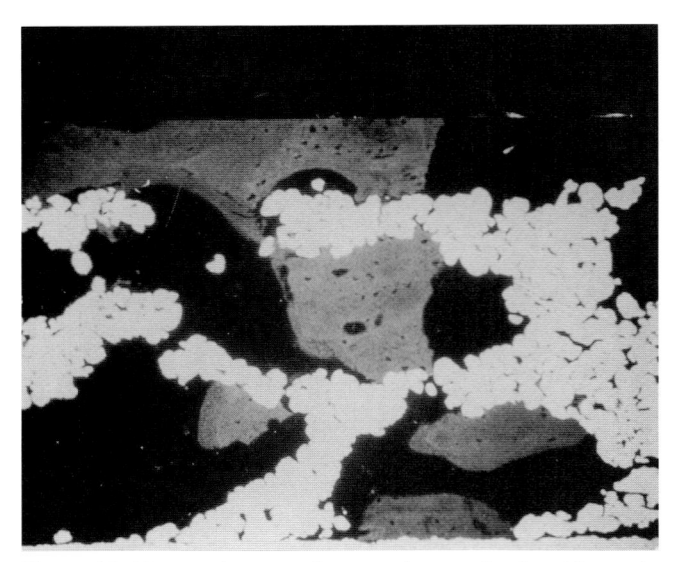

Figure 23–20. Backscatter electron micrograph of an 18-month specimen showing mature osteon formation within the porous coated, cancellous structured titanium ingrowth substrate.

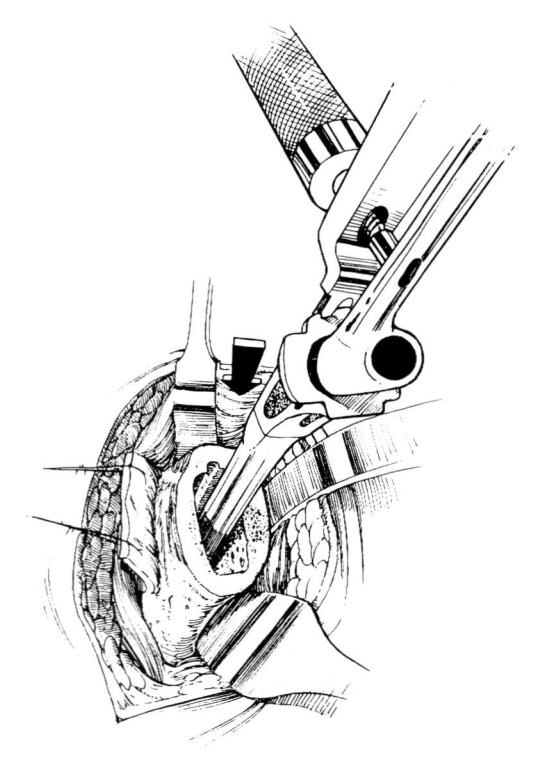

Figure 23–22. The Select Shoulder System implant impacted into place with version control guide impactor. An additional 1-mm press-fit is present in the proximal one-third of the prosthesis to promote proximal fixation.

interference fit by providing three-point fixation and ensures valgus positioning of the stem. Six stem sizes, with matching broaches, increase from 7 to 14.5 in 1.5-mm increments to ensure early stability and apposition, important factors for biologic fixation (Figure 23–21). There is a 1-mm press-fit provided by the proximal body of the implant compared to the broach (Figure 23–22). A medial suture hole in addition to two lateral suture holes provides for quadrilateral fixation of fracture fragments (Figure 23–23). A conventional Morse taper provides secure fixation for a cobalt chrome modular head, which is short enough to allow for glenoid or humeral head revision and oversized and bipolar heads for revision situations.

The polyethylene glenoid component utilized in the majority of patients is designed to be utilized with PMMA. However, in an effort to perform cementless fixation, a

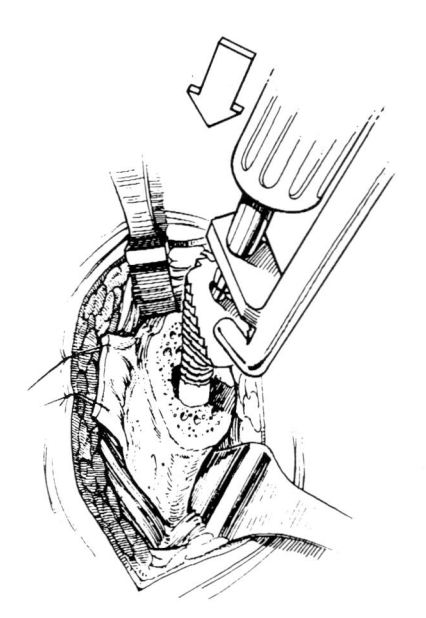

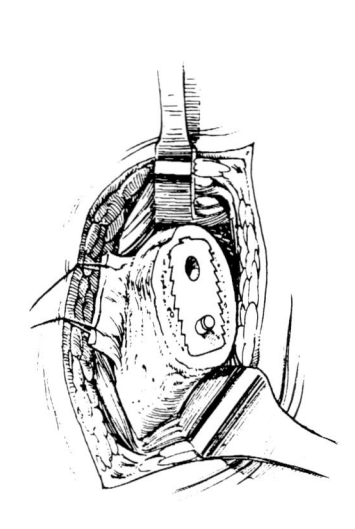

Figure 23–21. Broach for the Select Shoulder System cuts a track through the cancellous and cortical bone of the proximal portion of the humerus.

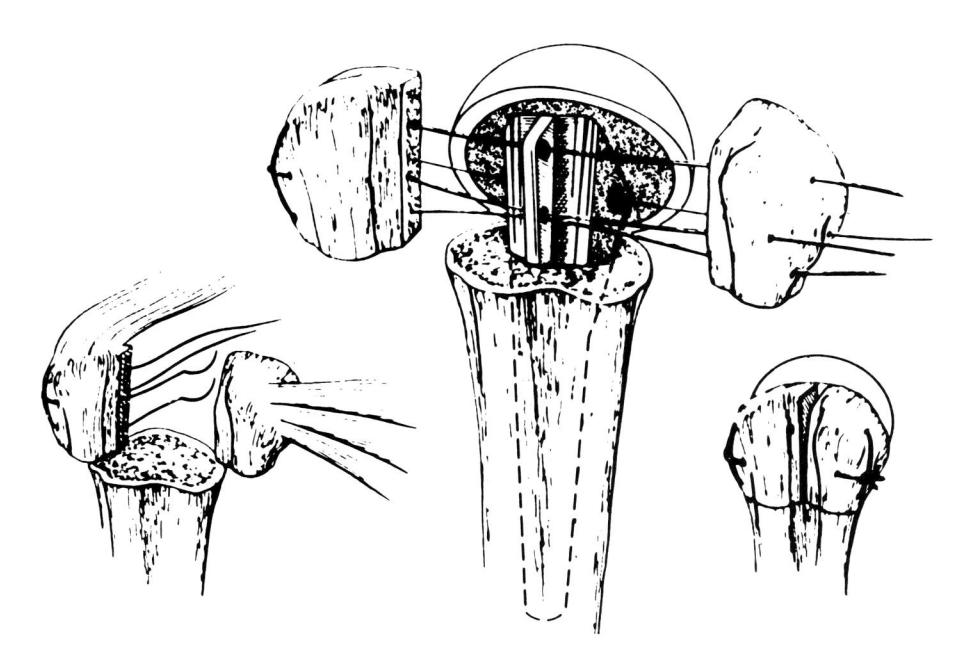

Figure 23–23. Suture technique for four-part fractures. This quadrilateral suture fixation pulls the tuberosity into the exposed cancellous structured, titanium porous surface. A second suture is placed through the shaft of the humerus and is used to repair the rotator interval. Medial and lateral suture holes allow a quadrilateral suture replacement, providing a very stable fixation for four-part fractures.

glenoid was designed with a flat back, three pegs for long-term stability, and a polyethylene component that snapped into place (see Figure 23–18C). A 6.5-mm fully threaded, central titanium screw was utilized along the lines of Kessel to secure the implant temporarily. The implant was reserved primarily for young active patients in whom a cemented glenoid might eventually loosen.

Since 1987, 140 humeral stems have been implanted by the author, with only 15% requiring cement to achieve stable fixation, mainly in patients with rheumatoid disease and rotator cuff tear arthropathy. No patient has undergone revision for humeral loosening. There have been 3250 humeral stems implanted as of May 1992, and only one report of a modular head dissociation in 1989.

Engh et al.[75] classified radiographic evidence of bone ingrowth as follows:

- Type I—Fixation by bone ingrowth. No subsidence with normal to no radiopaque line formation around the stem. Most of the bone implant interface should appear stable.
- Type II—Fixation by stable fibrous ingrowth. No progressive migration, extensive radiopaque line formation that is parallel and separated by a space no greater than 1 mm.
- Type III—Unstable implant. Progressive subsidence or migration with divergent radiopaque lines.

In uncemented stems with longer than 2 years of follow-up, 69% had no lucent or sclerotic lines. Radiographic evidence for ingrowth, as defined by densification around porous coated pads and an absence of lucent lines (Engh I), occurred in 69% (Figure 23–24).[75] A fine radiodense line, separated by a lucent zone less than 0.5 mm (Engh II), was seen around the nonporous stem in 31%. No component migration or Engh type III radiographs have occurred.

Retrieved specimens for instability revealed ingrowth over a significant portion of the porous coating in the proximal body and undersurface of the collar (see Figure 23–19). Backscatter electron microscopy[76–82] (see Figure 23–20)

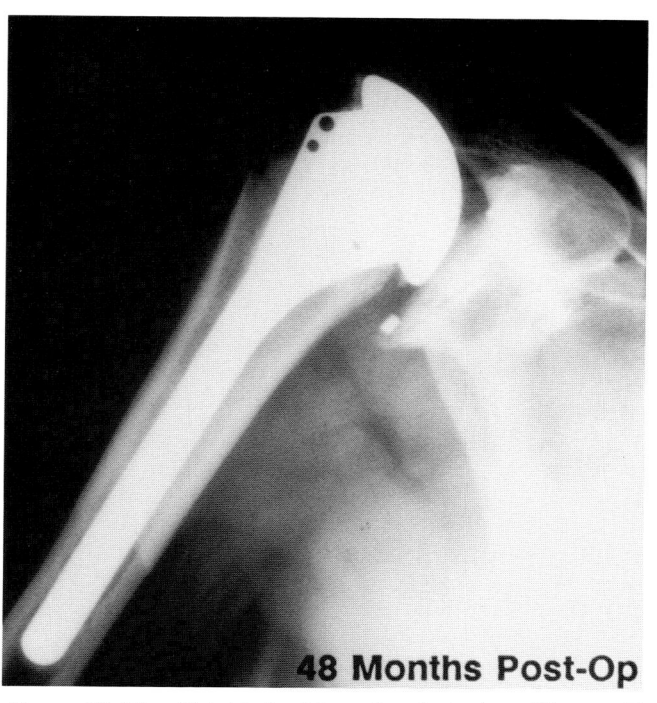

Figure 23–24. Hybrid shoulder arthroplasty in a 75-year-old white male, 4 years after implantation. Clinical result was excellent. The humeral stem was rated Engh I (i.e., direct abutment and densification proximally) and there were no lucent or sclerotic lines distally.

revealed mature bone with osteon formation deep within the porous coating. The fact that the stem is only coated in patches over the proximal one-third and not fully coated, and that fixation is largely cancellous in nature, made the specimens relatively easy to retrieve without disastrous loss of proximal humeral bone.

Of 49 patients with osteoarthritis, only 6 patients underwent cementless total shoulder arthroplasty.[83] These patients were younger (ranging in age from 48 to 64 years; mean, 54 years) than those who underwent a hybrid total shoulder arthroplasty with an uncemented humeral component and cemented glenoid component (mean age, 65.4 years; range, 60 to 78 years). Of the six porous coated glenoids done without PMMA, one became grossly loose 3 months postoperatively and the polyethylene dislocated superiorly (Figure 23–25). Postoperative radiographs revealed that the screw fixation did not reach the cortex of the scapula, leading to the screw backing out and dissociating the polyethylene from the metal shell. A second patient sustained a traumatic dislocation of his shoulder while wrestling with his teenage son. Upon relocation of his shoulder the polyethylene component dissociated from the glenoid prosthesis. This was treated by replacing the polyethylene component. At the time of surgery, the metal base plate was well fixed, and the patient continued to do well. The remainder of the patients appeared to have solid ingrowth radiographically (Figure 23–26).

The results, based on Neer's criteria, were excellent in two, satisfactory in three, and unsatisfactory in one. However, there were five cases of polyethylene dissociation by 1 year postoperatively in 89 components, and therefore the design was discontinued. A review of the retrieved specimens and examination of the clinical histories revealed that all of these were associated with instability, with selective wear on the thin polyethylene in the area of the fixation device, leading to failure. Bone ingrowth into the glenoid component was suggested by the radiographs.

The problem of thin polyethylene components dissociating from metal-backed trays has been reported for the hip, knee, and shoulder. The problem in the shoulder is that with a polyethylene liner 6-mm thick coupled with a metal backing of at least 4 mm, the component is thick enough to displace the center of rotation laterally, stress the anterior soft tissues, and predispose to instability. While more bone can be resected from the tibia, the same is not true of the glenoid.

A description of osteolysis behind screw-in acetabular components and total knee components raises concerns about long-term osteolysis problems in glenoid components with similar designs. Theoretically, polyethylene wear debris is pumped through the screw holes, setting up a macrophage reaction at the bone-implant or bone-cement interface.

Failure of the metal-backed glenoids in the series coupled with findings of fibrocartilaginous tissue on the resurfaced glenoid behind the titanium implant has led to a series with biologic resurfacing of the glenoid.

HEMIARTHROPLASTY COMBINED WITH BIOLOGIC RESURFACING OF THE GLENOID

Based on the experience with metal-backed glenoids and concerns regarding polyethylene wear, glenoid loosening, and osteolysis, the author has performed biologic resurfacing of the glenoid since 1989 as an adjunct to uncemented hemiarthroplasty.[83] Eight male patients, ranging in age from 36 to 68 years, were followed longer than 2 years. The technique involves reaming or sawing the glenoid surface down to bleeding subchondral bone and then covering it with either capsular flap tissue (Figure 23–27) or fascia lata (Figure 23–28). Four patients have undergone resurfacing

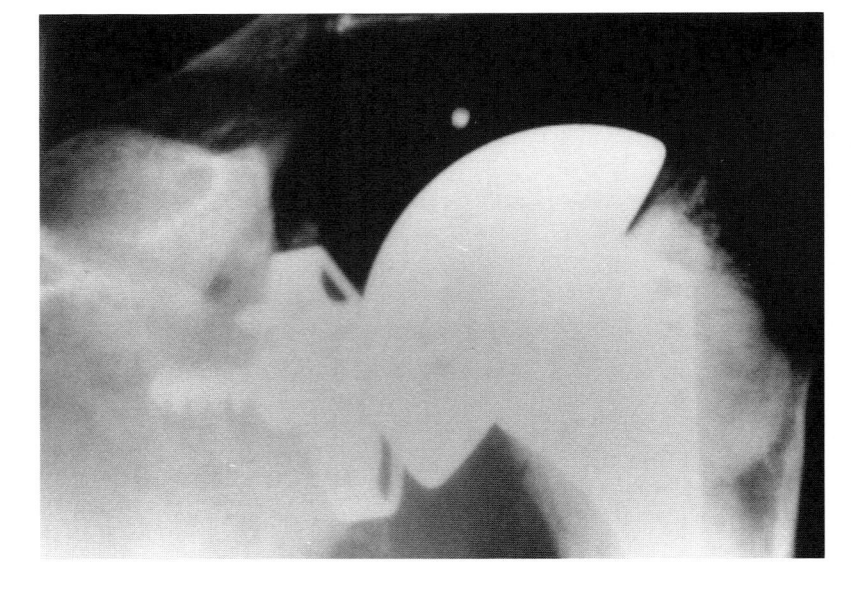

Figure 23–25. Dissociation of polyethylene component superiorly (metal marker in polyethylene superior to the head) 3 months after porous coated glenoid fixation. The screw did not engage the cortex of the scapula. The glenoid component rotated and eventually the polyethylene dissociated, requiring revision to hemiarthroplasty.

Cementless Shoulder Arthroplasty   297

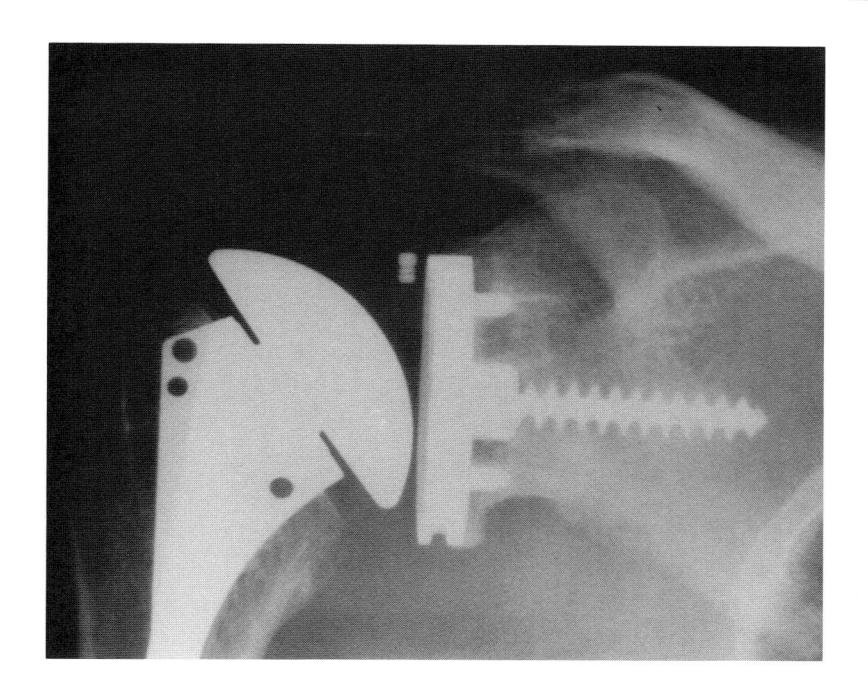

Figure 23–26. Well-fixed metal-backed component of a cementless total shoulder arthroplasty. Note the densification on the undersurface of the glenoid component and the solid screw fixation. There are no lucent lines.

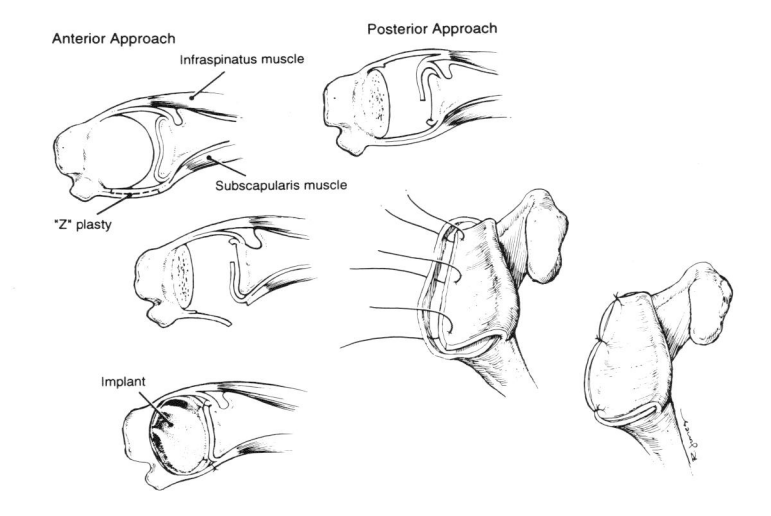

Figure 23–27. Biologic resurfacing of the glenoid. In patients with a thick anterior capsule complex (i.e., after Putti-Platt reconstruction), a layer of anterior capsular tissue can be created and laid over the glenoid surface after debridement down to bleeding subchondral bone. (Reproduced with permission from Burkhead and Rusty Jones.)

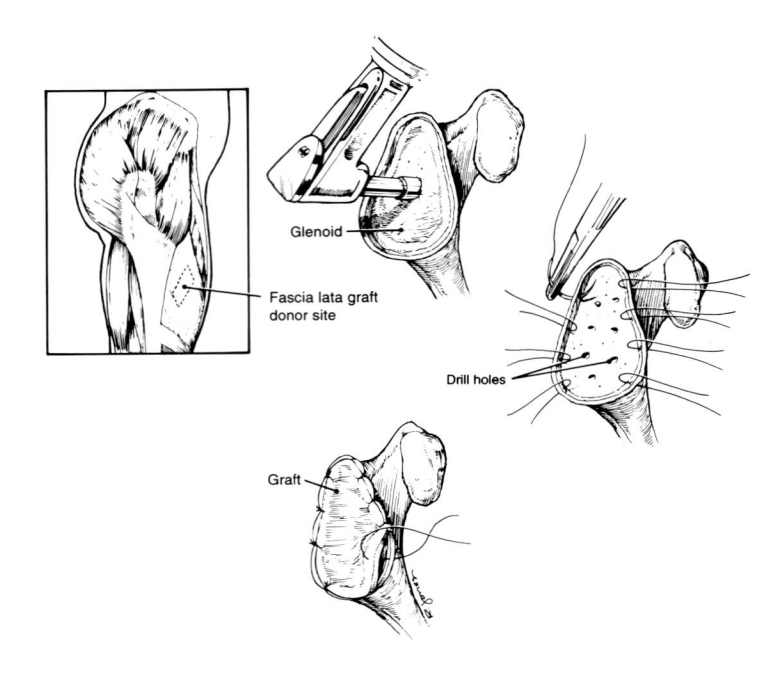

Figure 23–28. Fascia lata graft for biologic resurfacing of the glenoid. The glenoid surface is debrided down to bleeding subchondral bone. Autologous fascia lata is harvested from the ipsilateral thigh and sutured to the glenoid rim labrum or capsular structures. This technique can be used when the anterior soft tissues are thin. (Reproduced with permission from Burkhead and Rusty Jones.)

with a capsular flap (three anterior, one posterior), and four with fascia lata reconstruction.

The results have been excellent in six and satisfactory in two, with no unsatisfactory results. One patient had persistent anterior pain in the region of the biceps tendon. At the time of biceps tenodesis, an arthroscopy and tissue biopsy of the resurfaced joint revealed fibrous rather than fibrocartilaginous tissue. Autopsy specimens are not available and the long-term fate of the graft is unknown. However, radiographs at 24 months (Figure 23–29) showed maintenance of the space between the glenoid surface and the humeral head prosthesis. Theoretically, the soft wettable surface of the graft will create less metallic debris when compared to an implant contacting subchondral bone and may protect the pleuripotential cells on the newly created bleeding surface from damage by direct contact with the metal. These patients have all been extremely enthusiastic about returning to active sports including polo, tennis, and golf.

CEMENTLESS FIXATION OF FOUR-PART FRACTURES

Trochanteric osteotomies in revision hip surgery heal faster, with a lower incidence of wire fracture and nonunion when cementless revisions are compared to cemented revisions.[84] It might be possible that tuberosity union rates in four-part fractures would be improved with cementless fixation.

From 1987 to 1989, 18 patients underwent humeral hemiarthroplasty for four-part fractures or fracture-dislocations of the proximal end of the humerus. Follow-up ranged from 2 to 4 years, with an average of 34 months. The prosthesis, with its trapezoidal proximal shape, is porous coated in its proximal segment to allow long-term bone ingrowth of the tuberosity and shaft fragments. In 10 patients (average age, 62 years), the prosthesis was implanted without PMMA (group I), and in 8 patients (average age, 68 years) PMMA was utilized (group II). The tuberosities were sutured to the shaft of the humerus and the prosthesis using 1-mm cottony Dacron suture. Radiographic evidence of healing of the tuberosities to the shaft and prosthesis was present in 9 of 10 patients in group I. Two of 8 tuberosities did not unite in Group II, and proximal migration with poor results occurred. Patients in group I rated higher in terms of patient satisfaction, range of motion, and strength testing than did group II patients. Radiographs at 3 weeks frequently showed exuberant callus formation (Figure 23–30) in patients with a cementless component, which has been utilized in patients as old as 92 years. The risk of hypotension associated with PMMA is eliminated, and excellent functional results with return to active independent living have been obtained (Figure 23–31).

POROUS COATED PROSTHESIS IN AVASCULAR NECROSIS

Six patients with avascular necrosis have been treated with porous coated prostheses. The porous coating extends past the area of necrotic bone in the humeral head. All six patients had excellent results, with no revisions for humeral loosening at an average 34 months of follow-up. All had densification proximally (Figure 23–32) without progressive lucencies distally.

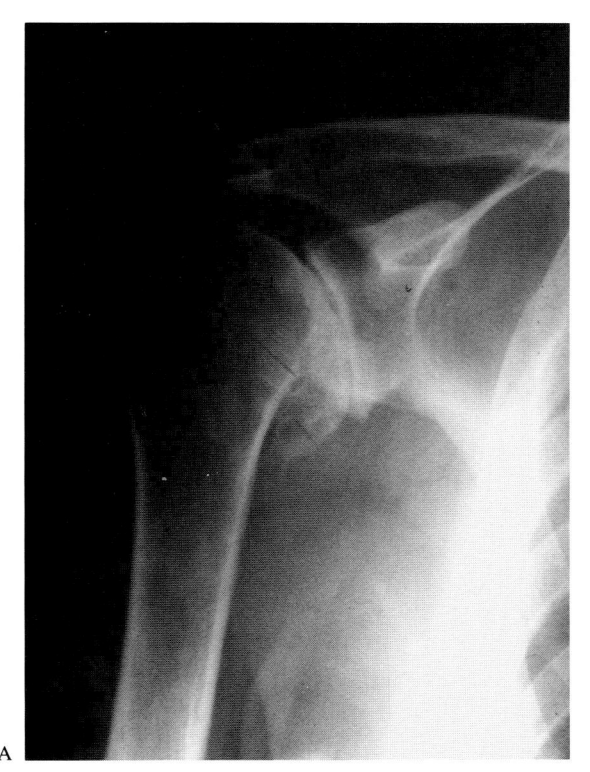

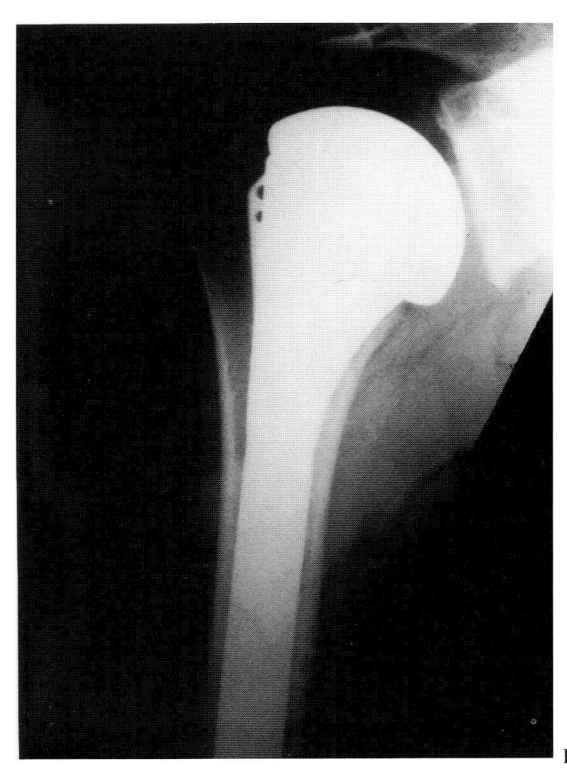

Figure 23–29. **A.** Postreconstruction osteoarthritis for a dislocating shoulder. **B.** Two years after biologic resurfacing, capsular flap–type with maintenance of the space between the implant and the resurfaced glenoid.

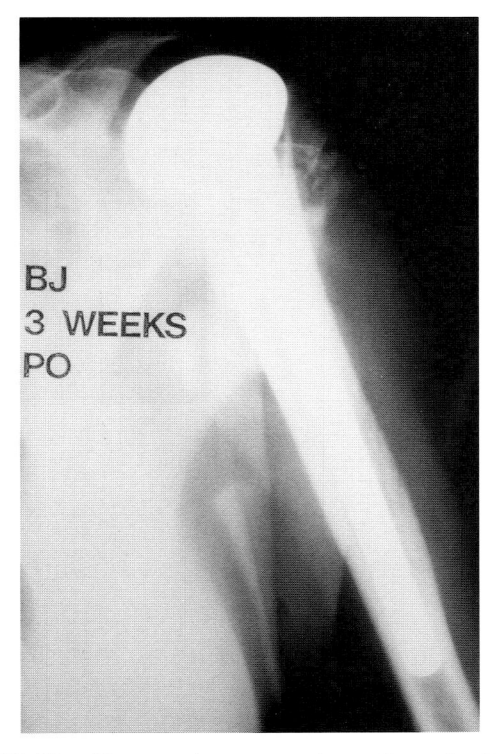

Figure 23–30. Three-week postoperative radiograph of a 65-year-old woman with a four-part fracture managed by an uncemented treatment. Note the exuberant callus formation, similar to what is seen in intramedullary rod fixation with reaming.

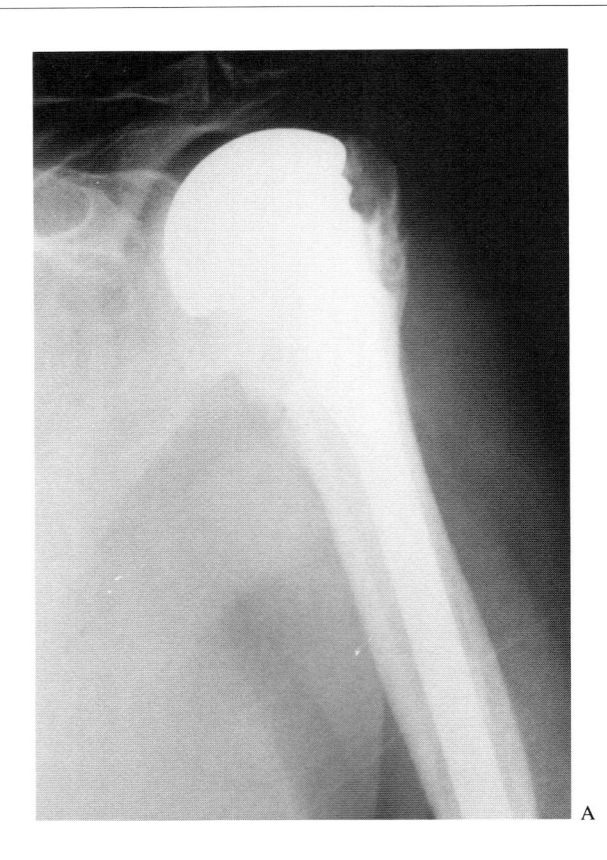

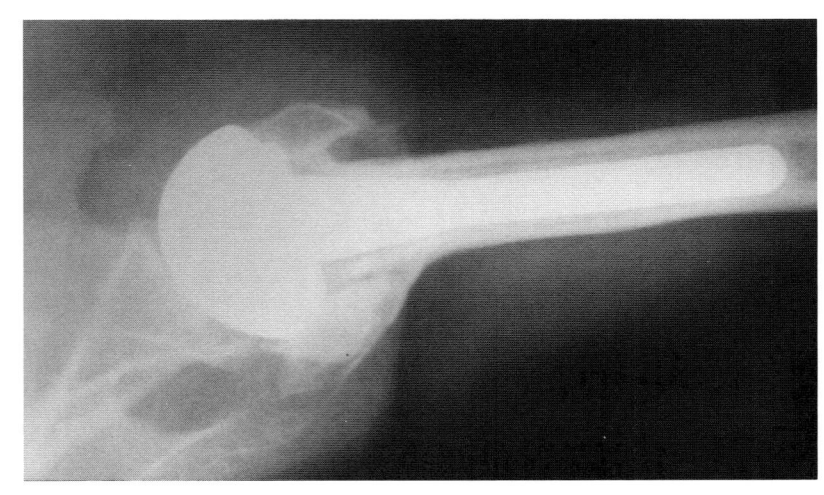

Figure 23–31. A and B. Anteroposterior and axillary radiographs of a 92-year-old after four-part fracture fixation with cementless implant, showing excellent tuberosity healing.

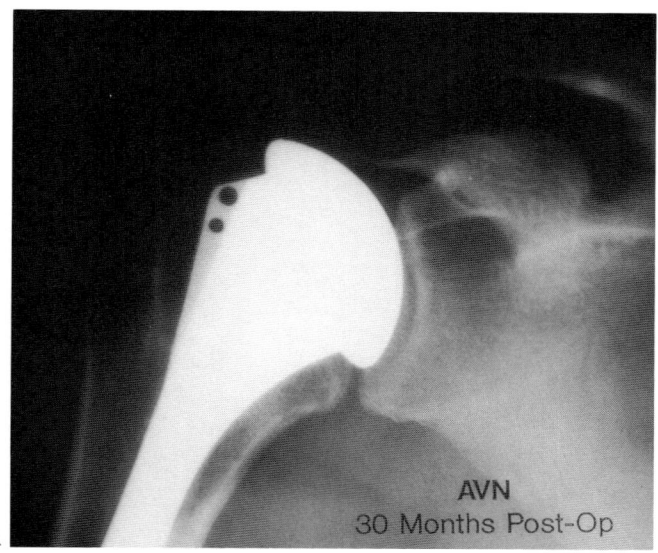

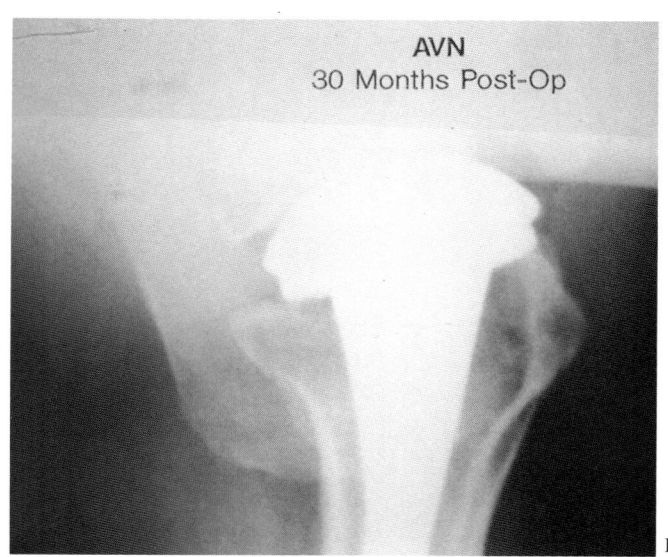

Figure 23–32. A and B. Anteroposterior and axillary radiographs of a patient with Avascular necrosis 30 months postoperatively. Engh type I radiograph.

HYBRID TOTAL SHOULDER ARTHROPLASTY

Most of the patients who are candidates for total shoulder arthroplasty are older, and the demands upon their shoulders are less. To subject these patients to the risk of cementless glenoid fixation seems unjustified. Therefore, in patients over 65 years old, hybrid total shoulder arthroplasty with an uncemented humeral stem and a cemented all-polyethylene glenoid component is indicated.

In order to lower the lucency rate, a flat-back design was developed to prevent the rocking-horse effect.[29] Two peg holes into the glenoid are connected beneath a bridge of subchondral bone (Figure 23–33A). This allows the surgeon to fill one peg hole while the other is plugged by the gloved finger, thus truly pressurizing the cement (Figure 23–33B, C). The holes are created to provide a cement mantle of 3 mm. A flat surface may be preferred, even in patients with rheumatoid arthritis, since this provides resistance to rocking and allows lateralization of the joint line, which has been shown to be of variable importance for a good result.[85] When used on a curved surface, it allows a cement mantle behind the glenoid component (Figure 23–34).

While Neer[86] and others[87] prefer no PMMA on the back of the glenoid, Wroblewski et al.[88] found that a lack of PMMA between the outside of polyethylene acetabular components and the bone led to areas of increased wear on the polyethylene socket. Wear particles from this area, not necessarily the articular bearing surface, may be partially responsible for the osteolytic response.

Plain radiographic results in 25 hybrid total shoulder arthroplasties for osteoarthritis were reviewed according to the classification of Franklin.[29] There were 13 patients with no lucencies (class 0), 8 patients with a lucency under the back of the implant (class I), and 4 patients with an incomplete lucency under the pegs (class II). There were no class III, IV, or V changes at an average 34-month follow-up.

SUMMARY

Unlike the history of shoulder arthroplasty in general and cemented total shoulder arthroplasty in particular, the history of cementless shoulder replacement is very short, sporadic, and still in its infancy. Biologic fixation of the humerus does not appear to be as big of a challenge as biologic fixation of the glenoid. Still, there is room for continued investigation and improvement. Friedman (personal communication, 1993) implanted six hydroxyapatite-coated humeral stems, with excellent clinical results and roentgenographic evidence of ingrowth in all.

The shoulder with its unique bony architecture demands a glenoid bearing surface that is thin enough not to interfere with the soft-tissue reconstruction. Unfortunately, the wear characteristics of polyethylene make this difficult to accomplish. Hopefully in the future, better bearing surfaces and better ways of securing these bearing surfaces to bone for the long-term will be developed. A truly anatomic glenoid with a soft but durable bearing surface and a low coefficient of friction seems an ideal goal. Until such time when a successful cementless glenoid arthroplasty that does not introduce the added complications of dissociation, metal-on-metal wear, and instability is available, hybrid total shoulder arthroplasty in the older patient and biologic resurfacing of the glenoid in the younger patient remain viable alternatives.

Acknowledgments. The author would like to thank Karen Lozano for her careful preparation of this manuscript; Stacy Johnson, Keith Shull, and the Medical Photography Depart-

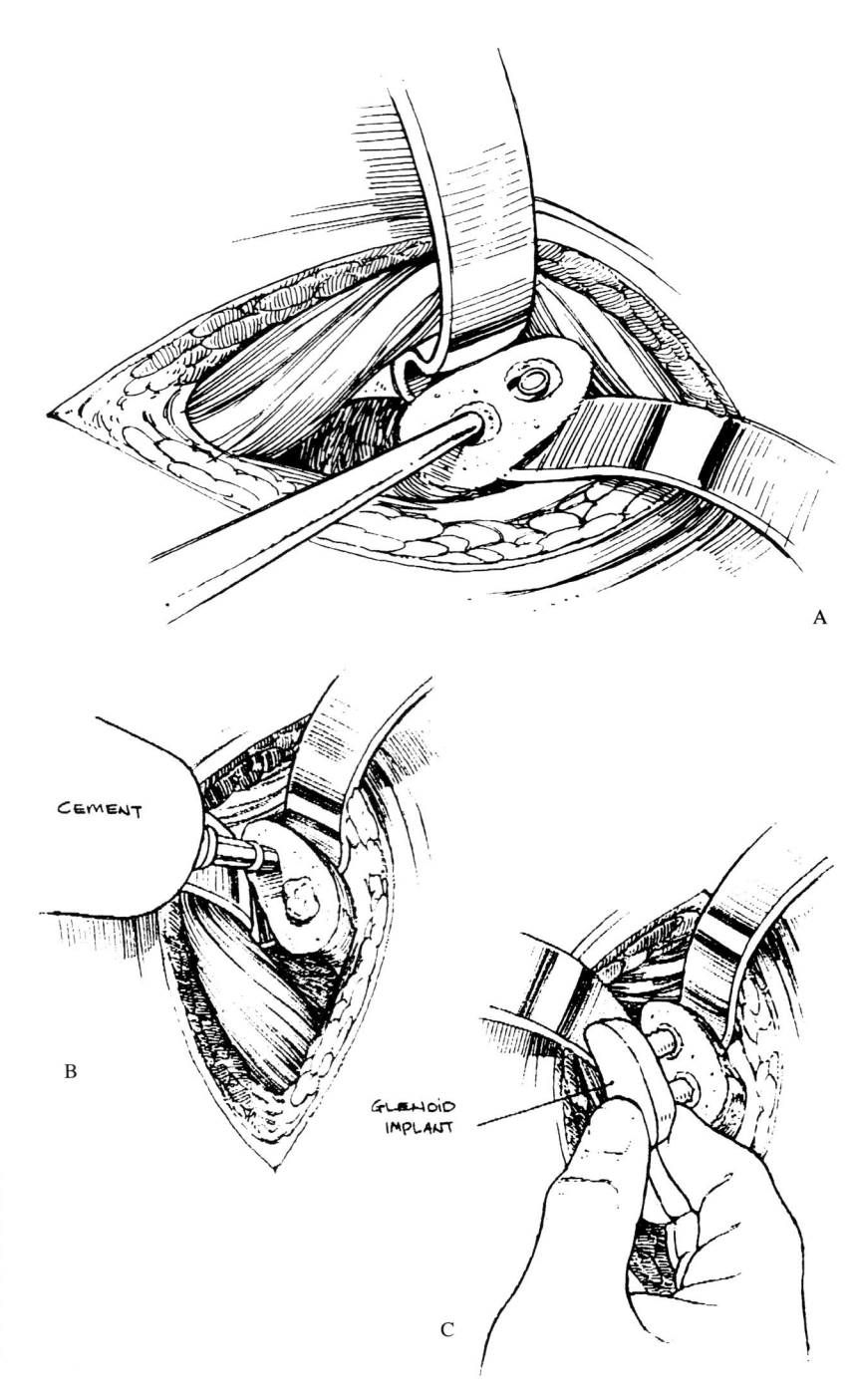

Figure 23–33. **A** and **B.** Cementing technique for glenoid in hybrid total shoulder arthroplasty, allowing pressurization of the cement into the glenoid vault. The cement is introduced through one hole while the other is plugged. **C.** Insertion of the glenoid into pressurized cement mantle.

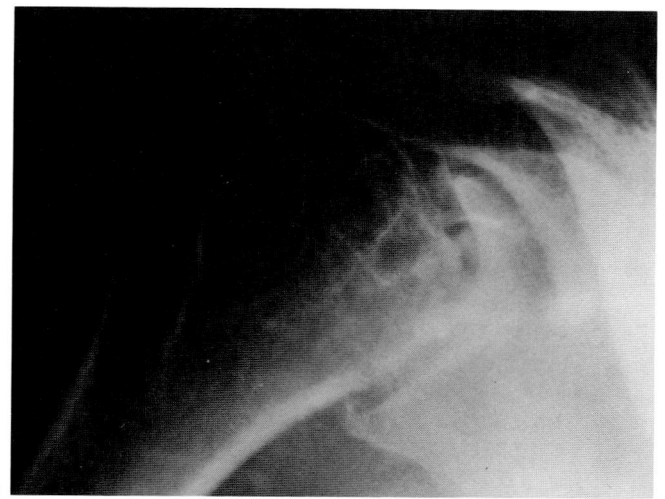

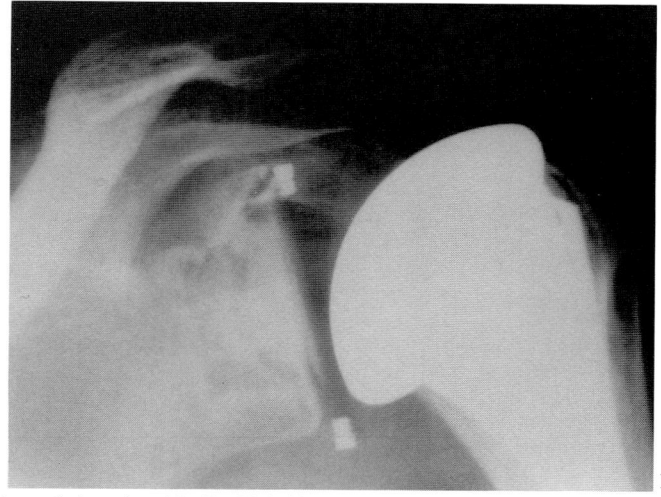

Figure 23-34. A. Rheumatoid arthritis with central erosion of the glenoid. **B.** Hybrid shoulder arthroplasty in rheumatoid arthritis with uncemented humeral component and cemented polyethylene component. Note that placement of a flat-backed prosthesis on this curved surface gives a 3-mm cement mantle. Note the absence of lucent lines around the pegs on the glenoid component at 4 years postoperatively. One-millimeter nonprogressive lucency is present in some areas under both of the components.

ment at Baylor University Medical Center; and my wife and children for their patience and understanding during the preparation of this manuscript.

REFERENCES

1. Venable CS, Stuck WG. Electrolysis controlling factor in the use of metals in treating fractures. *J Am Med* 1938;15:1349–1352.
2. Smith DC. The acrylic denture base. Some effects of residual monomer and peroxide. *Br Dental J* 1959;106:331–336.
3. Charnley J. Anchorage of the femoral head prosthesis to the shaft of the femur. *J Bone Joint Surg [Br]* 1960;42:28–30.
4. Charnley J. The bonding of prostheses to bone by cement. *J Bone Joint Surg [Br]* 1964;46:517–529.
5. Charnley J. *Low Friction Arthroplasty of the Hip.* New York: Springer-Verlag, 1979.
6. Gruen TA, McNeece GM, Amstutz HC. Modes of failure of cemented stem type femoral components. *Clin Orthop* 1979;141:17–27.
7. Goodman SB, Carter DR. Acetabular lucent lines and mechanical stress in total hip arthroplasty. *J Arthroplasty* 1987;2:219–224.
8. Goldring SR, Schiller AL, Roelke M, Rourke CM, O'Neill DA, Harris WH. The synovial-like membrane of the bone-cement interface in loose total hip replacements and its proposed role in bone lysis. *J Bone Joint Surg [Am]* 1983;65:575–583.
9. Anderson GBJ, Freeman MAR, Swanson SAV. Loosening of the cemented acetabular cup in total hip replacement. *J Bone Joint Surg [Br]* 1972;54:590–599.
10. DeLee JG, Charnley J. Radiological demarcation of cemented sockets in total hip replacement. *Clin Orthop* 1976;121:20–32.
11. Chambers TJ. The cellular basis of bone resorption. *Clin Orthop* 1980;151:283–293.
12. Jones LC, Hungerford DS. Cement disease. *Clin Orthop* 1987;225:192–206.
13. Howie DW, Vernon-Roberts B, Oakeshott R, Manthey B. A rat model of resorption of bone at the cement-bone interface in the presence of polyethylene wear particles. *J Bone Joint Surg [Am]* 1988;70:257–263.
14. Howie DW, Cornish BL, Vernon-Roberts B. Resurfacing hip arthroplasty. Classification of loosening and the role of prosthetic wear particles. *Clin Orthop* 1990;255:144–159.
15. Jatsy M, Floyd WE III, Schiller AL, Goldring SR. Localized osteolysis in stable, nonseptic total hip replacement. *J Bone Joint Surg [Am]* 1986;68:912–919.
16. Lennox DW, Schofield BH, McDonald DF, Riley LH. A histologic comparison of aseptic loosening of cemented, press-fit, and biologic ingrowth prostheses. *Clin Orthop* 1987; 225:171–191.
17. Linder L, Lindberg L, Carlsson A. Aseptic loosening of hip prostheses. A histologic and enzyme histochemical study. *Clin Orthop* 1983;175 93–104.
18. Maloney WJ, Jasty M, Harris WH, Galante JO, Callaghan JJ. Endosteal erosion in association with stable uncemented femoral components. *J Bone Joint Surg [Am]* 1990;72:1025–1034.
19. Buchert PK, Vaughn BK, Mallory TH, Engh CA, Boby JD. Excessive metal release due to loosening and fretting of sintered particles on porous-coated hip prostheses. Report of two cases. *J Bone Joint Surg [Am]* 1986;68:606–609.
20. Cheng CL, Gross AE. Loosening of the porous coating in total knee replacement. *J Bone Joint Surg [Br]* 1988;70:377–381.
21. Cofield RH. Degenerative and arthritic problems of the glenohumeral joint. In Rockwood, CA and Matsen FA III. *The Shoulder.* Philadelphia, W.B. Saunders Company, 1990;678–742.
22. Engelbrecht E, Heinert K. More than ten years' experience with unconstrained shoulder replacement. In: Kolbel R, Helbig B, Blauth W, eds. *Shoulder Replacement.* Berlin: Springer-Verlag, 1987:234–239.
23. Barrett WP, Franklin JL, Jackins SE, Wyss CR, Matsen FA III. Total shoulder arthroplasty. *J Bone Joint Surg [Am]* 1987;69:865–872.
24. Cofield RH. Total shoulder arthroplasty with the Neer prosthesis. *J Bone Joint Surg [Am]* 1984;66:899–906.

25. Cofield RH. Total shoulder arthroplasty: Associated disease of the rotator cuff, results, and complications. In: Batemen JE, Welsh RP, eds. *Surgery of the Shoulder*. St. Louis: CV Mosby, 1984:229–233.
26. Cofield RH. Arthrodesis and resectional arthroplasty of the shoulder. In: EC McCollister, ed. *Surgery of the Musculoskeletal System*. New York: Churchill-Livingstone, 1983:109–123.
27. Cofield RH. Unconstrained total shoulder prostheses. *Clin Orthop* 1983;173:97–108.
28. Freeman MAR, Bradley GW, Revell PA. Observations upon the interface between bone and polymethylmetahacrylate cement. *J Bone Joint Surg [Br]* 1982;64:849–493.
29. Franklin JL, Barrett WP, Jackins SE, Matsen FA. Glenoid loosening in total shoulder arthroplasty. *J Arthroplasty* 1988;3:39–46.
30. Schmalzried TP, Kwong LM, Jasty MJ, et al. Mechanism of loosening of cemented acetabular components in total hip arthroplasty. Analysis of specimens retrieved at autopsy. *Clin Orthop* 1992;274:60–78.
31. Keller JC, Lautenschlager EP, Marshall GW Jr, Meyer PR Jr. Factors affecting surgical alloy bone cement interface adhesion. *J Biomed Mater Res* 1980;14:639–651.
32. Barb W, Park JB, Kenner GH, von Recum AF. Intramedullary fixation of artificial hip joint with bone cement precoated implant. *J Biomed Mater Res* 1982;16:459–469.
33. Harris WH. The first 32 years of total hip arthroplasty: One surgeon's perspective. *Clin Orthop* 1992;274:6–11.
34. Burke DW, Gates EI, Harris WH. Centrifugation as a method of improving tensile and fatigue properties of acrylic bone cement. *J Bone Joint Surg [Am]* 1984;66:1265–1273.
35. Bobyn DJ, Miller JE. Features of biologically fixed devices. In: Morrey BF, ed. *Joint Replacement Arthroplasty*. New York: Churchill-Livingstone, 1991:61–80.
36. Bobyn JD, Pilliar RM, Cameron HU, Weatherly GC. The optimum pore size for the fixation of porous surfaced metal implants by the ingrowth of bone. *Clin Orthop* 1980;150:263–270.
37. Bobyn JD, Pilliar RM, Cameron HU, Weatherly GC. osteogenic phenomena across endosteal bone-implant spaces with porous-surfaced intramedullary implants. *Acta Orthop Scand* 1981;52:145–153.
38. Bobyn JD, Wilson GJ, MacGregor DC, et al. Effect of pore size on the peel strength of attachment of fibrous tissue to porous-surfaced implants. *J Biomed Mater Res* 1982;16:571–584.
39. Galante JO, Rostoker W, Lueck R, Ray RD. Sintered fiber metal composites as a basis for attachment of implants to bone. *J Bone Joint Surg [Am]* 1971;53:101.
40. Klawitter JJ, Hulbert SF. Application of porous ceramics for the attachment of load bearing internal orthopaedic applications. *J Biomed Mater Res Suppl* 1971;2:161–229.
41. Bloebaum RD, Campbell PA, Reid S, Dorr L. Backscattered electron imaging of clinically retrieved porous coated implants. Presented at *Proceedings of the Uncemented Total Joint Replacement Symposium, Nov. 22–26, 1986*. Salt Lake City, Utah, USA.
42. Clemow AJT, Weinstein AM, Klawitter JJ, et al. Interface mechanics of porous titanium implants. *J Biomed Mater Res* 1981;15:73–82.
43. Hurlbert SF, Young FA, Mathews RS, et al. Potential of ceramic materials as permanently implantable skeletal prostheses. *J Biomed Mater Res* 1970;4:433–456.
44. Nilles JL, Lapitsky M. Biomechanical investigations of bone-porous carbon and porous metal interfaces. *J Biomed Mater Res Suppl* 1973;4:63–84.
45. Peterson CD, Miles JS, Solomons C, et al. Union between bone and implants of open pore ceramic and stainless steel. A histologic study. *J Bone Joint Surg [Am]* 1969;51:805.
46. Pilliar RM, Cameron HU, Macnab I. Porous surface layered prosthetic devices. *J Biomed Eng* 1975;10:126–131.
47. Spector M, Michno MJ, Smarook WH, Kwiatkowski GT. A high modulous polymer for porous orthopaedic implants. Biomechanical compatibility of porous implants. *J Biomed Mater Res* 1978;12:665–677.
48. Spector M, Harmon SL, Kreutner A. Characteristics of tissue ingrowth into proplast and porous polyethylene implants in bone. *J Biomed Mater Res* 1979;13:677–692.
49. Welsh RP, Pilliar RM, Macnab I. Surgical implants: The role of surface porosity in fixation to bone and acrylic. *J Bone Joint Surg [Am]* 1971;53:963–977.
50. Ypma JFAM. *Strength and Ingrowth Aspects of Porous Acrylic Bone Cement*. Nijmegen, The Netherlands: Catholic University, 1981. PhD thesis.
51. Hofmann AA, Rudman MH, Bloebaum RD, Bachus KN. Effect of autograft bone chips applied at the bone/implant interface of porous coated devices in human cancellous bone. *Trans Orthop Res Soc* 1991:16, 546.
52. Geesink RGT, de Groot K, Klein CPAT. Chemical implant fixation using hydroxyl-apatite coatings. *Clin Orthop* 1987;225:147–120.
53. Geesink RGT, de Groot K, Klein CPAT, Serekian P. Bone bonding to apatite coated implants. *J Bone Joint Surg [Br]* 1977;70:17–22.
54. Bobyn JD. *The Strength of Fixation of Porous Metal Implants by the Ingrowth of Bone*. Montreal: McGill University, 1977. MSc Thesis.
55. Brooker AF, Constable D. Bone ingrowth into titanium grooves: A comparison of surfaces for biologic fixation. *Adv Orthop Surg* 1986;10:125.
56. Oh I. Design rationale of interference-fit total hip prostheses. In: Fitzgerald R Jr, ed. *Non-Cemented Total Hip Arthroplasty*. New York: Raven Press, 1988:365.
57. Blaha JD, Enzler HP, Freeman MAR, Rovelle PA, Todd RC. The fixation of a proximal tibial polyethylene prosthesis without cement. *J Bone Joint Surg [Br]* 1982;64:326–335.
58. Magee FP, Longo JA, Hedley AK. The effect of age on the interface strength between porous coated implants and bone. *Trans Soc Biomat* 1989;12:85.
59. Collier JP, Mayor MB, Chae JC, Suprenant VA, Suprenant HP, Dauphinais LA. Macroscopic and microscopic evidence of prosthetic fixation with porous-coated materials. *Clin Orthop* 1988;235:173–180.
60. Collier JP, Bauer TW, Bloebaum RD, et al. Results of implant retrieval from postmortem specimens in patients with well functioning long-term total hip replacement. *Clin Orthop* 1992;274:97–112.
61. Orr TE Carter DR. Stress analyses of joint arthroplasty in the proximal humerus. *J Orthop Res* 1985;3:360–371.
62. Kessel L. *Clinical Disorders of the Shoulder*. Edinburgh: Churchill-Livingstone, 1982:94–102.
63. Kessel L, Bayley JIL. The Kessel total shoulder replacement. In: Bayley JIL, Kessel L, eds. *Shoulder Surgery*. New York: Springer-Verlag, 1982:160–164.
64. Wallensten R, Brostrom LA, Olson E. Kessel total shoulder arthroplasty in rheumatoid arthritis. In: *Proceedings of the 3rd International Conference on Surgery of the Shoulder, Fukuoka, Japan*. Professional Post Graduate Services, October 1986.
65. Bayley JIL. Total shoulder arthroplasty. Presented at the Closed Meeting of the American Shoulder and Elbow Society; 1990; Chicago, IL.
66. McElwain JP, English E. The early results of porous-coated total shoulder arthroplasty. *Clin Orthop* 1987;218:2317–224.

67. Faludi DD, Weiland AJ. Cementless total shoulder arthroplasty. Preliminary experience with 13 cases. *Orthopedics* 1983;6:431–437.
68. Cofield RH. Preliminary experience with bone ingrowth total shoulder arthroplasty. *Orthop Trans* 1986;10:217.
69. Cofield RH. Total shoulder arthroplasty with bone ingrowth fixation. In: Kolbel R, Helbig B, Blauth W, eds. *Shoulder Replacement*. Berlin: Springer-Verlag, 1987:209–212.
70. Cofield RH, Daly PJ. Total shoulder arthroplasty with a tissue ingrowth glenoid component. *J Shoulder Elbow Surg* 1992; 1:77–85.
71. Cofield RH. Total shoulder arthroplasty. Instructional Course Lecture. The Ninth Combined Meeting of the Orthopaedic Associations of the English Speaking World; June 22, 1992; Toronto, Ontario, Canada.
72. Copeland S. Cementless total shoulder replacement. In: Post M, Morrey BF, Hawkins RJ, eds. *Surgery of the Shoulder*. St. Louis: Mosby-Year Book, 1990:289–293.
73. Roper BA, Paterson JMH, Day WH. The Roper-Day total shoulder replacement. *J Bone Joint Surg [Br]* 1990;72:694–697.
74. Zweymuller KA, Lintner FK, Semlitsch MF. Biologic fixation of a press-fit titanium hip joint endoprosthesis. *Clin Orthop* 1988;235:195–206.
75. Engh CA, Bobyn JD, Glassman AH. Porous-coated hip replacement. The factors governing bone ingrowth, stress shielding, and clinical results. *J Bone Joint Surg [Br]* 1987;69:45–66.
76. Bloebaum RD, Campbell PA, Dorr L, Conaty JP. Analysis of retrieved clinical bone ingrowth TKR and THR implants. *Trans Soc Biomater* 1985;8:51.
77. Bloebaum RD, Campbell PA, Reid S, Dorr L. BSE imaging analysis of retrieved clinical prostheses. *Trans Soc Biomater* 1987;10:16.
78. Bloebaum RD, Gruen T, Campbell P, Dorr L. Backscattered electron imaging of retrieved clinical prostheses. *Trans Orthop Res Soc* 1988;13:366.
79. Bloebaum RD, Sanderson C, McCarvill S, Campbell P. Plastic slides in the preparation of implant and tissue for interface analysis. *J Histotechnol* 1989;12:307.
80. Bloebaum RD, Bachus KN, Boyce TM. Backscattered electron imaging: The role in calcified tissue and implant analysis. *J Biomater Appl* 1990;5:56.
81. Bloebaum RD, Merrell M, Gustke K, Simmmons M. Retrieval analysis of a hydroxyapatite coated hip prosthesis from a human donor. *Clin Orthop* 1991;267:97–102.
82. Bloebaum RD, Rubman MH, Bachus KN, Dorr LD. Comparison of hydroxyapatite coated and porous coated femoral hip implants retrieved from the same patient. *Trans Soc Biomater* 1991;14:14.
83. Burkhead WZ. Design rationale and clinical application of the Select Shoulder System in glenohumeral arthritis. Presidential Guest Lecturer. Presented at 18th Annual Meeting of the Japanese Shoulder Society; 1991; Kobe, Japan.
84. Rasmussen LJ, McGann WA, Welch RB. Trochanteric ostotomies: A comparison of cemented vs. cementless revision total hip arthroplasties. *Orthop Trans* 1991;15:39.
85. Figgie HE III, Inglis AE, Goldberg VM. An analysis of factors affecting long-term results of total shoulder arthroplasty in inflammatory arthritis. *J Arthroplasty* 1988;3:123–130.
86. Neer CS II. *Shoulder Reconstruction*. Philadelphia: WB Saunders, 1990.
87. Rockwood CA, Matzen FA. *Global Shoulder Surgical Technique Manual*. Warsaw, IN: DePuy, 1992.
88. Wroblewski BM, Lynch M, Atkinson JR, Dowson D, Isaac GH. External wear of the polyethylene socket in cemented total hip arthroplasty. *J Bone Joint Surg [Br]* 1987;69:61–63.

24 Glenoid Resurfacing in Shoulder Arthroplasty

Allen D. Boyd, Jr., M.D., and Thomas S. Thornhill, M.D.

The era of modern shoulder arthroplasty began in the 1950s with the introduction by Neer[1] of a metal device for replacement of the humeral articular surface. This prosthesis was initially used for fracture-dislocations of the humeral head, and later was implanted for painful osteoarthritis. In 1974, Neer[2] published the first extensive report on his results with this device in 48 shoulders with degenerative arthritis. Rheumatoid arthritis patients were excluded. The satisfactory results led to the conclusion that hemiarthroplasty would remain useful as the treatment for painful degenerative arthritis of the shoulder. In that series, the articular surface of the glenoid was smooth but usually consisted of eburnated bone devoid of cartilage. Neer proposed that the articular surface of the glenoid did not appear to be a significant source of pain.

Resurfacing of the glenoid with a cemented polyethylene device was introduced in the early 1970's for patients with significant glenoid erosion. Neer et al.[3] reported their results with total shoulder arthroplasty in 1982, which included 273 shoulders treated with metal-to-plastic glenohumeral units. This patient population comprised a mixture of diagnostic categories including osteoarthritis, rheumatoid arthritis, posttraumatic arthritis, cuff tear arthropathy, revision arthroplasty, and miscellaneous. Again, the results were satisfactory in most patients and total shoulder arthroplasty was recommended for painful arthritis of the glenohumeral joint.

Numerous investigators have reported similar results with the Neer device, and with other prostheses as well.[4-29] The results of shoulder arthroplasty continue to improve with refinements in surgical technique, prosthetic design, and postoperative rehabilitation. In many cases, this evolution has left the indications for glenoid resurfacing unclear. The surgeon must weigh the risks of increased operative time and long-term glenoid complications against the increased incidence of pain reported following hemiarthroplasty.[1-34] The preoperative decision to resurface the glenoid is usually based on patient diagnosis and radiographic evidence of glenoid erosion confirmed at the time of surgery. Severe erosion of the glenoid articular surface is thought to be a contributing factor towards the production of pain in symptomatic shoulders. It is still unclear whether glenoid resurfacing is indicated in osteoarthritic patients with a smooth eburnated glenoid surface.

The technical difficulties and potential complications of glenoid replacement are significant and require the risks and benefits of this procedure to be precisely identified. Glenoid resurfacing requires increased tissue dissection and exposure for component implantation, with a corresponding increase in operative time, blood loss, and anesthesia. Technical considerations with resurfacing include bone grafting for glenoid deficiency, and complex soft-tissue reconstructions for instability or rotator cuff tears. Potential complications include glenoid fracture, neurovascular injury, structural failure, component loosening, and dislocation.

The incidence of radiolucency at the glenoid bone-cement interface is high, ranging from 30 to 89% in several reported series.[3,7,8,12,14,28] These findings have not proved to be clinically significant but the long-term consequences are unknown. In cases requiring revision, the results have been inferior to index total shoulder arthroplasty procedures in limited reports.[35] Unnecessary glenoid replacement could contribute to the subsequent need for revision. The counterargument against hemiarthroplasty suggests that replacement of the humeral surface alone results in incomplete pain relief and progressive erosion of the glenoid, making future replacement even more difficult. Articular cartilage histologically will undergo accelerated wear when bearing against metal.[36-39] Moreover, late glenoid resurfacing is technically difficult when a nonmodular humeral component is well fixed. The risks and benefits of additional surgery and the technical difficulties of potential revision procedures must be considered in the long-term planning for patients with shoulder arthropathy. Conditions and circumstances in which shoulder arthroplasty may be indicated are listed in Table 24–1.

In this chapter, the established record for hemiarthroplasty and total shoulder arthroplasty is examined, specifically looking for data comparing these procedures. Shoulder biomechanics, design concepts, and clinical data are included. In addition, guidelines are offered regarding hemiarthroplasty versus total shoulder arthroplasty for the conditions noted in Table 24–1.

ANATOMY AND BIOMECHANICS

The glenohumeral joint is a skeletal mismatch in terms of bone mass and surface area. The humeral head has approximately four times the surface area of the glenoid and represents one-third of an irregular sphere.[40] The humeral

Table 24–1. Conditions with Potential Requirement for Shoulder Arthroplasty

Rheumatoid arthritis
Osteoarthritis
Avascular necrosis
Posttraumatic arthritis
Chronic dislocation
Cuff tear arthropathy
Systemic lupus erythematosus
Hemochromatosis
Ankylosing spondylitis
Psoriatic arthritis
Calcium pyrophosphate deposition disease
Gout
Hemophilia

head is inclined 130 to 150 degrees relative to the shaft and retroverted approximately 30 degrees relative to the distal end of the humerus.[40–42] The glenoid and its subcortical vault form a small, lateral expansion of the flat-shaped, predominantly cortical scapula. The vault itself is covered with thin cortical bone and surrounds cancellous bone of variable density (Figure 24–1), which is greatest beneath the glenoid cortical plate and diminishes from lateral to medial. The glenoid surface is retroverted approximately 7 degrees relative to the body of the scapula and faces 5 to 10 degrees upward.[40–42]

The stability of the glenohumeral joint is highly dependent upon soft-tissue integrity. The glenoid labrum is composed of dense, fibrous connective tissue and enhances the containment function of the relatively shallow glenoid fossa.[43] Anterior thickenings of the capsulolabral complex form the superior, middle, and inferior glenohumeral ligaments, which provide some degree of static stability to the joint and restrict abnormal translation of the humeral head.[44] The deltoid and rotator cuff musculature surround the humeral head and provide dynamic restraint as well as motor power. In abduction, the rotator cuff depresses and fixes the humeral head against the glenoid fossa, enabling the deltoid to elevate the arm. Without rotator cuff function, attempted abduction results in proximal subluxation of the humerus, shortening of the deltoid lever arm, and limited ability to abduct the arm.

Normal shoulder motion and glenohumeral loading are dependent on synchronous function of the deltoid and rotator cuff muscles. Poppen and Walker[45] have shown the average excursion of the humeral head on the face of the glenoid to be less than 1.5 mm between each 30-degree arc of motion. In the presence of a shoulder disorder such as degenerative joint disease, rotator cuff tear, or instability, the muscle envelope does not center the humeral head and abnormal gliding occurs throughout the arc of motion. Barrett et al.[7] reported increased glenoid component loosening in shoulders with a massive rotator cuff tear and attributed this finding to eccentric loading of the glenoid. The glenoid component is clearly subjected to abnormal loads under these circumstances, but a direct correlation between rotator cuff tears and glenoid component loosening has not been reported in other series.[12,22,30–32]

The compressive force of the glenohumeral joint is maximal at 90 degrees of abduction and may rise to one times the body weight, or approximately 7 to 10 times the weight of the extremity (see Figure 2–5).[46] The shear force is maximal at 60 degrees of abduction and can equal 40% of body weight. These forces will be active at the articulation between nonconstrained metal-to-plastic glenohumeral prostheses and therefore introduce issues of polyethylene wear, component loosening, and mechanical failure when performing total shoulder arthroplasty. Glenoid resurfacing must address these known mechanical parameters for successful results. The loading response of the glenohumeral joint with hemiarthroplasty presents different problems with metal-to-bone and/or metal-to-cartilage reactions. Glenoid erosion and incomplete pain relief are potential complications with repetitive or excessive loading. The clinical significance of these problems in total shoulder arthroplasty and hemiarthroplasty are addressed in the following sections.

SOURCES OF SHOULDER PAIN

Pain relief is the primary goal of shoulder arthroplasty and a successful surgical result must address the specific source of pain in each case. The source of pain may be secondary to the disease process, surface incongruity, mechanical impingement, or soft-tissue deficiency. The diagnostic category, physical examination, radiographic picture, and intraopera-

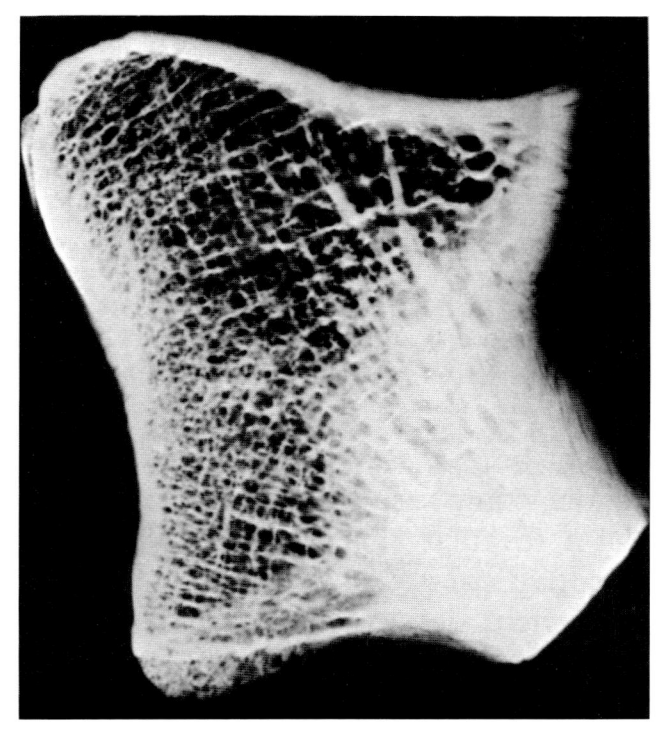

Figure 24–1. Photograph of a cross section of the glenoid showing cancellous bone structure.

tive findings should be considered in selecting appropriate treatment.

The disease process is an important element in predicting the natural history of the shoulder arthropathy and clinical outcome. Patients with intrinsic cartilage abnormalities such as hemochromatosis and calcium pyrophosphate deposition disease, or extrinsic cartilage abnormalities such as rheumatoid arthritis, ankylosing spondylitis, and systemic lupus erythematosus will often present with reactive synovitis and abnormal glenoid anatomy. Failure to remove remaining cartilage may perpetuate the inflammatory response and subsequent pain. Osteoarthritis and osteonecrosis often demonstrate relative sparing of the glenoid and preservation is an appropriate option.[2] The source of pain, however, may be secondary to glenoid incongruity and resurfacing will require an intraoperative decision.

In some cases, mechanical pain has been attributed to proximal migration of the humerus and impingement under the acromion (Figure 24–2).[47,48] Several authors suggested that the presence of preoperative proximal migration indicates a torn or incompetent rotator cuff.[7,49,50] Pain may be due to the tear, impingement, or both. This finding alone is not an indication for glenoid resurfacing. The preceding algorithm that considers diagnosis, surface congruity, and intraoperative findings must be included in treatment selection.

In a previous study of 131 Neer total shoulder arthroplasties, the authors[31] did not find a correlation between postoperative proximal migration and pain. There was a lack of correlation between progressive proximal migration and a documented tear in the rotator cuff. Moreover, there was no correlation between major rotator cuff tears and component loosening, but an association was noted between proximal migration of the humerus and loosening of the glenoid component that was not statistically significant (Figure 24–3). It was not possible to establish a definite or statistically significant connection between proximal migration and any single anatomic or operative variable.

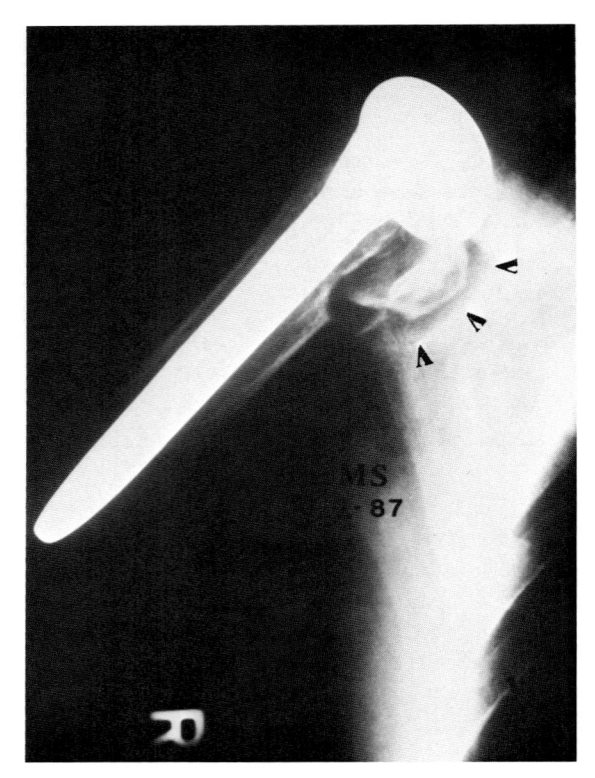

Figure 24–3. Total shoulder arthroplasty with proximal migration and complete radiolucency larger than 2 mm at the glenoid component bone-cement interface.

The authors believe that the development of postoperative proximal migration most likely requires a combination of several factors that may include (1) an increase in the glenoid component facing angle; (2) release of the coracoacromial ligament; (3) an irreparable rotator cuff tear; (4) placement of the humeral component in a proud position; (5) muscle imbalance between a thin, poorly functioning rotator cuff and a strong deltoid; (6) preoperative proximal migration; and (7) diagnosis of cuff tear arthropathy. Proximal migration and massive rotator cuff tears are not absolute indicators for failure in total shoulder arthroplasty. These data do not support routine glenoid resurfacing or the use of a constrained prosthesis for irreparable rotator cuff tears or proximal migration of the humerus.[31]

Periarticular soft-tissue integrity and function are critical for hemiarthroplasty or total shoulder arthroplasty, and soft-tissue reconstruction is an integral part of the operative procedure. Shoulder arthroplasty should be considered before the patient develops end-stage soft-tissue contractures that are not amenable to reconstruction.

HEMIARTHROPLASTY

Glenoid Response to Humeral Prosthesis

The most direct way of monitoring the glenoid response to a humeral prosthesis is following a hemiarthroplasty longitu-

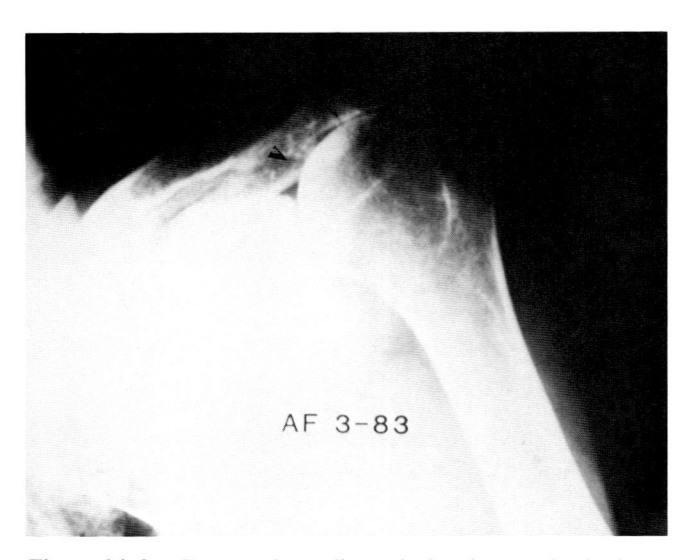

Figure 24–2. Preoperative radiograph showing proximal migration of the humeral head.

dinally with serial radiographs, and looking for sclerosis or erosion that would indicate wear. Topographic changes in the glenoid surface may lead to translation of the humeral head and migration from its normal position in relation to the glenoid. The significance of such findings depends on a corresponding increase in pain, loss of function, decreased implant survivorship, and the prospect of a complex revision procedure. Although these clinical factors have been noted in retrospective reviews of shoulder hemiarthroplasty, no human pathologic specimens or animal models have been studied that would allow assessment of histologic changes at the glenohumeral interface.

An analogous situation is found in hemiarthroplasty of the hip where the problems of pain, erosion, and revision have been studied both in clinical trials and in animal models.[36-39] The femoral head is contained in a true ball-and-socket configuration that is far less dependent on soft-tissue function than the shoulder. Forces across the hip joint reach three to five times the body weight with single-leg stance, which are similar multiples of the peak forces recorded at the glenohumeral joint.[10,46,51,52] Despite these differences, useful information can be extrapolated for shoulder hemiarthroplasty. Cruess et al.[36] evaluated the response of articular cartilage to weight-bearing against metal in hemiarthroplasty of the hip using a dog model. There was an early loss of proteoglycan, followed by surface damage to the cartilage, progressive degenerative changes, and growth of pannus from the articular margins. No normal cartilage was present after 6 weeks and complete cartilage loss was noted after 24 weeks (Figure 24-4). Remodeling of the subchondral bone that conformed to the shape of the prosthesis was found.

The reported incidence of acetabular erosion in humans ranges from 0 to 11%, with variable follow-up. In a review of 258 Thompson hemiarthroplasties, Phillips[39] reported that the level of physical activity and duration of follow-up had the highest correlation with acetabular erosion. The severity of the erosion increased with time only in active patients, but was associated with pain and disability during walking. Bipolar hemiarthroplasty of the hip attempts to reduce the forces at the prosthesis-acetabulum interface but the degree of functional improvement with this modification is uncertain.

The direct application of this information to shoulder arthroplasty may not be biomechanically valid but the following assumptions can be made: (1) Weight-bearing against metal results in breakdown and loss of articular cartilage. (2) The presence of cartilage is not necessary for a satisfactory result with hemiarthroplasty of the hip. (3) Bony erosion is a function of activity level and duration of follow-up. (4) The relatively low incidence of clinically significant erosion with major load-bearing forces in the hip suggests that progressive glenoid erosion may not be a frequent problem.

Clinical Results With Hemiarthroplasty

The early results with prosthetic replacement of the humeral head were documented by Neer in several reports between 1955 and 1964.[1,53-55] As noted previously, the report in 1974[2] represents the first extensive review of this procedure with careful follow-up (average follow-up was 6 years, with a range from 1 to 20 years). Relief of pain and restoration of function were noted in nearly all patients. The success of this study established shoulder hemiarthroplasty as an appropriate and predictable procedure for patients with degenerative arthritis of the shoulder. The use of this device was extended to patients with rheumatoid arthritis and the early reports on a limited number of patients were encouraging. Neer and Cruess[56] reported 26 cases of humeral head replacement for rheumatoid arthritis in 1971, with satisfactory results. Clayton and Ferlic[57] evaluated seven patients with shoulder arthroplasty for rheumatoid arthritis in 1975 and noted success with this treatment, but the average follow-up was less than 1 year. In 1977, Marmor[21] reviewed 10 rheumatoid arthritis patients with shoulder hemiarthroplasty at an average follow-up of 4.5 years. Pain relief was good and preoperative proximal subluxation of the humeral head was not a contraindication to surgery.

More recent studies by numerous authors have evaluated shoulder hemiarthroplasty as the treatment for a variety of shoulder arthropathies.[8,9,11,19] The average follow-up in these studies ranged from 16 months to 3 years, with fewer than 20 patients in each study available for review. In 1990, the results of 64 Neer hemiarthroplasties in 59 patients with an average follow-up of 44 months (range, 24 to 124 months) were reported.[30] The average age was 58, with a range from 29 to 85 years. The diagnoses were rheumatoid arthritis (27 patients), osteoarthritis (10 patients), osteonecrosis (7 patients), and fracture (15 patients). Good pain relief was achieved in 92% of the patients and range of motion improved in all diagnostic categories. The presence of a rotator cuff tear did not significantly alter the results in this review. With longer follow-up the patients with hemiarthroplasty tended to develop increasing pain and the radiographic appearance of subchondral sclerosis and joint space narrowing (Figure 24-5).

A bipolar shoulder implant was developed by Swanson in 1975 and long-term results with this device were reported in 1989.[27] As in the hip, the device is designed to decrease wear between bone and the implant by allowing motion to occur between both the glenoid and bipolar cup and the bipolar cup and humeral head. Swanson et al.[27] reported no glenoid erosion with an average follow-up of 63 months, but progressive superior subluxation of the prosthesis was noted over time. Pain relief was good to excellent in 31 of 35 shoulders and all patients reportedly had improved function postoperatively.

The existing literature on shoulder hemiarthroplasty is limited in terms of both patient numbers and follow-up.[2,8,9,11,19,27] Early results have been uniformly good in all reports. Postoperative motion has been better in the absence of acute trauma in some studies.[19] Incomplete pain relief with hemiarthroplasty in the rheumatoid arthritis population has been noted.[30] Loosening of the humeral prosthesis has

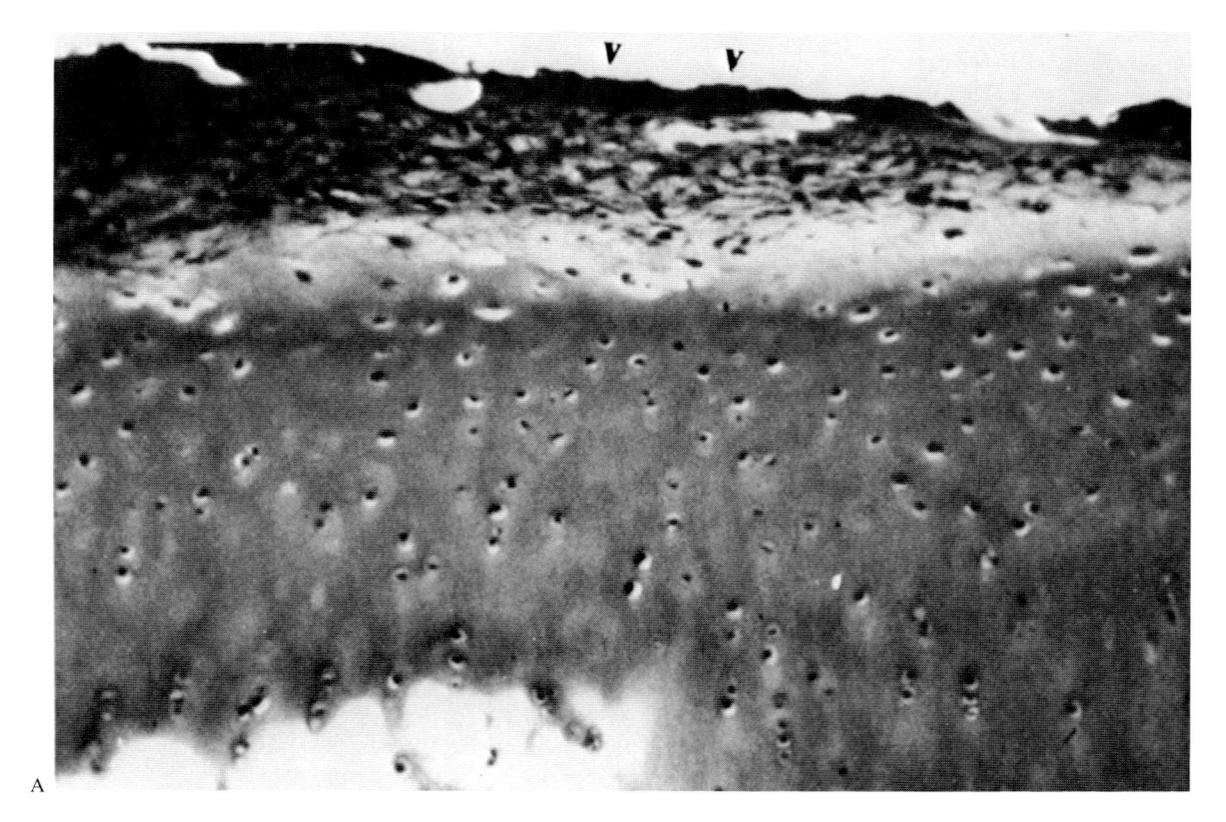

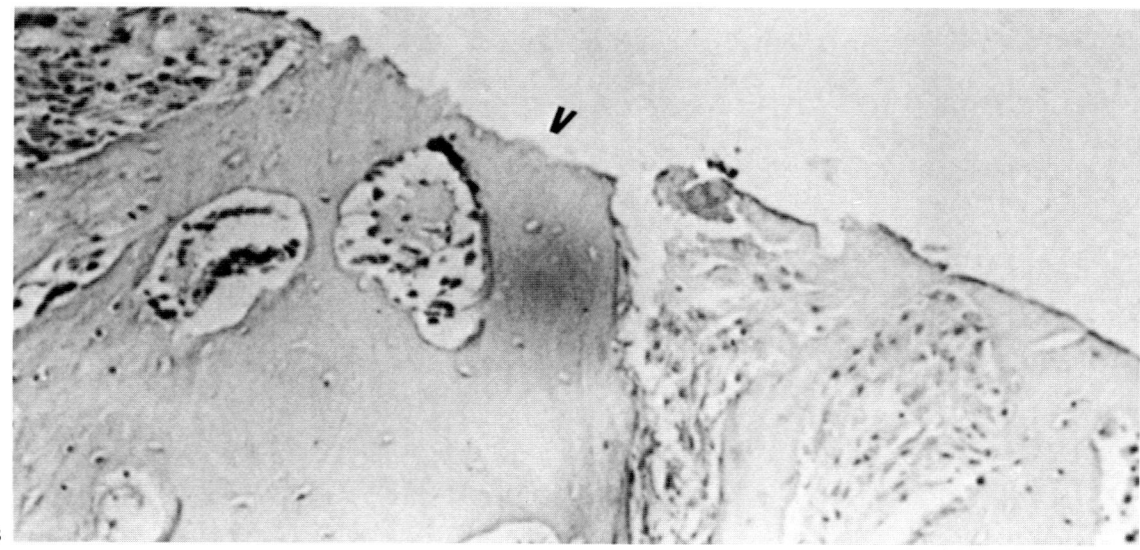

Figure 24-4. Histologic pictures of canine hip cartilage in contact with metal prosthesis. **A.** Pannus overgrowth and underlying cartilage changes at 12 weeks following hip hemiarthroplasty. **B.** Complete cartilage loss and exposed bone in hip harvested at 24 weeks. (Reproduced with permission from Cruess et al.[36])

not been a significant problem with either cemented or uncemented components, although incomplete radiolucent lines have been observed in up to 31% of humeral implants in total shoulder arthroplasty.[18,22] Radiographic evidence of humeral component loosening ranges from 0 to 4% in larger reviews of total shoulder arthroplasty, but this finding has not been reported with hemiarthroplasty.[2,4,8,9,11,12,18,19,26,30] Technical factors that may be important in overall results include (1) maintenance of humeral length, (2) soft-tissue tension, and (3) version of the prosthesis. It is not clear at this time whether issues related to current prosthetic design and modularity are important factors in long-term results.

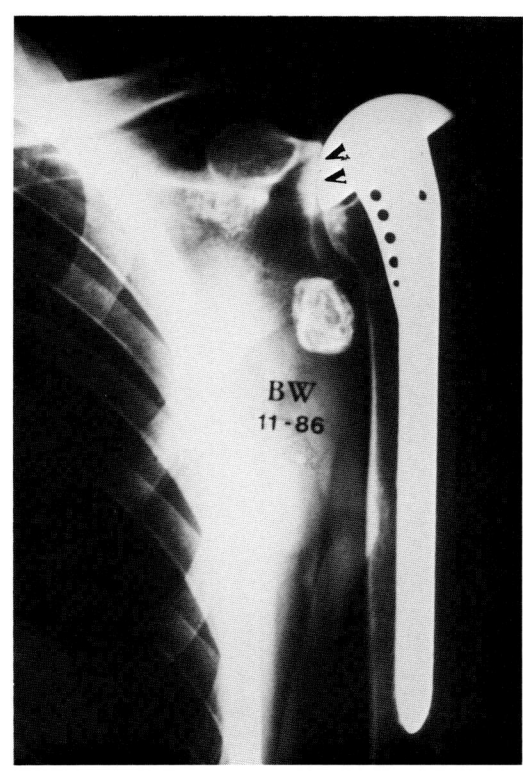

Figure 24–5. Radiograph showing erosion and sclerosis of the glenoid with hemiarthroplasty.

TOTAL SHOULDER ARTHROPLASTY

Glenoid Design

Component fixation remains the primary technical problem in resurfacing the glenoid. The limited depth and cross-sectional area of the glenoid vault restrict the options for mechanical fixation to the scapula. The original design by Neer of an all-polyethylene component with a wedge-shaped keel secured to the glenoid by methylmethacrylate has remained the most commonly used type of implant since its introduction in 1974.[3,12,18,28] The surface area of the glenoid component approximates the size of the natural glenoid, and the radius of curvature is the same as that of the humeral head component, in order to provide slight constraint. Modifications of this design include a metal backing with optional screw fixation and variations in size, shape, and curvature of the polyethylene surface.[4,26,35]

In an extensive finite element analysis of glenoid component designs, Orr et al.[58] reported that with all-polyethylene components, the load was transmitted centrally, and the stresses in the bone near the edges of the component were decreased from those calculated for the natural joint. The metal backing of the component was found to distribute the forces more evenly to the underlying bone and prevent deformation of thin polyethylene. It is unclear if this stress distribution provides significant benefit, as it is not markedly different from the pattern with plastic components. The trade-off is that the metal backing limits the thickness of polyethylene and increases wear at the polyethylene interface and the subsurface areas. In addition, stress shielding of cancellous bone beneath the tray was noted with firm fixation of the metal keel to surrounding bone. In some cases, limited glenoid bone stock may prevent the use of a standard-size metal-backed component and require intraoperative alteration of an all-polyethylene implant to obtain a satisfactory fit. Modification of the polyethylene surface to provide additional constraint and superior coverage of the humeral component has been shown to adversely affect the loading characteristics of the implant and cause loosening.[58,59] The indications for fully constrained total shoulder arthroplasty have been limited by frequent complications that include glenoid loosening, traumatic dislocation, and component failure.[23]

Radiographic evaluation of the glenoid component in total shoulder arthroplasty frequently demonstrates the presence of radiolucent lines at the bone-cement interface. It is important to distinguish between radiolucent lines and true component loosening. As noted previously, the incidence of radiolucent lines ranges from 30 to 89% in different reports but the incidence of radiographically loose glenoid components ranges from 0 to 12% in the same reports.[3,7,8,12,14,28] Loosening is usually defined as definite by the presence of one or more of the following radiographic findings: (1) a complete radiolucent line of 2 mm or more at the bone-cement interface, (2) fracture of the cement mantle, (3) any radiolucent line at the implant-cement interface, and (4) component migration on serial radiographs. It remains speculative if the presence of radiolucent lines less than 2 mm at the bone-cement interface indicate probable loosening (Figure 24–6). Barrett et al.[7] distinguished between radiolucent lines around the flange and those around the keel, and noted that radiolucent lines around the flange alone were not associated with loosening of the component. Migration or dislocation of the component may occur in cases with documented loosening (Figure 24–7).

In most cases the presence of radiolucent lines has not correlated with clinical symptoms in any context. Follow-up beyond 10 years is limited but these findings have not proved to be significant in available reports.[6,30,32,59] An extensive review of these findings with long-term follow-up is necessary to establish the true significance of early radiolucencies surrounding the glenoid component.

The option for using an uncemented glenoid component is provided by some types of metal-backed implants using screw fixation (Figure 24–8). The use of this device requires sufficient bone stock that allows firm purchase with cancellous screws, and in most designs, only two screws can be used for fixation. A glenoid component that relies on a press-fit concept has not been introduced for clinical application at this time. Preliminary results with the uncemented glenoid and screw fixation have been good but insufficient information is currently available to fully evaluate this device. Additional concerns with screw-fixated metal-

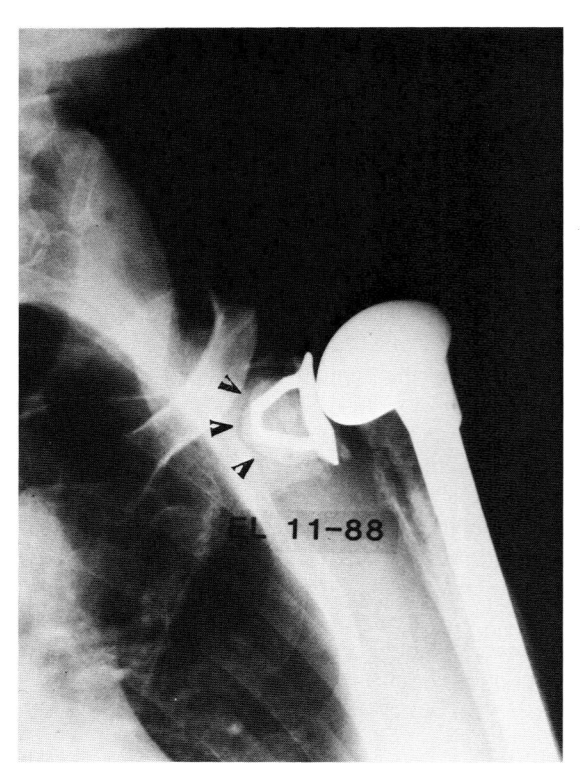

Figure 24–6. Radiograph showing complete radiolucent line less than 2 mm at the glenoid bone-cement interface.

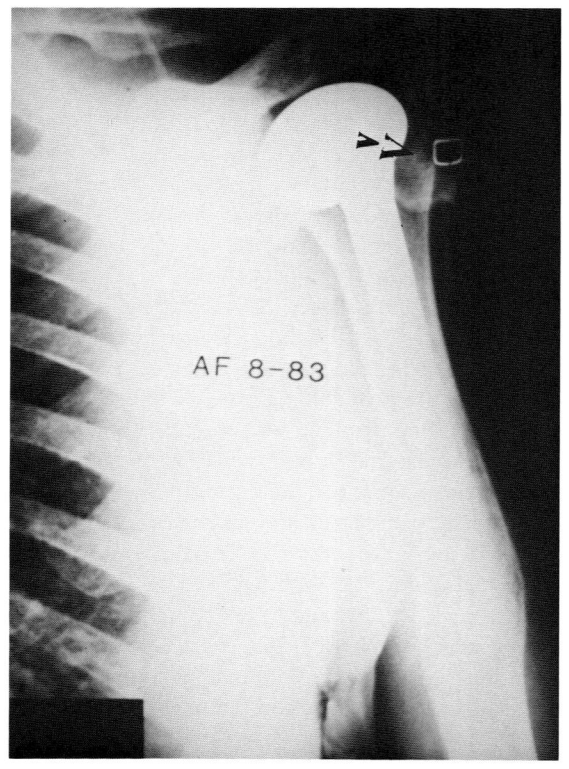

Figure 24–7. Radiograph showing dislocation of a loose all-polyethylene glenoid component in a patient with a preexisting radiolucency greater than 2 mm at the bone-cement interface.

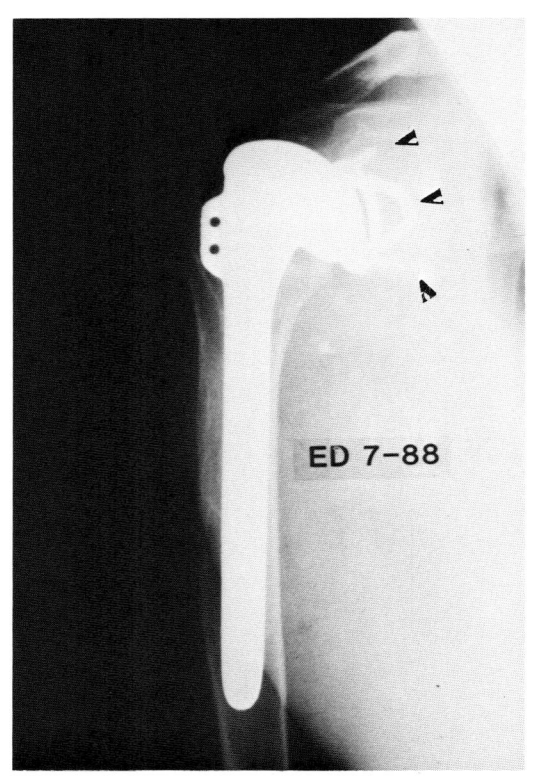

Figure 24–8. Radiograph showing uncemented metal-backed glenoid component implanted with screw fixation.

backed glenoid components include screw osteolysis, component fracture through the screw hole, and accelerated polyethylene wear. Malposition of the glenoid component with subsequent subluxation or dislocation of the humerus has been reported as an infrequent complication in several reports.[4,7,15,25,26,31,32]

Clinical Results with Total Shoulder Arthroplasty

Experience with total shoulder arthroplasty in this country now approaches 20 years. Early designs by Neer, Bickel, Buechel, Post, Amstutz, Gristina, and others were introduced in the 1970s with variable degrees of success. Some of these devices provide mechanical constraint at the glenohumeral joint, but subsequent problems with loosening, material failure, and dislocation led to the use of nonconstrained prostheses in most cases.[60] The initial reviews of total shoulder arthroplasty most often contained patients from multiple diagnostic categories with shoulder arthropathy, but mainly rheumatoid arthritis, osteoarthritis, and posttraumatic arthritis were included.[5,11,14,25,35]

In a report from the Hospital for Special Surgery, Ranawat et al.[25] reviewed 27 patients with 31 total shoulder arthroplasties using four different types of prostheses implanted between 1973 and 1979. Pain relief was good in 22 patients (82%) and functional improvement was noted in 23 patients (85%). Complications included malposition (1), dislocation (3), and glenoid loosening (2).

Amstutz et al.[5] reviewed 11 shoulders using the UCLA total shoulder arthroplasty implanted from 1976 to 1978, and reported excellent pain relief in 9 patients and improved function in 10. Two patients with extensive preoperative soft-tissue deficiencies required reoperation and 1 patient with unrelieved pain was not treated. Technical problems included penetration of the glenoid wall with extravasation of cement in several patients. Shallow glenoid cavities required trimming of the glenoid keel to allow seating of the component.

Coughlin et al.[15] reviewed 16 Stanmore total shoulder arthroplasties in 1979 and reported complete pain relief in only half the patients. There was one recurrent dislocation postoperatively and a loose glenoid component was found on reexploration.

An extensive review of 194 Neer total shoulder arthroplasties was reported by Neer et al. in 1982, with follow-up ranging from 24 to 99 months.[3] A subgroup of patients from this population was assigned to a separate "limited goals" category because of severe bone or soft-tissue deficiencies. Of the 150 patients in the regular rehabilitation program, 129 (86%) achieved an excellent or satisfactory rating. Only 4 patients from the total group thought that they had not benefited from the procedure. The authors concluded that neither bone loss nor a deficient rotator cuff was a contraindication to nonconstrained total shoulder arthroplasty. Complications included infection (1), dislocation (4), subluxation (2), and malposition (2).

Cofield[12] compared his results with Neer in a review of 73 Neer total shoulder arthroplasties implanted at the Mayo Clinic between 1975 and 1979. Forty-eight (73%) of 66 patients in the regular rehabilitation program had an excellent or satisfactory result. Complications included axillary nerve laceration (1), reflex sympathetic dystrophy (2), wound hematoma (1), pulmonary embolism (1), nonunion of tuberosity osteotomy (1), and symptomatic loosening of the glenoid (4). In contrast to the study by Neer, Cofield[12] had no shoulders with instability, but 80% showed a radiolucent line at the glenoid bone-cement interface. Eight glenoid components were definitely loose by roentgenographic criteria and three required revision for pain.

In 1983, Thornhill et al.[28] reviewed 140 Neer total shoulder arthroplasties performed between 1974 and 1981 and reported good pain relief in 91% of patients. Range of motion and function improved in nearly all patients. The complications were dislocation (4), humerus fracture (4), and axillary nerve palsy (1). Radiolucent lines were noted around 80% of the glenoid components but none were clinically symptomatic.

In 1987, Barrett et al.[7] reported a prospective study of 50 Neer total shoulder arthroplasties with an average follow-up of 3.5 years (range, 2.0 to 7.5 years). Forty-four shoulders (88%) had no significant pain and 48 (94%) had improved function. Reported complications included malposition (1), subluxation (1), intraoperative humerus fracture (2), axillary nerve injury (1), and cement extrusion with decreased motion (1). In 4 shoulders, the glenoid component shifted position and required revision for pain. The presence of a massive rotator cuff tear in these 4 shoulders and subsequently in 3 additional shoulders led Barrett et al. to relate the rotator cuff tear and altered shoulder kinematics to glenoid component loosening.

Hawkins[18] reviewed 70 Neer total shoulder arthroplasties in 1989 that were performed between 1975 and 1983 with an average follow-up of 48 months (range, 24 to 103 months) and reported satisfactory pain relief in 91% of the shoulders. No difference in pain relief was noted between patients with osteoarthritis and those with rheumatoid arthritis, but improvement in postoperative motion was significantly better in the osteoarthritis group. Complications included two intraoperative glenoid and two intraoperative humerus fractures. Symptomatic glenoid loosening requiring revision occurred in two patients.

In most reviews, rheumatoid arthritis is the largest diagnostic category requiring total shoulder arthroplasty for end-stage shoulder arthropathy. Several authors have specifically addressed total shoulder arthroplasty in the rheumatoid population, which often includes patients with complex bone and soft-tissue deficiencies.[6,20,22] Pain relief has been excellent in most reports, and functional activity often improves after total shoulder arthroplasty despite small changes in range of motion.

Kelly and Foster[20] reviewed 42 Neer total shoulder arthroplasties in rheumatoid arthritis patients and found good pain relief in 88% of the shoulders. Subjective improvement was reported by most patients despite modest gains in motion. Glenoid bone stock deficiencies were found in 26 shoulders (62%) and rotator cuff disease in 34 shoulders (81%). The authors concluded that there was a poor correlation between range of motion and functional recovery. In addition, neither the state of the rotator cuff at surgery nor the recorded quality of rotator cuff repair predicted a poor result. Complications included one intraoperative fracture of the glenoid and one of the humerus.

McCoy et al.[22] evaluated 29 Neer total shoulder arthroplasties in rheumatoid arthritis patients performed between 1975 and 1983, and found significant pain relief in 93% of the patients. Pain relief was not significantly affected by the presence of rotator cuff disease, which was found in 38% of the patients. Full-thickness tears were found in 7 patients (24%). Postoperative motion and function were limited compared to other disease states. Radiographs demonstrated nonprogressive radiolucent lines around 86% of the glenoid components and 31% of the humeral components, but no clinically significant loosening was noted.

Barrett et al.[6] reviewed 140 total shoulder arthroplasties in patients with polyarticular rheumatoid arthritis performed between 1974 and 1984 at the Robert Breck Brigham and Brigham and Women's Hospital, with an average follow-up of 5 years (range, 2 to 11 years). A Neer humeral component was used in 133 shoulders and a Gristina monospherical component in 7. Standard plastic glenoid components were used in 121 shoulders and metal-backed components in 19. All glenoid components were cemented. Rotator cuff abnormalities were found in 80% of the shoulders and 45% (62 shoulders) had either a moderate-size or massive tear. Excellent pain relief was reported in 93% of the patients. Average preoperative forward elevation was 56 degrees and improved to 90 degrees postoperatively. A press-fit of the humeral component was used in 95 shoulders and subsidence ranging from 4 to 7 mm was noted on follow-up radiographs in 5 shoulders (5%). No long-term symptoms were associated with this degree of subsidence and no humeral components were revised. Radiolucent lines were found around 82% of the glenoids with 2-year follow-up. Two glenoids migrated secondary to loosening, and 10 were thought to be loose based on the width and progression of radiolucent lines. There were two dislocations, two malpositions, two axillary nerve palsies, and one intraoperative cardiac arrest.

Thomas et al.[59] reviewed 30 DANA total shoulder arthroplasties performed in rheumatoid arthritis patients from 1976 through 1988 with an average follow-up of 46 months (range, 24 to 120 months). Pain and function improved but motion remained unchanged. Two glenoid components were revised for loosening.

HEMIARTHROPLASTY VERSUS TOTAL SHOULDER ARTHROPLASTY

Extensive reviews of total shoulder arthroplasty are currently available, with average follow-ups ranging from 37 to 60 months.[3,6,7,11,18,22,29] The results with hemiarthroplasty have most often been derived from early reviews of small series with average follow-ups ranging from 36 to 72 months.[2,9,21] Clinical findings to date indicate that good results can be achieved in 82 to 93% of patients treated with hemiarthroplasty or total shoulder arthroplasty. More recent data have allowed accurate comparison of hemiarthroplasty with total shoulder arthroplasty in patient populations similar in age, gender, rotator cuff function, preoperative range of motion, and diagnostic category.[30]

Replacement of both the humeral and glenoid surfaces provides excellent pain relief in more than 90% of patients in all diagnostic categories. In the absence of glenoid surface incongruity and synovitis, hemiarthroplasty provides levels of pain relief similar to those after total shoulder arthroplasty in patients with humeral head fractures, osteoarthritis, and osteonecrosis. Smooth, eburnated bone devoid of cartilage does not compromise the results with hemiarthroplasty.[2,30] Hemiarthroplasty does not appear to provide pain relief comparable to total shoulder arthroplasty in patients with inflammatory arthropathies, intrinsic cartilage abnormalities, or severe glenoid erosion.[8,11,30] Residual pain in rheumatoid arthritis patients with hemiarthroplasty may be secondary to retained cartilage and ongoing synovitis or the articulation of metal against abnormal bone stock.

A comparison of postoperative motion in patients with hemiarthroplasty and total shoulder arthroplasty parallels the results with pain relief.[7,11,12,27,30] Patients with osteoarthritis, osteonecrosis, or posttraumatic arthritis obtain comparable postoperative motion and function with either hemiarthroplasty or total shoulder arthroplasty. In the rheumatoid arthritis population, preoperative motion is often severely limited and subsequent postoperative gains are proportionately reduced with any type of arthroplasty.[59] In most studies, rheumatoid arthritis patients obtain slightly better motion with total shoulder arthroplasty than hemiarthroplasty.[6,11,21,30] The improved pain relief may allow for easier rehabilitation and greater use of the extremity. With effective pain relief, functional improvement may be secondary to increased scapulothoracic motion in addition to gains at the glenohumeral joint. The presence of a rotator cuff tear, with or without preoperative proximal migration, does not dictate the type of prosthesis to be used. The diagnostic category and condition of the glenoid remain the most significant factors in selecting hemiarthroplasty or total shoulder arthroplasty. An irreparable tear or incompetent rotator cuff will compromise the functional result, but pain relief is unaffected in most cases.[3,12,18,20,22,31,59]

The authors believe that overall pain relief, range of motion, and patient satisfaction are better with total shoulder arthroplasty than hemiarthroplasty in the rheumatoid arthritis population. Total shoulder arthroplasty with glenoid resurfacing is the recommended procedure of choice in patients with intrinsic cartilage abnormalities and inflammatory arthropathies, except in cases with inadequate bone stock to support a glenoid component. Significant glenoid erosion may require bone grafting and resurfacing in selected cases. Anecdotal evidence from several authors suggests that hemiarthroplasty may be a satisfactory salvage procedure in patients with massive loss of glenoid bone stock.[6,59] In this situation, the humeral component serves as a spacer that improves the kinematics of the shoulder and often provides some degree of pain relief.

Hemiarthroplasty is recommended for osteoarthritis, osteonecrosis, and acute three- and four-part fractures of the humeral head with relative preservation of glenoid congruity and absent synovitis. Patients with normal muscle strength and function will experience significant compressive forces at the glenohumeral joint approaching one times the body weight. With follow-up longer than 5 years, patients with hemiarthroplasty may develop increasing pain and the radiographic appearance of subchondral sclerosis and joint space narrowing of the superior portion of the glenoid.[11,30] Reoperation with glenoid resurfacing may be indicated under these conditions. Recent component designs with modular humeral heads may facilitate exposure for late glenoid resurfacing. The development of these signs and symptoms is a factor of muscle strength, activity level, and length of follow-up. Young, active patients with hemiarthroplasty are more likely to demonstrate glenoid erosion over time.

The incidence of symptomatic glenoid loosening ranges from 0 to 12% in reviews, with average follow-ups ranging from 37 to 55 months.[3,7,8,12,14,28] The significance of nonprogressive radiolucent lines at the bone-cement interface is unknown, but no consistent correlation has been shown with pain relief, range of motion, motor power, or functional improvement. Radiographic lucencies, however, have not proved to be reliable indicators of clinically significant loosening. In a review of failed total shoulder arthroplasty by Boyd et al.,[32] only four of seven grossly loose glenoids revised for pain demonstrated a complete radiolucency greater than 2 mm at the bone-cement interface. Five of 16 humeral components were grossly loose at surgery, yet none demonstrated this roentgenograpic finding.

The causes of glenoid loosening are thought to be multifactorial and include (1) poor-quality and deficient bone stock, (2) technical limitations in fixation, and (3) proximal migration. A statistically significant correlation between rotator cuff tears and glenoid component loosening has not been conclusively demonstrated. Post et al.[24] showed that compressive forces at the glenohumeral joint are greatly diminished where muscle power is weak. The combination of decreased loads across the glenoid component and limited activity levels in rheumatoid arthritis may contribute to the increased survivorship of these components in this group as reported by Brenner et al.[61]

In conclusion, the benefits of preserving the glenoid include (1) shorter operative time, (2) elimination of potential component loosening and polyethylene wear, (3) a bone-sparing procedure, (4) a functional result equal to that after total shoulder arthroplasty, and (5) a greater functional activity range. Disadvantages of this procedure include (1) incomplete pain relief in specific patient populations, and (2) long-term effects of progressive cartilage wear. The underlying diagnosis and glenoid surface features should guide the selection of hemiarthroplasty or total shoulder arthroplasty. Parallel survivorship analysis studies are needed to compare the relative complication of progressive glenoid erosion in hemiarthroplasty versus glenoid component loosening in total shoulder arthroplasty.

REFERENCES

1. Neer CS II. Articular replacement of the humeral head. *J Bone and Joint Surg [Am]* 1955;37:215–228.
2. Neer CS. Replacement arthroplasty for glenohumeral arthritis. *J Bone Joint Surg [Am]* 1974;56:1–13.
3. Neer CS, Watson KC, Stanton FJ. Recent experience in total shoulder replacement. *J Bone Joint Surg [Am]* 1982;64:319–337.
4. Amstutz HC, Thomas BJ, Kabo JM, Jinnah RH, Dorey FJ. The DANA total shoulder arthroplasty. *J Bone Joint Surg [Am]* 1988;70:1174–1182.
5. Amstutz HC, Sew Hoy AL, Clarke IC. UCLA anatomic total shoulder arthroplasty. *Clin Orthop* 1981;155:7–20.
6. Barrett WP, Thornhill TS, Thomas WH, Gebhart EM, Sledge CB. Nonconstrained total shoulder arthroplasty in patients with polyarticular rheumatoid arthritis. *J Arthroplasty* 1989;4:91–96.
7. Barrett WP, Franklin JL, Jackins SE, Wyss CR, Matsen FA. Total shoulder arthroplasty. *J Bone Jont Surg [Am]* 1987;69:865–872.
8. Bell SN, Gschwend N. Clinical experience with total arthroplasty and hemiarthroplasty of the shoulder using the Neer prosthesis. *Int Orthop* 1986;10:217–222.
9. Bodey WN, Yeoman PM. Prosthetic arthroplasty of the shoulder. *Acta Orthop Scand* 1983;54:900–903.
10. Buechel FF, Pappas MJ, DePalma AF. "Floating-socket" total shoulder replacement: Anatomical, biomechanical, and surgical rationale. *J Biomed Mater Res* 1978;12:89–114.
11. Clayton ML, Ferlic DC, Jeffers PD. Prosthetic arthroplasties of the shoulder. *Clin Orthop* 1982;164:184–191.
12. Cofield RH. Total shoulder arthroplasty with the Neer prosthesis. *J Bone Joint Surg [Am]* 1984;66:899–906.
13. Cofield RH. Unconstrained total shoulder prostheses. *Clin Orthop* 1983;173:97–108.
14. Cofield RH. Total joint arthroplasty—The shoulder. *Mayo Clin Proc* 1979;54:500–506.
15. Coughlin MJ, Morris JM, West WF. The semiconstrained total shoulder arthroplasty. *J Bone Joint Surg [Am]* 1979;61:574–581.
16. Friedman RJ, Thornhill TS, Thomas WH, Sledge CB. Nonconstrained total shoulder replacement in patients who have rheumatoid arthritis and class IV function. *J Bone Joint Surg [Am]* 1989;71:494–498.
17. Gristina AG, Romano RL, Kammire GC, Webb LX. Total shoulder replacement. *Orthop Clin North Am* 1987;18:445–453.
18. Hawkins RJ, Bell RH, Jallay B. Total shoulder arthroplasty. *Clin Orthop* 1989;242:188–194.
19. Kay SP, Amstutz HC. Shoulder hemiarthroplasty at UCLA. *Clin Orthop* 1988;228:42–48.
20. Kelly IG, Foster RS. Neer total shoulder replacement in rheumatoid arthritis. *J Bone Joint Surg [Br]* 1987;69:723–726.
21. Marmor L. Hemiarthroplasty for the rheumatoid shoulder joint. *Clin Ortop* 1977;122:201–203.
22. McCoy SR, Warren RF, Bade HA III, Ranawat CS, Inglis AE. Total shoulder arthroplasty in rheumatoid arthritis. *J Arthroplasty* 1989;4:105–113.
23. Post M, Jablon M. Constrained total shoulder arthroplasty: Long-term follow-up observations. *Clin Orthop* 1983;173:109–116.
24. Post M, Haskell SS, Jablon M. Total shoulder replacement with a constrained prosthesis. *J Bone Joint Surg [Am]* 1980;62:327–335.
25. Ranawat CS, Warren R, Inglis AE. Total shoulder replacement arthroplasty. *Orthop Clin North Am* 1980;11:367–373.
26. Roper BA, Paterson JMH, Day WH. The Roper-Day total shoulder replacement. *J Bone Joint Surg [Br]* 1990;72:694–697.
27. Swanson AB, de Groot Swanson G, Sattel AB, Cendo RD, Hynes D, Wei JN. Bipolar implant shoulder arthroplasty: Long-term results. *Clin Orthop* 1989;249:227–247.
28. Thornhill TS, Thomas WH, Averill RM, et al. Total shoulder arthroplasty: The Brigham experience. *Orthop Trans* 1983;7:497.
29. Weiss AC, Adams MA, Moore JR, Weiland AJ. Unconstrained shoulder arthroplasty: A five-year average follow-up study. *Clin Orthop* 1990;257:86–90.
30. Boyd AD, Thornhill TS, Thomas WH, Scott RD, Sledge CB. Total shoulder replacement vs. hemiarthroplasty: Indications for glenoid resurfacing. *J Arthroplasty* 1990;5:329–336.
31. Boyd AD, Thornhill TS, Ewald FC, Scott RD, Sledge CB. Post-operative humeral migration in total shoulder replacement: Incidence and significance. *J Arthroplasty* 1991;6:31–37.

32. Boyd AD, Thomas WH, Sledge CB, Thornhill TS. Failed shoulder arthroplasty. *Orthop Trans* 1990;14:597.
33. Franklin JL, Jackins SE, Matsen FA. Glenoid loosening in total shoulder arthroplasty: An association with rotator cuff deficiency. *Orthop Trans* 1987;11:466.
34. Driessnack RP, Ferlic DC, Wiedel JD. Dissociation of the glenoid component in the Macnab/English total shoulder arthroplasty. *J Arthroplasty* 1990;5:15–18.
35. Neer CS, Kirby RM. Revision of humeral head and total shoulder arthroplasties. *Clin Orthop* 1982;170:189–195.
36. Cruess RL, Kwok DC, Pham Ngoc D, Lecavalier MA, Geng-Ting D. The response of articular cartilage to weight-bearing against metal: A study of hemiarthroplasty of the hip in the dog. *J Bone Joint Surg [Br]* 1984;66:592.
37. Devas M, Hinves B. Prevention of acetabular erosion after hemiarthroplasty for fractured neck of femur. *J Bone Joint Surg [Br]* 1983;65:548–551.
38. Leyson RL, Matthews JP. Acetabular erosion and the mong "hard top" hip prosthesis. *J Bone Joint Surg [Br]* 1984;66:172–174.
39. Phillips TW. Thompson hemiarthroplasty and acetabular erosion. *J Bone Joint Surg [Am]* 1989;71:913–917.
40. Sarrifian SK. Gross and functional anatomy of the shoulder. *Clin Orthpo* 1983;213:11.
41. Saha AK. Dynamic stability of the glenohumeral joint. *Acta Orthop Scand* 1971;42:491.
42. Saha AK. Mechanics of elevation of glenohumeral joint. *Acta Orthop Scand* 1973;44:668.
43. Galinat BJ, Howell SM. The containment mechanism: The primary stabilizer of the glenohumeral joint. *Orthop Trans* 1987;11:458.
44. Hollinshead WH. *Anatomy for Surgeons: The Back and Limbs.* 3rd ed. 1982:300. Harper and Row, Philadelphia.
45. Poppen NK, Walker PS. Normal and abnormal motion of the shoulder. *J Bone Joint Surg [Am]* 1976;58:195–201.
46. Poppen NK, Walker PS. Forces at the glenohumeral joint in abduction. *Clin Orthop* 1978;135:165–170.
47. Ozaki J, Fujimoto S, Nakagawa Y, et al. Tears of the rotator cuff of the shoulder associated with pathological changes in the acromion. A study in cadavera. *J Bone Joint Surg [Am]* 1988;70:1224–1230.
48. Weiner DS, MacNab I. Superior migration of the humeral head. A radiological aid in the diagnosis of tears of the rotator cuff. *J Bone Joint Surg [Br]* 1970;52:524–527.
49. Neer CS II. Impingement lesions. *Clin Orthop* 1983;173:70–77.
50. Rockwood CA. The role of anterior impingement syndrome to lesions of the rotator cuff. *J Bone Joint Surg [Br]* 1980;62:274–275.
51. McLeish RD, Charnley J. Abduction force in the one-legged stance. *J Biomech* 1970;3:191–209.
52. Crowninshield RD, Johnston RC, Andrews JG, Brand RA. A biomechanical investigation of the human hip. *J Biomech* 1978;11:75–85.
53. Neer CS II. Prosthetic replacement of the humeral head. Indications and operative technique. *Surg Clin North Am* 1963;43:1581–1597.
54. Neer CS II. Articular replacement of the humeral head. *J Bone Joint Surg [Am]* 1964;46:1607–1610.
55. Neer CS II. Degenerative lesions of the proximal humeral articular surface. *Clin Orthop* 1961;20:116–125.
56. Neer CS II. The rheumatoid shoulder. In: Cruess RE, ed. Surgery of rheumatoid arthritis. Philadelphia: JB Lippincott, 1971:117.
57. Clayton ML, Ferlic DC. Surgery of the shoulder in rheumatoid arthritis: A report of nineteen patients. *Clin Orthop* 1975;106:166–174.
58. Orr TE, Carter DR, Schurmann DJ. Stress analyses of glenoid component designs. *Clin Orthop* 1988;232:217–224.
59. Thomas BJ, Amstutz C, Cracchiolo A. Shoulder arthroplasty for rheumatoid arthritis. *Clin Orthop* 1991;265:125–128.
60. Neer CS II. Unconstrained shoulder arthroplasty. *Instr Course Lect* 1985;34:278–286.
61. Brenner BC, Ferlic DC, Clayton ML, Dennis DA. Survivorship of unconstrained total shoulder arthroplasty. *J Bone Joint Surg [Am]* 1989;71:1289–1296.

Index

(Italic page numbers indicate a table or a figure.)

Abduction, 106–107
Achilles tendon allograft, 256, *257*
Acromial fixation, 13
Acromioclavicular joint, 27, 145, 268
Acromion, 80
Acromionectomy, 5
Acromioplasty, 4
Acropole prosthesis, 16
Acrylic prosthesis, 5, *6*
Acute fractures, 46
Age, patient's, 197, 200, 207, 283
Allografts, 222, 255, *257*
American Shoulder and Elbow Surgeons form, *42*, *43*, 159
Anatomy, 27–29
    and bipolar shoulder arthroplasty, 263
    surgical, 80
    and unstable shoulder arthroplasty, 254–255
Anesthesia, 70–78
    general *see* General anesthesia
    local, 76
    regional *see* Regional anesthesia
Anterior humeral circumflex vessels, 83
Anterior instability, 237, 254–255, 256, 260
Apatite-associated destructive arthritis, 204
Arm elevation, 32, 104–106
Arthritis
    apatite-associated destructive, 204
    glenohumeral, 8, 41, 46, 194–213, 234, 238
    idiopathic destructive (IDA), 204
    posttraumatic, 46, *47–48*, *50*, 278
    see also Arthritis of dislocation; Rheumatoid arthritis
Arthritis of dislocation, 194–203
    clinical presentation, 197–198
    diagnosis failure, 194–195
    etiology, 194–197
    nonsurgical factors, 194
    physical examination, 198
    radiologic evaluation, 199–200
    rehabilitation, 202
    summing up, 202–203
    surgical considerations, 194, 200–202
    tumors, 218–223
Arthrodesis, 134–145, 150, 207
    arthroplasty versus, *135*
    complications, 143–144
    contraindications, 141
    extra-articular, 134
    indications, 137–141
    intra-articular, 134–135
    optimum position, 136–137
    pain, 145
    preoperative diagnosis, *138*
    reconstruction, 139
    results, *140*, 144–145
    shoulder joint destruction, 139–140
    technique, 134–136, 141–143
Arthropathy, 204
Arthroplasty *see* Shoulder arthroplasty
Arthroscopy, 196–197, 236
Articular cartilage, 147, 205
Aspirin, 77
Assisted stretching exercises
    abduction, 104, 106–107
    elevation, 104–106
    external rotation, 104, 106
    internal rotation, 105, 106
    supine elevation, 103
Axillary nerve, 80, 84
Axiohumeral muscle group, 29
Axioscapular muscle group, 29

Ball and socket prosthesis, 9–10, *11*, *12*, 36, 266
Basic calcium phosphate (BCP) crystals, 204, 206
BCP *see* Basic calcium phosphate (BCP) crystals
Biangular prosthesis, 19, 22, 289, *293*
Biceps muscle, 219–220, *221–222*
Bimodular prosthesis, 19, *21*, 22, 289
Biologic fixation, 282–283
Biopsy, 217–218, 236
Bipolar prosthesis, 17–18, 309
Bipolar shoulder arthroplasty, 265–279
    advantages, 266–267
    anatomic considerations, 265
    definition of, 266
    history, 266
    implants, 265–267
    results, 272–279
        complications and revisions, 278–279
        evaluation methods, 272–277
    surgical procedure, 267–272
        contraindications, 267
        indications, 267–268
        postoperative care, 267–272
        technique, 268, 269–271, 272
Bone
    cement interface, 62–63, *312*, 315
    cysts, 158, 165
    grafting, 145, 257, *259*, 260, 261
    heterotopic new formation, 67
    hook, *86*, 87, *88*
    ingrowth, 66, 281, 285, *289*, 295–296
    in rheumatoid arthritis, 158
    subchondral, 36, 158
Brachial plexus, 70, 74–76, 153
Bristow procedure, 196
Bursa, 119, 123, *124*, 207, 263

Callus formation, 298, *299*
Capsular flap tissue, 296, *297*, *299*
Capsule, 29, 85, *86*, 165, 200–201
Cardiac disease, 77–78
Cemented components, 64
Cemented prosthesis, 10
Cement fixation, 19, 281–282

317

Cementless shoulder arthroplasty, 281–303
   avascular necrosis, 298
   biologic fixation, 282–283
   cement fixation, 281–282
   clinical results, 284–289
   component loosening, 281
   four-part fractures, 298, *300*
   hemiarthroplasty and biologic resurfacing of glenoid, 296–298
   hybrid, 301, *303*
   remodeling, 283–284
   stable fixation, 283
   summing up, 301–303
   technique, 289–296
Cephalic vein, *82*, 83, 165
Cervical plexus, 70, 76
Chondrosarcoma, 215
Chronic fractures, 190
Clavicle, 80, 219, 221
Complications, 242–253
   arthrodesis, 143–144
   bipolar, 265–279
   constrained surgery, 232, 242
      non-rheumatoid, 250
      rheumatoid arthritis, 245
   hemiarthroplasty, 242, *243*
   of metal, 195–196
   Neer II Total Shoulder, 229–231
   nonconstrained surgery, 242
      non-rheumatoid, 242–245
      rheumatoid arthritis, 245, 250
   summing up, 252–254
Component
   cemented, 64
   constrained arthroplasty, 35
   dissociation, 67
   failure, 155, 234
   fixation, 311
   fracture, 67
   glenoid, 9–10, 19, *21*, 22, 37, 45, 208, 231, *252*
      loosening, 14, 64, *65*, 66, 155, 168, 229, 234–236, 238, 251, 314–315
      resurfacing, 311–312
      retroverted, 257, *258*, 260, *261*, 281
   humeral, 19, *20*, 37, 61–62, 95, 152–153, 237, *244–245*, 266, 289
      loosening, 64, *65*, 66, 190, 208, 281
   polyacetal, 22, *23*
   polyethylene, 282, *283*, 285, 289, 294, 296, 306
   uncemented, 63
Computerized tomography (CT), 53, 63, 162, 199, 201, 217
Constrained arthoplasty, 266
   components, 35
   nonrheumatoid, 250
   results, 207–208, 227–233
   rheumatoid arthritis, 245
Constrained prosthesis, 10, 14, 36–37, 45
Continuous passive motion, 110–111
Coracoid, 80
Core depression, 174–175
Corticosteroids, 77, 207
Crystal induced theory, 206
CT *see* Computerized tomography
Cuff tear arthropathy, 204–205
Cysts, 165

DANA (designed after natural anatomy) total shoulder, 13, 208, 233, 314

Débridement, 150, 164, 206
Deltoid muscle, 29, 83, 165, 187, 200, 202, 221, 265
Dislocation, 63–64, 194–203, 254–255
   see also Arthritis of dislocation
Displaced fractures, 183
Dissociation of components, 67
Drill, 91–92, *93*
Drugs *see* Medications; Narcotics

Elevation, 32, 100, 103, 104–106, 159
External fixation, 136
External rotation, 100–101
Extra-articular arthrodesis, 134

Facing angle, 61, *62*
Fascia lata graft, 296, 298
Fibula autograft, 1, *3*, *4*
Fixation
   acromial, 13
   biologic, 282–283
   cement, 19, 281–282
   component, 311
   external, 136
   internal, 135–136, 144
   scapular, 10, *11*, 12, 284–285, *286*
   screw, 10, *11*, 13, 22, *23*, 311, *312*
   stable, 283
Flail shoulder, 138, *139*
Forces, across glenohumeral joint, 29–32
Four-part fracture, 183, 184, *186*, *187*, 289, *295*, 298, 300, 314
Fractures, 67, 294
   acute, 46
   chronic, 190
   component, 67
   displaced, 183
   four-part, 183, 184, *186*, *187*, 289, *295*, *298*, *300*, 314
   head impression, 184
   head-splitting, 184
   humerus, 144, 155–156, 239
   proximal humeral, 1, 170–171, *172*, 183–193
   three-part, 184, 314
   valgus impacted four-part, 183, *186*
Functional improvement, 227–228, 275

General anesthesia, 76–78, 219
   cardiac disease, 77–78
   coexisting disease, 77
   joint and inflammatory disease, 77
   perioperative considerations, 76–77
   pulmonary disease, 78
Glenohumeral joint, 27, 29–35, 306–307
   arthritis, 8, 41, 46, 115, 194–213, 234, 238
      see also Rotator cuff
   arthrodesis, 143–144, 164
   dislocation, 194–203
   function, 265
   instability, 43, 237
   osteoarthritis, 147–157
      arthritis comparison, 149
      clinical presentation, 147–150
      complications, 154–155
      conservative treatment, 150
      contraindications, 153–154
      débridement, 150, 164
      difficulties, 155–156
      operative treatment, 150–153
      pathophysiology, 147

rehabilitation, 156–157
results, 157
Glenoid, 45, 153, 178, 201–202, 307
arthritis, 234, 238
bone deficiencies, 238
cavity, 27–28, 165
component, 9–10, 19, *21*, 22, 37, 45, 208, 231, *252*
loosening, 14, 64, *65*, 66, 155, 168, 229, 234–236, 238, 251, 314–315
retroverted, 257, *258*, 260, *261*, 280
design, 311–312
prosthesis, 19, *20–21*, 22, 91–92, *93–96*
response to humeral prosthesis, 308–310
resurfacing, 306–315
anatomy and biomechanics, 306–307
biologic, 296–298
clinical results, 312–314
component design, 311–312
hemiarthroplasty, 296–298, 308–310, 314–315
pain sources, 307–308
tilt, 53, *56*
Global Shoulder System, 22, 288
Greater tuberosity, 201, 234, 265, 268

Hand function, 224
Hardware, 195–196, 202
Head impression fractures, 184
Head-splitting fractures, 184
Hemiarthroplasty, 164, 190, 242, 265, 306
biologic resurfacing of glenoid and, 296–298, 308–310, 314–315
complications, 242, *243*
humeral, 234–240
rehabilitation, 212
rotator cuff defects and arthritis, 208–212
technique, 209, *210–211*, 212
total shoulder arthroplasty versus, 314–315
Heterotopic new bone formation, 67
High-grade tumors *see* Tumors
Hip joint, 29
Humeral region, 239–240
anterior circumflex vessels, 83
component, 19, *20*, 37, 61–62, 95, 152–153, 237, *244–245*, 266, 289
loosening, 64, *65*, 66, 190, 208, 281
fractures, 1, 144, 155–156, 170–171, *172*, 183–193, 239
head, 1, 15, 27–32, 34, 37, 44, 86–98, 165–166, *174*, 178–179, 183, *191*, 265, 268
hemiarthroplasties, 234–240
humerus, 91, 144, 201, 219, 221, 239, 284
prosthesis, 19, *20*, 96, 242, 266, *293*, 295, 310–311
retroversion, 53, *55*, 61–62
Hydroxyapatite, 280, *283*

Idiopathic destructive arthritis (IDA), 204
Imaging studies, 44–45
see also Radiology
Implant *see* Prosthesis
Infection, 46, *50*, 143, 153–154, 163, 239, 279
Inferior instability, 237, 254, 262
Inflammatory disease, 77
Instability, 43–44, 140, 154, 238, 254–262
anterior, 237, 254–255, 256, 260
classification and pathologic anatomy, 254–255
degree and direction, 194–196
evaluation and treatment, 257–262
inferior, 237, 254, 262

posterior, 237, 255, 256, 260–261
superior, 237, 254, 261–262
Internal fixation, 135–136, 144
Internal rotation, 101–102
Interscalene block, 74–75, 115, 187
Interscapulothoracic resection, 215
Intra-articular arthrodesis, 134–135

Joint
acromioclavicular, 27, 145, 268
disease, 77
glenohumeral, 27, 29–35, 306–307
scapulothoracic, 27, 32–35
shoulder, 27, 139–140
sternoclavicular, 27
see also Motion
Juvenile rheumatoid arthritis, 118, *119*

Kessel, Lippman, 284–285

Laboratory studies, revision shoulder arthroplasty, 236
Local anesthetic agents, 76

Magnetic resonance (MR) imaging, 53–55, 57, 217, 257, *259*
Magnuson-Stack procedure, 196
Malposition, 143–144
Malunion, 140, 190, *191*
Medications, 77
Methylmethacrylate, 10, 95, 166, 188, 237
Milwaukee shoulder, 204, 206
Modular endoprosthesis, 43, 222–223
Motion, 32–35, 167–168, 275, 314
continuous passive, 110–111
evaluation of, 100–102, 159
range of, 119, *122–123*, 130, 178, 189, 197–198, 202, 206–207, 237, 260
MR *see* Magnetic resonance (MR) imaging
Muscle
biceps, 219–220, *221–222*
deltoid, 29, 83, 165, 187, 200, 202, 221, 265
examination, 42
groups, 29
Musculocutaneous nerve, 80, 84

Narcotics, intravenous, 74
Neer, Charles S., II, 1, *2*, 7–19, 285, 296, 301, 306, 308, 313
Neer II total shoulder arthroplasties, 227–231
Neer prosthesis, 7, *8*, 9, 227–231, 282, 289
Nerve, 80–81
axillary, 80, 84
blockade, 75
musculocutaneous, 80, 84
stimulators, 73
Neurovascular region
bundle, 219, 223
exploration, 219
injuries, 190, 193
Nonconstrained arthroplasty, 265
nonrheumatoid, 242–245
results, 152, 208, 227–231, 234, 256
rheumatoid arthritis, 245–250
Nonunion, 143, 190, *192*

Osteoarthritis, 45–46, 56, *59*, 119, *120–121*, 140–141, 296, 314
see also Glenohumeral joint, osteoarthritis
Osteolysis, 296

Osteonecrosis, 46, 170–180, 314
  approach, 177–178
  classification, 172–174
  etiology, 170–172
  summary, 178–180
  treatment, 174–178
Osteophyte, *87, 90*, 91
Osteosarcoma, 215
Osteotome, 87, 89, *90*
Osteotomy, 126–127, 164
  indications, 126
  results, 126–127
  surgical technique, 126

Pain, 41, 197–198, 205–207, 275
  arthrodesis, 145
  relief, 162–164, 167–168, 175, 227–233, 236, 313–314
  sources of, 307–308
Paralysis, 138–139
Paresthesias, 73
Pean, Jules E., 1, *2*
Pectoralis major tendon, 83, 115, 165, 223
Pendulum exercise, 103
Peptococcus, 279
Physical therapy, 99–100, 162, 189–190, 198, 202
PMMA *see* Polymethylmethacrylate
Polyacetal component, 22, 23
Polyethylene component, 282, *283*, 285, 289, 294, 296, 306
Polymethylmethacrylate (PMMA), 281–282, 289, 294, 296, 298, 301
Posterior instability, 237, 255, 256, 260–261
Postoperative activities *see* Rehabilitation
Posttraumatic arthritis, 46, *47–48*, 50, 278
Preoperative clinical evaluation, 41–51, 257
  imaging studies, 44–45
  indications, 45–51
  patient history, 41
  physical examination, 41–44
Prosthesis
  acromial fixation, 13
  Acropole, 16
  acrylic, 5, *6*
  ball and socket, 9–10, *11, 12*, 36, 266
  biangular, 19, 22, 289, *293*
  biomodular, 19, *21*, 22, 289
  bipolar, 17–18, 309
  cemented, 10
  constrained, 10, 14, 36–37, 45
  cup, 18–19, 266, *267*
  DANA, 13, 208, 233, 314
  design, 35–39
  first, 1, *2*
  glenoid, 19, *20–21*, 22, 91–92, *93–96*
  Global Shoulder System, 22, 289
  humeral, 19, *20*, 96, 242, 266, *293*, 295, 310–311
  loosening of, 64–66, 190
  modular, 43, 222–223
  monospherical, 17
  Neer I, 7, *8*
  Neer II, 227–231, 282, 289
  Neer Mark III, 9
  nonconstrained, 37–38, 45, 166–168
  osteonecrosis, 176
  placement of, 188
  porous coated, 285, *287–288*, 289, *290*, 298
  replacement, 190
  reverse ball and socket, 12–13, *286*
  scapular fixation, 10, *11*, 12, 284–285, *286*
  Select Shoulder System, 19, *293–294*
  semiconstrained, 38–39, 45
  Silastic, 15
  trispherical, 13, *14*, 37
  vitallium, 7
Proximal humeral fractures, 1, 170–171, *172*, 183–193, 234
  complications, 190, 193
  evaluation, 183
  prosthetic replacement for, 190
  rehabilitation, 189–190
  surgical indications, 183–184
  surgical technique, 187–189
Proximal migration, 308
Pulmonary disease, 78
Putti-Platt procedure, 196, *199*

Radiology, 53–68
  arthritis of dislocation, 199–200
  complications, 63–67
  normal appearances, 61–63
  postoperative, 61–67
  preoperative planning, 53–61, 199–200, 235–236, 257
  radiographs, 53, 216, 260, 275
  results, 228–229
  rotator cuff, 205–206
Radiolucent lines, 155, 242, *244*, 306, 311, 314, 315
Range of motion, 119, *122–123*, 130, 178, 189, 197–198, 202, 206–207, 237, 260
Reamer, 89
Regional anesthesia, 70–76
  brachial plexus block, 74–76
  contraindications, 72
  equipment, 73
  indications, 72
  intraoperative management, 73–74
  paresthesias versus nerve stimulators, 73
  postoperative management, 76
  premedication, 72–73
  preoperative evaluation, 72
Rehabilitation, 99–111
  arthritis of dislocation, 202
  continuous passive motion, 110–111
  evaluation of motion, 100–101
  hemiarthroplasty, 212
  osteoarthritis, 156–157
  postoperative, 102–110, 202, 272, *273*
  preoperative, 99–100
  proximal humeral fractures, 189–190
  rotator cuff disease, 212
  tumors, 224
Resection, 14, 127–132, 165
  humeral head, 86–98
  interposition arthoplasty, *129*, 130–132
  interscapulothoracic, 215
  operative technique, 128–130
  results, 130–131
  shoulder girdle, 215–216
  tumors, 218–219
Retroversion, 61–62, 257, *258*, 260, *261*, 268, 281
Revision surgery, 234–240, 251
  pathogenesis of failure, 234–235
  preoperative evaluation, 235–236
  principles of, 236–239
  summary, 239–240
Rheumatoid arthritis, 45–46, 56, *58–59*, 113–115, 141, 158–168, 313
  alternative procedures, 163–165
  clinical examination, 159–160

complications, 245–250
conservative treatment, 162–163
features of, 158–159
juvenile, 118, *119*
nonconstrained arthroplasty, 245–250
radiographic evaluation, 160
results, 166–168
surgical considerations, 163, 165–166
Rheumatoid synovitis, 158
Rolling, 34
Rotation, 34
external, 100–101, 104, 106
internal, 101–102, 105, 106
Rotator cuff, 43, 46, 56–61, 140, 159, 200–201, 204–213, 237
diagnosis, 206–207
etiology, 205–206
historical review, 204–205
postoperative rehabilitation, 212
radiology, 205–206
results, 212–213
surgical management, 207–212
tear, *49*, *60*, 140, 205–206

Sarcoma, 215–218
Scapula, 27, 218–221
Scapular fixation, 10, *11*, 12, 284–285, *286*
Scapulectomy, 215–216
Scapulohumeral muscle group, 29
Scapulothoracic joint, 27, 32–35, 265
Screw fixation, 10, *11*, 13, 22, *23*, 311, *312*
Select Shoulder System, 19, *293–294*
Semiconstrained arthroplasty, 265
results, 208, 227–233
Shoulder arthroplasty
anesthesia, 70–78
arthritis of dislocation, 194–203
arthrodesis, 134–145
biomechanics and design, 27–39
bipolar, 265–279
cementless, 281–303
complications, 242–253
glenohumeral osteoarthritis, 147–157
glenoid resurfacing, 306–315
high-grade tumors, 215–226
history and development, 1–23
long-term results, 227–233
massive rotator cuff defects and glenohumeral arthritis, 204–213
osteonecrosis, 170–180
osteotomy and resection, 126–132
preoperative clinical evaluation, 41–51
proximal humeral fractures, 183–193
radiology, 53–68
rehabilitation, 99–111
revision, 234–240
rheumatoid arthritis, 158–168
surgery, 80–98
synovectomy, 113–125
unstable, 254–262
Shoulder evaluation form, *42*, 43
Shoulder girdle resections, 215–216
Shoulder joint, 27
Shoulder score, 272, 275, 277
Silastic prosthesis, 15
Sizer discs, 91
Skin, in rheumatoid arthritis, 158
Sling, 189
Soft tissue, 139, 158, 217–218, 224, *225*, 237, 308

Stability, 29
see also Instability
Stable fixation, 283
Staphylococcus aureus, 154
Sternoclavicular joint, 27
Stiffness, 155
Strengthening exercises, 108–110, 190
Stretching exercises, 103–108, 190
see also Assisted stretching exercises
Subchondral bone cysts, 36, 158
Subdeltoid bursa, 123, *124*
Subluxation, 63–64, 254–257, *259–260*, 260–262, 265, 278, *279*, *296*
Subscapularis tendon, 85, 166, 178, 224
Superficial cervical plexus block, 76
Superior instability, 237, 254, 261–262
Supraclavicular block, 75–76
Surgery, 80–98
arthritis of dislocation, 194, 200–202
arthroplasty *see* Shoulder arthroplasty
bipolar, 267–272
failed, 46, 51, 140
osteotomy, 126
proximal humeral fractures, 183, 184, 187–189
rotator cuff, 207–212
tumors, 218–234
see also Revision surgery
Survivorship, 229–231, 234
Synovectomy, 113–125, 164, 268
incidence and technique, 115–116
materials and methods, 116, 118
rationale for, 113–115
results, 118–125
Synovial membrane, 113
Systemic diseases, 171–172

Therapy, 99–100
Three-part fracture, 184, 314
Tissue *see* Soft tissue
Translation, humeral head, 34
Trauma, 147
Tuberosity, 188–190, *191–192*, 201, 234, 265, 268, 289
Tumors, 215–226
anatomic considerations, 218
biopsy technique, 217–218
historical background, 215
postoperative management, 225
resection, 218–219
axillary exploration, 219, *220*
bony defect reconstruction, 222–224
clavicle, 221
humerus, 221–222
neurovascular exploration, 219
posterior incision and lateral skin flap, 220–221
scapula, 219–221
shoulder girdle, 215–216
soft-tissue reconstruction, 139, 224, *225*
staging studies, 216–217
surgical technique, 218–224

Uncemented components, 63
Unstable shoulder arthroplasty, 254–262
see also Instability

Valgus impacted four-part fracture, 183, *186*
Vitallium prosthesis, 7

Z-plasty lengthening, 200, *201*, 237